THE CHIROPRACTIC ASSISTANT

THE CHIROPRACTIC ASSISTANT
Second Edition
Formerly Titled: Basic Chiropractic Paraprofessional Manual

R. C. SCHAFER, DC, FICC

Developed by
Associated Chiropractic Academic Press

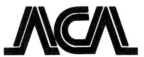

Published by
THE AMERICAN CHIROPRACTIC ASSOCIATION
1701 Clarendon Boulevard, Arlington, Virginia 22209

PUBLISHER'S POLICY

This manual has been developed for use as a basic instructional guide. The information concerning case management contained herein is based on sources believed to be generally correct within the United States. However, due to variances in state statutes, local codes, and court opinions, the publisher assumes no responsibility as to the accuracy or scope of the suggestions offered in individual circumstances.

The statements expressed herein are either of the author or the authorities cited. The publisher, its contractors, officers, or personnel neither endorse or approve any statements of fact or opinion expressed herein, nor are they responsible for the information presented in these pages.

When various apparatus and products are shown in this book as a general example of what is being used in the field, such illustrations should not be construed to be an endorsement of any particular instrument, modality, or product.

Library of Congress Catalog Card Number 90-83645

ISBN: 0-9606618-6-7

Copyright © 1991
The American Chiropractic Association
1701 Clarendon Boulevard
Arlington, Virginia 22209

Printed in the United States of America

COOPERATING ORGANIZATIONS

American Chiropractic Association
Associated Chiropractic Academic Press
Behavioral Research Foundation
Bibbero Systems, Inc.
Chattanooga Corporation

Colwell Systems, Inc.
Histacount, Inc.
Retrieval Business Systems
Safeguard Business Systems, Inc.
STC, Inc.

CREDITS

Unless credited to other sources, all drawings, photographs, and tables incorporated in this book have been produced with the permission of the Associated Chiropractic Academic Press (ACAP).

FOREWORD TO FIRST EDITION

In this decade, the practice of chiropractic health care has become too complex for the physician to operate an office without assistance. The doctor's time is far too valuable to be occupied with anything but health care. Responsibilities of receiving the patient, filing and record keeping, patient preparation, routine therapy and laboratory procedures, secretarial and clerical work, billings and receipts, and numerous other responsibilities are performed by a chiropractic assistant under supervision of the physician. Assistance must be at hand to maintain a sparkling office, to perform routine tests, to gather routine information, and to attend to the varied duties that reflect a well managed practice. These vital administrative and management functions place on the chiropractic assistant considerable responsibility. It is a responsibility clearly felt especially by the person new to the career of being a chiropractic assistant. For this reason, and to introduce the chiropractic student to the nonclinical aspects of conducting a successful practice, this manual has been developed.

A registered nurse has a certain degree of knowledge of medical practice, yet the nurse is not expected to practice medicine. Likewise, the chiropractic assistant must have a basic understanding of chiropractic health care to help her understand what is expected in the way of duties, responsibilities, and limitations. The information contained in this manual will be most helpful in this regard.

The chiropractic assistant is often called on to be the functional link between the clinical and the business side of practice. She must understand the basic principles on which chiropractic procedures in the doctor's practice are founded. Naturally, the gap between the knowledge of the doctor of chiropractic and his assistant(s) is vast. Yet without a basic understanding of the principles underlying consultation, examination, therapy, and rehabilitation, full assistance cannot be offered. The doctor and assistant(s) must function as a well organized health team. To achieve this, the assistant and doctor must be aware of mutual goals and motives. When this awareness is obtained, both will be in a position to achieve competency in their chosen careers.

The role of a chiropractic assistant is acquiring increasing professional recognition. In years past, the career rarely extended from that of a receptionist, secretary, and aide. Today, the career can be considered that of a paraprofessional. The ambitious and intelligent assistant will want to develop her capabilities and talents so that the full extent of personal potential can be realized. The American Chiropractic Association hopes assistants will find this manual a guide in achieving their career aspirations.

—Robert B. Jackson, D.C.
Development Director

Important note: While most doctors of chiropractic are males, the number of female practitioners is growing. Likewise, while the majority of chiropractic assistants are female, an increasing number of males are assuming the role of chiropractic assistant. For the sake of simplicity and not sexual bias, the pronoun "he" is used throughout this manual when referring to the doctor of chiropractic, and the pronoun "she" is used when referring to the chiropractic assistant. This is solely to avoid the redundant "he or she" or "he/she" when referring to the doctor or assistant.

PREFACE TO SECOND EDITION

The original edition of this manual was designed to offer both the chiropractic para-professional and the student doctor of chiropractic a comprehensive overview of the major aspects of practice administration and the management of the business side and technical-assistance aspects of health-care practice in the profession. In 1983, it was decided that this broad audience was no longer efficient. It was felt that a better solution would be to (1) develop a text specifically for the chiropractic student or recent graduate, and (2) revise this manual specifically for chiropractic paraprofessionals.

The first phase of this project was completed with the development of the text titled *Developing a Chiropractic Practice*. The second phase is now completed with the development of this revised edition—designed specifically to meet the needs of today's chiropractic assistants. This second edition is a completely updated and enhanced text. In addition, it includes a new chapter on office computers and word processors.

—RCS

PREFACE TO FIRST EDITION

This manual has been designed to offer the chiropractic paraprofessional a comprehensive overview of the major aspects of practice administration and the management of the business side and technical assistance aspects of health care practice in the profession.

Because the practice of chiropractic is regulated in all states and a number of foreign countries, the present scope of practice for doctors of chiropractic is necessarily determined locally by existing statutory enactment and judicial determination in the separate jurisdictions. The same is true for chiropractic assistants: scope of duties and responsibilities are determined locally by existing statutory enactment and/or judicial determination. Thus, the procedures and standards herein described are general. They may or may not be applicable in a specific state at this time.

In past years, courses conducted by individuals unaccountable to institutional chiropractic (courses which were sometimes in conflict with ethical, professional, or quality performance) have been severely criticized as being a forum for personal opinion or gain rather than a reference to contemporary thought of the vast majority in the profession. Thus, the basic motivation for writing this manual has come from many of the profession, within both clinical practice and chiropractic education, who stressed the need for a thorough work on the subject that was within generally accepted ethical and professional parameters. This was the challenge—one naively accepted the author soon learned once development was initiated.

The text is based on notes and tested policies from personal practice experience, advice from chiropractic leaders and authorities, extensive state-of-the-art research, sundry consultations and interviews, and contributions and counsel from recognized authorities, organizations, and agencies respected in their field. The author, therefore, makes no claim of originality but is grateful to all contributors, advisors, and experiences.

No text is a substitute for actually doing. To the reader inexperienced in the role and function of chiropractic practice administration and management, this manual will offer guidelines on which more meaningful and rapid on-the-job training can be conducted. To the experienced assistant, the text will serve as a reference to strengthen weak areas in career development and to broaden skills.

Health-personnel enthusiasm is not something that can be learned in the classroom. It is the effect of working each day in a practice—witnessing results first hand and becoming absorbed in the professional atmosphere and its contributions to the community. As one who performs an important job in an important field, the chiropractic paraprofessional has a right to be enthusiastic about her occupation and the people with whom she is associated. The word *enthusiasm* comes from the German *enthousiazein* (to be inspired, embedded with spirit). The author has attempted to impress students of this manual so that they may express greater personal potential.

Thousands of suggestions are offered within this manual. No one doctor will desire his assistants to accept all of them as we each have our individual genetic makeup, experiences, behavioral conditioning, prejudices, and preferences. Thus, the suggestions herein are but guidelines to common opinion that must be adapted to a specific practice. The reader should view these guidelines as a banquet of ideas and select those that are in harmony with your nature and environment.

In describing chiropractic paraprofessional disciplines, procedures, and practices, the manual will serve as a basic reference to both introductory seminar type courses and extensive resident programs. In the shorter courses, the instructor need only highlight the more important points and allow the text to serve as a future reference for greater detail. In the more sophisticated programs, this basic manual should be supported by discussion, supplemental texts, lectures, films, laboratory work, and field assignments.

A respectful tribute must be extended to the Board of Governors of the American Chiropractic Association. Without their recognition of need and support, publication of this manual would not have been authorized. Special thanks are also extended to Dr. Robert H. Jackson for his astute leadership and counsel in the preparation of the manuscript, to Dr. Louis G. Gearhart for his alert review of final drafts, and to the author's capable associate, Barbara Joann Ozimek, for typing and proofing the seemingly endless drafts required during research and development.

—RCS

CONTENTS

THE CHIROPRACTIC ASSISTANT

Chapter 1

Introduction to a Rewarding Career

To enter the health-care field as a chiropractic assistant is an adventure for the qualified individual. The nationwide trend in the primary care professions is not only to provide qualified health-care professionals but also to assure that assistants are qualified to carry out their duties and responsibilities in caring for the health needs of patients. To achieve this goal, (1) chiropractic physicians are encouraged to use assistants to increase personal efficiency, and (2) chiropractic organizations are encouraged to sponsor legislation establishing a nationwide accredited chiropractic assistants program.

All states and Puerto Rico have statutes recognizing and regulating the practice of chiropractic as an independent health service because the profession has proven its value as a public service. On foreign shores, the practice of chiropractic is officially recognized and regulated in Canada, Switzerland, Germany, New Zealand, Western Australia, Bolivia, and is acknowledged and accepted in the British Isles, South Africa, Zimbabwe, Japan, France, Denmark, Belgium, Italy, and Egypt. Official recognition is being initiated in scores of other countries.

WHO IS INVOLVED IN ADMINISTERING CHIROPRACTIC HEALTH CARE?

The Doctor of Chiropractic. The titles *doctor of chiropractic (DC)*, *chiropractic physician,* and *chiropractor* are synonymous. A doctor of chiropractic is a physician concerned with the health needs of the public as a member of the healing arts who gives particular attention to the relationship of the structural and neurologic aspects of the body in health and disease. The basic and clinical sciences as well as related health subjects prepares the chiropractic student as a primary health-care provider. As a portal of entry to the health delivery system, the chiropractic physician must be well educated in diagnosis and case management to care for the human body in health and disease and to consult with or refer to other health-care providers.

The Chiropractic Assistant. The terms *chiropractic assistant (CA)* and *chiropractic paraprofessional* are synonymous. A chiropractic assistant is a professional aid to the doctor of chiropractic under whose direct guidance and supervision performs various technical duties, office and business functions, and/or assists in the preparation, control, and care of patients. The term *chiropractic assistant* may refer to either an administrative assistant or a clinical assistant.

Administrative Assistant. An administrative assistant is one whose major duties and responsibilities concern basic office administrative, business, and other nonclinical procedures.

Clinical Assistant. The terms *clinical assistant* and *technical assistant* are synonymous. A clinical assistant is one whose major duties and responsibilities are related to helping with supervised diagnostic and therapeutic procedures.

Certified Chiropractic Assistant. Certification is awarded to an assistant who has received education in chiropractic philosophy, terminology, various physical diagnosis procedures, anatomy and physiology, clinical laboratory procedures, ethics and jurisprudence, radiologic technology, adjunctive therapy, and basic office procedures, *and* who has been examined by a credible agency (eg, Chiropractic Board of Examiners) and found worthy to carry out the duties and responsibilities of a chiropractic assistant in harmony with legislated, professional, ethical, hygienic, and safety standards.

Certification is a form of licensure. It allows an assistant to a primary care physician to perform certain diagnostic, therapeutic, and rehabilitative services that are beyond the legal scope of an uncertified assistant. There is a growing trend to have assistants obtain specific certification and continuing education in the application of roentgenographic equipment, physiologic therapeutics, and other clinical procedures. These requirements vary from state to state. For example, assistants can be certified in Oklahoma to administer vitamin/mineral supplements by injection.

HOW CHIROPRACTIC IS SIMILAR TO OTHER HEALTH-CARE PROFESSIONS

The federal government along with every state legislature recognizes three major professions as primary health provider groups. These healing arts in order of both number of practitioners and public utilization are the allopathic, chiropractic, and osteopathic branches of generic medicine. Governmental recognition, licensure in all states, educational standards maintained by an agency recognized by the U.S. Department of Education, inclusion in health-care programs, and utilization of standardized diagnostic procedures are but a few of the common factors among all recognized healing professions.

As explained above, practitioners of allopathic medicine (MDs), chiropractic (DCs), and osteopathic medicine (DOs) are the three types of primary health-care providers licensed in all states. Licensure is granted by state boards of examiners according to state statutes.

A listing of subjects common to all health sciences is shown in Table 1.1. It is an advantage of the aspiring chiropractic assistant to become quickly acquainted with these terms because they are commonly used.

As with other major health-care professions, chiropractic health care is provided for in such federal programs as Medicare, Medicaid, the Government Employees Hospital Association Benefit Plan, the Mailhandlers Benefit Plan, and the Postmasters Benefit Plan, along with other programs. It is included in the policies of virtually every major health-insurance carrier and in federal and state Worker's Compensation Acts. In addition, a substantial number of major international and local labor unions provide for chiropractic services in their health and welfare plans, and many industrial employers include chiropractic care in the health plans for their employees.

Table 1.1. Areas of Common Study and Specialties Among Primary Providers

Anatomy. The science that studies the structure of the organism and the relation of its parts.

Angiology. The study of blood and lymph vessels.

Bacteriology. The study of microscopic organisms. A specialist is called a microbiologist or a bacteriologist.

Cardiology. The study of the heart. A specialist is called a cardiologist.

Dermatology. The study of the skin. A specialist is called a dermatologist.

Diagnosis. The art or act of determining the nature of disease. A specialist is called an internist.

Dissection. The cutting of tissues of the body for the purpose of anatomical study or during autopsy to determine the cause of death.

Embryology. The study of the embryo and the origin and development of life.

Endocrinology. The study of ductless glands and hormones. A specialist is called an endocrinologist.

Gastroenterology. The study of the stomach and intestines. A specialist is called a gastroenterologist.

Gynecology. The study of diseases peculiar to women. A specialist is called a gynecologist.

Histology. The study of the microscopic structures of tissues.

Hygiene. The study of the rules of health. A person who emphasizes this aspect of health care is called a hygienist.

Kinesiology. The study of motion. A specialist is called a kinesiologist.

Myology. The study of muscles.

Neurology. The study of the nervous system. A specialist is called a neurologist.

Obstetrics. The care of the woman during pregnancy, parturition, and the puerperium. A specialist is called an obstetrician.

Ophthalmology. The study of the eye and vision. A specialist is called an ophthalmologist.

Orthopedics. The study of diseases of bones, joints, and related structures. A specialist is called an orthopedist.

Osteology. The study of bones and the morphology of bony parts.

Otolaryngology. The study of diseases of the ear, nose, and throat. A specialist is called an otolaryngologist.

Pathology. The study of the nature of disease. A specialist is called a pathologist.

Pediatrics. The study and treatment of children's diseases. A specialist is called a pediatrician.

Physiologic therapeutics. The application of natural forces (eg, light, heat, cold, electricity, vibration, massage, exercise, rest, supports) to assist in normalizing function and enhance recuperation. A specialist is called a physiatrist.

Physiology. The study of the functions of the living body or its parts. A specialist is called a physiologist.

Proctology. The study and treatment of diseases affecting the rectum and anus. A specialist is called a proctologist.

Psychiatry. The study and medical treatment of abnormal psychologic disorders. A specialist is called a psychiatrist.

Psychology. The study of the functions of the mind, the relation of behavior to the environment, and the nonmedical treatment thereof. A specialist is called a psychologist.

Radiology. The study of x-rays and their therapeutic application. A specialist is called a radiologist.

Roentgenology. The study of the diagnostic application of x-rays. A specialist is called a roentgenologist.

Spanchnology. The study of viscera; organs of the thorax, abdomen, and pelvis.

Syndesmology. The study of ligaments.

Terminology. The study of health-care terms.

Toxicology. The study of poisons. A specialist is called a toxicologist.

Urology. The study and treatment of diseases of the urinary system. A specialist is called a urologist.

HOW CHIROPRACTIC DIFFERS FROM OTHER HEALTH-CARE PROFESSIONS

Doctors of chiropractic are physicians who consider the human body an integrated being and give special attention to spinal mechanics and neurologic, osseous, muscular, and vascular relationships. The three types of primary health-care providers essentially differ in their philosophy of and approach to health care, emphasis, and legislated scope of practice (services).

The Chiropractic Approach

While facts are unalterable, viewpoint and emphasis can be different in an approach to health care. Disease, for example, is abnormal function, and abnormal function is function out of time and phase with environmental need. Disease does not involve a new function. It is only the consequence of change—change in quality, frequency, and/or channeling of nerve impulses and metabolism in terms of cellular nutrition, waste removal, and repair. Sickness is not the result of what something does to the body but what the body does about it because existing mechanical, chemical, and/or psychic impairment of the nervous system prevents adaptation. In other words, disease follows when environmental disturbances disturb the nervous system and prevent a normal adaptive response.

Environmental Irritants

Commonly encountered mechanical irritants include physical injuries, gravitational and occupational overstress, postural defects and faults, developmental asymmetries, prolonged unbalanced work or play, and deforming changes in the articular beds of joints. In the latter, spinal and extraspinal changes often are sites of insult difficult to detect by those untrained in chiropractic methods.

Other potential environmental irritants include the toxins of pathogenic microorganisms; drugs, pesticides, and other chemicals; radiation, noise, and metabolic wastes or other pollutants. Of these, the metabolic wastes of cellular activity probably tax the adaptability of cells the most. The emotional and mental disturbances arising from the effect of hostile human relations and blocked self-actualization are the principal psychic irritants encountered in our society today. Rarely does an organic disease not have a psychic component that adds to the clinical picture.

It has been erroneously reported that chiropractors do not believe in germs. Nothing is farther from the truth. It is a basic chiropractic precept that both internal and external environmental factors (and germs are an inescapable component of our environment) decide one's potential for health and disease. Further, this is not a matter of belief or disbelief but a realistic scientific appraisal of the germ theory.

Summary. Any undue hindrance to nerve function can produce dysfunction and thus initiate disease in the susceptible individual. Pathology (disease) is always preceded by dysfunction. In broad terms, disease is the product of abnormal function and abnormal function is the effect of the body's inability to cope with overstress. Such stress may result from one or a combination of irritations—mechanical, thermal, chemical, hormonal, bacteriologic, viral, parasitic, psychologic, and so forth. Susceptibility is also determined by many factors. A common external factor is the degree of noxious environmental demands, and a common internal factor is the body's resistance. The quality of the latter is essentially determined by neurologic, nutritional, and hereditary factors.

The Nervous System: Primary Regulator of Function

Why do some get sick and not others during an epidemic? Freedom from infectious disease does not solely depend on the absence of microorganisms—a condition never realizable because bacteria are ubiquitous—but on maintenance of normal function (physiologic activity) despite their presence. The body tries to protect itself against noxious microorganisms by producing antibodies and other defense mechanisms to destroy invading microbes and/or their products. The production of antibodies and other pertinent cells is regulated both directly and indirectly by the nervous system. Hence, the most fundamental therapeutic approach (and protection) is to assure undisturbed function of the nervous system.

Many potentially dangerous microorganisms are normally found within the healthy body but their growth is held in check. However, an excessive environmental irritation of the nervous system can disturb this symbiotic balance and permit microorganisms already present to initiate the infectious process. This is why chiropractic has emphasized the importance of human ecology in relation to the nature of disease.

The physiologic integrity of the host is usually more important than the microorganisms that invade it because progressing infection results from an inadequacy in natural defense mechanisms. Again, this inadequacy is due essentially to (1) one or more noxious environmental forces affecting the nervous system (by whatever means) or (2) unusual resilience or strength of the invading organism.

Contemporary medical practice emphasizes disease and the results of disease. After proper diagnosis, attention is given to relieve pain and other overt symptoms, neutralize chemical imbalances, and remove diseased tissues and organs. While such an approach has led to brilliant discoveries, much remains unchallenged. Chiropractic, in contrast, emphasizes health and the results of normal structure and balanced function.

Chiropractic: Often a Conservative Alternative

Little in life can be logically discussed in polarized terms of black or white. This is especially true within the healing arts. The chiropractic profession openly recognizes the positive results obtained in the cautious use of chemotherapy, but it also holds a concern over rigid rituals that fail to consider undesirable side effects. The profession also recognizes the need for necessary surgery, yet it is conscious of its dangers. Thus, the chiropractic profession feels that its more

conservative approach should be offered objective appraisal before the patient is subjected to potent drugs or risks the dangers involved in surgical intervention. While potentially dangerous measures may be necessary, they should be considered as the last resort and not as the only alternative available in health care.

It has been explained that infection represents the change from an uneasy truce into a state of open warfare between microorganisms and host when a lowered resistance arises primarily from a morbid irritation to the nervous system. Therefore, the role of chiropractic therapy is to relieve irritation of the nervous system and restore optimal function.

Antibiotics and other potent drugs have certain beneficial effects in reducing bacterial populations. However, it must not be forgotten that chemotherapy may enhance other latent microorganisms. As a chemical irritant to the nervous system capable of upsetting functional equilibrium in minor infections, the antibiotic could trigger an unfavorable reaction and thus produce iatrogenic complications. Therefore, drugs should not be indiscriminately used in infections of a minor or moderate character. While chiropractic has voiced its concern of the indiscriminate use of "miracle" drugs for several decades, it has only been in recent years that the scientific community and governmental agencies have also become openly concerned.

Only unbiased judgment and clinical experience can help the physician in making the decision to chance the beneficial effects of a therapy as opposed to the possible detrimental effects it could or might produce. Pathologist William Boyd emphasized the importance of such judgment when he reported that "Old diseases are disappearing, but new ones are taking their place which are often man-made, the result of injudicious use of therapeutic agents." Here we should realize that the disappearance of many diseases common in the past cannot be credited exclusively to the healing arts; the disappearance is due largely to accomplishments in sanitary engineering.

Chiropractic's approach establishes and maintains optimal physiologic activity by correcting abnormal functional and structural relationships. Its goal is to help the body in using its own biologic resources for a return to normal function. Its focal point of concern is with the integrity of the nervous system because it is the nervous system that is responsible for integrating and coordinating the major functions in the body responding to internal and external change—normal and abnormal.

Rational thinking concludes that a comprehensive health-care system must be more than an attempt to hide symptoms or remove diseased organs. While a drug may be helpful in easing pain, it may not rectify the *cause* of the pain. While surgery may be necessary to remove a diseased organ, it may not address itself to why the organ did not function normally. The suppression of symptoms or the removal of disease by-products cannot be considered actions that automatically return a person to optimal health. Chiropractic physicians are convinced that a comprehensive health-care system must be a great deal more than recipe, relief, repair, or removal.

Social Concerns

The position of the chiropractic profession is not negative. It is realistic and positive—compatible with the most advanced facts bearing on problems of human disease and disability. The encouragement of optimal nutrition, fresh air, sunlight, exercise, and personal hygiene long ago became an established routine of practice. The chiropractor is a champion of slum clearance and adequate housing who advocates working conditions avoiding unnecessary stress and an environment as free from pollution as possible. But he is not a radical. He considers fear campaigns and overly publicized situations leading to psychic stress a disservice to general health. He encourages the assurance of the highest level of efficiency of the nervous system and natural immune mechanisms and hence the best level of health and resistance to infection and tissue degeneration. He therefore encourages every effort that will decrease poverty or raise the level of living standards, general health, and physical fitness.

Interprofessional Concerns

Because a basic cause of disease is adverse environmental irritation of the nervous system, it is apparent that any measure that will help relieve such irritation, despite its nature, constitutes indicated therapy. At times, the source of nerve irritation is obvious, simple, and accessible—making the therapeutic approach easy. Then again, the irritating factors may be complex, obscure, manifold, and inaccessible or longstanding and thus pose a more complicated therapeutic problem.

Obviously, no single therapy offers a panacea. However, one approach may be better suited to a particular problem than another, or a combined effort might be advisable. This places an enormous responsibility on the physician because he has to decide which therapy or therapies are indicated for an individual patient's status. There might be a case in which the patient's disorder may be cared for by the therapeutic competency of one specific school of healing and other instances where the skill and wisdom of an alternative profession or more than one discipline of the healing arts is required. Principles oblige all physicians to discern according to their best ability which path of treatment should be followed. This obligation presents one of the most difficult tasks confronting practitioners of the healing arts.

Examples of Professional Recognition

In 1974, the Department of Family and Community Medicine of the University of Utah College of Medicine compared the effectiveness of the allopathic physician to that of chiropractic care. The study showed, in terms of both patient perception of improvement in functional status and patient satisfaction, that chiropractors are as effective if not more effective with the patients they treated as were the allopathic physicians. This conclusion has been arrived at by many similar studies since then.

The treatment of on-the-job injuries has not been avoided. Studies of worker's compensation records in several states provide objective evidence of the efficacy of chiropractic care. Comparisons of chiropractic and medical treatment demonstrate dramatically that cases under chiropractic care show reduced treatment costs, reduced compensation costs, reduced work-time losses, and reduced worker disability and suffering.

Because chiropractic offers a more conservative approach, possibly a more humanized approach to health care, it is no wonder that this form of therapy is rapidly gaining in recognition and acceptance.

The Philosophy of Chiropractic

It would be extremely rare if not impossible to find a person ill from a single specific disease entity such as a stomach ulcer. Is not the ulcer the result rather than the cause of the disorder? While surgical removal may be advisable in advanced cases, it does not mean that conditions allowing the formation of the ulcer in the first place have been removed. Yet, referred postoperative chiropractic therapy has not been used to its maximum. This is unfortunate—reducing the level of public health. It underscores that a change of attitude in the medical establishment is needed.

It is the rare neighborhood, for example, that does not have its number of people who have had numerous operations by numerous surgeons who have made numerous incisions resulting in numerous adhesions to remove the numerous by-products of failing organs—while the cause of the failure continues in its nefarious path to be displayed in numerous types of adverse symptoms, signs, and syndromes. For this reason, chiropractors believe there should be more to health care than the numbing of pain, the camouflaging of symptoms, and the removal of pathologic tissue.

The relationship of biomechanics (structure) to biodynamics (function) has been emphasized by the chiropractic profession for almost a century. Evidence of the importance of removing and preventing spinal impairments is growing each year—a recognition that the nervous system maintains a primary role in integration of all body systems.

The central nervous system (CNS) origi-
nates in brain centers and extends down through the spinal column, ultimately reaching every part of the body through the peripheral nervous system. Interference anywhere in the nervous system impairs bodily function and induces disease. One common site of insult is that point where nerves exit or enter the spinal column. Such insults often result from what chiropractors call *subluxations* (partly displaced vertebrae) or *fixations* (partly restricted vertebrae) that cause or contribute to neurologic disorders altering both structural balance and functional tone.

Articular Injury

The mechanical lesion (subluxation or fixation) is an attending complication of those structural, chemical, and/or psychic environmental irritations of the nervous system producing muscle contraction sufficient to cause dysfunction of spinal articulations. Once produced, the lesion becomes a focus of sustained irritation. It irritates nerves in the articular capsules, ligaments, tendons, and muscles of the involved spinal segment. A barrage of impulses stream into the spinal cord where they are relayed to motor and sensory pathways for control of muscles and glands. The contraction originating the lesion is thereby re-enforced, thus perpetuating both the subluxation and the pathologic process engendered. This vicious cycle is commonly recognized in clinical chiropractic. Not all the spinal irritation originates this way, however.

Intervertebral Foramen Impairment

Other complications involved include the effect on vessels and nerves as they enter or exit the spine through distorted "open doorways" called foramina. The injury (often microtrauma) attending the vertebral subluxation may set off an inflammatory reaction with swelling or bony compression that tends to encroach on the portion of the spinal nerves and attending vessels contained within the intervertebral channel. The process may terminate in adhesions. Greater encroachment may occur on the foraminal contents (such as the soft tissues, nerve trunk, and other elements) with the presence of developmental defects, congenital anomalies, osseous asymmetries, and degenerative and proliferative changes such as on the circumference of the channel or in the fibrocartilaginous discs between the spinal segments.

Intervertebral Disc Disorders

Each vertebra is separated from neighboring segments by a spinal disc. These 23 padlike structures not only cushion the 24 movable spinal vertebrae but also make possible the flexibility of the spine that is so essential to normal bending movements. Disc disorders can lead to irritation of the spinal nerves directly or indirectly. With the contributory factor of the subluxation, such complications may trigger a fullfledged syndrome of severe nerve root compression or irritation. Because almost all spinal nerves pass through movable passageways (the foramina), such contingencies are by no means rare. The validity of this approach is attested by millions of chiropractic patients each year.

While such mechanical lesions are frequently associated with the spine, they also can exist in other parts of the musculoskeletal system (eg, articulations of extraspinal joints). As disturbances in one area may produce disorders in other areas, the accurate determination of cause and effect of a patient's problem often involves detailed complicated analysis. The musculoskeletal system is intimately connected with all other body systems through the nervous system.

Chiropractic Adjustments

A corrective structural adjustment by a chiropractic physician (spinal or extraspinal) should not be confused with other forms of manipulation. Manipulative therapy in one form or another is used somewhat in all the healing arts. Allopathic manipulation is usually little more than a therapist putting a patient's joint through its normal range of motion to stretch muscles and break adhesions. Osteopathic manipulation is designed to increase joint motion and relieve fixa-

tions. On the other hand, a chiropractic corrective adjustment is made only after careful analysis and delivered in a specific manner to achieve a specific predetermined goal. It is a precise delicate maneuver requiring special bioengineering skills and a deftness not unlike that required by a neurosurgeon. The effect is stimulating but seldom painful.

Most chiropractic corrective adjustments are made upon the joints, especially those of the spinal column. Some techniques, however, are light touch reflex techniques that involve the neurovascular, neurolymphatic, and neuromuscular systems—much akin to the systems involved in Oriental meridian therapy. These surface techniques, often applied remote from the spine, are far more than massage or trigger point releases because they involve prudent diagnosis and can be scientifically applied only after comprehensive training.

BRIEF HISTORY OF HEALTH CARE

Although the exact origin of therapeutic manipulation is lost in antiquity, anthropologic findings show that this health approach has existed throughout the world since the beginning of recorded time. Some of the earliest indications of manipulation are demonstrated by the ancient Chinese *Kong Fou* document written about 2700 BC. Greek papyruses dating back to at least 1500 BC gave instructions on the "maneuvering" of the lower extremities in the treatment of lowback disorders. There appears no single origin of the art. Therapeutic manipulation was practiced by the ancient Japanese, Chinese, Indians of Asia, Egyptians, Babylonians, Syrians, Hindus, Tibetans, Tahitians, and American Indians.

Early Records

Records from as long ago as 5000 BC show that ancient societies had some type of standard of care for the sick and injured. Their theories were based on the religion and myths prevalent at the time. Around 2000 BC, certain men developed occupations as physicians in Egypt, Babylonia, Assyria, and the Orient. Moses, an advocate of preventive medicine and hygiene, incorporated rules of health into the Hebrew religion around 1205 BC.

Hippocrates

Hippocrates, the Father of Medicine, recognized the importance of spinal manipulation. Little was known at the time of human anatomy, physiology, and pathology, and there was no knowledge of biochemistry. Yet, despite these handicaps, he did much to separate medicine from mysticism and founded the first steps in giving it a crude scientific basis. Many of his classifications of diseases and descriptions of symptoms are still being used today.

A prolific writer, Hippocrates wrote at least 70 books on healing. They included *Manipulation and Importance to Good Health* and *On Setting Joints by Leverage.* Emphasizing the importance of the spine, he said, "Get knowledge of the spine, for this is the requisite for many diseases." *Summum bonum*—the highest good is to remove the cause, taught Hippocrates: "Nature must heal; the physician can only remove the obstruction." He taught that the body tends to heal itself and it is the physician's responsibility to help nature.

Herodicus

Herodicus, a contemporary of Hippocrates, earned wide fame by curing diseases by correcting abnormalities in the spine, which he did in the relatively healthy through therapeutic exercises and in the weak by manipulations with his hands. The early Greeks also used a multitude of mechanical devices for stretching the spine and setting dislocations. A variety of crude traction devices was invented.

Galen

In later Greece, Claudius Galen (AD 131–201) was the most distinguished practitioner of his time. He studied, practiced, and taught in Rome. There he wrote over 500 treatises on health care and conducted research in experimental physiology and neurology. It was he who first taught the proper positions and relations of the vertebrae and the spinal column. He was the first to describe the cranial nerves and the sympathetic nervous system.

Galen was given the title "Prince of Physicians" after he corrected a paralysis of the right hand of Eudemus, a prominent Roman scholar. He did so by treating the patient's neck, apparently by adjusting the cervical vertebrae interfering with normal nerve transmission to Eudemus' hand.

Like Hippocrates, Galen recognized the importance of the nervous system. He taught his students to "Look to the nervous system as the key to maximum health."

Resistance to New Thought by the Medical Establishment

During the Dark Ages, public opinion was thwarted by religious and political leaders who believed that all what could be learned was known. They held ancient religious teachings and the historic theories of Hippocrates and Galen as law. Thus, innovation was considered highly questionable behavior. It was not until universities formed in the 16th Century that the observation of the sick began to evolve as a study of theories of disease.

Throughout this period, the tendency to deviate from orthodox teachings was ridiculed. The Belgian anatomist, Vasalius (1514–1564), now considered the Father of Modern Anatomy, broke with many of Galen's teachings and was severely persecuted. This was also true for studies by William Harvey (1578–1657) on the heart and circulation—brilliant reasoning that was not fully recognized by the medical establishment until 200 years later.

The Hungarian physician, Philipp Semmelweis (1818–1865) recognized that some diseases were transmitted by physical contact. He ordered students and colleagues entering his wards directly from autopsy and dissecting rooms to wash their hands with a disinfectant (a solution of chloride of lime). Although this practice greatly reduced the spread of puerperal fever (that following childbirth), his hygienic measures were met with violent opposition. Later, Louis Pasteur (1822–1895), the Father of Bacteriology, and Joseph Lister (1827–1912), the Father of Sterile Surgery, proved Semmelweis correct, but they too suffered years of humiliation by the establishment who believed that infection and pain were Godgiven and inevitable.

Even Florence Nightingale (1820–1910), the creator of the Women's Nursing Service during the war in Crimea, was regarded as a "troublesome female intruder" when she advocated hygienic practices and that nurses receive special training and experience. The same was true for philanthropist Clara Barton (1821–1912) when she tried to improve medical record keeping and the recruitment of supplies and to organize a Red Cross Committee during the Civil War.

During the Middle Ages and Renaissance, the art of manipulation (often called "bonesetting") was handed down from father to son or mother to daughter and practiced by at least one supposedly "gifted" person in most communities of Europe, North Africa, and Asia. Because of the archaic state of medical practice in those days, the results obtained by these individuals were so unusual to traditional thinking that the people believed that the manipulators had inherited a divine gift to heal the sick. All but a few medical practitioners considered them "quacks."

Highly skilled but without the benefit of formal education, the bonesetters of Europe, particularly in England, met with flourishing success. Because of their eclat with many patients labeled hopeless by traditional physicians, early manipulators were inspired to exaggerate claims of cure that further alienated the "orthodox" medical community. Gradually, succeeding manipulators became more clinically and scientifically oriented and less prone to rash claims. But unpalatable memories remained, and the establishment kept their minds closed to any scientific advances made by the manipulators. Other physicians, though realizing the merit of manipulation, selfishly rationalized by rejecting it under the guise of "scientific unacceptability."

This bias has remained for centuries. Despite mounting scientific evidence to the contrary, political medicine has been stubborn in maintaining a monopoly in health care.

Birth of Modern Chiropractic

Modern chiropractic reflects the rediscovery of therapeutic manipulation. It was revealed, improved, and founded in the United States by Dr. D. D. Palmer in 1895. In his first book, he wrote: "I am not the first person to replace subluxated vertebrae, but I do claim to be the first person to replace displaced vertebrae by using the spinous and transverse processes as levers ... and to develop the philosophy and science of chiropractic adjustments."

By the late 19th Century, many basic concepts and clinical principles of modern day usage had been established. It seems probable that the genesis of modern theory and practice of manipulative therapy used by chiropractors and osteopaths arose from concepts generally acceptable to many 19th Century medical practitioners and scientists because it was during this period that the role of the spinal cord in health and disease was being vigorously explored and discussed.

The Effect of Poor Cooperation

However, the three contemporary clinical professions (MDs, DCs, DOs) have developed in relative isolation from one another. Each group evolved primarily in a clinical setting with a selfgenerated terminology specific to the history of their particular clinical school of thought. Individuals from each philosophy of therapy have crossed professional lines as students or instructors, but this has not been done openly or in large numbers. As a result, a major problem is the difficulty of sharing clinical experiences and scientific results because of self-developed terminology and interprofessional isolationism. In recent years, this barrier has begun to weaken.

The Dawn of a New Approach

Since its inception, chiropractic has felt that health is the result of the body's remaining in harmony with the principles of nature. Chiropractic pioneers were severely attacked for their criticism of drug overutilization, involuntary immunization programs, the perversion of food during processing, and the neglect of physical fitness. Today we realize the validity of such criticism. Both society and science now realize that we have placed too much attention on prescription rather than prevention, too much attention on weakening invaders rather than on strengthening their host. Concern for both the internal and external environments should be kept in balance. Ecology concerns our total environment—both within and without.

Scope of Chiropractic Practice

Spinal analysis and adjustment have always been emphasized within the practice of chiropractic, but they by no means constituted the sole scope of practice used by the majority of practitioners. In fact, several forms of therapy now gaining popularity within all the healing arts can thank chiropractic pioneers for their development in this country. Many physiotherapy modalities, for example, were perfected by DCs and their use taught in chiropractic colleges long before the profession of physiotherapy was created. History records that the use of physiologic therapeutic devices within the healing arts was initiated and developed in this country by nonallopathic professions, with pioneer chiropractors offering major leadership in both application and development.

Therapeutic nutrition also has been an important subject within the chiropractic curriculum for decades. Unfortunately, even during the enlightenment of today it is allowed only a few hours of instruction in medical schools. Emphasis is locked on chemotherapy and surgery.

While Oriental acupuncture and acupressure have received much publicity within the popular press and interest within the majority profession since the late 1960s, the use of peripheral stimulation to elicit certain physiologic reactions has been known and commonly applied within chiropractic since the turn of the century. It has always been an attribute of chiropractic to seek and develop conservative health-care measures.

HEALTH-CARE EDUCATION IN AMERICA

Medical Education

Few realize that it only has been in this century that medical education has been refined. During the early years of this country, the typical medical doctor had little formal education. In the western states, a candidate would observe a recognized doctor's work until that physician thought that the candidate was ready for solo practice. State licensure did not become widespread until after the turn of the century.

In 1893, John Hopkins University Medical School in Baltimore was the first medical college to require entrants to have a year's training in the natural sciences. It also established the first teaching hospital. However, it was not until an educator, William Flexner (1866–1959), received a commission from the Carnegie Foundation to study the quality of medical education that substantial improvement in medical education was made. The Flexner Report of 1910 resulted in many of the 155 medical schools rated to be closed because of their extremely poor quality of instruction and teaching facilities.

Modern Chiropractic Education and Professional Development

State licensed and regulated, the chiropractor is a valuable member of the health-care professions. Six years or more of college study and internship go into the making of a doctor of chiropractic—more if the DC selects a special area of interest (eg, orthopedics, roentgenography, etc).

The doctor of chiropractic has at his disposal modern x-ray, laboratory, and other diagnostic instruments and is thoroughly trained and skilled in orthopedic and neurologic procedures. Chiropractic examinations seek to determine what is causing the patient's body not to function properly. If the problem is one for which recognized chiropractic methods of treatment are applicable, the chiropractor will recommend a treatment plan.

Professional Requirements

A minimum of 2 years of prechiropractic college work are required for admission to an accredited chiropractic college. After that, 4 academic years of resident study at a chiropractic college, including practice in a teaching clinic, are required for the Doctor of Chiropractic degree. Courses are offered in a wide range of scientific areas such as human anatomy; biochemistry; physiology; microbiology; pathology; public health; physical, clinical, and laboratory diagnosis; gynecology; obstetrics; pediatrics; geriatrics; dermatology; otolaryngology; roentgenology; psychology; dietetics; orthopedics; physical therapy; first aid; spinal analysis; principles and practice of chiropractic; adjustive technic; and other appropriate subjects.

Clinical Experience. In the teaching clinics of chiropractic colleges, advanced students obtain experience in diagnosis, followed by treatment or referral. This represents the culmination of the academic learning experience and the transition from students to chiropractic physicians.

Academic Accreditation

The primary professional accrediting agency for chiropractic colleges is the Commission on Accreditation of the Council on Chiropractic Education (CCE). The Council has advocated and established high standards of quality in chiropractic college education and in postgraduate or continuing education programs. The CCE dates from 1947. Its work, including that of predecessor groups, dates from 1938.

The Commission on Accreditation of the Council on Chiropractic Education was added to the United States Commissioner on Education's list of Nationally Recognized Accrediting Agencies and Associations in 1974. In 1976, the Commission was officially recognized by the Council on Postsecondary Accreditation (COPA) as the accrediting agency for chiropractic educational institutions and programs.

Postgraduate Continuing Education

Most states require attendance at approved postgraduate educational programs as a prerequisite to annual license renewal. The chiropractic profession was pioneer in requiring practitioners to attend approved postgraduate programs as a prerequisite to annual license renewal. The state of Colorado adopted the first requirement in 1933.

FCER

The Foundation for Chiropractic Education and Research (FCER) is a nonprofit organization established by the profession. It makes direct grants to colleges, grants for scholarships and faculty assistanceships, grants for research projects, and grants for support of the CCE. The most important source of FCER funds is a percentage of the dues paid by the general members of the American Chiropractic Association. Other sources include memberships in the FCER itself, memorial giving, annual giving, donations earmarked for scholarships, interest on the FCER endowment fund, and bequests and wills.

FCER funds have been allocated directly to colleges for research, upgrading programs, and assisting in progress toward CCE accreditation goals. These programs benefit the public through progressive improvement of chiropractic care.

BASIC PRINCIPLES OF CLINICAL CHIROPRACTIC

Diagnosis plays the same role in chiropractic as in all the healing arts: the basis for determination of the treatment. A chiropractic diagnosis is usually arrived at after an interview, physical examination, and the use of necessary diagnostic aids and laboratory tests.

Chiropractic, regardless of jurisdiction, is built upon three related scientific theories and clinically established principles. Although these have been refined over the years, they represent in essence the basic concepts established by chiropractic pioneers early in the century. Today, they are accepted premises throughout the scientific community.

1. *Disease may be caused by disturbances of the nervous system.* While many factors impair health, disturbances of the nervous system are among the most important factors of disease etiology. The nervous system coordinates cellular activities for adaptation to external or internal environmental change. Environmental agents and conditions unduly impairing the nervous system and to which the body cannot successfully adapt produce fluctuations in the pattern of nerve impulses deviating from the norm. Thus originate many disease processes.

2. *Disturbances of the nervous system may be caused by derangements of musculoskeletal structures.* Subluxations and fixations of vertebral and extraspinal articulations represent a common clinical finding. Extended abnormal involvement of the nervous system may result from disturbances arising within the neuromusculoskeletal system due to the body's attempt to maintain an erect posture. The mechanical lesion (subluxation) is a common result of gravitational strains, asymmetrical activities and efforts, developmental defects, or other mechanical, chemical, or psychic irritations of the nervous system. Once produced, the lesion becomes a focus of sustained pathologic irritation that may trigger a full-fledged syndrome of severe nerve root irritation.

3. *Disturbances of the nervous system may cause or aggravate disease in various parts or functions of the body.* Vertebral and extraspinal subluxations may be involved in common functional disorders of a visceral and vasomotor nature and at times may produce phenomena relating to special organs. Under predisposing circumstances, almost any component of the nervous system may directly or indirectly cause reactions within any other component by reflex mediation.

No scientist, pathologist, physiologist, or clinician with good conscience can find fault with these established principles. They are a matter of everyday occurrence in health science and of much more frequent incidence than commonly realized by those not directly involved in their study.

A human being is a total integrated entity. A disorder in a specific organ or tissue will have its affect on other organs and tissue function. In addition, we must realize that summation of independent causes of dysfunction may jointly have more serious debilitating effects than these causes might have separately. For example, subluxation or fixation may be a contribution to the "triggering" or exacerbating of migraine types of headaches, asthmatic syndromes, indigestion, and certain types of neurovascular and neurovisceral instabilities though they may not be the sole cause of the illness. Correction of spinal lesions often is an imperative toward the effective total management of the case.

FORMS OF CHIROPRACTIC PRACTICE

Solo Practice

As with medical physicians, most DCs establish an unincorporated sole proprietorship in which an individual doctor holds the rights and title to all aspects of the practice and may or may not employ others to participate in the practice. In a solo practice, the owner is potentially liable for all acts of his employees but is not entitled to employee fringe benefits. Due to the increasing complexity of health-care practice and the necessity of carrying the burden of expensive equipment singularly, the number of solo practices has begun to diminish in recent years.

Specialty Practice

A specialty practice is one in which a doctor voluntarily narrows the practice to a special area of interest. In chiropractic, specialty councils have been established in (1) Diagnosis and Internal Disorders, (2) Mental Health, (3) Neurology, (4) Nutrition, (5) Orthopedics, (6) Chiropractic Physiological Therapeutics, (7) Diagnostic Imaging, (8) Sports Injuries and Physical Fitness, and (9) Technic. Doctors who advertise as specialists are required to attain a higher level of certified education in a certain field and are held to a higher standard of care than general practitioners.

Partnership

A partnership is a legal contract between two or more doctors in which all rights, obligations, and responsibilities of each partner are defined. Each partner is liable for the acts and conduct of the other partners unless otherwise specified in the partnership agreement.

Associate Practice

An associate practice is one in which two or more doctors agree to share office space in the same building and possibly certain equipment facilities (eg, x-ray department, clinical laboratory) and certain employees (eg, receptionist, bookkeeper) but conduct their practices as sole proprietors. Sometimes a doctor-employer will refer to an employed colleague as an *associate*, but this should not be confused with the legal definition of the term.

Corporate Practice

A professional corporation (PC) is composed of one or more doctors who serve as shareholders of the corporation. The practice is an artificial entity having a legal and business status that must meet strict state regulations. The doctors involved are considered employees of the corporation and liable only for their own acts. There are certain tax advantages in this legal entity, and the practice does not terminate with a change in shareholders. However, the legal and administrative complexities of a professional corporation discourage this type of arrangement for most physicians.

Group Practice

A group practice has three or more physicians engaged in a mutually agreeable, formally organized, and legally recognized contract in which each member of the group attends assigned patients and shares in the group's expenses, receipts, personnel, facilities, equipment, and records involved in patient care and business management of the group practice. Most small group practices consist of doctors with complementary specialties.

CLOSING REMARKS

Attention is given in this chapter to the chiropractic profession in general: its history, approach to health care, and standard office routines so that a perspective chiropractic assistant may better appreciate her role within the office as part of the health team. In the next chapter, an overview of office philosophy and practice goals is given, along with general business aspects of practice, assistant qualifications, duties and responsibilities, the essentials of professionalism, and office policies.

Chapter 2

The Important Role of the Chiropractic Assistant

Health is frequently front-page news and a common topic throughout the communications media because self-preservation is one of the strongest instincts. Thus, the high interest in this field will never cease. The struggle to defeat illness and degeneration is a never-ending quest.

More assistants are employed by physicians than any other type of allied health-care personnel. Doctors involved in solo practices, group practices, or associate practices all need qualified assistance. And the need for capable CAs is on the rise.

The number of graduating DCs is increasing, thus the need for skilled assistants is accelerating. The field offers many personal rewards such as sustained joy of service, abundant opportunities for growth and advancement, and above average financial reward. Other considerations are that it is one field where mandatory retirement is not required and the job turnover rate among assistants is surprisingly low. Many CAs have been known to remain with the same doctor from the beginning of his practice to his retirement.

Although doctors in private practice have employed assistants for many years, the paraprofessional profession was slow to grow until about 15 years ago. It is now rapidly accelerating. Most DCs employ two CAs, and many have five or more. The primary reasons for this accelerated need are advancing technology requiring skilled assistance, the administrative complexities involved in helping patients with insurance claims, computerization, and rising hospital costs that encourage more services to be performed "in-office."

BASIC QUALIFICATIONS OF A CHIROPRACTIC PARAPROFESSIONAL

In your function as a chiropractic assistant, the doctor will delegate many duties to you. However, the final responsibility for any decision is that of the doctor. It is therefore necessary that the DC be looked to for leadership and policy. It is the role of the chiropractic assistant to administer this policy. This is not so much a superior/subordinate relationship as it is a health-team approach composed of a team leader and staff working together toward common goals.

The chiropractic assistant is involved in two basic but often neglected phases of work: human relations and economics. All her experience and ability should be directed toward these aspects of the practice. Many attributes of an efficient assistant are not taught in a classroom; they are basic personality traits. For example, to perform her job successfully, especially in the one-doctor office, the productive assistant is

Intelligent	Cooperative
Courteous	Honest
Able to supervise	Ethical
A self-starter	Loyal
Neat and tidy	Industrious
Well groomed	Tactful
Understanding	Reliable
Gracious	A good executive
A good manager	Enthusiastic
Empathetic	Resourceful
Decisive	

Outward appearance as reflected in good grooming is a necessary qualification. The importance of personal appearance cannot be overemphasized. Give full attention to details.

As a matter of ethics, never masquerade as a registered nurse. Do not wear a nurse's type cap or mislead patients into believing you are a nurse. You will gain respect, stature, and prestige just by being yourself and doing your job well.

The doctor's patients will readily read your attitude in your posture, vocal tones, facial expressions, and gestures. Win friends through a pleasing, confident, clear, soft voice. Also keep in mind that silent body language can speak louder than what you say.

Good posture, emphasized in chiropractic, not only suggests good health, it also in reflects your temperament. Poor posture reduces the effectiveness of attractive clothes. Stand and walk and sit with grace, dignity, and charm.

Tact and understanding are basic qualifications, as are discretion and good judgment. It is important to known when to talk and when to listen. Your personality should be cheerful and respectful—radiating inter-

est in patients' concerns. However, relating *your* personal life's troubles has no place in communications with patients.

Trustworthiness, loyalty, and honesty are other basic qualifications. The doctor must be able to have full trust and confidence in your actions. Greater responsibilities cannot be given to you unless minor responsibilities are held with respect.

An assistant must be loyal to the doctor, the practice, and the profession. Indiscreet criticisms always have a way of coming home to roost. An honest, straightforward manner is necessary. The doctor should never have a reason to question your truthfulness as he may have cause to act quickly on your word without further investigation.

Accuracy, good business sense, and efficiency are also basic qualifications. Skill in recording the doctor's instructions, instrument readings, and a patient's vocal and nonvocal communications is a necessary qualification for every assistant. Accuracy in administrative routines, diagnostic procedures, and therapeutic procedures is essential in health care.

Common sense and good judgment are two more fundamental qualifications in instances where professional advice is not at hand. The doctor should feel that office procedures will be carried out effectively in minimum time and according to high standards without a great deal of direct supervision.

Versatility Is Often Necessary

Bookkeeping and Secretarial Abilities. An administrative assistant will not be asked to have CPA abilities, but a fundamental knowledge of record keeping and secretarial routines is often required. You may be asked to maintain accurate and detailed daily and summary records, as well as to develop monthly analyses of practice data required by the doctor.

Hostess Attitude. A friendly, pleasant disposition is as necessary to the administrative assistant as it is to the clinical assistant. Hostess abilities include the art of treating patients as invited guests and showing them the courtesy, grace, and social consideration necessary in a professional environment. Sincere concern, empathy, and respect for a patient's comfort, welfare, and feelings are paramount. Such an attitude is expressed in exceptional kindness and gentleness to the elderly or suffering. Remember that the *manner* in which a service is performed can affect its response and thus the health and welfare of the patient.

Housekeeping Consciousness. An assistant's housekeeping ability is expressed in her concern that the office is not only clean but sparkling clean. Spotlessness and necessary sterilization of equipment is the assistant's responsibility even if general office cleaning may be delegated to others.

Technical Skills. The need for versatility is especially necessary in smaller offices where the absence of one staff member must be assumed by one or more others. While you will not be asked to perform a duty for which you are not trained, you will likely be requested to perform certain basic tasks under the doctor's supervision. The most versatile CA is one who can handle any responsibility that does not require certain licensure or certification which has not been obtained.

Not Everyone Can Qualify

A doctor requires a reliable assistant—one who arrives for work on time and has the practice and patient's interests sincerely at heart. He prefers an assistant who desires to make a career out of this important work. He likes enthusiasm, cooperation, a spirit of self-confidence and satisfaction. He needs an assistant that is willing to act responsibly when he is not in the office. A dependable assistant will accept the responsibility to tend to routine functions and know how to handle any emergency that may arise.

How can you tell whether this career is for you? Besides the basic qualifications previously discussed, if you like people, enjoy being busy, are willing to learn new things, are adaptable to change, respect leadership, can remain calm in emergencies, are well organized, can follow instructions,

have a positive personality, are willing to admit your shortcomings and strengthen your weaknesses, and can keep your personal life to yourself while in the office, then you are probably the type who will find this career exciting and rewarding. However, if you would rather work alone, have a strong tendency to procrastinate, would rather avoid responsibilities, prefer the *status quo* to challenging changes, have difficulty following orders, get "uptight" in emergency situations, are undisturbed by uncleanliness, are a highly critical nature, and have the habit of excusing your shortcomings, you probably will not find this career to be of lasting interest.

The able assistant is one who learns to view a specific situation through the eyes of the patient involved. Only in this manner can proper attention be given. Some people, despite how hard they try, cannot develop this perspective.

The chiropractic assistant is an integral part of a well-managed practice. The opportunity to exercise independence and authority plus execution of many diversified duties makes chiropractic an extremely interesting and rewarding field. For the right person, the role of a CA is not just a job—it's an adventure in health care.

Salary

Assistant salaries vary depending on the size, activity, and age of the practice. There also are, as with most occupations, regional differences and differences between rural and urban areas. Most doctors respect the work done by assistants and will base the assistant's salary on the practice's net income and assistant's talent contribution. Experience has taught physicians that cheap help is the most expensive.

Most DCs have the reputation of paying their assistants fairly. Many offices have a "Position Classification System" that defines salary scales and ranges and differentiates among position responsibilities, experience, and practice contribution so that individual differences in value to the practice can be considered.

Salary Reviews

Most doctors review a new employee after the first 6 months and then on an annual basis. Both cost-of-living and merit increases are considered. Each position is rated on the degree of knowledge required, amount of formal education required, skill, independent judgment, performance attitude, weight of responsibility, and other traits necessary. Each job classification usually has a minimum and maximum rate through which an employee may be advanced.

Opportunity for Growth

The experienced assistant is often in a position to serve as the general business agent or office manager for her employer. If you can control general office routines, you can help the doctor run his practice in line with good business policies. The result of your efficiency will no doubt affect the doctor's income, and therefore will have a bearing on your position as well. You will find that as you become more proficient in your work, you, too, will reach new levels of income and satisfaction. The opportunities are many, as are the challenges.

DUTIES AND RESPONSIBILITIES

In the well-managed office, an assistant serves as another brain and another pair of hands. She does those duties that do not require the special knowledge, skill, or training of the doctor. In a sense, the assistant acts as a partner, performing details and office functions that the DC does not have the time to provide.

Each practice reflects the individual personality or personalities of the doctor or doctors involved. As humans vary in genetic and conditioned personality structure, it is unlikely that the duties of an assistant in one practice will be identical with those in another even if several other major practice characteristics are similar. Duties of any given assistant thus will be determined as much by the personality and goals of the doctor in charge as they will by the type and size of the practice itself.

The Practice Plan

Typically, the average health practice grows from the one doctor and one assistant operation with changes made to meet growth problems. Often organizational changes are made from time to time to meet emergency situations without regard to future plans. Unfortunately, this has led to some internal problems and personnel frustrations in the past. Today, however, the average DC is cognizant of the necessity of sound organization and planning.

The basic practice plan must first meet the needs of the doctor's practice philosophy and objectives. To achieve this, the ideal organizational plan will define and identify all functions that must be performed successfully if the practice is to develop as intended.

Assigned Duties

Each practice, regardless of size, has certain functions that must be performed by an assistant, and these functions will be assigned. Specific assignments vary from office to office and are determined by the size of the practice involved, the number of doctors involved, the number of assistants involved, the established relationships between doctor(s) and assistant(s), the laws of the state, and the individual talents and personalities of the people involved.

As previously explained, although duties of the assistant vary from practice to practice, all personnel except licensed DCs who assist in a chiropractic office are called chiropractic assistants or parachiropractic personnel. All such personnel must be keenly aware of their individual responsibilities, where these responsibilities may overlap with those of other personnel, and where (and to what degree) one may be required to substitute for an absent employee. Despite assigned duties, all office personnel are expected to perform their duties cheerfully and to the best of their abilities. Assistants are the office's front-line good will ambassadors and public relations representatives.

As duties vary from office to office, job descriptions and classifications of functions differ from office to office. However, to obtain an overview of the work of the chiropractic assistant, we will, for simplicity, divide the duties into two large and frequently overlapping classifications: (1) an assistant generally serving as a receptionist/secretary, and (2) an assistant generally serving as a clinical aide.

Administrative Assistant

Reception and secretary personnel carry out many functions of a nontechnical nature such as receptionist, executive secretary, file and billing clerk, telephone operator, typist, and all-around girl friday. A pleasant personality, a gift for cordial human relations, tact and neatness, and a willingness to help whenever and wherever are essential qualifications.

Below is a listing of general duties that might be assigned. The duties are not listed in priority, as priority varies from office to office and the needs of the moment.

- Opens office
- Contacts the doctor's answering service
- Attends the telephone
- Receives and dismisses patients
- Schedules appointments
- Sends appointment reminder cards to or telephones patients
- Screens nonpatient office visitors
- Explains general office procedures to patients
- Answers questions about procedures
- Explains doctor's fees to patients
- Obtains basic new-patient information
- Pulls scheduled patients' charts
- Escorts patients to appropriate office area
- Attends to special needs of youth and elderly
- Assists patients in completing office forms
- Receives payments and give receipts
- Files records and other materials
- Types correspondence
- Transcribes the doctor's dictation
- Opens, sorts, and distributes office mail
- Prepares correspondence for doctor's signature
- Prepares referral letters and forms

- Prepares and oversees doctor's calendar
- Prepares periodic examination reminders
- Answers mail not requiring the doctor's signature
- Performs general office management
- Keeps daily bookkeeping records
- Maintains employee payroll records
- Balances checkbooks and checks bank statements
- Controls accounts receivable and sends reminders
- Prepares and mails statements to patients
- Processes insurance claim forms
- Controls accounts payable and pays bills
- Maintains office business supplies and inventory
- Maintains office petty cash account
- Supervises office community and public relations programs
- Distributes educational office mailings
- Sends birthday, anniversary, congratulatory, and thank-you notes
- Maintains cross-indexed bibliography of articles in professional journals that the doctor has marked
- Assists in maintaining the doctor's personal library and office lending library
- Maintains laundry control
- Keeps office conditioned for proper heating and cooling; ventilates and deodorizes when necessary
- Oversees office housekeeping and general facilities
- Maintains periodic equipment service records
- Other administrative responsibilities as necessary

Clinical Assistant

Technical personnel perform many functions of a clinical nature such as assisting in physical diagnostic procedures, x-ray film processing, in-office laboratory tests, auxiliary therapeutic applications, massage and muscle therapy, rehabilitative procedures, posture training, explanation and distribution of diet and exercise regimens, recording of basic case history data, and other paraprofessional functions. These duties are performed under close supervision of the doctor-employer.

Below is a listing of general duties that might be assigned after training and possibly certification. Again, the duties are not listed in priority, as priority varies from office to office and situation.

- Records general body measurements (eg, height, weight)
- Records such signs as temperature, pulse, respiratory rate, and general vision
- Conducts general posture analyses with instrumentation
- Records routine re-evaluation data
- Dispenses diet regimens and supplements
- Teaches good health habits, personal hygiene
- Assists DC in certain therapeutic applications
- Conducts certain auxiliary therapeutic applications; eg, physiotherapy
- Records clinical findings for DC during examinations
- Orients patient to equipment to be used during office therapy
- Conducts therapeutic massage and passive exercises
- Teaches prescribed home-therapy techniques
- Teaches home rehabilitative equipment care and maintenance
- Explains necessity of patient cooperation for optimal recovery
- Processes laboratory prescription orders
- Assists in administering first aid
- Assists during gynecologic examinations
- Prepares pap specimen slides
- Prepares patient x-ray identification markers
- Conducts assigned x-ray patient positioning, exposure, processing, and film-filing functions
- Performs assigned counsel to patient's family when necessary
- Collects specimens from patients
- Performs in-office hematologic tests
- Performs in-office urinalyses
- Prepares patient for metabolic and electrocardiogram tests
- Checks outside laboratory and clinical supply invoices
- Maintains inventory control of clinical supplies
- Checks arriving shipments of clinical supplies
- Maintains cleanliness and sanitation of clinical areas and equipment
- Cleans and sterilizes laboratory and other diagnostic instruments
- Maintains cleanliness of darkroom and laboratory
- Other technical responsibilities as necessary

As can be seen, the duties of a chiropractic assistant are broad and varied. The assistant may be called on to carry out numerous secretarial functions, serve as business manager, prepare examination and therapy setups, conduct laboratory tests, and help the doctor during various parts of the examination and treatment procedure. Some doctors feel strongly that there is much routine work that can be delegated to a well-trained assistant, thus allowing the doctor to see more patients or spend more time with patients. On the other hand, some doctors are against delegating any work of a clinical nature to their assistants.

The work a chiropractic assistant is called on to do is thus determined by the office's needs and the assistant's ability. Another factor is that of legal requirements. In some states, well-trained assistants are permitted to conduct x-ray exposures, apply physiotherapeutic applications, withdraw blood samples, and administer injections under the direct supervision of a licensed doctor of chiropractic. In other states, the assistant must be personally licensed or certified in the state to conduct such applications.

THE ATMOSPHERE OF A PROFESSIONAL OFFICE

People, especially sick people, warrant alert attention from anybody engaged in offering a service. There should never be shown a lack of interest. Privacy is also important. When the doctor is with a patient, all avoidable interruptions should be prevented. Health service is a private service.

Regardless of assigned duties and responsibilities, the doctor is responsible for employee actions. When chiropractic ethics are offended, the assistant may subject her doctor-employer to embarrassment and even a lawsuit. She must therefore be confident in what she is doing and know her limitations. The following points should always be kept in mind.

General Ethical Standards

Privileged Information. All knowledge of a patient's life, personal or clinical, learned within the office is strictly confidential. Nothing learned from doctor or patient conversations, case histories, telephone messages, or correspondence must ever be divulged. The doctor-patient relationship is *protected by law.* No one may pass information about the patient or the care utilized to an attorney, an insurance company, a relative, etc, without the personal authorization of the patient.

Referral Limitations. It is customary that a referred patient be treated only for the condition for which he was originally sent to the doctor. If a referred patient does not wish to return to the referring doctor, the assistant should mention this to her employer so that the matter can be discussed in private with the patient.

Health Education. All doctors are prohibited from making false claims. Therefore, the chiropractic assistant must be careful not to say anything that could be interpreted as soliciting patients in such a manner. However, an assistant may praise her doctor-employer and/or the office in a professional, dignified manner. It is not unethical for an office to distribute health education information and materials, but a chiropractic assistant must never give specific health advice to a patient. She may, however, relay the doctor's instructions to a patient and discuss procedures that the doctor wishes explained. Offering professional advice to a patient may subject an assistant to being accused of practicing chiropractic without a license. Likewise, an assistant must never attempt to interpret laboratory reports, diagnostic x-ray films, or any other type of clinical data, though she may be involved in the data-gathering process.

Derogatory Remarks. Another doctor, regardless of which healing branch is involved, should never be criticized in front of a patient even if your doctor-employer has expressed certain opinions in private.

Professional Availability. According to codes of professional conduct, the doctor should hold himself in constant readiness to respond to calls of the sick from established patients. Thus, the assistant should be aware that emergency situations may frequently arise which will sometimes extend normal office hours.

Prohibited Actions. In a few states, it is against the law for an unlicensed person to make x-ray exposures, conduct an invasive diagnostic test, or apply certain physiotherapeutic instruments or measures. The assistant should be fully informed by her doctor-employer of the various practice acts of the state in which she is employed.

Professional Courtesy. According to professional standards, chiropractors and their immediate dependents are entitled to the gratuitous services of any one or more of the profession. Doctors of chiropractic are unable to care for themselves in full when ill. The anxiety and solicitude felt when a member of the immediate family is ill may render them incompetent to care for that family member. In these circumstances, chiropractors are especially dependent on each other, and professional aid is always cheerfully and gratuitously offered. The assistant thus should be careful that colleagues of the doctor or the colleagues' immediate family are not billed for services rendered. However, this policy is changing because many DCs now have broad health-insurance coverage.

Staff Adaptability

The office health-team relationship requires a great deal of harmony and mutual dependability. An unwillingness on the part of an assistant to be punctual or to work overtime will disrupt this harmony. Doctors often take for granted that the assistant knows what she is expected to do and is willing to work long hours when the office requires it. The assistant, as the doctor, must plan her personal life according to patient needs and emergency situations.

While practices vary with the individual office, chiropractic assistants are often called on to perform every service that does not require a professional license. Every service performed by the doctor but which could be done by his assistant is an expensive service as far as the patient and practice are concerned.

The Business Aspect of Health Practice

Today's doctor of chiropractic invests at least 6 years in formal education learning to provide a unique health-care service. Both the doctor's education and priorities are of a clinical nature. This is proper, but a health practice cannot be run successfully without good administrative and management systems.

While chiropractic is not a business, there *is* a business aspect to practice. Good business sense is fundamental to provide good clinical service. Unless sound business judgment is used, the practice will be unable to finance optimal services, equipment, or maintain a compensatory lifestyle for either the doctor or personnel.

Increasing Administrative Complexities

Thirty years ago many health practitioners could operate the business side of their practice from a roll-top desk and a few file cards. This is not so today. An increasing amount of health care is involved with third-party payors such as insurance companies and Worker's Compensation Boards and Funds. As many offices do not accept cases "on assignment," patients today require accurate, detailed, rapidly prepared records and forms to collect on their coverage. Yesteryear's simplistic, often haphazard and erratic, record and billing systems cannot be

tolerated. Poor office administration and management will unfairly reflect on the doctor's clinical competency.

The care of the sick, by itself, offers a "pressure" situation for doctor and staff. Paperwork pressure is an added burden if efficient administrative and management procedures are not implemented. Good organization and alert assistance are important in freeing the doctor from the less vital yet time-consuming tasks that can keep him from his main objective of caring for patients in need of his services.

Three decades ago, emphasis on peer review and concern over malpractice were extremely rare. Today they are concerns necessitating accurate clinical and financial records, along with good patient rapport.

The importance of detailed record keeping is paradoxical to the average doctor. On one side, the typical doctor of chiropractic was drawn into the profession for idealistic reasons and a desire to practice health care. On the other side, the doctor was neither educated nor motivated to be a good businessman. This underscores the necessity of good office assistance.

The Human Relations Element

Good human relations is good business, and good human relations is a primary concern of the chiropractic assistant just as it is of the doctor. When the doctor is busy with other patients or duties, it is the assistant who first meets the patient entering the office. First impressions are lasting impressions. Thus the attitude of the assistant is the attitude of the office as far as the patient is concerned.

The first responsibility of the office is the responsibility of the assistant in greeting the patient, welcoming the patient, and putting the patient at ease. Sick people are apprehensive, nervous, and often extremely sensitive. An assistant's friendly, professional attitude will help create an atmosphere helpful to the situation.

Initial Data Gathering

Another responsibility of the assistant is in obtaining certain basic information from the patient before the patient personally consults with the doctor. Basic records must be filled out. In some instances, the assistant also may record the basic case history and possibly take some measurements. The clinical assistant will frequently be at the doctor's side during examination procedures, helping in the process so that the doctor's time and motions will be most efficient.

Foresight

Even before the first patient of the day is greeted, the efficient assistant has been busy behind the scene. Consultation, examination, and therapy rooms have been inspected for neatness, cleanliness, and organization. Supplies have been checked. Equipment has been checked. Instruments have been checked. Nothing is left to chance. Everything the doctor will need will be at hand where he will expect to find it. Carelessness cannot be tolerated in health care, and disorganization cannot be tolerated in a businesslike operation. Without capable, sincere assistance, the doctor is severely handicapped.

To do good work, you need good equipment and working conditions. However, do not expect the doctor to check on the condition of your typewriter or know if your desk's lighting is insufficient. It will be up to you to bring such situations to his attention. Requisition supplies before you run out, and try to anticipate future needs the best you can rather than waiting until the last minute.

Fees for Services

Every doctor must charge and collect for his services if the practice is to survive and grow. There is nothing unprofessional or unethical about applying sound business techniques to operating a health-care practice. The more sound management principles are applied within a practice, the more time the doctor will have to spend with his patients. The challenge, of course, is in arriving at a proper balance between clinical and business concerns. Neither aspects should be ignored, as both are needed to achieve practice goals.

Community Relations and Involvement

It is well, personally and professionally, to build stature and respect by becoming a willing worker in your community. Professional status grows as the community looks to you for aid and advice. For these reasons, doctors of chiropractic encourage their employees to practice good citizenship and become actively involved in their community. However, care should be taken that such involvement does not interfere with one's work responsibilities.

Organizations such as political groups, charitable organizations, the PTA, the Boy and Girl Scouts, civic organizations, women's clubs, church groups, and so forth, offer many social and community service benefits. You may, of course, support any cause of your choice, but do not carry your interest or enthusiasm into the office.

Never burden patients or fellow employees for contributions, to sign a petition, to support your political candidate, or to purchase raffle tickets unless you have gained permission from the doctor. Your personal opinions on politics and religion should be kept to yourself. Avoid any topic that may be considered controversial.

On-the-Job Conduct

All office personnel have a part to play in developing a professional office atmosphere. Health care is a serious business. Patients should not be likened to customers. Professionalism must be conveyed to patients in a subtle manner through office routine, office appearance, and personnel appearance and attitudes. Smoking, gum chewing, eating, drinking, reading newspapers and popular magazines, and the like should be confined to a designated area and never done before patients.

Experienced assistants should help orient new assistants to the office's team approach to patient care. Use the editorial "we" frequently in talking with patients. References to the office as "our office" becomes automatic when the paraprofessional becomes truly team oriented.

Regulation of an employee's after-hours activities is not the prerogative or intention of the employer-doctor. However, keep in mind that the office has many patients and personnel are frequently observed both within and without the office. Actions of staff help develop the public image of the office. Likewise, the "dating" of patients is usually frowned on as such practice frequently leads to embarrassing if not extremely delicate situations. Office personnel are requested to avoid any personal relationships that might cause patients to feel uncomfortable when returning to the office. Serious indiscretions may be considered cause for dismissal, as would unethical conduct, alcoholism, or drug abuse.

Emergency Situations

The need for adaptability has been previously described. Even if regular working hours are established, most doctor-employers will expect their assistants to be on hand during emergency situations. If another job is desired for extra income or if organizational work may conflict with work requirements, such matters should be discussed with the doctor before a final commitment is made. Many people find that holding two jobs leaves them physically unable to perform efficiently. Working for another health practitioner may be considered a conflict of interest.

Personal Conversations

Limit discussions with patients to office matters, and do this in a friendly manner. This does not mean you cannot be a good listener. Conversations with fellow staff members also should be limited to office-related matters during office hours. Habitual chatting reduces the time and opportunities for self-development in your career.

The office telephone is the practice's primary link with the community. Personal telephone calls during office hours should be brief and limited to the needs of the situation.

Professional Appearance

A practice concerned with health care should reflect a healthy appearance of personnel. CAs should get plenty of rest so they will be alert and efficient during working hours. A well-balanced nourishing diet should be followed because nutrition is a basic factor in radiant health. Cosmetics should be used sparingly; a glowing, fresh appearance is evidence of good health. A sparkling smile should also show the world well cared for teeth.

Personal Attire

What could be more important to the appearance of the office than you? If you look neat, the office will look neater. If you are dressed as a professional, you will help give the office a professional atmosphere.

Staff Uniforms. Most DCs prefer that their assistants wear white uniforms. However, colored uniforms coordinated with those of the doctor and other personnel are also acceptable. White is commonly used because it symbolizes cleanliness and is associated with the health professions. A white uniform is dignified and commands respect because of the authority it represents. In addition to a clean white uniform, it is recommended that the chiropractic assistant groom herself conservatively. It is better to lean to the simple and tailored side during selection than to overdress. In the office, conservatism displays good taste and dignity.

Besides its practical application, a uniform has a decided psychologic effect as patients feel more at ease with an assistant dressed in a uniform—they feel less embarrassment in answering personal questions and in disrobing, and are more willing to cooperate.

Uniforms of good quality look better and last longer than the more economical brands, although they may need ironing despite what it says on the label. A good uniform is never transparent. The nylon uniform is usually avoided as it is commonly associated with beauty parlor attendants or restaurant waitresses. When pastel colors are used for assistant uniforms, the doctor also should consider using the same color for his clinic jacket as it enhances the team concept and indicates concern for harmony, thoroughness, and detail.

Hands and Nails. Hands should always be well washed, and the nails should be well kept and trimmed moderately short. Colorless nail polish is preferred to bright red. Never use exotic colors during office hours.

Hair Styling. A CA's hairstyle should be neat, conservatively styled, and well brushed. Elaborate or unusual hair styles are out of place in the professional office. Long flowing hair is inconsistent with the professional uniform and offensive to many patients. It should be pinned up during office hours.

Hosiery. Hose should be of a neutral color with standard mesh. Bare legs, colored hosiery, and unusual weave or embroidery are inappropriate in a professional office, especially with a uniform.

Shoes. Wear comfortable, well-made shoes (preferably, white) because aching feet and calf muscles will be reflected in your attitude. Shoes should be coordinated with the uniform, comfortable, of conservative style, and may be of the assistant's personal selection. Excessively soiled or worn shoes should be replaced regardless of age.

Overgarments. In late spring or early fall when the building temperature is not always consistent, a sweater or light jacket can be coordinated to the basic uniform. Such covering should be kept clean and used only when necessary.

Only jewelry suitable with a uniform should be worn. Use only a reasonable amount of perfume. Bathe or shower daily, and use deodorant as necessary. Breath sprays and mouthwash should be used as needed. Strongly spiced foods and alcoholic beverages should be avoided during the working hours.

The Professional Image

The assistant's part in the chain of public relations starts when a patient opens the door to the office. First impressions made on the patient because of office appearance and staff behavior are lasting impressions to be conveyed to others. The power of speech can be to an office's advantage or disadvantage, depending on how much it is human relations oriented.

A first in-office public relations function is to make the office comfortable, appealing, efficient, and professional in every respect. Another important task is to develop an ability to make friends, gain the confidence of patients quickly, work efficiently, and act professionally. These qualities must become second nature to every member of the staff. A third important public relations effort should be one of public education. To be effective, health education must be centered in the office and expanded in scope to touch every contact of all personnel.

People tend to generalize and stereotype. You represent all chiropractic assistants, the chiropractic profession, and especially your office outside the office, at work, or at play. You have a responsibility not only to your doctor-employer but also to yourself to be a good courier of public relations.

Your every act as a chiropractic assistant, your every word, your every letter, your touch and gentleness, and your every contact with the public should "breathe" prestige, restraint, good manners, and professionalism. This is the image you should want to build and strengthen. It starts in the morning when you arise from sleep; it stops when you go to bed at night.

Thus, to many patients and acquaintances, you represent the office. Since you are building an image every minute of every day, your duty to yourself and your profession is to build an image of friendliness, sincerity, professional "know-how," and respect. Your image should be one of pride in accepting a responsibility and fulfilling a need. Be recognized as a community-minded citizen who aids in the health and welfare of human beings. It's a giant step toward a positive self-image and success.

Essentials

Chiropractic assistants should keep in mind a few essential responsibilities:

• Be aware that you are a professional. Use the highest level of ethics in dealing with patients and the public. Assure that your services are of the highest professional caliber and unquestionable merit. Indicate confidence in every way possible, but with dignity and tact.

• Be sincerely interested in every patient who enters the office. Also be interested in the physical well-being of America's citizens and interested in chiropractic as a profession. Do your part to inform and educate the public, thereby advancing the reputation of chiropractic.

• Work diligently toward increasing respect for your profession. The public is always conscious of a professional person's appearance and behavior and the appearance of the office. As a professional, you are constantly under the public's microscope to be analyzed and critiqued. What you say, what you do, and how you act and react are important. Never let your community lose confidence in you. Practice good public relations in everything you do.

Your personal public relations, the public relations of your office, and national and state chiropractic public relations all have the same objectives: respect, understanding, recognition, and favorable comment. To help you achieve these goals, note the following five rules for dealing with people.

1. Meet new people, and show an interest in them. Learn of their interests, hobbies, likes and dislikes: find out what motivates them. One of the best ways to do this is to become a good listener. By seeking to understand others, you will cause others to understand you.

2. Treat people with respect. Be courteous; be understanding; be patient. Acknowledge the rights and opinions of others. Treat all as you would like to be treated, and you then have every right to expect the same in return.

3. Don't force yourself on people. Whenever possible, try to be professional in your approach. Don't be "pushy." Aggressive social behavior does not fit the dignified image of a professional.

4. Truly welcome the stranger. Make the welcome cheerful but to the point. Be friendly and a good listener. Be down to earth and practical in your conversation, and give others a chance to voice their views. Develop the ability to know when to terminate a conversation tactfully and leave.

5. Use a giving rather than a taking approach. Build respect by becoming a contributor of your time, effort, ideas, empathy, and understanding. Don't become burdensome with your conversations or requests. People should be happy to see you, knowing that the visit will have purpose and meaning. If you accept a job or a project, do it. Don't expect someone else to carry you.

ACQUAINTING YOURSELF WITH OFFICE POLICIES

Keeping in mind that it would be impossible to prepare a list of pertinent policies that would be germane to every office, the following section describes topics of which most offices will have either a written or informal policy to meet the needs of the practice involved. Typical office policies concerning uniforms, grooming, attire, personal habits, and general attitudes are not described here as they have been explained previously in this chapter.

Policies vs Procedures

It is important as an assistant to recognize the difference between an office *policy* and an office *procedure*. A policy is a statement or principle on which the practice operates. A procedure indicates the method or system by which the policy will be administered. For example, a credit *policy* (principle) establishes whether cash only payments will be accepted for services or if credit will be extended and under what circumstances and to what limits. A credit *procedure* (mechanics), on the other hand, defines the methods and systems by which the credit policy will be executed such as how charges will be recorded, how and when statements will be processed, how records will be filed, how overdue accounts will be handled, and other management and administrative methods.

Again we must be aware of the varying scope of office policies—depending on the size of the practice staff, and personal philosophy of the doctor-employer involved. A policy that might be vital to the successful operation of a large office may be quite unnecessary to a small office. In this book, we have tried to take the middle road—describing policies that are common to the majority of established practices. Keep in mind, however, that any particular office may greatly reduce or expand the areas of policy described.

Practice Policies vs Employee Policies

An assistant, even prior to entering the staff, should be aware of what is established in the way of practice and employee policies. *Practice policies* relate to office hours, collections, billings, inventory control, bulletin boards, etc. *Employee policies* concern personnel policies such as salary, holidays, overtime, uniforms, vacations, insurance, and so forth. Many practice and employee policies overlap. For instance, tardiness, attitude, attire, and grooming are policy areas that directly concern the practice and the individual involved.

Personnel Records

Each assistant should see to it that her personnel records reflect accurate and current information. Changes in tax exemptions affect payroll deductions. Address and telephone number changes are important to keep current.

Payroll Deductions

Deductions for federal and state income taxes, social security, and required city or county taxes are made automatically on employment. Deductions for such voluntary items as savings plans, insurance programs, etc, are made only on employee request. Any changes in your number of exemptions should be reported to your employer or the person in charge of payroll.

Pay Advances

Except in rare circumstances, most offices refuse to make advances. In cases of severe financial emergency, pay advances are usually limited to the amount of the next check. An assistant in financial embarrassment should seek the aid of her bank or a loan company.

Absenteeism

It is assumed when you are hired that you will be available for work on a regular basis. Absenteeism, tardiness, attitude, and performance are important factors in determining advancement in terms of both increasing responsibilities and salary.

Chronic or unexplained absenteeism may be cause for dismissal. Most offices will have a policy for granting reasonable requests for time off when justifiable. Absences during the probationary period of employment are usually without pay, and irregularity in attendance during this period may be cause for termination. Unjustifiable chronic absenteeism of any employee may be cause for discharge because efficient operation of an office requires the presence of a full staff. Periodic contact with the doctor-employer should be made during prolonged absences such as those caused by sickness. Infrequent excusable absences of salaried employees do not as a rule reduce their compensation, but hourly employees will likely be affected.

Election Service

Most office policies do not allow absence from work with pay to serve as an election official during election time. Before an employee makes plans to work at the polls, authorization for absence from work should be obtained from your doctor-employer.

Some offices recognize such work as a civic duty and may pay the difference between your regular rate and the pay received.

Holidays

The number of observed holidays in chiropractic offices varies in different communities and offices. Most offices observe Christmas Day, New Year's Day, Memorial Day, Independence Day, Labor Day, and Thanksgiving. Other holidays such as Presidents Day, Columbus Day, Veterans Day, Good Friday, First Day of Passover, Jewish New Year, Yom Kippur, etc, may be observed.

Working Hours

A CA's hours vary according to personal responsibilities, type of practice, patient load, community custom, and emergency situations. Each office has its own policy. Some offices have evening hours; others do not. Hours may vary according to the day, but the total during a week rarely exceed 40 hours. For instance, you may be required to work 10 hours on certain days and 6 hours on others. Hours for administrative assistants may vary from those of technical assistants. Administrative functions proceed even if patients are not in the office. Most technical functions cease soon after the last patient leaves.

Rest Periods

Because of the nature of health care practice, it is difficult if not impossible to establish fixed rest periods. Rest periods and coffee breaks must be considered relative to the needs of the office so that absence from duties will not interfere with efficient doctor-patient relations or patient flow.

Personal Leaves of Absence

When justifiable, most offices will allow personal time off and charge this time to either the employee's vacation credit or deduct it from the next payroll. The method applied is often at the employee's option. Personal leaves of absence are not charged against sick leave credits. Many offices will allow an authorized personal leave of absence of less than 4 hours to be made up at a future date or dates rather than charging the time against vacation time or payroll.

Jury Duty

Because many injury trials go on for several weeks or months, most DCs request that the employee be excused from duty as such absence would have an adverse affect on efficient patient care. When jury duty is approved in office policy for established employees, their income is usually not affected; ie, the office will likely reimburse the difference between jury payment and regular income.

Witness Service

A call to duty as a court witness as a result of a subpoena issued by the court is usually considered a justifiable absence with no loss in pay.

Sick Leave

Most offices are willing to consider salary continuation for assistants during a period of short disability. Such consideration is usually reserved for permanent full-time assistants who have a good work record and are employed in practices that can afford to pay for nonperformance. The policy should never be abused, when offered, by considering it as extended earned vacation time. Sick leave only refers to an illness of the employee, not a member of the employee's immediate family in which case the employee is required to be absent. The benefits are not usually cumulative from calendar year to calendar year. That is, they cannot be converted into cash or vacation allowance at the time of termination or resignation.

Accidents

Every working environment contains some degree of hazard, thus safety procedures must be observed at all times. If you become injured during working hours, even slightly, report the fact to your doctor-employer immediately. Most employees will be covered under the State Worker's Compensation Plan to cover the cost of work-related injuries. You will be treated within the office or referred to another physician, depending on the nature of the injury. The doctor involved in treatment will complete the necessary report form and determine necessary time off from work on approval of the accident insurance carrier.

Accident and Health Insurance

The purpose of this type insurance is to protect employees against loss of income during periods of nonwork-related disability. Premiums for this type of insurance are usually paid by the employee. As office policy and coverage vary, the employee should discuss this with her employer and personal insurance agent when optimal coverage is desired.

Maternity Leave

During pregnancy, the common practice is for the employee to leave around the 6th month of term or earlier on the obstetrician's recommendation. State laws supersede office policy. Time of leave and return in most practices is often a matter of mutual agreement between employee and employer. Earned seniority and benefits are not affected by most offices' maternity leave policies.

Vacations

Doctors realize that everyone needs to get away from the job occasionally. Most doctors require that employees earning 2 or 3 weeks vacation take no more than 1 week at a time unless advanced authorization has been made for an extended trip. Vacation time is usually extended when a recognized holiday falls within a scheduled vacation. Staff seniority usually determines who will receive first choice for a requested vacation period.

As health-care practices operate the year around, there is usually no good time or no bad time to take a vacation. Normally, permanent full-time employees are granted, with pay, a 1-week vacation after the first year of employment, 2 weeks after the 2nd year, and 3 weeks after the 5th year of employment. Unused vacation time, if so chosen by the employee, is usually not compensated in cash, but it may be extended from one year to the next if agreed on in advance.

Voting Time

Most doctors recognize that voting is a basic responsibility of good citizenship. While it is preferred that voting not be done during regular working hours, the doctor-employer will likely authorize time off with pay when necessary if the absence does not interfere with normal office function.

Bonding

Many practices carry a bond on employees handling large sums of cash. Such insurance protects the office against possible loss. When a bond is required, the employee should not consider the fact as a question of personal honesty. It is a standard business procedure. The cost of bonding is a responsibility of the office, not the employee. If an employee cannot be bonded for some reason and it is office policy that the position requires bonding, the inability to obtain bonding may be cause for termination.

Medical, Dental, and Optometric Appointments

Except in emergencies, exterior health-care appointments should be made on the CA's personal time so that they will not interfere with work responsibilities. However, periodic health-care examinations are encouraged as the doctor-employer desires all his employees to be in the best of health.

Time off will usually be permitted during working hours if a more advantageous time cannot be obtained. The appointment should be scheduled during the least busy time of your office as possible. Employees abusing such privileges may be asked to subtract the time from their vacation allowance.

Funeral Leave

Most chiropractors allow salaried employees time off to attend funerals of the immediate family without loss of income. Exact definition of immediate family varies with the office, as does the maximum number of days allowed. Funeral leave with pay is usually restricted to full-time, nonprobationary employees on salary.

Resignation

In cases of resignation, most offices require 2–4 weeks' notice so that a replacement can be hired and indoctrinated. An employer's "letter of recommendation" is determined by the circumstances involved in the resignation and the employee's work history. Accrued benefits are compensated according to state law and office policy.

Dismissal

When an employee does not perform as expected after customary training, dismissal may be in the best interests of both the employee and the practice. To reduce the probability of such an occurrence is the reason for the common 3-month probationary period on initial employment. Usually, several warnings are given an employee prior to actual dismissal. Theft, failure to execute policy, insubordination, unacceptable attitude, etc, are causes for immediate dismissal. Inefficiency or inability to perform as required, chronic absenteeism, excessive tardiness, poor personal hygiene, and the like, also may be cause for dismissal.

If an employee is dismissed for the convenience of the office such as when the position is no longer required, it is said that the employee is "terminated without prejudice." In such case, the employee is usually given a 2-week notice or 2-weeks' pay in lieu of notice, and accrued sick leave, vacation benefits, and other compensation earned. If an employee is dismissed for gross neglect, severe infraction of employment standards, immoral conduct, antisocial behavior, conviction of a felony, or an act that adversely affects the practice's image, it is said that the employee is "terminated for cause." In such case, dismissal may be immediate and without notice, but accrued benefits will be compensated.

Judicial Incarceration

When an employee is found guilty of violating the law and detention prevents coming to work, it is cause for immediate dismissal. Employees detained and awaiting trial may be granted absences unless the length of detention requires the vacancy to be filled for the good of the practice.

Drug Abuse and Use

Use of nonprescribed controlled drugs is a criminal offense and cause for immediate dismissal—as would be the sale, distribution, or possession of illegal or addictive drugs by an employee. The employee likely would be referred to proper authorities for further action. This policy does not refer to drugs specifically prescribed for the employee by a medical physician. However, any employee under the care of a medical physician and who is using narcotics in the treatment of an ailment should so advise her employer.

Alcohol Use

While usually an unwritten policy, drinking on the job or working under the influence of alcohol is cause for immediate dismissal.

Most employers have no objection to social drinking as long as it is not on office premises and its effects do not affect performance. Alcoholism, however, is considered a progressive illness whose adverse affects on work are cause for discharge. The doctor is restricted in his flexibility in such matters by terms of his malpractice insurance policy.

Educational Assistance

Attendance at seminars, workshops, and other educational activities required by your doctor-employer is an office expense as far as tuition, parking, and registration, fees are concerned. Incidental expenses such as meals are not usually reimbursed unless previously authorized. Some offices will encourage employees to take adult education courses designed to enhance improvement in patient care. In such situations, the office may pay all or part of the expenses involved. This benefit is usually limited to permanent employees who are taking a course having a direct or indirect effect on personal performance or the practice in general.

Housekeeping Control

Although housekeeping is usually considered an uninteresting subject, its importance should not be de-emphasized. Most office policies state that housekeeping is a responsibility shared by the entire staff even if janitorial services are provided. In a professional health-care facility, spotlessness is essential, supplies must be kept in order, equipment must shine, and all tabletops and traffic areas must be free of clutter. Office housekeeping requirements are not just periodic cleanups, they mean constant survcillance by the entire team.

Confidential Information

Information about a patient or a member of the staff should never be discussed except in the line of professional conduct. Gossip displays poor judgment and adversely affects employee reviews. A severe breach of confidence, especially if it concerns a patient, is cause for immediate dismissal. Patient information is guarded by law from disclosure unless prior authorization is received from the patient. It is also considered unprofessional to make derogatory remarks about the practice, office personnel, or another practice either within or without your office.

Smoking

The trend today is toward prohibiting smoking in poorly air-conditioned or ventilated health-care offices among visitors, patients, and staff unless special areas are provided (eg, a staff lounge).

Personal Telephone Calls

Assistants should realize the importance of keeping office telephone lines open to professional needs. Personal telephone use should always be restricted to emergency use. When calls are necessary, they should be limited to periods when incoming and outgoing calls are infrequent.

Bad Weather

If the weather is so bad that assistants cannot come to work, it usually is so bad that patients will be unable to keep their appointments. If the patient load is normal and the employee is unable to come to work because of poor road conditions or a stalled car, time lost is usually charged to earned vacation credit. During winter months in northern offices, a serious storm may make it advisable to close the office. In this event, employees and patients should be notified as soon as possible. Such a closing would not adversely affect an employee's salary.

Parking

Your doctor-employer cannot be responsible for damage to your car while parked in the office parking area, nor can he be responsible for theft from your vehicle while it is parked on the premises. Report such theft to the police and your insurance agent immediately. If you damage another car while entering or leaving the premises, report the accident to the owner and your insurance company. Never park blocking a driveway or loading zone, or leave your car in a "No Parking" area. When certain areas are reserved for doctors and/or patients, respect this need.

Grievances

Grievances, complaints, and employee dissatisfactions are rare in a team-oriented staff. When and if they arise, most gripes can be satisfied within the periodic review consultation. However, if a situation arises needing immediate attention, feel free to arrange a conference with your doctor-employer. Clear and open expression is encouraged in most offices.

Let the "Golden Rule" be the basis of your patient relations. Personnel policies of the office mandate that fairness, kindness, and empathy be given to all. Do what you can at every opportunity to build a pleasant atmosphere in which to work.

ACQUAINTING YOURSELF WITH THE DOCTOR'S PRACTICE GOALS

The primary purpose of a DC's practice is to strive to provide the highest possible quality of chiropractic health care to every patient. All other goals are secondary. If this major purpose is satisfied, almost all other goals must be satisfied. To understand this is to grasp an understanding of several secondary goals.

The typical practice functions within the provisions of the rules of the State Board of Chiropractic Examiners and Code of Ethics of the State Chiropractic Association. By adhering to these tenets, the practice is enabled to fulfill its fundamental responsibilities and simultaneously do the most possible for the patients, the community, and the profession. It therefore is important that day-to-day decisions be made within an ethical and professional framework. Be mindful in your function as a chiropractic assistant that a patient's health needs should always be met in the best way possible so that each patient may have the opportunity to obtain the finest chiropractic care.

If you are one who feels that patients are cases, you are in the wrong profession. Patients are people: people who have feelings, emotions, and personal burdens. People with health problems especially must be considered in this light. Patients are not there to serve the practice; the practice is there to serve the patients.

The office needs patients. Patients do not need a particular office. They could go elsewhere. However, without patients, there is no practice.

All office employees are expected to be alert to the doctor's office philosophy, to work in its spirit, and to share its spirit for patient service. If you ever have any doubt about the goals, policies, and procedures of the office, discuss it with the doctor. Take nothing for granted. Be confident that your function is in tune with both the needs and philosophy of the office. The doctor will appreciate your questions for they suggest your sincerity to do a good job and render a meaningful contribution. Most doctors will hold periodic staff meetings in which a review of policies and procedures of the practice will be made.

By learning of the doctor's background, the "spirit" of the office will be understood. Learn of the doctor's educational background, licenses and professional certificates, clinical experience, professional activities and memberships, community involvement, personal interests, family, and philosophic viewpoints. By so doing, you will be in a better position to anticipate needs and add to your helpfulness.

DEVELOPING YOUR CONTRIBUTION AND ASSURING CAREER GROWTH

To maintain maximum quality of health service, the doctor attends several postgraduate educational programs each year. The goal of these programs through continuing education is constantly to upgrade services by implementing new and proved chiropractic and office procedural techniques. As the doctor is expected to keep abreast with the latest developments in clinical chiropractic, the chiropractic assistant is expected to be alert to developments in her role.

Health-Team Consciousness

The chiropractic assistant will be required to assume many roles and do many tasks. Among them may be telephone operator, hostess, nurse, business manager, bookkeeper, technical assistant, even baby-sitter. Whatever her specific duties, harmony between assistant and doctor is paramount. An atmosphere of friendly cooperation is essential to the successful care of the sick and disabled.

A good assistant considers no job too large, too small, or too burdensome. In a small office where responsibilities are broad, a spirit of support and mutual respect must prevail. There is no room for "prima donnas." The goal for both assistant and doctor should be a smooth flow of patient care with as little loss of time and effort as possible. As a valuable member of the health team, the assistant is in a key position to make each work day a pleasant and rewarding experience rather than an ordeal.

Creativeness and Adaptability

Each doctor of chiropractic, of course, selects office procedures that lend themselves best to his training, hours, and work habits. He will no doubt explain from several viewpoints more than once a general outline of the organization of his rationale, the routine he prefers, and the duties expected to be performed. Each assistant will be given instructions for handling patients, telephone calls, and personal calls.

The DC will no doubt familiarize employees with pertinent instruments, equipment, and laboratory and chiropractic procedures used in his practice. It also would be wise for him to establish mutually acceptable and easy to execute policies relating to care and arrangement of furniture, ordering of supplies, and general administration of the office. An assistant's alertness, efficiency, and desire to learn will pay dividends for her, the doctor, and the practice as a whole.

From time to time, every CA will see the opportunity for improvement on established methods used by her employer. While she is urged to keep her eyes open to potential betterment, she should use care and caution in making changes in office routine, arrangement, or appearance. A change should not be made without first offering the suggestion to her employer. Discuss it thoroughly, and obtain consent.

Every doctor has certain likes and dislikes. He must gain confidence in you before complying with your suggestions for change. Initially, the doctor may feel strongly about his preferences; in which case, you should learn and follow his ways graciously. The wise assistant, through diligent effort and diplomacy, proves that her suggestions are of value to the team before she attempts to remake an office system in her image. Both doctor and assistant should be receptive to change, provided it will result in improvement.

Efficiency Consciousness

When walking into a professional office, the patient expects to enter a calm atmosphere. He expects it to be as well managed, efficient, and capable as the professional service he seeks. It is up to the chiropractic assistant to create and maintain this atmosphere. An efficient assistant tries to expedite the flow of patients without advertising any form of "rush." She tries to assign appointments and rooms so efficiently that waiting time is kept to a minimum. She tries to arrange that patients do not cross each other's paths.

There is no more certain sign of inefficiency than a hectic office, regardless of the size of practice. And there is no more certain way of losing patients than to keep them waiting for unreasonable lengths of time or have them embarrassed by coming into contact with each other after treatment has begun.

Before a CA becomes a dependable and capable member of the team, she must first learn certain tasks that are routine. These must be completed each day without fail. Once she has mastered daily duties, she will find that her background in chiropractic procedure and office management has become strong enough to allow pursuit of additional tasks to be done on a weekly or monthly basis. With daily tasks falling into a pattern, she will have more time and freedom to concentrate on special projects.

Emergency Situations

In the performance of everyday duties, you probably will be required at times to make special decisions. For example, you may find it necessary to work in an unscheduled patient for emergency treatment. In handling the situation, you must bear in mind that the person requiring emergency treatment believes that his case is the only important case. To the person who has a standing appointment, his case is of equal importance. Your job is to handle both as diplomatically and efficiently as possible.

When a patient enters for emergency treatment, it is best to place him immediately in a spare or alternate room. The doctor should then be informed immediately by intercom, office phone, buzzer system, written note, or verbal message. The doctor should be advised of the extent of the injury or gravity of the emergency so he can be guided accordingly. Take care, however, to inform the doctor discreetly. The object is to avoid having another patient being treated feel as if he is being slighted should the doctor take a few moments to attend to the urgent needs of the emergency case. By work-

ing-in the unscheduled emergency this way, neither the patient being treated nor those waiting to be treated will feel alienated. In situations where more serious cases of emergency require considerable more time, the doctor will decide how the daily schedule is to be handled.

Developing Your Initial Contribution

It is important to learn rapidly about the doctor's interpretation of chiropractic fundamentals. Sit with your employer, discuss them with him, let him discuss his approach and application of the principles of chiropractic so that you will develop the background to act and talk intelligently, harmoniously.

Next, learn established procedures and be guided by them, even if they seem unnecessary at times. Remember, you must crawl before you can walk; walk before you can run. Policies and standards of practice are your guidelines. As you begin to understand your duties and the routines of the office, you will notice much of your work follows a pattern. As a result, your responsibilities and decisions will come easier. Rapid learning is based on close observation, intelligent questioning, interest in the work, alert follow-through, and adaptation to the results obtained.

One of the best ways to learn is the age-old method of keeping your eyes open, keeping your brain fertile, and asking questions. Whenever you have a question, ask the doctor when he is not busy with patients. He will feel that you are comfortable in what you are doing if you do not ask questions.

Ask the doctor for pertinent literature that would be helpful and informative. Be sure to acquaint yourself thoroughly with all literature available to patients. With study and sincere application, your contribution will increase steadily. Your importance will multiply. Adult education programs at local schools may help you to strengthen some weaknesses that you feel should be enhanced for career development.

Your job as an assistant or business manager is extremely important to strengthen your employer's practice. Whether it operates at a profit or loss often depends on you. In addition, you are in a position of direct patient contact which gives you the opportunity to enhance and build the doctor's image with his patients. An image of efficiency and respect reflects on the practice by affecting patient confidence and office income. It also has a psychologic effect that has shown to enhance a patient's healing rate.

When dealing with patients, be businesslike but friendly on every occasion. When time permits conversation, make it significant by steering the discussion toward your belief in the doctor's skill and in the principles of chiropractic. Coming from a third party, it will enhance the confidence of the patient.

In recording clinical data or matters of finance, be businesslike and thorough. Have a clear understanding of office bookkeeping and help develop accurate records of all services performed and payments made. Do not become delinquent in record keeping and bookkeeping or let it get away from you. Once it does, it can become a hodgepodge of data that are neither profitable nor interpretable. A large amount of information or money can be lost in the professional office if all services are not clearly and accurately recorded at the time they are performed.

In the beginning of your career, you will be called on to carry out whatever system of record keeping is presently being used. As you learn and progress in the performance of your tasks, you may be able to suggest improvements. It may be wise as time goes on to review the entire system with a public accountant to gain even greater efficiency.

Learn to be a "stickler" for detail. In the area of financial matters, let nothing slide to another time. Assure every patient gets a statement at the first of every month and that every service is shown, if this is your responsibility. Do not allow accounts to become delinquent for several months before an attempt at collection is made. When attempting collection, be tactful, but also be consistent. Reliable records will greatly aid you in your job.

FINDING THE RIGHT POSITION

Seeking optimal employment requires more than searching the want-ads and arranging an interview if you wish to find a position that will hold long-term satisfaction.

Develop a General Plan

Initial planning is a must. An effective plan can be constructed by asking and answering several points such as listed below.

1. List the skills of which you are most proud. List your weaknesses. Be honest. No one will see this list but you. What weaknesses can be changed and which cannot? Are the reasons for inflexibility based on facts or opinions (eg, fear, misconceptions)? Emotional blocks can be overcome. Have others with handicaps greater than yours overcome them to attain success?

2. Write a paragraph describing the ideal practice in which you would want to work and develop for many years.

3. What region of the country do you prefer? Why? Are the seasonal changes satisfactory? What advantages and disadvantages do the states in this region have on others (eg, taxes, housing/rental costs, recreational facilities)? Have you contacted various State Chambers of Commerce for their literature?

4. Do you prefer an urban or a rural community? Why? If rural, how far are you willing to commute for the advantages of a metropolitan area (eg, shopping, airport, etc)? Have you contacted various City Chambers of Commerce for their literature?

5. In which type of work do you think you would function best? That is, do you prefer the duties of an administrative assistant over those of a clinical assistant? If so, why? Is this a preference based on personality and character or one that could be changed with training?

6. What priority do you give salary, hours, and location? Define minimums and maximums.

7. Would you prefer the atmosphere of a small intimate office or that of a large group practice? Why?

8. List those things you learned during previous employment that you wish avoided in the future.

Interview Preparation

Check your personal employment inventory. It should include copies of pertinent diplomas, certifications, and a carefully prepared updated resumé. Miscellaneous data should include your social security number and driver's license. Check your local library for a current book on preparing a resumé, for modern style is rapidly changing. Be concise (no more than two or three single-spaced *typed* sheets) and stress your best points and accomplishments. See Figure 2.1. Briefly list EMPLOYMENT DATA, EDUCATIONAL DATA, EXTRACURRICULAR INTERESTS AND ACTIV ITIES, and pertinent MEMBERSHIPS (if any). Points should be listed in reverse chronological order. End the resumé with a heading titled PERSONAL GOALS in which you define your immediate goals and long-term objectives. The final line of the resumé should state that references will be provided on request. If references are requested, always gain permission before you use a name. Preferred salary, benefits, hours, and office policies should be discussed during the interview but not delineated in the resumé.

Keep in mind that resumés do not get jobs. People get jobs. Resumés and other supporting literature get interviews and help to justify a hiring decision.

Locating Prospective Employers

Few DCs advertise for assistants in local newspapers or professional journals. Most place announcements in district newsletters and state journals. The American Chiropractic Association can provide you with the addresses of state chiropractic associations, and the associations, in turn, can provide you with addresses of district newsletter editors. Request a sample of their latest edi-

tion. There may be a small charge. Call various offices in the community of your choice and ask the CAs there if they know of any DC seeking an assistant. Avoid employment agencies except as a last resort. Take charge—it's your future.

Requesting an Interview

If you find an announcement that lists an address and telephone number, view the location, building, and parking facilities to assure your satisfaction before you make a telephone call to request an interview. If only a PO box number is given, respond with a brief request for an interview that includes your short-term and long-range objectives and mention that you will bring your credentials and resumé with you during the meeting. This letter should be concise, neat, orderly, enthusiastic, and professional so that it will stand out from other letters that might be received. Thank the reader for considering your request, and be sure to list prominently a telephone number at which you can be reached.

Triple check all correspondence for accuracy, completeness, and attractive format. Once you are satisfied, have a competent friend review it and seek their suggestions. Seek someone willing to play a devil's advocate, not someone that will be afraid to hurt your feelings by pointing out area for improvement.

Actions During the Interview

Plan your appearance carefully so that you will look well groomed, conservative, well pressed, and professional. Keep in mind that first impressions are lasting impressions. Recheck your personal inventory folder to assure it is in order and complete. Arrive 5 minutes prior to your appointment and go alone. Introduce yourself to the receptionist with a confident smile. Do not sit until requested. Express appreciation when asked to be seated. Sit with good posture while waiting and during the interview. Do not smoke or chew gum. Never interrupt.

Your first job is to sell yourself. When

VITA

Name: _____

Address: _____   Bus. Telephone: _____

_____   Res. Telephone: _____

Personal Data

Birth date _____   Hobbies: _____

Height/Weight _____   Marital Status: _____

SS#: _____   Dependents: _____

Employment History

_____
_____
_____

Education

_____
_____
_____

Additional Seminars and Courses

_____
_____
_____

Memberships and Affiliations

_____
_____
_____

Offices Held

_____
_____
_____

Credit References

_____
_____
_____

Personal References

_____
_____
_____

Figure 2.1. Sample format for preparing an autobiographical sketch.

asked, explain how your skills and character will be a positive influence on the doctor's practice and that you are very adaptable in working with various types of personalities. Explain indirectly what type of employee you would be: dependable, loyal, versatile, trustworthy, dedicated, willing to accept responsibility, etc. During this time, the doctor will be observing your friendly manner, communication skills, directness, mannerisms, poise, sense of humor, level of common sense, etc.

Do not speak or listen to the wall. Look at the doctor. Make occasional eye contact, but do not firmly stare into his eyes.

Once you feel the doctor is pleased with your credentials and personality, now is the time you may wish to inquire casually into concerns of hours, salary, benefits, office policy, potential for advancement, etc., if any of these subjects have not been brought up voluntarily by the doctor. Become informed. Listen, but neither agree nor disagree if possible.

The best time to mention your needs is *after* the doctor has made a job offer. That is your best time to negotiate special priorities. The timing of this is very important to your best interests.

On leaving the interview, note any interesting subjects that might be placed on the doctor's desk or on the walls. They would not be there if the doctor did not have some pride in them (eg, pictures, plaques, diplomas, awards, etc). Your comments should be guided accordingly.

If you are introduced to any personnel, try to remember their names so that you can thank them later for their friendliness. The doctor will likely ask them of their impressions of you after you have left.

If the doctor states that he has others to interview and will contact you later, delay discussion of your special needs until a firm job offer is made. If an offer is made, arrange a second appointment to discuss details of your potential position and have a tour of the office. By making a firm job offer, the doctor has overcome any potential obstacles to your employment in his mind. Now is the time to resolve any questions *you* may have.

If you are not contacted after a few days, call the office to determine if the position has been filled. Regardless, express that you enjoyed meeting the doctor and having the opportunity for the interview.

If you do not get the job, ask yourself why. Did you look your best, show friendly professionalism, listen carefully, answer frankly with tact? No interview is a waste of time. Each is a learning experience. Avoid rationalizing the rejection with such ideas as "I really didn't want to work there, for him, anyway." That's just self-defeating mind talk. Correct any mistakes and go on. It is the rare person in any field that is hired on the first interview.

CONTINUING EDUCATION

Administrative assistants should keep abreast with good business practices, techniques, and evolving methodology with computerization. State laws are constantly changing that affect insurance claim processing, and diagnostic and therapeutic codes are frequently revised.

Clinical assistants should keep current with the rapid changes within the profession and in health-care technology in general. In fact, many states mandate this for certified CAs. State chiropractic associations conduct periodic classes and seminars for this purpose. These courses should be supplemented with reading appropriate literature, attending local CA meetings, and otherwise keeping abreast with events concerning the profession. An inquisitive mind is a positive attribute in health care.

There is also a national association of chiropractic assistants that helps to inform members of current events and changing trends. As explained above, many states have extremely active CA organizations. Participation is important as it is estimated that health-care knowledge doubles in less than 5 years.

CLOSING REMARKS

The doctor of chiropractic extends to his patients his knowledge, skill, time, and responsible care. All professional functions of the DC depend on these and can only be performed by the chiropractor. Practice success, clinically and economically, depends on the extent to which these factors can be applied to the patient's health needs. Optimum chiropractic health care is therefore the maximum application of the doctor's skills to the patient's condition. Optimal performance by the doctor can only be achieved when he is supported in all areas that do not require appropriate professional licensure.

Good management often requires good delegation. Maximum delegation means maximum utilization of the doctor's time and energy. Whenever the doctor can delegate a duty or responsibility to an assistant, he is more able to apply his professional skills to more patients. To do this efficiently, careful planning, organization, administration, and management of the practice are necessary. Logical policies and efficient procedures offer the framework of a successful health-care practice.

Chapter 3

The Health-Service Role of the Doctor of Chiropractic

This chapter briefly describes the role of the doctor of chiropractic in the health care of the nation. It also introduces the reader to the rationale of clinical diagnostics, therapeutics, rehabilitation, and counseling in the chiropractic approach. Some particular areas of special interest are also described.

DIAGNOSTICS: THE ART OF DECIDING WHAT IS WRONG

The diagnostic process of a patient's disorder begins with the recording and interpretation of the patient's medical history. Thus, the initial interview and consultation with the patient is of utmost importance. It will direct the examinations and tests that are to follow. Every measure of observation that will substantially profile the patient is employed and recorded. A systematic and thorough physical examination is conducted using the methods, techniques, and instruments that are standard with all health professions. In addition, the doctor of chiropractic will include a postural and spinal analysis, an innovation in the field of physical diagnosis and examination.

Background

The chiropractic physician uses the standard procedures and instruments of physical and clinical diagnosis, and he is well acquainted with the need for differential diagnosis. Diagnostic radiology, especially as it pertains to the skeletal system, is a primary clinical diagnostic aid in chiropractic and has been since the early 1900s.

In addition, doctors of chiropractic are knowledgeable in the standard and special clinical laboratory procedures and tests usual to modern diagnostic science. Facilities for roentgenography (x-ray), thermography, electrocardiography (ECG), and electromyology (EMG) are standard among many other technologic advancements. Each accredited chiropractic college has a laboratory licensed to carry on clinical laboratory examinations, including such fields as cytology, chemistry, hematology, serology, bacteriology, and parasitology.

After experiencing a diagnostic evaluation from a doctor of chiropractic, many patients report that it was the most thorough examination of their lifetime. The reason for this is that the chiropractic physician views each patient as an individual who has been subjected to both unique outside and inside forces, who is interested in both correction and prevention, and who is interested in the preservation of both the quantity and the quality of life. Thoroughness is a necessity to achieve such goals.

Overview of the Diagnostic Process

Any professional therapy administered ethically, professionally, and legally must be based on the doctor's diagnosis of the patient's condition. That is, the diagnosis must direct the treatment. By understanding why the doctor does what he does during the diagnostic process, the CA will be in a better position to answer patient questions.

Diagnosis (determining the cause of the patient's complaint) involves the use of inductive and deductive logic. This process can be divided into two major divisions: data gathering and data interpretation (Table 3.1).

Once the initial collection of facts has been completed, the patient's complaint will tend to fall into one or more of 13 general etiologic classifications: (1) traumatic (extrinsic or intrinsic), (2) inflammatory, (3) neurologic, (4) vascular, (5) endocrine, (6) metabolic, (7) neoplastic, (8) degenerative, (9) deficiency, (10) congenital, (11) allergic, (12) autoimmune, or (13) toxic. Each of these general classes contains scores of specific disorders. The suspicions obtained at this point will then be either confirmed or rejected by the results or further examination and test data until only one likely cause remains.

The above process is aided by determining whether the patient's symptoms are arising from physiologic, structural changes, or mental/emotional changes. This process is often called *problem group analysis.*

1. Functional. A physiologic disorder; a pathophysiologic disease process without overt structural changes. Symptoms resulting from physiologic changes arise from

Increased function: eg, hypertrophy, spastic paralysis, anxiety, tachycardia, diarrhea, pain, edema, fever, and articular instability.

Decreased function: eg, atrophy, flaccid paralysis, depression, bradycardia, constipation, numbness, dehydration, hypothermia, and articular fixation.

Altered function: eg, convulsions, tremors, arrhythmias, various visual disturbances, paresthesia, and aberrant articular movement.

2. Structural. An organic disorder, with or without signs of overt pathology. Symptoms resulting from structural changes arise from (a) *bone and joint infection* with resultant soft-tissue reactions, subperiosteal

Table 3.1. Elements of Diagnostic Logic

1. Collect the Facts (Data Gathering)

Clinical history	Laboratory data
Physical examination	Ancillary examinations
Orthopedic examination	Progress reports
Neurologic examination	Periodic re-examination

2. Analyze the Facts (Data Interpretation)

Critical evaluation of data
List of reliable symptoms, signs, and findings in order of their apparent importance
Exclude disorders that might produce similar data
Select disease(s) or disorder(s) that best fit the facts at hand
Continually verify the current diagnosis

calcification, decalcification, bone destruction, and infiltration processes; (b) *congenital anomaly;* (c) *deformity*—witnessed as abnormal changes in angularity, displacement, or loss of continuity; (d) *degenerative process;* (e) *endocrine and metabolic imbalance;* (f) *tumor* (malignant or benign); (g) *trauma.*

3. Mental/emotional. A neurosis or psychosis; a predominantly psychosomatic or somatopsychic disturbance. Symptoms resulting from mental/emotional changes may be the result of either a physiologic or structural lesion.

It is often most difficult to draw the line between functional and organic illness. In functional disorders, there is undoubtedly a degree of chemical and intracellular alterations preceding gross structural (organic) manifestations. In addition, nontraumatic altered structure and its gross signs and symptoms are inevitably preceded by altered function and its more subtle symptoms. A clinical sign or a symptom is never an isolated phenomenon. It has multiple interrelationships, some physiologic and some psychologic, that can be of a major or minor importance.

THERAPEUTICS: THE ART OF CORRECTING WHAT IS WRONG

Chiropractic treatment methods are determined by the scope of practice authorized by state law. In all areas, however, these methods do not include the use of prescription drugs or major surgery, thus avoiding the dangers therein. Essentially, treatment methods include the chiropractic adjustment when indicated and, according to the doctor's judgment, such ancillary services as necessary dietary advice, nutritional supplementation, physiotherapeutic measures, and professional counsel.

The most characteristic aspect of chiropractic practice is the release of one or more hypomobile (fixated) and possibly subluxated spinal or extraspinal articular surfaces by making a specific predetermined adjustment. The purpose of this correction and its determination is to normalize the dynamic relationships of segments within their articular range and thus associated neurologic, muscular, and vascular disturbances.

Physiotherapy or Physical Therapy. Physiotherapeutic methods and procedures are frequently used as adjunctive therapy to enhance the effects of the chiropractic adjustments. Such procedures may include the use of diathermy, galvanic current, infrared and ultraviolet light, ultrasound, paraffin baths, hot or cold compresses, acutherapy, hydrotherapy, heel or sole lifts, foot stabilizers, and other commonly used modalities. Taping, strapping, and other forms of minor surgery are sometimes used in injuries of the spine or extremities. Neck, lower back, elbow, knee and ankle injuries may require supportive collars or braces to enhance the effects of corrective treatments during recuperation to help tissue healing and strengthening.

Nutrition. The adequate intake and assimilation of essential nutrients is necessary to maintain health, and tissue demands increase during illness and stress. Vitamin, mineral, enzyme, and tissue (eg, protein) supplementation can, if professionally supervised, serve to prevent the onset or assuage the existence of some types of dysfunction of the nervous system and other tissues. If deemed necessary in case management, dietary regimens and nutritional supplementation are often advised.

Patient Counsel. Rehabilitative exercises, as a physical therapy, compose an important aspect of professional counsel to aid recovery and prevent further strain.

An assistant may be asked to record in a patient's entering data a few words that would describe the patient's common exercise level. Descriptors are shown in Table 3.2.

Advice is often given in such areas as dietary regimens, physical and mental attitudes affecting health, personal hygiene, occupational safety, life-style, posture, rest, work, and the many other activities of daily living that would enhance the effects of chiropractic health care. Chiropractic is truly

Table 3.2. Descriptors in Recording a Patient's Exercise Level

Light	Light means light office work, auto driving, desk work, typing, slow walking, sewing, cooking, riding lawn mower, piano playing, golf with a cart, etc.
Light-moderate	Light-moderate includes the light construction trades, welding, cleaning windows, truck driving in traffic, fast walking, golfing without a cart, small boat sailing, bowling, friendly volleyball, touch football, pushing a light lawn mower, pitching horseshoes, house cleaning, etc.
Moderate-heavy	Moderate-heavy effort includes soft-soil digging, splitting wood, tennis, skating, bicycling, square and disco dancing, cross-country skiing, etc.
Heavy	Heavy effort includes activities such as digging ditches, aerobic dancing, sawing hardwood by hand, jogging, basketball, hockey, mountain climbing, weight lifting, and other activities requiring much energy.

concerned with the total individual: the patient's health, welfare, and survival.

Nutrition and counseling will be described further in the following sections of this chapter.

REHABILITATION: THE ART OF AIDING NATURAL HEALING PROCESSES

The human body is a complex, integrated organism. It has been explained how spinal disorders may cause or contribute to disease processes and/or how these processes may cause or contribute to spinal disorders. While the nervous system influences the glandular system, for example, hormones in turn have a great influence on the nervous system. A digestive disturbance may result in spinal pain, and a spinal disorder may result in digestive dysfunctions. A heart condition may send shooting pain down the arm, and a spinal or rib joint disorder may mimic a heart condition. The cycles are endless. The processes are one of life and dynamic motion and reaction that, unfortunately, cannot be truly identified by static x-ray studies or even an autopsy. It can only be witnessed in life by thorough examination.

The name given to a disease process does not negate the chiropractor's duty to correct the anatomical disrelationship and/or the neuromechanical disorders that are caus-

ing, maintaining, or associated with the disease process. Through the ages, the musculoskeletal system has been cooled, heated, massaged, stretched, cut, and injected, yet never truly considered of primary importance until the birth of chiropractic concepts.

Today this is changing as witnessed by publicity for external heart massage and the diaphragm "lift" to dislodge a food bolus. Both procedures are adaptations from chiropractic techniques developed many decades ago. Publicity reflecting the chiropractic care of various athletes, that enable several world records to be broken, is also a compliment to the chiropractic approach.

The concept that mechanical spinal disorders such as subluxation-fixations may cause functional abnormalities is the basis of chiropractic thought and one of its major contributions to generic medicine. Continuous research in this area must be made for this precept promises to answer many unsolved problems facing health science today.

Nutritional Considerations

Besides the correction of localized biomechanical faults, the development of good posture habits, and the necessity for regular exercise, nutrition plays an important role. Nourishing food that builds bone and muscle and maintains nerve and blood integrity is essential to good health and repair mechanisms.

Autointoxication

Too often in our society a well-balanced diet has been replaced by manufactured sweets, snack foods, TV dinners, and other "junk" foods. While four fifths of our daily foods should consist of alkaline-forming vegetables, raw salads, and fresh fruits, most American tables display four fifths acid-forming concentrated proteins, starches, and sugars.

Autointoxication, which weakens natural resistance forces, results from an accumulation of acidic by-products of digestion, metabolism, and cell decomposition. Most pathogenic microorganisms prefer an acidic environment, and calcium will not abnormally deposit in tissues (eg, arthritis, gallstones, kidney stones) except in an acidic environment. Thus, anything that burdens the body's alkaline reserves depletes its functional potential.

Moderate exercise helps to speed metabolism and to oxidize and eliminate excessive amounts of protein by-products. However, the products of muscle fatigue from excessive exercise are acid ash. Also, comparatively speaking, many people avoid regular exercise because we are twice as efficient mentally as we are physically. While a diet rich in fruits and vegetables would be of benefit, processing and cooking minimize their potential. The doctor is therefore confronted with adapting his advice from the *ideal* to the life-style the patient lives.

Food Alteration

Although all natural foods contain the micronutrients necessary for their metabolism, they seldom have their original spectrum of vitamins when they reach the table. While caloric values and the quantity and quality of protein, carbohydrate, and fat are relatively unchanged, at least six vitamins can be lost or partly destroyed by steaming, frying, roasting, boiling, freezing, drying, storage, or irradiation. Industrialized food processing often results in a deficiency in vitamins and elements necessary for metabo-

lism. Many trace elements that were once plentiful in American soil and necessary for optimal health and resistance have been grossly depleted by the use of commercial fertilizers. Dietary supplementation is the price we must pay for wide distribution of purified, stored, and processed foods. Without supplementation, we run the risk of unbalancing the diet in terms of essential micronutrients.

While meat is the common source of protein, it must be kept in mind that meat is commonly ingested with an array of antibiotics, hormones, and scores of additives designed to preserve, age, cure, tenderize, color, flavor, season, and scent to satisfy the consumer's interest and producer's profit. Fruits and vegetables commonly purchased at the corner supermarket contain a degree of pesticide residue. Without question, many common food processing techniques and additives have a nefarious effect on our natural resistance and recuperative powers.

Physiologic Needs

Maintaining cellular homeostasis of biochemical equilibrium by supplying proper nutrients is the purpose of nutrition and a primary basis of good health. Yet, a number of authorities claim that Americans are the most overfed and undernourished people in the world. Thus, dietary management under chiropractic care is often necessary to see that a patient's diet provides balanced meals made of proteins, carbohydrates, fats, and other micronutrients necessary for proper metabolism.

The subject of nutrition is an important part of the curriculum at each accredited chiropractic college. It is unfortunate for the public that most medical schools do not list the subject in their catalogs.

Posture and Physical Fitness

Americans lag behind many countries of the world in physical fitness. Easier living caused by space-age developments has encouraged a life-style of minimal physical effort. A society of button pushers neglects its physical fitness, however. Nature is not

Table 3.3. Systemic Changes of the Inactivity Syndrome

System	Pathophysiologic Manifestations	
Cardiovascular	Decreased cardiac reserve	Postexercise angina
	Excessive adrenal reaction	Sympathicotonia
	Increased BMR	
Central nervous	Altered sensory perception from decreased sensory input	Demoralized personality
		Disturbed sleep patterns
	Anxiety/depression syndrome	Impaired learning ability
	Autonomic imbalance leading to poor exercise level adaptation	
Digestive	Altered eating habits	Decreased GI motility
	Constipation	Decreased GI secretions
Immune	Diminished resistance	
Musculoskeletal	Activation of latent trigger points	Muscle mass atrophy
		Osteoporosis
	Fatigue (general)	Reduced coordination
	Fibrositis	
Respiratory	Decreased respiratory muscle strength	Dyspnea upon mild exertion
Urinary	Bacteriuria	Urine retention
	Hypercalcemia	Urgency

wasteful; what is not used, degenerates. Physical fitness is no exception. Table 3.3 lists the major systematic changes associated with physical inactivity.

Since its development, the chiropractic profession has offered national and community leadership in encouraging parents and teachers to support physical fitness programs in schools. Youngsters should be encouraged by their parents to develop good fitness and health habits at an early age. Fitness is a family affair.

From birth, the biped human being enjoys an architectural *opus magnum* that allows for agility, leverage, mobility, and balance against gravity's constant pull. When biomechanics are disturbed through stress and strain even slightly, distortion results because of the close interrelationship of our structural and functional systems: the body is a whole. Posture not only has a direct bearing on comfort and work efficiency, it is also a factor determining resistance to disease or disability.

The chiropractic profession is uniquely attentive to the importance of nerve integrity and body mechanics for good health. The doctor of chiropractic is most concerned with the effects of and prevention of spinal defects affecting physical fitness. He is skilled to treat health problems, and his treatment is aimed at maintaining joint integrity by correcting spinal and extraspinal mechanical defects and postural distortions.

The need for good posture is far more significant than an attractive appearance. To assure health our bodies must be free from structural distortions and our functions must operate at peak efficiency. Any activity in which the structure of the human frame is thrown out of normal balance can cause distortion of the spine. The spine not only supports the weight of the entire body above the pelvis, it also protects the spinal cord which connects the higher brain centers with nerves to and from the vital organs.

Too often we think of our spine as a flexible rod that moves only on the command of our will. Yet man is a dynamic creature, structurally as well as functionally. Movement never ceases. Motion is constant. With every breath the spine, ribs, and their attachments are in motion. Add this small movement to the gross movements of daily living and we can appreciate the persistent motion, constant stress, and necessity for proper alignment.

When disorders occur to our normal musculoskeletal system, we see the rise of sore backs and stiff necks, aching joints and easy fatigue, headaches and nervous tension, and scores of other complaints so common to our time. Such structural abuses and their frequently painful effects are an important area in chiropractic counsel and care for both prevention and treatment.

As early as 1930, the White House Conference on Child Health recognized the importance of spinal integrity and body mechanics in relation to health. The report showed that correct posture is essential to proper development, balance, coordination, rhythm, and timing—body efficiency. Distortions not only affect comfort but also the function of major organs and systems. Thus, there is an undisputed relationship between good posture and health, and poor biomechanics and the ability to cope with a variety of diseases. Again, this shows how the body operates as a complex yet synchronized unit, how structural defects may result in functional disturbances, and how functional disorders may result in structural impairment.

To be physically fit is to bring the efficiency level of the body to a point where it can meet the demands of everyday living. This requires the building of stamina. The rewards are greater energy, greater resistance to disease and disability, and greater mental potential. People with good posture are generally more physically fit, mentally alert, and emotionally adjusted—three characteristics that lead to happier and more productive lives.

A spinal injury or mechanical defect that may occur may not have dramatic effects initially. It may occur subtly and grow worse with time. Unless trained in the health sciences, most people do not usually recognize subtle health problems. Rather, they learn to adapt and suffer in silence. As a result, many spinal defects are unknown until the prob-

lem grows more serious and pain is felt. To add to the mystery, symptoms often occur in a part of the body not ordinarily associated with the spine. For this reason, chiropractic care is attentive to the cause.

The spinal subluxation and the extraspinal mechanical lesion are yet only partially understood. Because of their observed importance in degenerative diseases and functional disorders, the chiropractic profession has sponsored and will continue to sponsor research in this area so that we may know more of the implications involved which have been demonstrated successfully with millions of patients in chiropractic offices since the turn of the century. It is unfortunate that the subluxation, and its attendant soft-tissue trauma, is one of the most commonly missed diagnoses within the healing arts. It is not only a mimic of many diseases, it also can be a causative or contributing factor in a variety of disorders.

Mechanical disorders and their functional alterations are probably the most common of man's ills today. Yet, this is not unusual when we consider that the body's response to gravity is a constant strain in the upright posture. Such stress must have a negative effect on the healing powers of our nature. We should be ever mindful that the musculoskeletal system comprises more than 60% of our body's total mass, yet this 60% is often overlooked within our healing arts.

COUNSELING: THE ART OF PREVENTIVE THERAPY AND ENHANCEMENT

In our era of rapidly advancing technology, we have attempted to adapt to both mental and physical stresses unknown by our forefathers. While it is commonly agreed that emotional disturbances may cause structural disorders, clinical observations verify that the reverse is also true. Structural faults may lead to a low stress threshold resulting in a variety of emotional illnesses.

It was the Father of American Psychology, Professor William James of Harvard, who insisted that while emotional disturbances can cause structural and functional disorders, so can structural and functional disorders also cause emotional disturbances. Thus, the structural neurologic approach of chiropractic may often benefit associated behavioral disorders. Several chiropractic papers report excellent results in handling many types of emotional disorders such as certain forms of hyperkinesis, anxiety, and depression. A monograph titled *Nervous and Mental Cases Under Chiropractic Care* describes 400 cases. This paper was written by a former president of the Council on Mental Health of the American Chiropractic Association, H. S. Schwartz, DC, in collaboration with G. W. Hartman, PhD, professor of psychology at Columbia University.

Increasing evidence of the serious consideration now being given to the chiropractic somatopsychic approach to many emotional illnesses is to be found in scientific literature. Several authorities have shown a distinct relationship between mental illness and vitamin deficiencies; others between mental illness and overconsumption of refined sugar or food additives. Still others show a definite relationship between the ingestion of lead or copper (with use of lead or copper plumbing) and zinc deficiency (with decreasing soil content). With these dietary factors removed and treatment directed to somatopsychic structural correction, a promise arises for the reduction of our nation's increasing mental health problem.

GENERAL PRACTICE AND SPECIALIZED INTERESTS

While chiropractors emphasize the importance of the correction of spinal and extraspinal mechanical lesions, no practitioner believes that these are the sole causes of disease. However, clinical chiropractic has shown repeatedly that neurologic aberrations originating from mechanical lesions are a contributing or inducing factor in many more dysfunctions than commonly realized. As has been shown, when combined

with poor nutrition, pollutants, physical and emotional overstress, germs, trauma, drug-related weaknesses, poor habits and addictions, and other common debilitating factors, such mechanical lesions become an important consideration far too often overlooked.

Pain and Preventive Care

In matters of health, a warning signal matters a great deal. Pain is such a warning. As nature's early warning signal, it is a message that tells us that our body is not functioning properly—that something serious may be wrong with our health. Pain of any kind is an alarm that nature uses to signal where there is a health problem that deserves attention. It is just as foolhardy to do no more than kill the pain with a pill or injection as it would be to silence a fire alarm and fail to seek its cause. To affect proper care, the cause must be treated—not just the symptom.

Common Complaints

Headaches are the most common complaint encountered in the healing arts today, and a common cause of headaches originates from a vertebral articular disorder in the spine. It is important that such mechanical lesions be recognized by a trained chiropractic physician. Unfortunately, sufferers of headaches are too often offered a generalized diagnosis such as sinus trouble, migraine, cluster headaches, and so forth. Because chiropractic care is attentive to the neurologic implications involved, headache sufferers have frequently found relief under chiropractic care where other forms of therapy have failed.

The second most common complaint is that of backache. Here again, lumbago, sacroiliac strains, and disc injuries are usually of a musculoskeletal nature having neurologic overtones. It is important that the cause be recognized and cared for before permanent damage is done. Because chiropractic care recognizes the structural/functional relationships involved, the profession has earned a respected reputation in handling cases of both acute and chronic back pain.

Remember that many pains remote from the spine originate from a spinal disorder. In the same manner, many pains that appear to be situated within the spine originate in some distant tissue. Differential diagnosis in such conditions requires a thorough holistic approach—an approach demonstrated under modern chiropractic care.

Resistance to Disease

Health science would be much simpler if a single disease could be attributed to a single cause. But this is not so. We all live in an environment of potential bacterial and viral invasion, but only a small minority of us become infected. Even many of the most virulent strains of pathogenic organisms do not infect every person exposed. Bodily resistance, acquired or inherited, and many other factors combine to decide whether an invading organism will result in noticeable infection.

Human ecology and economy are complex considerations. The cause of disease is not singular, neither is the response to disease singular. Thus the logic of a health care that considers a person as a total being. Any illness affects the total person, and any disease is multicausal. The total person is affected because illness is not a thing, it is a process.

Chiropractic's emphasis on the importance of body resistance is a contribution that has yet to realize its full potential. Every person is an individual from his fingerprints to his structure, functions, responses, adaptability, habits, and addictions. All logical theory and therapy should be directed to recognition of individual differences and supportive of one's peculiar nature.

It is unfortunate that the health sciences traditionally have not emphasized the importance of the nature of health as it has the nature of disease. In recent years, L. J. Rather, MD, a Stanford University pathologist, reminded the International Congress of Logic, Methodology and Philosophy of Science that "If we measure interest by activities rather than by protestations, physicians have been and are, for the most part, as little interested in health as soldiers in peace."

Sports Injuries

Because of chiropractic's emphasis on structural/functional relationships in health and disease processes, it is logical that there is much attention within the profession given to therapeutic kinesiology. One purpose of the ACA Council on Sports Injuries and Physical Fitness is to seek improvement in the prevention and correction of sports and recreational problems. Because of chiropractic input, counsel, and ingenuity, several contributions have been made regarding protective gear and shoes in contact sports, athletic health maintenance, and therapy and enhanced rehabilitation after injury.

While chiropractic contributions in this area have been made for many years, the public press has brought increasing attention to the profession's unique approach. Much publicity surrounding chiropractic care with Olympic athletes and professional athletes has been given in recent years. Football, baseball, basketball, and most other sports can be thankful for chiropractic's advanced approach to the care of sports injuries.

Prenatal and Postnatal Care

During pregnancy, there is a natural change within the mother's pelvic structure along with an accompanying change in weight distribution. Health disorders such as headache, backache, leg pains, and lower extremity circulation disturbances often can be attributed solely to the strain on the neuromusculoskeletal system involved. In association with regular obstetrical care, periodic chiropractic spinal analysis and adjustments throughout the course of pregnancy show excellent clinical results in either reducing or eliminating such disorders as well as easing the labor of delivery.

Spinal examination and necessary correction after delivery is a positive step toward preventing potential lower back and sacroiliac disorders that may have been initiated during pregnancy or delivery. Correction of these often minor disorders at this time may serve as a positive deterrent against possible structural/functional gynecologic problems of later years.

Pediatric Care

The strain of delivery plus the disproportionate weight of the child's head upon yet to be fully developed neck structures may result in insults to the child's upper cervical vertebrae, effecting a variety of dysfunctions. Chiropractors recommend a spinal examination of the child shortly after birth so that proper corrections can be made if problems exist. Only a chiropractic physician has been trained to make such determinations. Clinical records show that chiropractic pediatric examination and care during the postnatal period have positive influence on reducing the possibility of colic, digestive sensitivities, allergies, and other common dysfunctions in the newborn—as well as remove predisposition to common childhood diseases.

Since it is impossible to restrain a normal child from participating in the many activities that may cause stress and strain, the early correction of faulty body mechanics is important. Active children are particularly prone to spinal subluxation because they are energetic and impatient, and have an innocent disregard of caution. Spinal disorders often are the result of twists, sudden turns, awkward lifts and postural positions, and shocking body contact and jolts during play and sports. If not corrected, spinal problems may lead to interference with nor-

mal function and body mechanics causing or contributing to severe illness.

Professional Groups

Various professional organizations are available in which a DC with a special area of interest may keep abreast with the latest research in that field. These groups are called *councils*, and members are encouraged to devote many hours of postgraduate study to prepare themselves, by examination, for *diplomate* status.

Professional councils on diagnostic imaging, orthopedics, and chiropractic diagnosis and internal disorders strive to keep the field abreast with the latest scientific and technologic advancements. Councils on nutrition, neurology, technic, physiologic therapeutics, and mental health also are continually investigating efficient methods. Some objectives of the Council on Sports Injuries and Physical Fitness have been described earlier in this chapter.

CLOSING REMARKS

Chiropractic is an exciting profession, and serving as a chiropractic assistant offers a stimulating and challenging career. This chapter has briefly described an overview of chiropractic health care. Most briefly, the profession's implementation of diagnosis, therapy, rehabilitation, and counseling have been explained. In addition, some important aspects of general practice and specialized interests have been defined so that the reader will have a better understanding of the profession. This will serve as a foundation for further study.

In the next chapter, the language of the health-care professions will be explained.

Chapter 4

The Language of the Health-Care Professions

When more than one person is involved in any task, good communication is basic for success. Thus, a sound foundation in chiropractic terminology is an important functional skill to be possessed by any chiropractic assistant. It is a requisite to becoming an important asset to the office.

If a CA's duties include taking dictation of case histories, examination findings, or narrative reports, she must know how to record scientific terms in shorthand and know how to spell them accurately. A good medical dictionary will be an important reference. Even if dictation is not required, she still must know what the doctor means when certain terms are used. He will expect his assistants to have a fundamental grasp of commonly used medical terms, abbreviations, and acronyms.

Do not enter this study lightly. On the other hand, do not let yourself be appalled by the formidable and specialized vocabulary used in health care. The learning of professional terms will not come overnight. It will extend the entire length of your career as new and unfamiliar words are confronted.

THE UNIVERSAL LANGUAGE OF HEALTH CARE: WHY IT IS NECESSARY

It would not be unusual if you found many words used in the first three chapters of this book strange or at least unknown. When you undertake the transposition from lay person to chiropractic assistant, you are faced with an entirely new language that must be mastered so the transition will be successful. The most efficient method to accomplish this is by securing an understanding of basic word roots, prefixes, and suffixes used in the formation of technical words and gaining an understanding of the meaning of commonly used abbreviations and acronyms. Study and repetitive use is the way to mastery.

A fundamental knowledge of anatomy (structure) and physiology (function) will be of great assistance in learning terminology. A basic understanding of human anatomy and physiology is offered in the following chapter. This chapter will prepare you for the terminology of those and other clinical subjects. While professional terms may

American Chiropractic Association

at first seem strange, you will see their purpose in this and following chapters.

PHONETICS: THE QUICK WAY TO GRASP MEANINGS

In studying the terminology of any science as in learning any language, phonetics or word sound plays an important role. While you will never need to know how to spell or pronounce every word in your reference dictionary, you will be required to be familiar with common terms and know where and how to look up unfamiliar terms. Phonetics and an understanding of prefixes and suffixes will be helpful, if not necessary, to do this.

There are two simple rules for correct pronunciation of scientific terms. They are based on the syllable breakdown of the word and the occurrence of vowels (a, e, i, o, u):

1. *If the vowel is not followed by a consonant in the same syllable, it has the long sound; eg, the word abdomen* (ab-do-men). Here the "o" in "do" has the long low sound.

2. If the vowel is followed by a consonant in the same syllable, it has the short sound; eg, the word *abdominal* (ab-dom-i-nal). Here the "o" in "dom" has the short higher sound as in "Tom."

HOW THE WORDS ARE FORMED

As chiropractic vocabulary is studied, the student will find it made largely of many variations of various roots, prefixes, and suffixes in different combinations. Thus the number of word parts necessary to learn is not so great as one would suspect.

Most technical words used in chiropractic terminology come from the root languages (Greek and Latin). Some are pure translations; others are combined forms of Greek and Latin. While the number of English words is enlarging, prefixes and suffixes usually remain Greek or Latin.

Besides Greek and Latin, other languages have had their influence. Words such as *alcohol, alkali, camphor,* and *tartar* are derived from Arabic. Many simple anatomical terms such as *arm, back, bladder, blood, finger, foot, gut, hair, hand, knee, liver, lung, mouth, neck, ache, fat,* and *sick* are Anglo-Saxon in origin. Other monosyllable terms such as *ill, leg,* and *skin* are of Scandinavian descent. Words such as *chancre, cretin, fontanelle, grippe, malaise, poison, role, cul de sac, grand* and *petit mal,* and *tic douloureux* come from the French, as do such Americanized terms as *goiter, gout, malinger, jaundice, ointment,* and *physician.* Some examples of Greek-French terms are *surgeon, plaster, migraine,* and *palsy.* From the Italian we have gained the words *influenza* and *malaria,* and from the Dutch, *cough, litmus,* and *splint.* The Germans, Persians, Chinese, and Spanish also have contributed their share.

It is not unusual for a student new to health science terminology to recoil in fright when confronted with a term such as *hemangioendothelioblastoma.* But once the roots, prefixes, and suffixes making such compounds are learned, what seems at first impression to be unintelligible soon becomes quite clear.

For this reason, commonly used prefixes, suffixes, and word elements should be studied diligently. The first step is to break a compound term into its parts. For example, view the example given above as hem + angio + endothelio + blast + oma. This aids spelling, pronunciation, and remembering. Once the definitions of these units are known, the meaning of the compound word is understood. *Hemangioendothelioblastoma* means a primitive cell tumor located in the endothelium of a blood vessel:

hem	-	blood
angio	-	vessel
endothelio	-	endothelium
blast	-	primitive cell (germ)
oma	-	tumor

Other examples of how words are made and their literal meanings are *cardiogram,* meaning tracing of heart action, from cardio (heart) + gram (picture); *colitis,* meaning inflammation of the lower intestine, from col (colon) + itis (inflammation); and *leukocytes*, meaning white blood cells, from leuko (white) + cytes (cells).

euphony, a vowel or a consonant is sometimes added to or subtracted from word elements in combination.

Refer to Table 4.1. The root is given first; then a brief definition follows.

COMMON LATIN AND GREEK WORD ROOTS

Table 4.1 lists many common Latin and Greek roots used in chiropractic terminology. Some word elements are frequently placed before other word elements as *prefixes* or after other elements as *suffixes*. For

COMMON LATIN AND GREEK PREFIXES

Table 4.2 lists common prefixes. Remember that a word element may be placed before or after another element or as the word denoting the meaning when used with another

Table 4.1. Common Latin and Greek Roots

Root	Definition	Root	Definition
abdominus	abdomen	astro	star
acantha	spine	atmo	vapor, air
acousia	hearing	atrophy	a wasting away
acro	extremity	audio	to hear
actin	ray	auris	the ear
acuo	sharp, sudden	auto	self
aden	gland	bacter	rod
adeps	fat	baro	weight
adit	entrance, approach	bary	heavy
aer	air	basis	foundation
ala	wing	bilis	bile
alba	white	blos	life
alex	to protect	blast	germ
algia	pain	bovine	cow, ox
ama	together	brachlon	arm
ana	to build up	brachium	arm
andro	man	brachys	short
anglo	vessel	bradys	slow
anima	soul	brevis	short
ankylo	loop, adherence	bromos	stench
anom	irregular	bronchus	bronchial tube
ansa	handle	bubon	groin
antero	before	bursa	sac, pouch
anthrop	man	caco	bad, poor, sick
antrum	cavity	calor	heat
anulus	circular	caput	head
aqua	water	cardio	heart
arche	beginning	carno	flesh
archo	anus	cartilago	gristle
arcus	bow, arc	cata	down
arthro	joint	cauda	tail
articulus	joint	cavum	cavity

Table 4.1. Continued

Root	Definition	Root	Definition
cele	hernia	esthesia	feeling, touch
celia	abdomen	eu	good, healthy
centesis	puncture	exo	outside, without
cephal	head	febris	fever
chir(o)	hand	femina	woman
chole	bile	fibra	fiber
chondra	cartilage	fila	thread
chroma	color	flex	bend
chyle	juice	galactia	milk
cide	to kill	gastr	the stomach
clast	breaking down	gen	to beget
color	hue	genu	knee
colp	vagina	germen	germ, sprig
cor	heart	gingiva	the gum(s)
corpus	body	glossa	tongue, speech
costa	rib, side	glyco	sugar
crico	ring	graph	to write, record
crucis	the cross	gravi	weight, serious
cry	cold	gyne	women
crypt	hidden	gyros	circle
cutis	skin	hala	breath, air
cyano	blue	helio	the sun
cyna	dog	hema	blood
cyte	cell	hepat	the liver
dacry	tear	heter	other, different
dactyl	finger	hidro	perspiration
deca	ten	histo	tissue
demo	people	homo	like, same
dens	tooth	humerus	shoulder
derma	skin	hydro	water
dexia	on the right	hygea	health
dexter	right	hypno	sleep
digit	finger, toe	hyster	womb
diplo	double	icthy	fish
dolor	pain	idio	self
durus	hard, lasting	ileum	distal small intestine
dynia	ache, pain	ilium	hip bone
dys	difficult, painful	intestinum	intestine, entrail
ectasis	dilatation of	ipso	same
ecto	without, outside	iso	equal
ectopy	displacement of	jecur	liver
embryo	to grow within	juxta	near
emia	blood	keras	horn, cornea
endo	within	kine	motion
ensis	sword	lachryma	tear
entero	intestine	lact	milk
equus	equal	later	side
erotic	pulsation	lati	broad
erythro	red	lave	wash

Table 4.1. Continued

Root	Definition	Root	Definition
lepid	scale, scaly	neuro	nerve
lepsy	spasm, seizure	nidus	nest
leuko	white	niger	black
lexia	word	nocte	night
lien	the spleen	nomen	name
lingua	tongue	nosto	to return, go
lipa	fat	novus	new
lith	stone, calculus	nychia	nail of finger, toe
logue	speech	ob	against, obstructive
luna	moon	odont	tooth
lysis	to dissolve, break down	odor	smell
macro	great, long	olig	little, sparse, few
mal	bad, painful	omni	all
malacia	softening	onoma	name
mamma	breast	oophor	ovary
mania	madness	ophthalma	the eye
mas	man, male	ora	mouth
mast	breast	orch	testicle
medicamentum	medicine	ortho	straight, regular
medio	middle	os	mouth
mega	large, great	osma	odor
megalo	large, great	osteo	bone
melano	black	ot	ear
meno	month	ovum	egg
mens	mind	pachy	thick
mensis	month	paleo	old, ancient, past
mentis	mind	pan	all
meso	middle	para	to bear
meta	between, after, beyond	paries	wall
meter	measure	partum	to give birth to
metro	the uterus	path	disease, disorder
micro	tiny, minute	pedi	child
mis	bad, poor, dislike	pedis	foot
mono	single, alone, one	penia	poverty, poorness
morbus	disease	pexy	fixation
mortis	death, dead	phagy	to eat
muco	mucus	pharmac	medicine, drug
multi	many	phil	to love
musculus	muscle	phleb	vein
myelo	marrow	phobia	morbid fear
myo	muscle	phone	voice, sound
nano	dwarf	photo	light
naso	nose	phrasia	utterance, speech
nasus	nose	phren	mind, head, skull
natus	birth	phylaxis	anti-infection
necro	death	physi	nature
neo	new	plasia	to form
nephr	kidney	pnea	to breathe, breath
nervus	nerve	pneumo	lung

Table 4.1. Continued

Root	Definition	Root	Definition
podia	foot	splanchna	organ, viscus
polio	gray	spondy	vertebra, spine
poly	many, excessive	squama	a scale
procto	anus	staphyl	grape
pseudo	false, mimic	stasis	stopping, checking
psyche	mind, soul, spirit	stere	solid
pteryg	wing	steth	chest
ptya	sputum, saliva	stoma	mouth
pulmo	lung	stomachus	stomach
pulsus	pulse, stoke, beat	sudor	perspiration
puter	rotten, putrid	super	over, abnormal
pyelo	trough, basin	supra	above
pyo	pus	tachy	swift
pyr	fire	tact	touch
pyreto	fever	tend	tendon
quadri	four	teno	tendon
rachis	spine	testis	testicle
ramus	branch	tetra	four
rar	thin, rare, sprase	thana	death
ren	kidney	thenia	strength, power
rheo	current	theo	god, deity
rhin	the nose	therapy	treatment
ruber	red	therm	heat, temperature
salping	tube	thorax	chest
salpinx	tube	thrombo	blood clot
sanguis	blood	thyro	shield, thyroid
sanitas	health	tocia	childbirth
sapro	putrid	toco	childbirth
sarco	flesh	tonus	tone, sound
sarx	flesh	tricho	hair
schist(o)	to separate, split	trophy	nutrition, growth
schiz	to divide, split	ula	gum
scler	hard	ultra	over, beyond, excess
scopy	observation of	unguis	nail
scota	darkness	unus	one, single
sect	to cut	uria	urine
sial	saliva	uter	womb
sito	food	vas	vessel
soma	body	ven	vein
somnus	sleep	vertebra	spine, backbone
spasm	seizure, convulsion	xanth	yellow
sphen	wedge	xero	dry
sphygma	pulse, throb	xylo	wood
spina	spine	zoo	animal
spiritus	spirit	zymo	to ferment

prefix or suffix. Also recall that a vowel or consonant is sometimes added or subtracted between combined word elements to obtain euphony.

Refer to Table 4.2. Prefixes are shown in the left column followed by their common definition. Examples and their definitions are shown in the columns on the right.

Table 4.2. Common Prefixes and Examples of Use

Prefix	Meaning	Example	Definition
a-	without, not, absence of	achromia	without color
ab-	from, away from, negative	abduct	draw away from
abdomin-	abdomen	abdominoscopy	direct stomach inspection
acid-	sour	aciduric	pertaining to acidic urine
acou-	hearing	acousma	auditory hallucination
acr-	extremity	acromegaly	enlarged extremities
acro-	extremity, apex, extreme	acromegaly	extremity hyperplasia
act-	do, drive, act	action	an act, deed, or performance
actin-	ray, ray like	actinoid	resembling a ray
acu-	needle	acupoint	meridian point
ad-	to, toward, on, near, by	adoral	toward the mouth
aden-	gland, glandular	adenoma	gland tumor
aden(o)-	gland, glandular	adenodynia	ache in a gland
adip-	fat	adipocellular	pertaining to fatty cells
aer(o)-	air	aerophagia	swallowing of air
alb-	white	albinism	whiteness
all-	other, different	allergy	induced sensitivity
alve(o)-	cavity, socket, channel	alveoalgia	dry socket pain (eg, tooth)
ama-	together	amarthritis	multijoint arthritis
ambi-	both, around	ambivalence	simultaneous opposites
amph(i)-	both	amphibolia	period of doubtful diagnosis
amyl(o)-	starch	amylosuria	amylase in the urine
an-	without, not, absence of	anorexia	absence of appetite
ana-	up, back again, increase	anabolism	constructive metabolism
andro-	man, male	androphobia	morbid fear of the male sex
angi(o)-	vessel (blood)	angiolith	stone in a blood vessel wall
anima-	life, spirit, soul	animate	to quicken, make alive
ankyl(o)-	loop, bend, adherence	ankylosed	joint immobility, consolidation
anomalo-	irregular	anomalotrophy	abnormality of nutrition
ante-	before in time or place	antepartum	before delivery (childbirth)
anter-	before, front	anteriorly	toward the front
anthrop-	man, mankind, humanity	anthropoid	resembling man, ape
ant(i)-	against, counter	antidote	against poison
antr-	cavern	antrodynia	pain from a cavity or viscus
apo-	separation, away from	apophysis	bone outgrowth or projection

Table 4.2. Continued

Prefix	Meaning	Example	Definition
aqua-	water	aquatic	inhabitant of water
arch-	beginning	archetype	original model or pattern
archi-	first	archineuron	first nerve starting an impulse
arch(o)-	rectum	archoptoma	prolapsed portion of rectum
arthr(o)-	joint, articulation	arthritis	inflammation of joint(s)
articu-	joint	articulation	union or junction between bones
astro-	star	astrocyte	star-shaped cell
atmo-	vapor, air, breath	atmosphere	mass of surrounding air
audi(o)-	to hear	auditory	pertaining to hearing
auri-	the ear	auriform	ear shaped
auto-	self	autotoxin	self-made organic poison
bacter-	rod	bacteria	rod-shaped microorganisms
baro-	weight	barograph	air weight or pressure chart
bary-	heavy	baryglossia	thick speech
basi-	base, lower part	basilar	pertaining to the foundation
bi-	two, twice, double	biceps	muscle with two heads
bili-	bile	bilirubin	ruby-colored bile pigment
bio-	life	biology	science of life
blast-	germ	blastolysis	destruction of germ substance
bovin-	cow, ox	bovinoid	resembling a cow or an ox
brachi-	arm	brachialgia	severe arm pain or ache
brachy-	short	brachydactyly	short fingers and toes
brady-	slow	bradycardia	abnormally slow heart beat
brevi-	short	breviflexor	any short flexor muscle
bromo-	stench, foul odor	bromopnea	foul breath, halitosis
bronch-	bronchial tubes	bronchitis	inflammation of the bronchi
bubon-	groin	bubonalgia	pain or ache in the groin
burs-	sac, pouch	bursitis	inflammation of a bursa
caco-	bad, ill	cacogeusia	a bad or poor taste
calor-	heat	calorie	a unit of heat measurement
capi-	head	capitate	head shaped
cardio-	heart	cardiostenosis	narrowing of heart chambers
carni-	flesh	carnivora	flesh-eating animals
cata-	down, lower, under	catarrh	a down-flow of mucus
caud-	tail, tail like	caudate	having a tail
cephal-	head	encephalitis	brain inflammation
cervic-	neck	cervicitis	inflammation of the cervix
chondra-	cartilage, gristle	chondralgia	pain in a cartilage

Table 4.2. Continued

Prefix	Meaning	Example	Definition
chromat-	color	chromatology	science of color
chylo-	juice	chylothorax	effused chyle in the chest
circum-	around, about	circumduction	circular movement of extremity
co-	together, with	coalesce	grow together
com-	together, with	combination	a united set of things
con-	together, with	congenital	existing since birth
contra-	against, counter, opposite	contraception	against conception, pregnation
cor-	heart	cordiform	heart shaped
crico-	ring	cricoid	resembling a ring
cry-	cold	cryesthesia	anesthesia produced by cold
crypt-	hidden	cryptorchidism	undescended testicle
cut-	skin	cutitis	inflammation of the skin
cyan-	blue	cyanosis	bluish skin
cyn-	dog	cynophobia	morbid fear of dogs
cyto-	cell	cytopenia	poverty of blood cells
dacry(o)-	tear	dacryorrhea	excessive tear discharge
dactyl-	finger	dactylogram	fingerprint
de-	down, away, from, removal	demote	lower in rank, class, or grade
deca-	ten	decameter	ten meters
deci-	one-tenth	decimeter	one-tenth of a meter
demo-	people	demotic	pertaining to people
dent-	tooth	dentoid	resembling a tooth
dermat-	skin	dermatitis	skin inflammation
dexio-	on or toward right side	dexiotropic	curving from left to right
dextro-	right	dextromanual	right-handed
di-	double, twice	dicrotic	double pulse beat
dia-	through, apart, between	dialysis	passing through a membrane
digi-	finger, toe	digital	pertaining to a finger or toe
diplo-	double, twin	diplopia	double vision
dis-	apart, away from	disease	no ease, away from ease
dolor-	pain	dolorus	painful, expressing pain
dors-	back, toward the back	dorsal	pertaining to the back
dura-	hard, solid, compact	dura mater	outermost tough meninges
dys	difficult, bad, painful	dysmenorrhea	painful menstruation
ec-	out of, from	eccentric	away from normal or average
ect(o)-	outside of, without	ectoderm	external layer of skin
electro-	electric	electrotheraphy	therapy by electric current
en-	in, within	encephalia	within the skull
end(o)-	within, in	endogastric	within the stomach
ensi-	sword	ensiform	sword shaped
enter(o)-	intestine	enteritis	intestinal inflammation

Table 4.2. Continued

Prefix	Meaning	Example	Definition
ento-	within, inner	entocyte	contents within the cell
epi-	on, over, upon	epicondyle	bony prominence on a condyle
equi-	equal	equilibrium	equally balanced
erythro-	red	erythrocyte	red blood cell
esthesio-	touch, sensation, feeling	esthesiogenic	producing sensation
cu-	good, well, pleasant	cuphoria	state of joy or well-being
ex-	away from, out, outside	excentric	away from the center
exo-	outside, out, without	exocardial	external to the heart
extra-	outside of, beyond	extraspinal	apart from the spine
febri-	fever	febriphobia	morbid fear of catching a fever
fil-	thread	filiform	thread-like shape or character
flex-	bend	flexure	curvature, bend of a part
galact-	milk	galactose	milk sugar
gastr-	stomach	gastritis	inflammation of stomach lining
gen-	to give birth to, beget	genetics	science of heredity
germi-	germ, sprig	germicidal	destructive to germs
gingi-	the gum	gingivitis	inflammation of the gums
gloss(o)-	tongue	glossolysis	paralysis of the tongue
glyco-	sugar	glycopenia	deficiency of sugar
gravi-	weight, serious, heavy	gravid	pregnant, heavy with child
gyn-	woman, female	gynecology	study of female diseases
gyr-	circle	gyrospasm	spasmotic rotary head motions
hali-	breath, air	halitus	an exhaled breath
helio-	the sun	heliotherapy	treatment by sun rays
hem-	blood	hemorrhage	gushing forth of blood
hemi-	half	hemiparesis	paralysis of half the body
hepat-	the liver	hepatitis	inflammation of the liver
hetero-	other, different	heterochromic	composed of various colors
hidro-	sweat	hidrosis	perspiration
hist(o)-	tissue	histolysis	destruction of tissue
homo-	same, like	homogenesis	of same character throughout
humer-	shoulder	humeral	relating to the shoulder
hydro-	water, fluid	hydrothorax	fluid in the chest cavity
hyper-	over, beyond, excess	hyperostosis	overgrowth of bone
hypno-	sleep	hypnosis	sleep-resembling state
hypo-	under, deficiency	hypoplasia	incomplete growth
hyster-	womb, uterus	hysterectomy	surgical removal of the uterus
icthy-	fish	icthyderm	scaly (fish-like) skin
idio-	self	idioneurosis	neurosis arising from nerves

Table 4.2. Continued

Prefix	Meaning	Example	Definition
ileo-	ileum	ileocecal	pertaining to ileum and cecum
ilio-	ilium, flank	iliospinal	relating to ilium and spine
im-	not	impermeable	unable to be permeated
in-	within, into, not	incise	to cut into
infra-	beneath, below	inframandibular	below the jaw
ino-	fiber, tendon	inopolypus	a fibrous polyp
inter-	between, among	intercostal	between the ribs
intestin-	entrail, intestine	intestinotoxin	interotoxin
intra-	within, into	intraspinal	within the spine
intro-	into, in, inward	introspect	to look within
ipsi-	same	ipsilateral	on the same side
iso-	equal	isotonic	of the same or uniform tone
jeco-	liver	jecoral	relating to the liver
juxta-	near, nearby, close to	juxtaspinal	near the spine
kerat-	horn, horny	cornea	similar to a horn
kinesi-	motion	kinesiology	study of motion
lachry-	tear	lachrymose	tearful, saddening, weeping
lact-	milk	lactose	milk sugar
later(o)-	side	lateroflexion	bending to the side
lati-	broad	latissimus	a broad muscle
lav-	wash	lavipedium	foot bath
lepid-	scale, scaly, fish-like	lepidosis	skin resembling that of a fish
leuko-	white	leukocyte	white blood cell
levo-	left, to the left	levorotation	turning to the left
lexi-	word	lexical	pertaining to the vocabulary
lien-	the spleen	lienocele	splenic hernia
lingu-	tongue	linguiform	tongue shaped
lip(o)-	fat	lipoma	fatty tumor
litho-	stone, calculus	lithotripsy	crushing of stones in bladder
luna-	moon	lunate	moon shaped
macro-	long, great, large	macrosis	increase in size, bulk, length
mal-	bad, painful, poor	malnutrition	poor nutrition
mamm-	breast	mammectomy	breast amputation
mas-	man, male	masculation	development of male features
mast-	breast	mastitis	inflammation of mammary gland
medi-	medicine	medicator	one who administers drugs
medi(o)-	mid, middle	mediolateral	relating to the center and side
mega-	large, great	megalosplenic	enlarged spleen
melan(o)-	black, ebony	melanocarcinoma	a black cancer

Table 4.2. Continued

Prefix	Meaning	Example	Definition
meno-	month	menopause	cessation of monthly menses
ment-	mind	mentality	mental power
mens-	month	menstruation	monthly discharge of menses
meso-	middle	mesocephalic	medium-sized head
meta-	beyond, change, between	metastasis	transition, going more
metro-	uterus	metroscope	intrauterine inspection device
micro-	small, minute	microorganism	organism invisible to naked eye
mis-	bad, dislike	misopedia	dislike of children
mono-	one, single, alone	monochromatic	of one color
morbi-	disease	morbific	disease producing
muco-	mucus	mucumembraneous	having a mucous membrane
multi-	many	multipara	woman who has had many children
musculo-	muscle	musculophrenic	pertaining to diaphragm muscle
myelo-	marrow	myelomalacia	softening of bone marrow
my(o)-	muscle	myotonia	muscle tone
nano-	dwarf	nanocephalous	dwarf-like crainum
nas-	nose	nasoseptitis	inflammation of nasal septum
necro-	death	necrosis	death of a part or tissue
neo-	new	neoplasm	new tissue formation, growth
nephr-	kidney	nephralgia	kidney pain
nervi-	nerve	nerviomtor	pertaining to a motor nerve
neuro-	nerve	neurocyte	nerve cell
noct-	night	noctambulism	sleepwalking
nomen-	name	nomenclature	classification by name
non-	not, anti, against	nonstriated	without striations
noso-	disease	nosogenesis	the progression of disease
nost	home, to go, to return	nostalgia	homesickness
nov-	new	novice	newcomer
ob-	against, in the way of	obdurate	stubborn
odont-	tooth	odontotechny	dentistry
olig-	little, few	oligocholia	insufficient bile
om-	shoulder	omarthritis	shoulder arthritis
omni-	all	omnifarious	of all types, classes, or kinds
onom-	name	onomatology	the study of names
oophor-	ovary	oophoritis	inflammation of an ovary
ophthalm-	the eye	ophthalmopathy	disease of the eye
opistho-	backward, behind	opisthoporeia	involuntary walking backward

Table 4.2. Continued

Prefix	Meaning	Example	Definition
orch-	testicle	orchiocele	hernia of the testicle
ortho-	regular, normal, straight	orthotonic	correct tone
ora-	mouth	orad	toward the mouth
oste(o)-	bone	osteomyelon	bone narrow
ot-	ear	otalgia	earache
evi-	egg	oviduct	Fallopian duct (egg canal)
pachy-	thick	pachyemia	thick blood
paleo-	old, ancient	paleogenetic	originated long ago
pan-	all, every	pandemic	widespread epidemic
para-	near, by the side of	parallel	side by side
pariet-	wall	parietal	pertaining to wall of a cavity
partu-	give birth to, bring forth	partuition	childbearing
path-	disease	pathology	the study of disease
ped-	child	pediatrics	science of childhood diseases
pedi-	foot	pediferous	having feet
per-	through, throughout	percussion	to strike through
peri-	around	pericanalicular	around a canal
phago-	to eat	phagocyte	cell that ingests bacteria
pharm-	medicine, drug	pharmacotherapy	treatment by medication
phleb-	vein	phlebitis	inflammation of vein lining
phon-	sound, voice	phonetic	relating to the voice
photo-	light	photophobia	morbid fear of light
phren-	mind, head	phrenopathy	any mental disease
physi-	nature	physiotheraphy	treatment by natural forces
pleuro-	side, rib	pleurocentrum	lateral part of the spine
pluri-	more, several	plurimenorrhea	increased menstrual frequency
pneumo-	lung	pneumopathy	any lung disease
pod-	foot	podarthritis	arthritis of the foot
polio-	gray	poliosis	premature gray hair
poly-	many, excessive	polyuria	frequent urination
post-	after, behind, late	posttherapy	after treatment
pre-	before, front of, early	prenatal	before birth or delivery
pro-	affirmative, according to	procreate	to generate
proct(o)-	rectum	protocele	rectal hernia
proto-	first	protoplasm	early form of living matter
pseudo-	false	pseudocyesis	false pregnancy
psych-	mind, soul, spirit	psychogenic	originating in the mind
pteryg-	wing	pterygoid	resembling a wing, wing shaped
ptya-	sputum, saliva	ptyalism	excessive flow of saliva
pulmo-	lung	pulmonary	relating to a lung
puls-	pulse, stroke, beat	pulsation	throbbing or rhythmical beat
putre-	putrid, rotten, decayed	putrefactive	relating to decomposition
pyelo-	trough, basin	pyelogram	kidney x-ray film
pykn-	thick, compact, frequent	pyknic	short, thick, stocky build

Table 4.2. Continued

Prefix	Meaning	Example	Definition
pyo-	pus	pyomyositis	purulent muscle inflammation
pyreto-	fever	pyretograph	fever chart
pyro-	fire, fever	pyrogenetic	fire- or fever producing
quadri-	four	quadrifid	separated into four parts
rach-	spine	rachioplegia	spinal paralysis
rami-	branch	ramiform	branch like, tree shaped
rar-	thin, rare, sparse	rarefaction	making thinner, less dense
re-	again, back, against	recreation	to create again, restore
reni-	kidney	renipuncture	surgical kidney puncture
retro-	behind, back, backward	retroflexed	bent backward
rhin-	the nose	rhinitis	nasal inflammation
rubi-	red	rubicund	blushing, reddish
salping-	tube	salpingitis	inflammation of fallopian tube
sangui-	blood	sanguinary	bloody
sanit-	health	sanitarian	a hygienist
sapro-	putrid	saprogenic	producing decay
sarco-	flesh	sarcoma	connective-tissue cancer
schiz-	to divide, split, fissure	schizophrenia	split personality
scler-	hard, indurated	sclerosis	condition of hardening
scoto-	darkness	scotophobia	morbid fear of the dark
sect-	to cut	sectile	able to be cut
semi-	half	semilunar	half-moon shape
sero-	serum	serous	watery, serum like
sial-	saliva	sialochesis	salivary flow suppression
sit-	food	sitology	study of food, nutrition
soma-	body	somatic	pertaining to the body
somni-	sleep	somnipathy	any sleep disorder
spasmo-	seizure, convulsion	spasmodyspnea	difficult or jerky breathing
sphen-	wedge	sphenoid	wedge shaped
sphygmo-	pulse	sphygometer	pulse-measuring instrument
spino-	spine	spinograph	spinal x-ray film
spondylo-	vertebra, spine	spondylosis	degeneration of the spine
squamo-	a scale	squamoid	scale like, resembling a scale
steno-	contracted, narrow	stenocoriasis	pupil contraction
stereo-	solid	stereodynamics	motion of solid bodies
steth-	chest	stetoscope	chest examination device
stomat-	mouth	stomatitis	inflammation of the mouth
sub-	less, under, below	subcutaneous	under the skin
sudor-	perspiration	sudorific	causing sweat
super-	over, above, excessive	supercilia	above the eyelid or eyebrow

Table 4.2. Continued

Prefix	Meaning	Example	Definition
supra-	above, upon, on	supraorbital	above the eye socket
sym-	together, with	symbiotic	living together
syn-	together, with	syndactylism	webbed fingers or toes
tachy-	swift, fast, rapid	tachycardia	abnormally rapid heart beat
tact-	touch, sensation	tactile	pertaining to touch
tend-	tendon	tendotomy	surgical cutting a tendon
test-	testicle	testitis	inflammation of a testicle
tetra-	four	tetragenous	separated into four parts
thana-	death	thanology	the study of death
theo-	god, deity	theomania	fanaticism
thera-	to heal, treat	therapeutics	the science and art of healing
thermo-	temperature, heat	thermometer	heat-measuring instrument
thoraco-	chest	thoracodynia	chest ache
thrombo-	blood clot	thrombostasis	circulation stopped by clot
thyro-	shield	thyroid	resembling a shield
toco-	childbirth	tocology	obstetrics
topo-	place, location, site	topogrpahic	describing a specific area
tox-	poison	toxemia	intoxication
toxi-	poison	toxipathy	toxicosis
toxic(o)-	poison	toxicogenic	producing toxins
toxo-	poison	toxophilic	susceptible to poison
trans-	across, through	transudate	fluid seeping through membrane
tri-	three, thrice	triad	group of three
tricho-	hair	trichopathy	any hair disease
ul-	gum	ulatrophy	shrinking of gum tissue
ultra-	over, excess, beyond	ultramarine	beyond the sea
un-	not	unconscious	not conscious
ungu-	nail	ungual	relating to nails
uni-	one	unilateral	one-sided, on one side
utero-	womb	uteroplasty	repair of the uterus
vaso-	vessel	vasoparesis	vasomotor paralysis
veni-	vein	veniplex	a venous plexus
ventro-	front, anterior	ventroptosis	falling abdomen
vertebr-	vertebra, spine	vertebrarium	vertebral column
vesic-	blister, bladder	vesicocele	hernia of the bladder
xanth-	yellow	xanthodont	yellowish teeth
xero	dry	xerosis	abnormal dryness
xyl-	wood	xyloid	resembling wood
zoo-	animal	zoology	the study of animals
zymo-	to ferment	zymogenic	producing fermentation

COMMON LATIN AND GREEK SUFFIXES

Table 4.3 lists common Latin and Greek suffixes used in health science terminology. Such word elements are not commonly used before other word elements as prefixes. However, when they are, for euphony, a vowel or a consonant is sometimes added or subtracted between word elements in combination.

Refer to Table 4.3. The suffix is given first, followed by its most common definition.

SINGULARS AND PLURALS

Traditional Style

Table 4.4 lists common word endings in singulars and plurals despite root. While there are some exceptions, this guide can be considered generally true in traditional health science usage.

Table 4.5 shows examples of common Greek and Latin singular and plural forms. Basic principles can be learned from a re-

Table 4.3. Common Suffixes and Definitions

Suffix	Definition	Suffix	Definition
-acusis	hearing	-kinetic	motion, dynamic
-age	to move	-logy	study of, science of
-agogue	inducing	-lysis	setting free
-agra	catching, seizure	-malacia	softening
-al	characterized by	-meter	measure
-algia	pain, ache	-odynia	pain, ache
-ase	enzyme	-oid	like, resembling
-atrics	the practice of	-ology	study of, science of
-cele	swelling, tumor, hernia	-oma	tumor, neoplasm
-cian	one who	-osis	condition, state, process
-cide	causing death, killer	-ostomy	opening into for drainage
-cle	little	-otomy	to cut into, incise
-cocle	chamber, ventricle	-ous	full of
-cosis	condition or state of	-pathy	disease of, feeling
-cule	little	-plasty	repair
-cyst	bladder, bag	-penia	lack or poverty of
-cyte	cell	-peutics	science of
-ectomy	excision, surgical removal	-phage	consuming, eating
-emia	blood	-plastic	molded
-en	in, into	-plegia	paralysis
-ence	condition, state of being	-practic	the practice of
-form	resembling, like, same	-ptosis	falling, prolapse
-fuge	driving away	-raphy	suture of
-genetic	origin, producing	-rrhagia	sudden flow
-genic	origin, producing	-rrhea	discharge, flow
-gram	tracing, picture	-rrhexia	rupture of
-graph	record, chart	-scopy	direct examination of
-iasis	condition of	-stomy	opening
-ic	pertaining to, relating to	-tomy	incision of, cut
-ical	pertaining to, relating to	-trophy	nutrition
-icosis	condition or state of	-tropy	a turning
-itis	inflammation	-uria	urine
-kinesis	motion, movement	-zyme	ferment

Table 4.4. Greek and Latin Singular and Plural Word Endings

Singular Word Ending	Plural Word Ending	Common Singular Example	Common Plural Example
a	ae	bursa	bursae
ad	ades	gonad	gonades
cus	cera	viscus	viscera
er	era	cadaver	cadavera
ex, ix	ices	apex	apices
ia	es	esthesia	estheses
is	es	axis	axes
is	ides	ascaris	ascarides
ma	mata	adenoma	adenomata
men	mina	sudamen	sudamina
s	sa	vas	vasa
s	des	glans	glandes
s	tes	albacans	albacantes
sis	ses	diagnosis	diagnoses
u	ua	cornu	cornua
um	a	bacterium	bacteria
um	i	dorsum	dorsi
us	i	bacillus	bacilli
us	ora	corpus	corpora
x	a	nox	noxa

Traditional Singular	Traditional Plural	Modern Plural
antenna	antennae	antennas
bursa	bursae	bursas
fossa	fossae	fossas
lamina	laminae	laminas
adenoma	adenomata	adenomas
enema	enemata	enemas
fibroma	fibromata	fibromas
pathema	pathemata	pathemas
antiad	antiades	antiads
gonad	gonades	gonads
monad	monades	monads

view of this list that will help you in applying the correct form.

Modern Style

The examples given in Tables 4.4 and 4.5 depict traditional usage. However, everything is subject to change. For example, we see with increasing frequency in modern writings that singular word endings of "a" are pluralized by adding the common "s" rather than the traditional "ae" (eg, antennas rather than antennae). In singular words ending in "ma," we see editors also using the common "s" rather than the traditional "mata" (eg, adenoma rather than adenomata). In the singular words ending in "ad," use of the common "s" is replacing the traditional "ades" (eg, gonads rather than gonades). Whichever form is used, consistency is the important consideration. A few examples are shown below.

COMMON ANATOMICAL TERMS

Terms of position, direction, and location are commonly used in reference to body parts. Following are some examples.

Terms of Patient Position

Adams position. Standing with the heels together, the knees locked, and the spine fully flexed forward.

Anatomical position. Standing erect with the arms at the sides and the palms of the hands facing forward. The anatomical position is the position of reference when terms of direction and location are used.

Antalgic position. Any physical attitude assumed to gain some relief of pain.

Knee-chest position. Resting on the knees and upper chest (also called the genupectoral position).

Knee-elbow position. Resting on the knees and elbows (also called the genucubital position).

Lateral recumbent position. Lying on either the right or left side, with one or both hips and elbows flexed.

Lithotomy position. Lying in a supine position with the hips and knees flexed at right angles, with the feet usually supported by stirrups (also called the dorsosacral position); a variant of Simon's position.

Physiologic position. Standing in the habitual posture.

Prone position. Lying face down.

Table 4.5. Examples of Traditional Greek and Latin Singular and Plurals

Singular	Plural	Singular	Plural
addendum	addenda	focus	foci
aden	adena	fornix	fornices
adenoma	adenomata	fossa	fossae
ala	alae	glans	glandes
albacans	albacantes	gonad	gonades
amygdala	amygdalae	gonococcus	gonococci
antenna	antennae	gyrus	gyri
antiad	antiades	ilium	ilia
antrum	antra	index	indices
apertura	aperturae	keratosis	keratoses
apex	apices	labium	labia
aponeurosis	aponeuroses	lamina	laminae
appendix	appendices	loculus	loculi
aqua	aquae	locus	loci
arcus	arcus	medium	media
ascaris	ascarides	mucosa	mucosae
ascus	asci	naevus	naevi
atrium	atria	nodus	nodi
axis	axes	nox	noxa
bacillus	bacilli	os	ora
bacterium	bacteria	ovum	ova
bronchus	bronchi	papilla	papillae
bulla	bullae	pathema	pathemata
bursa	bursae	pes	pedes
cactus	cacti	petechia	petechiae
cadaver	cadavera	pilula	pilulae
calcaneum	calcanea	polypus	polypi
calculus	calculi	ramus	rami
calis	calices	septum	septa
cantharis	cantharides	sequestrum	sequestra
canthus	canthi	serosa	serosae
cornu	cornua	spasmus	spasmi
corpus	corpora	spectrum	spectra
crisis	crises	speculum	specula
cuniculus	cuniculi	stoma	stomata
dens	dentes	sudamen	sudamina
diagnosis	diagnoses	sulcus	sulci
diaphoreticus	diaphoretici	tarsus	tarsi
diastema	diastemata	tela	telae
digitus	digiti	tinctura	tincturae
dorsum	dorsi	toxicosis	toxicoses
echolatus	echolati	typha	typhae
enema	enemata	ulcus	ulcera
ensis	enses	varix	varices
epididymis	epididymides	vas	vasa
esthesia	estheses	vesicule	vesiculae
fibroma	fibromata	vis	vires
filix	filices	viscus	viscera
filum	fila	vomica	vomicae
flagellum	flagella	zygoma	zygomata

Simon's position. Lying supine with the hips slightly raised and flexed, the knees flexed, and the thighs widely separated.

Sims' position. Lying in a lateral recumbent position with one arm behind the back; the thighs are flexed, the upper more than the lower (also called the semiprone or English position).

Supine position. Lying on the back, face up (also called the dorsal position).

Terms of Direction and Location

- *Anterior.* Toward or nearer the front or belly side of the body; ventral.
- *Caudad.* Toward the feet.
- *Cephalad.* Toward the head or cranial vertex.
- *Contralateral.* On the opposite side.
- *Distal.* Away from the point of reference or origin.
- *Dorsal.* Posterior.
- *Inferior.* Situated or directed below; caudad.
- *Ipsilateral.* On the same side (homolateral).
- *Lateral.* Away or farther from the median or midsagittal plane, right or left of the midline; toward the side.
- *Medial.* Toward or nearer the midline, median, or midsagittal plane.
- *Palmar.* Referring to the palm or volar surface of the hand.
- *Plantar.* Referring to the sole or volar surface of the foot.
- *Posterior.* Toward or nearer the back or backside of the body; dorsal.
- *Proximal.* Near the point of reference or origin.
- *Superior.* Situated or directed above; cephalad.
- *Ventral.* Anterior.
- *Volar.* Referring to the palm of the hand or sole of the foot.

The Planes of the Body in Biodynamics

Motion occurs in a plane. The question arises: What is a *plane?* Simply put, a plane is any real or theoretical flat surface containing all the straight lines required to connect any two points on it.

Many chiropractic hypotheses derive from the science of biomechanics, and many basic considerations in biomechanics involve time, mass, center of mass, movement, force, and gravity—which operate according to the laws of physics. However, while numerous parameters of movement are interrelated, no one factor can completely describe movement by itself.

Because a force, either traumatic or therapeutic, may act along a single line in a single plane or in any direction in space, this factor must be considered in any reference system. Such a reference system is necessary if we are to communicate effectively with each other about joint position and motion. Thus, the following sections will review pertinent terms and principles that will enhance your communicative skills as well as deepen your understanding of *spinal dynamics.*

Structural Motion

From a clinical viewpoint, structural motion can be defined as any body part's relative change of place or position in space within a timeframe and about some other object in space. Thus, motion may be determined and illustrated by knowing and showing the body part's position before and after an interval of time. While linear motion is readily demonstrated in the body as a whole as it moves in a straight line, most joint motions are combinations of translation and angular movements that are more often than not diagonal rather than parallel to the cardinal planes of the body. For example, a vertebra cannot move in the anterior-posterior (A-P) plane because its articulating facets are slanted obliquely. Besides muscle force, joint motion is governed by factors of movement freedom, axes of movement, and range of motion.

The force of gravity is always directed toward the earth's center. Thus, the gravity lines of action and direction are constants. In the upright "rigid" body posture, the gravitational force on the entire body can be considered a single vector through the center of mass that represents the sum of many parallel positive and negative coordinates (Fig. 4.1).

Describing Positions in Space

In a two-dimensional reference system, the plane is simply divided into four quadrants by a perpendicular vertical ordinate line (Y axis) and a horizontal abscissa line (X axis). A third axis (usually labeled Z) can be used to locate points in three dimensions. The Z axis crosses the origin and its perpendicular to planes X and Y.

There are several reference systems. This particular system is the *Cartesian coordinate system* in which (1) flexion/extension rotation is rotation about the X axis, (2) axial rotation is rotation about the Y axis, and (3) lateral flexion rotation is rotation about the Z axis. All Z points in front of the X-Y plane are called positive, while those behind are called negative (Fig. 4.2). By using X, Y,

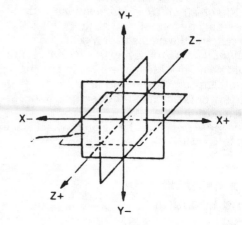

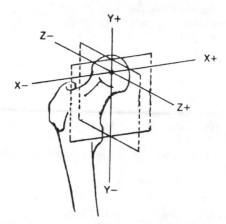

Figure 4.2. Top, positive and negative X, Y, and Z axes. Bottom, system of coordinates pertinent to the mechanical axis of the hip.

and Z coordinates, any point in space can be located and depicted. However, a minimum of six coordinates is necessary to specify the position of a rigid body (eg, a vertebra).

In biomechanics, the body's reference origin is at the body's center of mass. When this point is known, gross body space can be visualized as in the sagittal (right-left) Y-Z plane, frontal or coronal (anterior-posterior) X-Y plane, or horizontal or transverse (superior-inferior) X-Z plane. With such a reference system, movement of any body segment in these planes can be described by placing a coordinate system at the axis of a joint and projecting the action lines of the muscles involved.

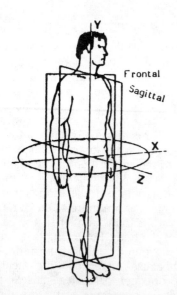

Figure 4.1. The planes of the body as related to the line of gravity. The X (frontal) axis passes from side to side (horizontally) and perpendicular to the sagittal plane. The Y (vertical) axis passes perpendicular to the transverse plane and the ground. The Z (sagittal) axis is perpendicular to the frontal plane, passing horizontally from front to back.

Axes

An axis is a straight line around which an object rotates, a line serving to orient a space or object (about which the object is symmetrical), or a reference line in a system of coordinates. Most body movements are rotations about joint axes and are rarely confined to a simple arc. Some motions vary to compensate for muscle/joint restrictions, bones twisting about their axes, and the transfer of power from one set of muscles to another within the range of movement. The joint surfaces of spinal joints are usually convexo-concave in design; ie, the convex (rounded) surface is larger than the concave (hollowed) surface. This relationship is exaggerated in all ball-and-socket joints.

If the anatomical position is used as a reference point, joint movements occur in a definite plane and around a definite axis. Flexion, extension, and hyperextension are movements in the sagittal plane about a frontal axis. Abduction and adduction are movements in the frontal plane about a sagittal plane about a vertical axis. Rotation, pronation, and supination are movements in the transverse axis. Circumduction is movement in both the sagittal and frontal planes.

Linear and Circular Motion

The two basic types of body motions are *linear movement* and *circular movement.* Linear motion occurs when the body as a whole or one of its parts is moved as a whole from one place to another in a straight line. An example of linear (sliding, gliding, translation) movement without any circular motion is long axis distraction of a finger joint.

Circular movement (angular, rotational) occurs when the body or a part is moved around the arc of a circle. An example of circular motion is seen between the long bones of the extremities and in the spinal column. Circular movements occur in definite planes and around definite axes (centers of rotation). They compose an important diagnostic viewpoint in musculoskeletal disorders, and, as previously described, each of these

three axes of rotation is perpendicular to the plane in which motion occurs.

Degrees of Joint Movement Freedom

The body is composed of many uniaxial, biaxial, and multiaxial joints. Joints with one axis have one degree of freedom to move in one plane such as pivot and hinge joints. Joints with two axes have two degrees of freedom to move in two different planes, and joints with three axes have three degrees of freedom to move in all three planes (eg, ball-and-socket joints). Thus, the potential motion in which an object (eg, a body part) may translate to and fro along a straight course or rotate one way or another about a particular axis equals one degree of freedom.

The degrees of freedom of a fingertip about the trunk, for example, are the sum of the degrees of freedom of all the joints from the distal phalanges to the shoulder girdle. While the distal phalanges have only one degree of freedom (flexion-extension), the entire upper extremity has 17 degrees totally. This summation process is an example of an *open kinematic chain.*

Combined Movements

Simple translatory motions of a body part invariably involve movements of more than one joint. This requires reciprocating actions of three or more segments at two or more joints if parallel lines are to be followed. For example, a fingertip cannot be made to follow the straight edge of a ruler placed in front when the wrist, elbow, and shoulder joints are locked. The fingertip then must follow an arc, not a straight line. Thus, human motion can be described as translation that gains major contributions from linear, angular, and curvilinear movements. The terms *general* or *three-dimensional body motion* infer that a body part may move in any direction by combining multidirectional translation and multiaxial rotation.

Plane Motion

Any motion in which all coordinates of a rigid body move parallel to a fixed point is called *plane motion*. Such motion has three degrees of freedom (ranges of motions); viz, (1) moving toward the anterior or posterior, (2) laterally moving toward the right or left, and (3) spinning in one direction or the other. In other words, plane motion has two translatory degrees of motion along two mutually perpendicular axes and one rotational degree of motion around an axis perpendicular to the translatory axes. Thus, when a person flexes his spine forward, the vertebrae flex and rotate in a single plane about an axis perpendicular to the sagittal plane. In such plane motion, various points on a particular vertebra will always move in parallel planes.

The Instantaneous Axis of Rotation

Plane motion is described by the position of its *instantaneous axis of rotation* and the motion's rotational magnitude about this axis. In the above example of spinal flexion, for instance, as a vertebra moves in a plane, there is a point at every instant of motion somewhere within or without the body that does not move. If a line is drawn from that point so it perpendicularly meets the line of motion, the point of intersection is called the instantaneous axis of rotation for that motion at that particular time. Most joint motions are largely rotational movements, but the axis of motion may change its location and/or its orientation during a complete range of motion.

Out-of-Plane Motion

As contrasted to plane motion, *out-of-plane motion* is a type of general body motion with three degrees of freedom: two rotations about mutually perpendicular axes and translation perpendicular to the plane formed by the axes. Thus, in out-of-plane motion, the body as a whole or a segment can move more than in a single plane. For example, if a person bends laterally, a mid-thoracic vertebral body translates from the sagittal plane toward the horizontal plane. This is not plane motion because various points on the vertebra do not move in parallel planes.

Terms of Motion

The mental picture of the spine being a straight, vertical, static structure is inaccurate. It is a living, dynamic, segmented organ that is in constant motion during locomotion, work, and every breath taken during rest. As most organs of the body during day or night, work or rest, the spine never rests—it is in constant motion, constantly *dynamic*.

The terms previously described in this chapter concerning position, direction, and location generally refer to static positions; ie, when the body is apparently still. Thus, additional terms are necessary to describe actions involved when body parts (eg, joint parts) move from one place in space to another such as during bending, lifting, walking, and running. Acquaint yourself with the following terms.

Motion. Movement refers to a continuous change (displacement) of position.

Coupling. Coupling is a motion of translation or rotation occurring along or about an axis as an object (eg, a vertebra) moves about another axis.

Kinetics. Kinetics is the study of the rate of change of a specific factor in the body that disregards the cause of the motion; ie, the study of the relationship between a force acting on a body or body segment and the changes produced in body motion. Kinetic actions are expressed in amounts per units of time.

Kinematics. Kinematics is the complex study of motions of body parts and forces causing motion (with emphasis on displacement, acceleration, and velocity) that is mainly the result of muscle activity.

Flexion and Extension. Generally, when the joint angle becomes smaller than when in the anatomical position, it is in *flexion*. For example, when the elbow is bent, it is flexed. The opposite of flexion is *extension*. Thus, when the elbow is straight, it is extended. Most joints can flex and extend. When motion exceeds the normal range, it is called hyperflexion or hyperextension; eg, as in instability of the elbow or knee.

Abduction and Adduction. When a part is farther away from the midline than it is in the anatomical (zero) position, it is an *abduction*. The opposite of abduction is *adduction*. Abduction and adduction occur at the shoulder, metacarpophalangeal, hip, and metatarsophalangeal joints.

Elevation and Depression. Raising a part from its normal (zero) position is called *elevation. Depression* means to lower a part from its normal position. Good examples of both show in the shoulder.

Circumduction. Movement of a bone circumscribing a cone such as at the shoulder or hip is called *circumduction*. Such motions usually comprise at least flexion, extension, abduction, and adduction.

Rotation. If a bone of a joint is capable of angular motion or turning on its longitudinal axis (spinning), the motion is called *rotation*. The motion of turning an anterior surface of a part toward the midline of the body is called inward or *internal rotation*. The motion of turning out is called outward or *external rotation*. The axis may be located outside or inside the rotating body. The classic example of internal-external rotation is at the shoulder.

Pronation. The word *pronation* refers to the act of assuming the prone position or the state or condition of being prone. When applied to the hand, it refers to the act of turning the hand backward, posteriorly, or downward by medial rotation of the forearm. When applied to the ankle or foot, it refers to a combination of eversion and abduction movements taking place in the tarsal and metatarsal joints that result in lowering the medial margin of the foot and thus the longitudinal arch.

Supination. *Supination* is the opposite of pronation. It is the act of turning the palm forward or upward or of raising the medial margin or longitudinal arch of the foot. Pronation and supination movements are seen at the forearm (rotation of forearm between the wrist and elbow, palm turning up or down, respectively) and in the foot. How-

ever, inversion and eversion are better terms to use for actions of the foot than pronation and supination.

Dorsiflexion and Plantar Flexion. Backward flexion or bending such as of the hand or foot is called *dorsiflexion:* movement toward the dorsal surface. *Plantar flexion* or *palmar flexion* is the opposite of dorsiflexion: movement toward the plantar surface or palm. In the hand or foot, the midline is an arbitrary line drawn through the middle finger or toe. Dorsiflexion movements are seen at the ankle and wrist, toes and fingers.

Inversion and Eversion. A turning inward, inside out, or other reversal of the normal relation of a part is called *inversion.* Inversion is a type of adduction of the foot where the plantar surface is turned inward relative to the leg. *Eversion* is the opposite of inversion, referring to a turning outward of a part. Eversion of the foot means to turn the plantar surface outward in relation to the leg.

Translation. Linear motion that occurs when all parts of an object at a given time have the same direction of motion about a fixed point is called *translation*. This commonly occurs in a train moving along a track, the body moving as a whole during gait, or a facet that glides or slips across a relatively fixed surface. Translation is measured in millimeters.

Degrees of Freedom. Vertebrae have six degrees of freedom (ranges of motions); ie, translation along and rotation about each of the three orthogonal axes. Any motion in which an object may translate back and forth along a straight course or rotate one way or another about a particular axis equals one degree of freedom. For example, joints with one axis have one degree of freedom to move in one plane (eg, pivot and hinge joints). Joints with two axes have two degrees of freedom to move in different planes, and joints with three axes have three degrees of freedom to move in all planes (eg, ball-and-socket joints).

Range of Motion (ROM). ROM refers to the difference between two points of physiologic extremes of motion. Rotation is measured in degrees. A vertebra has six degrees of freedom as it moves in three-dimensional space; eg, translations along and rotations about each of the three cardinal axes (X, Y, and Z). If passive distraction is considered a motion, seven degrees of freedom exist.

Instantaneous Axis of Rotation (IAR). The IAR is that fixed point which does not move but about which rotation occurs. It can exist inside or outside the object moving and is subject to change at any given instant.

Closed Kinematic System. This phrase refers to a series of body links or a chain of joints in which segments are interdependent on each other for certain movements so each joint can function properly in a co-ordinated movement; eg, the movement of the first costotransverse joint necessary for the cervical spine to extend and laterally flex.

COMMON DIAGNOSTIC AND PROCEDURAL TERMS

Health is a state of physical and mental well-being in which the body can function fully with comfort and the ability to renew and restore itself. On the other hand, disease is any departure from health. It is any disorder that interferes with the normal operation of a body process. In broad terms, disease (sickness) can be considered any departure from health that is caused by pathogenic organisms OR any other factor not involving an external physical force. An injury, in broad terms, is any departure from health due to an external physical force or environmental condition (eg, a wound, strain, or sprain).

Background Review

Certain points previously made deserve review here. First, the CA should realize that disease depends on irritations from the environment overcoming the body's resistance and the nervous system acting as the mediating factor between. Whereas life is a stimulus-response phenomenon in the normal state, disease is an abnormal response to stimuli which in turn may be beyond the capacities of the body to adapt physiologically. The cause of disease is broadly considered an irritation caused by either *environmental* or *constitutional* factors.

Major environmental factors are physical injury; various parasitic, bacterial, fungi, viral infections, etc.; harmful inanimate objects such as inert foreign bodies or chemical toxins; and nutritional abnormalities from either cellular deficiency and/or excess in various food substances or deficiency in a local tissue from impaired blood supply or drainage.

The major constitutional factors are inheritance of genetic abnormalities such as cleft lip, congenital heart disease, or malformed bones and articulations. Nongenetic factors also may lower a person's resistance to disease by impairing his constitutional health, particularly as a by-product of previous disease.

Many diseases, dysfunctions, and disabilities leave a "memory" on the nervous system that tends to perpetuate the process after the cause has been removed. This finding is motivating considerable research.

Terminology

Some conditions may attend, be associated with, pre-exist or predispose to, disease or musculoskeletal injuries. These may exist as separate entities, the aftermath of previous injury or disease, or complicate a more recent affection and form a large category. Common examples are spinal distortions and subluxations, local disease of vertebrae and pelvis, and malformations such as developmental anomalies of a bone or joint.

Proper procedural and diagnostic terminology contains statements of being as they exist in logical sequence. The most recent (or important) conditions are given first consideration, other involvements following, and qualified by proper descriptive terms. Examples of these descriptors include:

• *Accompanying:* denoting companionship with, but not dependent on or necessarily closely joined (ie, may be coexisting but possibly independent)
• *Associated:* closely joined, but not necessarily dependent on
• *Attendant:* following as consequential
• *Concomitant:* that which accompanies or is attendant with
• *Consequent:* following as a result of (because)
• *Predisposing:* giving a tendency toward
• *Pre-existing:* existing before, but not necessarily giving a tendency to

While not limited to injuries, chiropractic care in musculoskeletal disorders is a major concern. Examples are *sprain,* an overstretching or overexertion of the ligaments of a joint (including capsular tissues); *strain,* an overstretching of muscular or tendinous tissues; *fracture,* a rupture of living bone; *dislocation,* and *subluxation.*

Common direct complications of a musculoskeletal injury include

• *Myositis:* inflammation of muscle
• *Muscular spasm:* an involuntary contraction of muscle
• *Tendinitis:* inflammation of tendons or muscle attachments
• *Tenosynovitis:* inflammation of tendon sheaths
• *Bursitis:* inflammation of a bursa
• *Capsulitis:* inflammation of a joint capsule
• *Synovitis:* inflammation of a synovial membrane
• *Fibrositis:* inflammation of fibrous tissue
• *Radiculitis:* inflammation of a nerve root
• *Paresthesia:* abnormal sensory awareness
• *Neuralgia:* ache or pain in a nerve
• *Neuritis:* inflammation of a nerve
• *Contusion:* a bruising of tissue

Spinal Distortions. Curvatures (abnormal bending of the spine) are classified as *kyphosis,* an abnormal flexion of an area of the spine; *lordosis,* an abnormal extension of an area of the spine; *scoliosis,* an abnormal lateral bending of an area of the spine with vertebral rotation; and *lateral curva-*

ture, an abnormal sideward bending of an area of the spine without vertebral rotation.

In terms of traditional medicine, the word *subluxation* means an incomplete or partial dislocation. However, in chiropractic, the word has a much deeper and complex meaning. Essentially, it means an alteration of the normal dynamics of a joint in which there is an alteration to structural and/or functional relationships. Quite frequently one sees the term subluxation used to refer to a *fixation,* a partially restricted joint; or to a *hypermobile joint,* a condition in which an articulating bone moves beyond its normal range of motion but there is no joint locking.

The immediate causes of subluxation may be divided into two major categories: the unequal or asymmetrical muscular efforts on the joint structures; and the inequality in the supporting tissues of a particular joint such as the cartilage, intervertebral disc, ligaments, etc. Inequality in muscular balance may be the result of injury (acute frank trauma or microtrauma), postural distortions, biochemical reactions, psychomotor responses, paralytic affects, or somatic and visceral responses. Abnormal structural support may be brought about by developmental abnormalities, various acquired disease processes within the joint, or the resolution of major injury or microtraumas or of other primary disease processes.

The importance of a subluxation depends on its clinical features and whether the subluxation and its influence on the nervous system are abnormally influencing the health of the individual to a significant degree. Minor mechanical errors in position and motion occur in all people and so, consequently, do neurologic irritations from these effects. We are all subject to environmental irritations and respond to these in a manner creating errors in musculoskeletal symmetry in the body. Thus, errors in position and mechanics occur. These, in turn, may cause abnormal responses within the body that may be of a temporary nature, for the body can correct mechanical faults within itself provided they are of a minor nature. On the other hand, certain subluxations cannot be corrected without proper professional attention. It is not so much the presence of a subluxation that is significant but how it is affecting the total economy of the body and how involved it is in the production of abnormal responses. These effects are determined by proper diagnostic procedures.

The next chapter will describe the basic parts and functions of the human body.

Chapter 5

Understanding the Human Body

This chapter provides a brief overview of major body systems and the basic terminology used in describing structure and function of these systems.

BODY SYSTEMS AND LANDMARKS

The science of *anatomy* is the study of body structure: its organs and the relation of its parts. There are many subdivisions or branches of this science. *Physiology* is the study of the functions and activities of the body. This science also has many subdivisions. In this chapter, both anatomy and physiology will be presented in a brief summary of the structure and function of the various systems of the human body—all of which are closely interrelated and interdependent.

The Ten Systems

The organs of the human body are arranged into major systems, each of which has its specific function to perform and all are in-terdependent. The body systems and their general functions are

1. The *skeletal system* (bones) gives the body framework, support, and protection, and furnishes a place of attachment for muscles.
2. The *muscular system* (muscles) moves and propels the body.
3. The *nervous system* (brain, spinal cord, nerves) gives the body awareness of its environment, enables it to react to stimuli from the environment, and allows the body to work together as a unit.
4. The *circulatory system* (heart and blood vessels) transports oxygen and nutrient materials in the blood to all parts of the body and carries away waste products formed by the cells.
5. The *respiratory system* (lungs) takes in air, delivers oxygen from the air to the blood, and removes wastes (eg, carbon dioxide) from the blood.
6. The *digestive system* (stomach and intestines) receives, digests, and absorbs food substances and eliminates waste products.
7. The *urinary system* (kidneys and uri-

nary bladder) filters waste products from blood and excretes waste products in urine.

8. The *endocrine system* (glands excreting hormones) controls many prolonged body activities by the manufacture of hormones that are secreted into the blood.

9. The *reproductive system* (genitals) produces and transports reproductive (sex) cells.

10. The *integumentary system* (skin) covers and protects the entire body surface from injury and infection, has functions of sensation reception (heat, cold, pressure, touch, and pain), and assists in regulation of body temperature and the excretion of wastes.

Terms of location in relation to body regions are shown in Figure 5.1.

Body Cavities

The major cavities of the body to hold organs are the *dorsal cavity* (toward the back part of the body) and the *ventral cavity* (toward the front part of the body). See Figure 5.2.

The dorsal cavity has a cranial area, which contains the brain, and a vertebral area, which contains the spinal cord. These areas are continuous.

The ventral cavity has a thoracic cavity and an abdominopelvic cavity. These areas are separated by the diaphragm.

In the thoracic cavity are two pleural cavities, each containing a lung. In the space between the pleural cavities is the pericardial cavity, which contains the heart, and the mediastinal region, in which are contained the trachea, esophagus, thymus gland, large blood and lymphatic vessels, lymph nodes, and nerves.

In the upper part of the abdominopelvic cavity are the stomach, small intestine, liver, gallbladder, pancreas, spleen, kidneys, adrenal glands, and ureters. The lower part of the cavity (pelvic cavity) contains the urinary bladder, the end of the large intestine (rectum), and parts of the reproductive system.

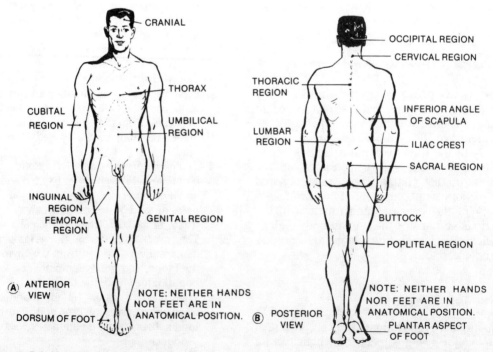

Figure 5.1. Names of body regions.

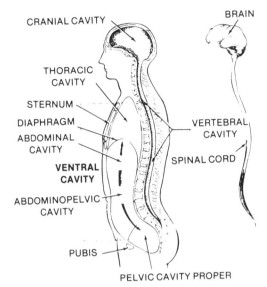

Figure 5.2. Main body cavities.

The Abdominal Quadrants

The large anterior area of the abdominopelvic cavity is divided into four parts or quadrants. The initials identifying quadrants are LUQ (left upper), RUQ (right upper), LLQ (left lower), and RLQ (right lower). These initials are often used to indicate on charts the approximate location of organic pain.

Besides identification by quadrants, the upper central abdominal region is called the *epigastric* area (over the stomach), and the lower central region is the *suprapubic* area (above the pubis). The rib area is called the *costal* area.

The Thoracoabdominal Membranes

Certain membranes are combined layers of tissue that form partitions, linings, envelopes, or capsules. They reinforce body organs and wall cavities. Others are a combination of only connective tissues; eg, the mucous, pleural, pericardial, and peritoneal membranes. Connective-tissue membranes are combinations of various connective tissue; eg, meninges, fascia, periosteum, and synovia.

Different types of membranes are associated with different body parts or systems such as the pleural membranes of the respiratory system; pericardial membranes of the heart and the circulatory system; peritoneal membranes of the digestive system; meningeal membranes of the nervous system; fascial membranes of the muscular system; and periosteal and synovial membranes of bone and joints.

THE SKELETAL SYSTEM

Skeletal Functions and Divisions

The skeletal system includes the bones and joints (articulations). See Figure 5.3.

The Skeletal System. The major functions of the skeletal system are to give support and shape to the body, protect internal organs, provide movement when acted on by muscles, manufacture blood cells, and store mineral salts.

Divisions of the Skeleton. For study purposes, the 206 bones of the adult are divided into the bones of the axial skeleton (80 bones) and the appendicular skeleton (126 bones). The axial skeleton includes the skull, vertebral column, ribs, and sternum. The appendicular skeleton includes the bones of the shoulder girdle, upper limb, pelvic girdle, and lower limb.

General Bone Structure and Classes

Bone is living tissue, containing blood vessels and nerves. The living cells that form bones are called *osteocytes.* Bone cells can select calcium and other minerals from blood and tissue fluid and deposit the calcium in the connective-tissue fibers between bone cells. With increasing age from childhood to adulthood, bones become harder; in old age, they become brittle because there are higher proportions of minerals and fewer active cells. *Periosteum,* the hard membrane covering bone surfaces, carries blood vessels and nerves to the bone

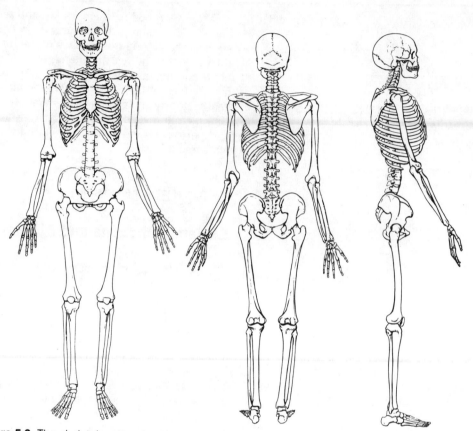

Figure 5.3. The skeletal system as viewed left to right from the front, back, and side.

cells. Bone-producing cells in periosteum are active during growth and the repair of injuries.

Two types of bone are formed by the bone cells—*compact* and *cancellous*. Compact bone is hard and dense, while cancellous bone has a porous structure. The combination of compact and cancellous bone cells produces maximum strength with minimum weight.

Shape

Bones are classified by their shape as long, short, flat, and irregular. *Long bones* are in the extremities and act as levers to produce motion when acted on by muscles. *Short bones*, strong and compact, are in the wrist and ankle. *Flat bones* form protective plates and provide broad surfaces for muscle attachments such as in the shoulder blades.

Irregular bones have many surfaces and fit in locations such as the facial bones, spine, and pelvic bones.

Long Bone Features

A long bone is used as an example of bone structure in Figure 5.4. The following should be noted:

1. *Long bones* have a shaft (the diaphysis) and two extremities (the epiphyses). The shaft is a heavy cylinder of compact bone with a central medullary (marrow) cavity. This cavity contains bone marrow, blood vessels, and nerves. Cancellous bone is located toward the epiphyses and is covered by a protecting layer of compact bone.

2. *Articular cartilage* covers joint surfaces at the ends of connecting bones. The

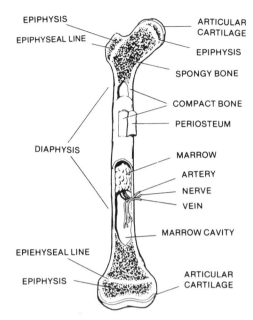

Figure 5.4. A long bone (femur).

cartilage provides a smooth contact surface in joint formation and gives some resilience for shock absorption.

3. *Periosteum*, the membrane covering the surface of compact bone, is anchored by strong connective-tissue fibers. Periosteum also is essential for bone nourishment and repair for it contains some blood vessels and is richly innervated. In severe bone injuries, the periosteum may be torn away or damaged, inhibiting repair of the bone.

Bone Marrow

Two types of marrow, red and yellow, are found in the cavities of bones. Red bone marrow is active blood-cell manufacturing material, producing red blood cells and many of the white blood cells. Deposits of red bone marrow in an adult are in cancellous portions of some bones—the skull, ribs, and sternum, for example. Yellow bone marrow is mostly fat and is found in marrow cavities of mature long bones.

Landmarks

Special markings and projections on bones are used as points of reference. Each mark-

ing has a function; eg, in joint formation for muscle attachments or as passageways for blood vessels and nerves. Terms used to refer to bone markings include:

- *Head*—a rounded ball end
- *Neck*—a constricted portion
- *Spine*—a sharp projection
- *Condyle*—a projection fitting into a joint
- *Crest*—a ridge
- *Foramen*—an opening, a hole
- *Sinus*—an airspace
- *Fossa*—a socket

The Skull and Face

The skull forms the framework of the head. It has 29 bones: eight cranial, 14 facial, six ossicles (the three tiny bones of the ear), and one hyoid (the single bone of the throat).

The Cranial Bones

The cranial bones support and protect the brain. They almost fuse after birth in joints called *sutures*. The eight cranial bones include one frontal, two parietal, one occipital, two temporal, one ethmoid, and one sphenoid. See Figure 5.5. The frontal bone forms the forehead, part of the eye socket, and part of the nose. The parietal bones form the dome of the skull and the upper side walls. The occipital bone forms the back and base of the skull. The foramen magnum, the large hole in the lower part of the occipital bone, is the passageway for the spinal cord. The temporal bones form the lower part of each side of the skull and contain the essential organs of hearing and balance in the middle and inner parts of the ear. The ethmoid and sphenoid bones complete the floor of the cranium: the ethmoid toward the front and the sphenoid toward the center. The air spaces (sinuses) are in the frontal, ethmoid, and sphenoid bones.

The Facial Bones

The 14 facial bones fit together like a complicated jigsaw puzzle; eg, part of seven different cranial and facial bones form each

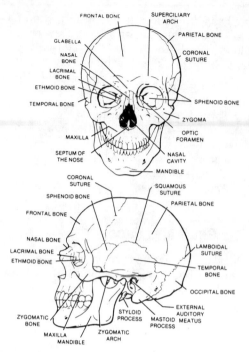

Figure 5.5. The skull.

eye socket: two maxillary bones, the upper jaw, two zygomatic, the upper cheek bones (maxillary), and one mandible (lower jaw). Refer to Figure 5.5. The maxillary bones support the upper teeth, and the mandible supports the lower teeth. The joints (TMJ) formed by the mandible of the face and temporal bones of the skull permit jaw movement. Nine smaller facial bones complete the nose and roof of the mouth.

The Vertebral Column

The 26 bones of the vertebral column form a flexible structure supporting the head, thorax, abdomen, and upper extremities. The arrangement of vertebrae provides a protected passageway for the spinal cord. Vertebral bones are classified into four regions: cervical (neck), thoracic or dorsal (chest), lumbar (lower back), and sacral-coccygeal (pelvic). See Figure 5.6.

Vertebral Structure

A typical vertebra has an anterior portion, a body, and a posterior arch. See Figure 5.7.

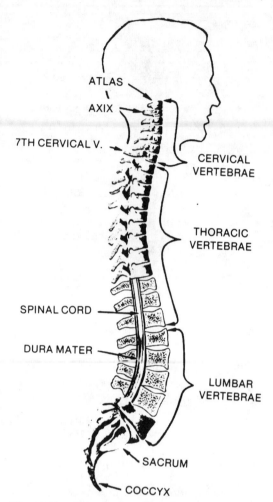

Figure 5.6. Side view of the vertebral column.

The body (centrum) and arch encircle the spinal canal, the opening through which the spinal cord passes. Between vertebral bodies are the intervertebral discs (IVDs), which are fibrocartilage structures serving as shock-absorbing connections between vertebrae. The irregular posterior projections from the arches are spinous processes. These are the projections felt when you run your fingers alone the midline of the back. Transverse processes project laterally. Intervertebral foramina open on either side of the arches for passage of spinal nerves to and from the spinal cord. It is this area where subluxations resulting in nerve insults often occur.

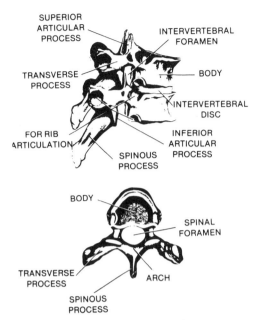

SUPERIOR ARTICULAR PROCESS

INTERVERTEBRAL FORAMEN

TRANSVERSE PROCESS

BODY

INTERVERTEBRAL DISC

FOR RIB ARTICULATION

INFERIOR ARTICULAR PROCESS

SPINOUS PROCESS

BODY

SPINAL FORAMEN

TRANSVERSE PROCESS

ARCH

SPINOUS PROCESS

Figure 5.7. Typical thoracic vertebra.

Spinal Curves

The vertebral column has four normal curves for strength and balance. The cervical curve in the neck and the lumbar curve in the lower back are concave; ie, curving inward. The midspine thoracic and bottom sacral curves are convex; ie, curving outward. Abnormal spinal curvatures often lead to disability.

Classification of Vertebrae

There are seven cervical vertebrae in the neck. The first cervical vertebra is called the *atlas;* the second, the *axis.* These are the only named vertebrae. All others are numbered according to region. The prominent knob at the base of the neck is formed by the spinous process of the last cervical (C7) or first thoracic (T1) vertebra. Twelve thoracic vertebrae form the posterior midline of the chest, and each thoracic vertebra articulates with one pair of ribs. The five lumbar vertebrae in the lower back support the posterior abdominal wall. The sacrum (a flat, spade-shaped bone) forms the posterior part of the pelvic girdle. The coccyx is the "tail bone"—the small curved end of the vertebral column. In the adult, five sacral

segments fuse to form one sacrum, and four coccygeal segments fuse to form one coccyx.

The Thorax

The thorax (chest cage) is formed by 25 bones: 12 thoracic vertebrae, 12 pairs of ribs, and the sternum. Rib cartilages (costal cartilages) complete the chest cage. The thorax contains and protects the heart, lungs, and related structures of circulation and respiration. The ribs curve outward, forward, and downward from their posterior attachments at the vertebrae. The first seven pairs of ribs are joined directly to the sternum by their costal cartilages. The next three pairs (numbered 8, 9, 10), are attached to the sternum indirectly each cartilage attaches to the one above. The last two pairs of ribs ("floating" ribs) are not attached to the sternum. The sternum (the anterior flat breastbone) and the ribs form the expandable chest cage wall.

The Shoulder Girdle and Upper Limbs

The shoulder girdle is a flexible yoke that suspends and supports the arms. Held in place by muscles, it has only one point of attachment to the axial skeleton—the joint between the clavicle and sternum.

The shoulder girdle is formed by the two scapulae posteriorly and two clavicles anteriorly. See Figure 5.8. The bones of the shoulder and upper limb include the scapula (shoulder blade), clavicle (collar bone), humerus (arm bone), radius and ulna (forearm bones), carpals (wrist bones), metacarpals (hand bones), and phalanges (finger bones).

1. The *scapula* is a large triangular bone extending from the second to the seventh or eighth ribs, posteriorly. The heavy ridge extending across the upper surface of the scapula ends in a process called the *acromion,* which anteriorly forms the tip of the shoulder and the joint with the clavicle. A socket for the head of the humerus is on the lateral surface of the scapula. Strong muscles at-

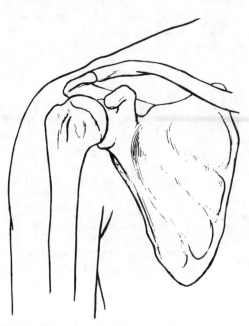

Figure 5.8. Front view of the right shoulder girdle.

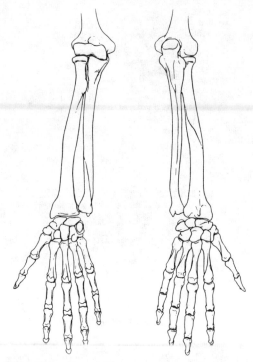

Figure 5.9. Bones of the forearm and hand. Left, front view; right, back view.

tach to the scapula for shoulder and arm movement.

2. The *clavicle* is a slender S-curved bone placed horizontally above the first rib. The lateral end of the clavicle forms a joint with the scapula (acromioclavicular joint). The medial end of the clavicle forms a joint with the sternum (the sternoclavicular joint), which can be felt as the knob on either side of the notch at the base of the throat. The clavicle acts as a shoulder brace, holding the shoulder up and back.

3. The *humerus* is the heavy long bone in the arm that extends from the shoulder to the elbow. The rounded proximal end fits into the scapula in a socket, the glenoid fossa. The distal end of the humerus forms the elbow joint, articulating with the ulna and radius. Strong muscles reinforce the shoulder joint and attach to the humerus, protecting the large blood vessels and nerves that extend along the bone.

4. The *radius* and *ulna* are the bones of the forearm. See Figure 5.9. The ulna, on the little finger side, forms the major part of the elbow joint with the humerus. A projection of the ulna, the olecranon, is the "funny

bone" at the point of the elbow. The radius, on the thumb side, forms the lateral part of the wrist joint. The action of the radius about the ulna permits rotation of the hand.

5. The *wrist* has eight small bones (carpals) arranged in two rows of four each. These ball-bearing-like structures articulate with each other and with the bones of the hand or forearm. Articulating with the carpals are the five metacarpals of the hand, which form the bony structure of the hand.

6. The *hand* includes the metacarpal of the thumb, whose muscular attachment allows the thumb to meet the other fingers of the hand, an action called opposing. The 14 phalanges in each hand are the finger bones: three in each of the four fingers and two in the thumb.

The Pelvis and Lower Limbs

The two hip bones form the pelvic girdle and provide articulation for the lower limbs.

The pelvis, jointed by the hip bones and sacrum, forms a strong bony basin supporting the trunk and protecting the contents of the abdominopelvic cavity. When the upright body is in proper alignment, the pelvis distributes upper-body weight evenly to both lower extremities. The bones of the pelvis and lower extremity are the os coxa (hip bone), femur (thigh bone), patella (knee cap), tibia and fibula (leg bones), tarsals (ankle bones), metatarsals (foot bones), and phalanges (toe bones). See Figure 5.10. In contrast to the shoulder girdle, the healthy pelvic girdle is strong for bearing weight.

1. The *hip bones* are formed by the fusion of three bones into one massive, irregular bone, the os coxa. The two hip bones are joined anteriorly in the symphysis pubis. Posteriorly, the hip bones articulate with the sacrum (sacroiliac joints). Each hip bone has three distinctive parts: the ilium, ischium, and pubis. See Figure 5.11. The ilium is the broad, flaring, upper part of the hip. The iliac crests are important landmarks. The ischium is the lower, posterior portion

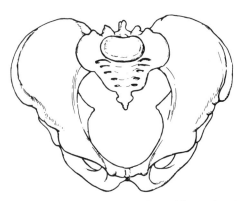

Figure 5.10. The pelvis as viewed from above.

on which one sits. The pubis is the anterior portion of the hip. A deep, cup-shaped socket, the *acetabulum*, is located on the lower lateral surface of each hip bone. The cup shape of the acetabulum fits the head of the femur to form the hip joint.

2. The *femur* (thigh bone) is the longest and strongest bone in the body. Refer to Figure 5.4. The head of the femur fits into the

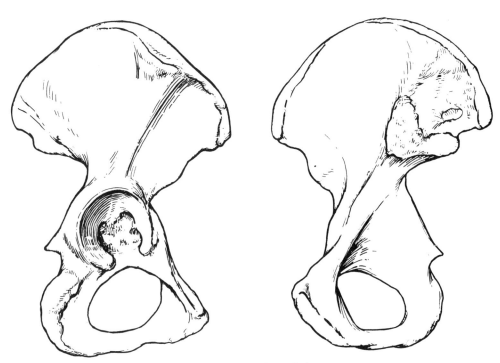

Figure 5.11. The hip bone. Left, medial view; right, lateral view.

acetabulum. The distal end of the femur articulates with the tibia to form the knee joint. A large prominent projection at the junction of the shaft and neck of the femur is called the *greater trochanter*. It is an important attachment point for the strong thigh muscles.

3. The *patella* (knee cap) is the bone protecting the front of the knee joint. It is a special type of bone embedded within the powerful tendon that extends from the strong anterior thigh muscles. The patella has an oval shape in cross-section and is classified as a *sesamoid* (bone embedded in tendon).

4. The *tibia* and *fibula* are the two bones of the leg. The tibia, which is thicker and stronger, is the shin bone. It supports body weight and articulates with the femur at the knee joint. The projection at its lower end is the medial *malleolus*, the inner ankle bone. The fibula, the lateral leg bone, articulates with the tibia at its distal and proximal ends but not with the femur. The projection at the distal end of the fibula is the lateral malleolus, the outer ankle bone.

5. The skeleton of the *foot* consists of the tarsals, metatarsals, and phalanges. Seven tarsals form the ankle, heel, and posterior half of the instep. The talus is the largest ankle bone, and the calcaneus is the heel bone. Five metatarsals form the anterior half of the instep. The tarsals and metatarsals together form the arch of the foot—a structure important in weight distribution to the foot. Muscles, tendons, and ligaments hold the tarsals and metatarsals in their arched position, and when this support is weak, the foot is flat. The 14 phalanges of the toes are similar to finger bones but are less important for foot function than fingers are for hand function.

Joints (Articulations)

A joint is a structure holding separate bones together. Joints are classified according to the amount of movement they permit: immovable, slightly movable, and freely movable. See Figure 5.12.

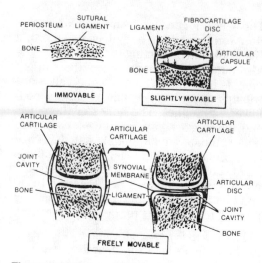

Figure 5.12. Types of joints.

1. *Immovable joints* have bone surfaces fused to prevent motion. At one time during skeletal development, these joints had some movement but as the bones matured they fused for stability. The sacral and coccygeal segments are examples of immovable joints in the adult. Some authorities consider adult skull joints as immovable but others find that they usually exhibit slight motion.

2. *Slightly movable joints* usually have fibrocartilage (discs) between the bones and are held in place by strong ligaments. The cartilage permits some give, and the ligaments prevent bone separation. The interface between the clavicle and sternum, the vertebral bodies, the two pubic bones (symphysis pubis), and the articulations between the sacrum and hip bones are examples of slightly movable joints.

3. *Freely movable joints* permit maximum motion. These joints have a complex arrangement because they have joint cavities. The major parts of a joint cavity include the joint capsule, the capsule lining (synovial membrane), and some lubricating fluid within the cavity. Ligaments are strong fibrous connective-tissue bands that hold the bones together. In some joints, the ligaments enclose the joint, forming the cover of the joint capsule.

Some joint disorders are mechanical: the

parts of the joints are displaced or dislocated. Another term for a type of partial dislocation is *subluxation*—a particular displacement of bone surfaces within the normal range of joint motion. When ligaments stabilizing the joint are partially torn but the joint is not displaced, the injury is called a *sprain*. When muscles are injured by overstretching, the injury is called a *strain*.

Joint Movements

Movable joints allow change of position and motion. Examples of joint movement are flexion (bending), extension (straightening), abduction (movement away from the midline), adduction (movement toward the midline), pronation (turning the forearm so that the palm of the hand faces downward), and supination (turning the forearm so that the palm of the hand faces upward).

Attempts to force joints to move beyond their normal limitations can be quite harmful. The structure of the joint determines the type of movement possible because the bone ends reciprocate (fit into each other) at the joint. Examples of joint structure permitting certain types of joint movement include:

1. *Ball-and-socket joints,* as in the shoulder and hip, permit the widest range of motion: flexion, extension, abduction, adduction, and rotation.

2. *Hinge joints,* as in the elbow and knee, allow flexion and extension. Elbow joints have gross forward movement only; ie, the anterior bony surfaces approach each other. Knee joints have gross backward movement; ie, the posterior bony surfaces approach each other.

3. *Pivot joints* such as found between the head and neck, and between the first and second cervical vertebrae. The distal ends of the radius and ulna also form a pivot joint for rotation of the wrist.

Bursae

At some joint locations, the tendon connecting muscle to bone passes over a joint; eg, at

the shoulder, elbow, knee, and heel. To reduce friction and pressure, small sacs containing fluid are formed over and around the tendon. The sac is called a *bursa,* and an irritated bursa results in *bursitis.* Bursitis may produce severe pain and restrict normal movement.

THE MUSCULAR SYSTEM

The muscles of the body include (1) smooth muscle in the walls of internal organs, arteries, and cardiac muscle in the walls of the heart, and (2) skeletal muscle attached to and causing movements of bones. Muscles have the ability to contract, and it is this power of contraction that produces movement.

Skeletal Muscle Function

Although skeletal muscles are called voluntary muscles, they require a functioning nerve supply and something to pull against for normal function. It is important to think of skeletal muscles as one part of a three-part neuromuscular skeletal unit. A functioning nerve supply (a motor nerve from the central nervous system) is needed to stimulate muscle contraction. The muscle must be able to contract and relax, and the power of contraction must be transmitted to a bone or other attachment to produce the desired movement. When any one part of this three-part unit cannot function normally, the other two parts also lose their ability to function normally. When all three parts (nerve, muscle, and bone) are intact, the many movements associated with skeletal muscles are possible.

Skeletal muscle movements provide locomotion (body movement from place to place), position changes, rhythmic breathing movements, blinking of eyelids, chewing and swallowing, coughing, and changes in facial expression. Many of these movements are essential for survival.

Muscle Structure and Motion

Long slender muscle cells form fibers. Muscle fibers are grouped in bundles; and the bundles are grouped together to form an individual skeletal muscle. Each skeletal muscle is wrapped in a connective-tissue sheath, a form of fascia. This muscle sheath encloses blood vessels and nerves that stimulate and nourish muscle cells. Connective tissue is opaque (dense white), while the muscle bundles are the lean red meat part of muscles. Individual muscles differ considerably in size, shape, and arrangement of muscle fibers. Fiber arrangement determines the line of pull of an individual muscle. The quantity of muscle does not vary after birth. Exercise increases muscle quality, not quantity.

1. *Muscle Attachments.* Extensions of muscle sheath become continuous with tough connective-tissue attachments such as tendons or aponeuroses that bind muscles to bones or adjacent muscles. Tendons are cord-like attachments of connective tissue that unite with the periosteum of bone. Aponeuroses are broad sheet-like attachments that unite with muscle sheaths of adjacent muscles. At the midline of the abdomen, where there are no bones for muscles to attach, abdominal muscles to the left and right of the midline attach to a central aponeurosis.

2. *Muscle-Bone Movements.* When muscle fibers are stimulated to contract by an impulse received from a motor nerve, the muscle shortens and pulls against its connective-tissue attachment. One attachment is sometimes a joint or fixed anchor. Then the direction of pull is toward it. The power of muscle contraction is transmitted to the bone or to an adjacent muscle. Movement then occurs.

3. *Muscle Tone.* Healthy muscle is characterized by active contraction in response to the reaction of the nervous system. This readiness to act (resulting in firing or motor units as stimuli from the environment impinge upon the nervous system) is called *muscle tone.* Muscles having lost their tone through lack of exercise, primary muscle disease, or nerve damage become flabby (flaccid). The tone of muscles is due to the steady contraction and relaxation of different muscle fibers in individual muscles, which help to maintain the "chemical engine" of muscle cells. Even minor exercise helps maintain tone by renewing blood supply to muscle cells.

4. *Muscle Activity.* Muscle contraction consumes food and oxygen and produces acids and heat. Muscle activity is the major source of the body's heat. Acids accumulating because of continued activity cause fatigue, which occurs most rapidly when contractions are frequent. It occurs slowly if rest periods are taken between contractions. Exercise causes muscle to become enlarged, stronger, and better developed. An increase in muscle size is called *hypertrophy;* diminished muscle size, *atrophy.* Physical exercise is necessary to keep muscles in good condition.

Principles of Skeletal Muscle Action

The three principles listed below will help associate muscle actions with normal body movements and patient-care activities.

1. Muscles produce movements by pulling on bones. Since bones move at joints, most muscles attach to bones just above and below a joint. One bone is stabilized while the other bone moves.

2. Muscles moving a part are usually proximal to the part moved. For example, muscles moving the humerus are in the shoulder, chest, and back. Muscles moving the femur are in the hip and lumbar region.

3. Muscles usually act in groups rather than singly. The coordinated action of several muscles produces movement. While one group contracts, an opposing group relaxes. The muscle(s) whose contraction produces the movement is called the *prime mover.* The muscle(s) that relaxes is called the *antagonist.* In bending (flexing) and stretching (extending) the forearm, the biceps and triceps in the upper arm are, alternately, prime movers and antagonists.

Principal Groups of Skeletal Muscle

Muscles are usually named for features such as their location, action, shape, or points of attachment. As there are more than 400 individually named skeletal muscles, only a few will be discussed in this chapter. Major muscles are shown in Figure 5.13.

Head and Face. Muscles of the head and face act in movements of the eye, facial expressions, talking, chewing, and swallowing. The orbicularis oculi closes the eyelid,

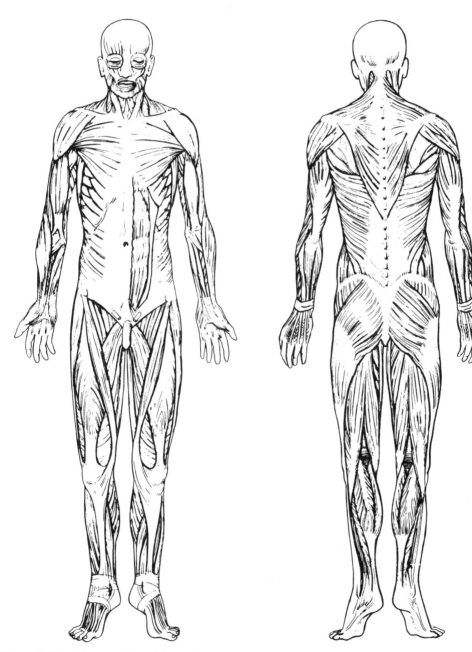

Figure 5.13. Major muscles of the body.

the obicularis oris closes the lips, and the masseter closes the jaw and clamps the back teeth together.

Arms. The major muscles producing movement of the arms are the deltoid, biceps, and triceps. The extensors and flexors cause hand and finger movement. The deltoid is a triangular-shaped muscle that caps the shoulder and upper arm. The deltoid lifts the arm forward, sideways, and to the rear. The biceps, a long two-headed muscle located in the anterior arm, flexes the forearm at the elbow. It also helps to turn the palm upward in supination. The triceps, a large three-headed muscle located in the posterior arm, extends the forearm at the elbow.

Back. The muscles of the back are large and some are very broad. Because they are attached to vertebrae and sometimes ribs, the back muscles keep the trunk in an erect posture and aid it in bending and rotating. In the thoracic region, these muscles assist in respiration and in movements of the neck, arms, and trunk. Although muscles of the midback are powerful, the thigh and buttock muscles should be used in lifting to avoid straining the bony and ligamentous structures of the spine.

Abdomen. The abdominal muscles form broad thin layers that support the internal abdominal organs, assist in respiration, and help in flexion and rotation of the spine. Their names indicate their line of pull: external oblique, rectus abdominis (straight up and down), and transverse. Abdominal muscles also aid urination and defecation.

Neck. The muscles of the neck move the head from side to side, forward and backward, and rotate it. Some also help in respiration, speaking, and swallowing. The bilateral sternocleidomastoideus muscle bends the head forward and helps to turn it to the side.

Chest. The strong chest muscles move the arm, brace the shoulder, and compress the chest for effective coughing. The diaphragm, the major muscle of respiration, separates the thoracic and abdominal cavities. This broad thin horizontal muscle is not shown in Figure 5.13. The pectoralis major on the front of the chest draws the upper arm forward across the chest. The latissimus dorsi and trapezius of the back are the largest muscles of the posterior thorax.

Perineum. The muscles of the perineum (bottom of groin) form the floor of the pelvic cavity and aid in defecation and in urination.

Buttocks. The thick, strong muscles of the buttocks help stabilize the hip. With the muscles of the posterior thigh, they distribute weight to the pelvis during lifting and relieve the strain on the back muscles. The gluteal group includes the gluteus maximus, gluteus medius, and gluteus minimus. These muscles extend and rotate the thigh.

Thighs. The muscles located on the anterior and posterior of the thigh cross two joints: those of the hip and knee. When they contract, they extend one joint and flex the other. The anterior thigh muscles are called the *quadriceps;* the posterior ones, the *hamstrings.*

Leg. The anterior muscle group of the leg includes the anterior tibialis, which flexes the foot on the leg to turn the foot upward (dorsiflexion). The largest posterior muscle of the leg is the gastrocnemius (the calf muscle), which attaches to the heel through the Achilles tendon.

THE SKIN

The skin is called the integumentary (covering) system and serves the body in many important ways. The most obvious feature of skin is its outward appearance. Indeed, the appearance and feel of the skin offer important indications of general health and hygiene. See Figure 5.14.

Function

The four primary functions of skin are (1) *protection* as a mechanical barrier to the entrance of bacteria; (2) *regulation of body temperature* through heat loss; (3) *sensory perception* through nerve endings that transmit sensations of touch, heat, cold, and pain; and (4) *excretion of body wastes*

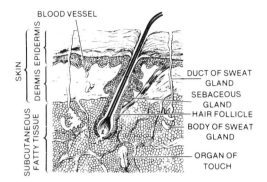

Figure 5.14. Structure of the skin.

through sweat. Although this is not one of its normal functions, the skin can absorb water, certain drugs, toxic agents, lead salts in gasoline, insecticides, and other substances.

Structure

The skin has two principal layers: the epidermis (outer layer) and dermis (inner layer). The epidermis and dermis are supported by a subcutaneous (under skin) layer that connects the skin to underlying muscle fascia. There are no blood vessels or nerve endings in the epidermis.

Skin pigment, found in the deepest parts of the epidermis varies in individuals. It determines the darkness or lightness of skin color. However, the color of the skin is also due to the quantity and state of the blood circulating in the dermis. Pinkness, blueness (cyanosis), or paleness (pallor) of the skin surface is due to the quantity and quality of circulating blood.

The dermis is the deep (main) layer of skin. Nerves, blood vessels, glands, hair roots, and nail roots in the dermis are supported by a connective-tissue meshwork of elastic fibers. Tiny involuntary muscle fibers in the dermis contract and account for the reactions described as "hair standing on end" or "goose pimples." Hair, nails, sebaceous (oil) glands, and sweat glands are accessory skin organs.

The layer of tissue beneath the dermis is not skin. It is superficial fascia, a connective tissue. Fat and other connective tissues in the subcutaneous layer round-out body surfaces and cushion bony parts.

Temperature Regulation

Skin helps regulation of body temperature by controlling heat loss in several ways. Blood vessels in the dermis can change size. For example, when blood vessels are dilated, warm blood is closer to the skin surface and heat is lost more rapidly. When blood vessels constrict, the amount of blood at the skin surface is decreased and heat is conserved. Because the surface of the skin is so large, heat loss by radiation is considerable. Added to this heat loss by radiation is the heat loss by evaporation of sweat. In humid weather, evaporation of sweat from the skin and saturated clothing decreases.

It is important to keep alert to skin structure and function whenever you are assisting the doctor in applying heat, cold, lotions, or ointments to a patient.

THE CIRCULATORY SYSTEM

The circulatory system has two major fluid transportation systems: the cardiovascular and lymphatic.

1. *The Cardiovascular System.* This system, which contains the heart and blood vessels, is a closed system that transports blood from the heart via arteries, arterioles, and capillaries to all parts of the body and then back to the heart via venules and veins. See Figure 5.15. Blood flowing through the circuit formed by the heart and blood vessels brings oxygen, food, and other chemical elements to tissue cells and removes carbon dioxide and other waste products produced by cell activity (metabolism).

2. *The Lymphatic System.* This system, which provides drainage and filtration (by lymph nodes) of intercellular tissue fluid, is an auxiliary part of the circulatory system. It returns an important amount of tissue fluid to the blood stream through its own

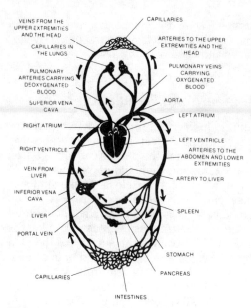

Figure 5.15. Schematic of blood circulation in the cardiovascular system.

system of lymphatic vessels. These vessels are closely aligned with but independent from peripheral cardiovascular vessels.

The Heart

The heart, designed somewhat to be a pump, is a four-chambered muscular organ lying within the chest. Although the heart is generally considered a pump, it serves more as a measuring cup. The "pumping" strength of the heart is not great enough to transport blood through the many miles of blood vessels within the body. Peripheral transportation (pumping) is aided by the alternating contraction and relaxation (pulsation) of the large arteries. Both heart and arterial muscle action are under the synchronized control of the autonomic nervous system and the effects of circulating chemicals.

Structure

About two-thirds of the mass of the heart is to the left of the midline. It lies in the pericardial space in the thoracic cavity between the right and left lungs. In size and shape, it resembles a person's closed fist. Its lower

point (the apex) lies just above the left side of the diaphragm. See Figure 5.16.

Heart Chambers

There are four chambers in the heart. The two upper chambers, called the *atria*, are smaller than the two lower chambers, the *ventricles*. The right atrium communicates with the right ventricle; the left atrium communicates with the left ventricle. The septum (partition) dividing the interior of the heart into right and left sides prevents direct communication of blood flow from adjacent chambers. This is important because the right side of the heart receives deoxygenated blood returning from systemic (body) circulation. The left side of the heart receives oxygenated blood returning from the lungs. This design of the heart keeps blood flowing in its proper direction to and from the chambers.

Each chamber of the heart is lined with endocardium. At each opening from the chambers this lining folds on itself and extends into the opening to form a valve. When healthy, the valves allow blood to pass from a chamber but prevent its return.

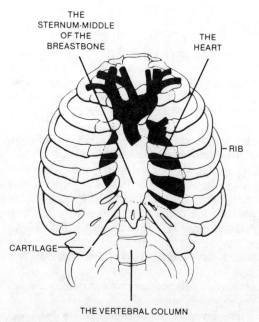

Figure 5.16. The heart (in black) and thoracic cage viewed from the front.

Function

The heart is the connection between general body circulation and pulmonary circulation. All blood returning from the systemic circulation must flow through the pulmonary circulation for exchange of carbon dioxide for oxygen. Returning blood from the upper part of the body enters the heart through a large vein, the *superior vena cava,* and from the lower part of the body by the *inferior vena cava* (Fig. 5.17).

Heart muscle gets its blood supply from the right and left coronary arteries. These arteries branch off the aorta just above the heart, then subdivide into many smaller branches within heart muscle. Blood from heart muscle is returned by coronary veins to the right atrium. If any part of the muscle tissue is deprived of its blood supply through interruption of blood flow through the coronary arteries and their branches, the tissues deprived of blood cannot function. This is called *myocardial infarction.*

Nerve Control

The nerve supply to the heart is from two sets of nerves originating in the medulla of the lower brain. These nerves are part of the involuntary (autonomic) nervous system. One set acts as an accelerator while the other acts as a brake.

Impulses within the heart muscle are mi-nute electric currents that can be recorded by an electrocardiograph (ECG). Their purpose is to initiate heart muscle contraction. Heart muscle has the special ability of contracting automatically, but nerve coordination is needed to provide a regulated contraction for optimal coordination between auricles and ventricles. When the nerve conduction system does not operate properly, heart contractions are uncoordinated and ineffective.

Blood Vessels

The blood vessels of the body are a closed system of tubes through which blood flows. The arteries and smaller arterioles are distributors. The capillaries are the minute vessels through which the exchange of fluid, oxygen, and carbon dioxide take place between the blood and tissue cells. The venules and larger veins are collectors, carrying blood back to the heart.

The system of arteries and arterioles resembles a tree, with the large trunk, the aorta, giving off branches that repeatedly divide and subdivide. Arterioles are very small arteries, having about the diameter of a hair. In comparison, the aorta is more than an inch in diameter. Figure 5.18 shows an overview of the arterial system.

Capillaries

The capillaries (precellular) and venules (postcellular) are the smallest of these vessels but are of the greatest importance functionally in the circulatory system. The larger vessels are essentially conduits.

Capillaries are the essential link between arterial and venous circulation. The vital exchange of substances from the blood in the capillary with tissue cells takes place through the capillary wall. Blood starts its route back to the heart once it leaves the capillaries.

Microscopic capillaries are so numerous that there is at least one or more near every living cell. A single layer of endothelial cells forms the walls of a capillary.

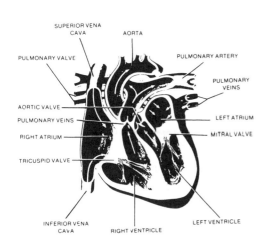

Figure 5.17. Schematic of heart chambers and blood flow.

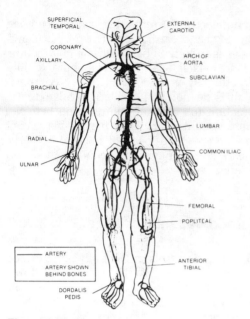

Figure 5.18. Diagram of the arterial system.

Veins

Veins have thin walls and valves formed from the inner vein lining. These valves prevent blood from flowing back toward the capillaries. Venules, the smallest veins, unite into veins of progressively larger size as the blood is collected to return to the heart. The superior vena cava, which collects blood from regions above the diaphragm, and the inferior vena cava, which collects blood from regions below the diaphragm, return the venous blood to the right atrium of the heart. See Figure 5.19. Superficial veins lie close to the surface of the body and often can be seen through the skin, especially the extremities.

Pulse

Pulse is a characteristic associated with the heartbeat and the subsequent wave of expansion and recoil produced in the wall of an artery. With each heartbeat (contraction), blood is forced into the aorta and subsequent arteries, causing them to dilate (expand). Then the arteries contract (recoil) in response to a nerve impulse as the blood moves further along in the circulatory system.

The nerves controlling arterial wall contraction are called *vasomotor* nerves. They are a part of the sympathetic division of the autonomic nervous system.

The pulse can be felt at certain points in the body where an artery lies close to the surface. The most common location for feeling the pulse is at the wrist, proximal to the thumb (radial artery) on the palm side of the hand. Alternative locations are at the side of the neck (carotid artery), in front of the ear (temporal artery), and on the top surface of the foot (dorsalis pedis).

Blood Pressure

An artery's wall has a layer of elastic muscular tissue that allows it to expand and recoil. When an artery is cut, the wall does not collapse but bright red blood escapes from the artery in spurts because of the pressure within the closed system. There is also pressure in veins, but it is fairly constant (does not pulsate).

The force that blood exerts on the walls of vessels through which it flows is called *blood pressure.* All parts of the blood vascular system are under pressure, but the term blood pressure usually refers to arterial pressure. Pressure in arteries is highest when the ventricles of the heart contract (systole) and lowest when the ventricles relax (diastole). The brachial artery, in the upper arm, is the artery usually used for blood pressure measurement. In certain disorders, blood pressure will be taken in both arms and/or both legs and compared.

The Lymphatic System

The lymphatic system consists of lymph fluid, lymph vessels, and lymph nodes. The spleen belongs, in part, to the lymphatic system. Unlike the cardiovascular system, the lymphatic system lacks a "pump" or vessel pulsations to move the fluid it collects, and there is little pressure in the lymph system. Lymph (the fluid found in the lymph vessels) is primarily transported by the massaging action of adjacent muscle contractions. Breathing movements also aid in the move-

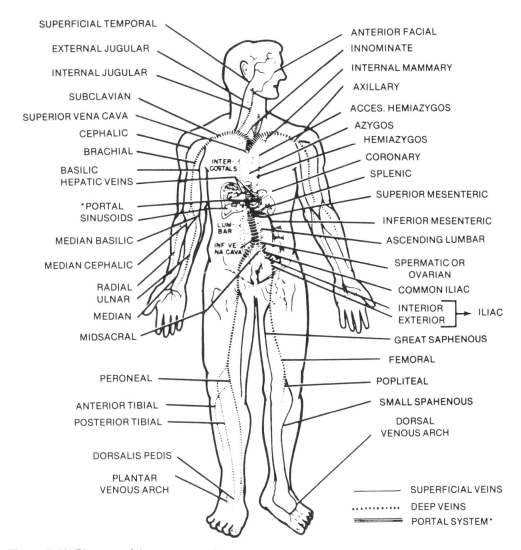

SUPERFICIAL TEMPORAL

EXTERNAL JUGULAR

INTERNAL JUGULAR

SUBCLAVIAN

SUPERIOR VENA CAVA

CEPHALIC

BRACHIAL

BASILIC

HEPATIC VEINS

*PORTAL

SINUSOIDS

MEDIAN BASILIC

MEDIAN CEPHALIC

RADIAL

ULNAR

MEDIAN

MIDSACRAL

PERONEAL

ANTERIOR TIBIAL

POSTERIOR TIBIAL

DORSALIS PEDIS

PLANTAR
VENOUS ARCH

ANTERIOR FACIAL

INNOMINATE

INTERNAL MAMMARY

AXILLARY

ACCES. HEMIAZYGOS

AZYGOS

HEMIAZYGOS

CORONARY

SPLENIC

SUPERIOR MESENTERIC

INFERIOR MESENTERIC

ASCENDING LUMBAR

SPERMATIC OR
OVARIAN

COMMON ILIAC

INTERIOR
EXTERIOR } ILIAC

GREAT SAPHENOUS

FEMORAL

POPLITEAL

SMALL SPAHENOUS

DORSAL
VENOUS ARCH

INTER-
COSTALS

LUM-
BAR

INF VE-
NA CAVA

————— SUPERFICIAL VEINS

··········· DEEP VEINS

═════ PORTAL SYSTEM*

Figure 5.19. Diagram of the venous system.

ment of lymph through its channels and its return to the blood stream.

Lymph is clear and watery. It is similar in appearance to tissue fluid that fills the spaces between tissues and cells. Tissue fluid serves as the "middleman" for the exchange between blood and body cells. Formed from blood plasma, it seeps through capillary walls and bathes the cells. The lymphatic system collects tissue fluid, and, as lymph, starts it on its way for return to circulating blood.

Starting as small blind ducts within the tissues, the lymphatic vessels enlarge to form lymphatic capillaries. These capillaries unite to form larger lymphatic vessels, which resemble veins in structure and arrangement. Valves in lymph vessels prevent backflow.

Superficial lymph vessels collect extracellular fluid from the lower skin and subcutaneous tissues. Deep vessels collect it from other parts of the body. The two largest collecting vessels are the thoracic duct and the right lymphatic duct (Fig. 5.20). The thoracic duct receives lymph from all parts of the body except the upper right side. The lymph from the thoracic duct drains into the

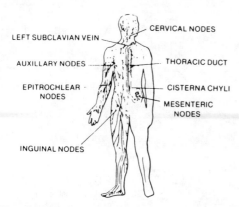

Figure 5.20. Diagram of the lymphatic system.

left subclavian vein, at the root of the neck on the left side. The right lymphatic duct drains into a corresponding vein on the right side.

Occurring in groups up to a dozen or more, lymph nodes lie along the course of lymph vessels and tend to group at certain locations. Although variable in size, they are usually small oval bodies of lymphoid tissue. Their purpose is to act as filters for removal of microorganisms and foreign materials from the lymph stream. Important groups of these nodes are located in the axilla (armpit), the cervical region, the submaxillary region (under the jaw), the inguinal (groin) region, and the mesenteric (abdominal) region.

Lymph vessels and nodes often become inflamed as the result of infection. When untreated, an infection in the hand may cause inflammation of the lymph vessels as high as the armpit, possibly the neck. A "sore throat" may cause inflammation and swelling of lymph nodes in the neck, submandibular nodes below the jaw, and cervical nodes posteriorly.

The largest collection of lymphatic tissue in the body is in the spleen. The spleen rests high in the abdominal cavity on the left side (LUQ), below the diaphragm and behind the stomach. It is somewhat long and oviformid (egg-shaped). Although it can be surgically removed without noticeable harmful effects, the spleen has useful functions in serving as a reservoir for blood and extra red blood cells.

The Blood

Blood varies in color from bright red (oxygenated blood) when it flows from arteries to dark red (deoxygenated blood) when it flows from veins.

Functions

The major functions of blood are (1) to carry oxygen from the lungs to tissue cells and carbon dioxide from the cells to the lungs; (2) to carry food materials absorbed from the digestive tract to the tissue cells and to remove waste products for elimination by excretory organs—the kidneys, intestines, and skin; (3) to carry hormones, which helps regulate body functions, from ductless (endocrine) glands to the tissues of the body; (4) to help regulate and equalize body temperature—body cells generate large amounts of heat, and circulating blood absorbs this heat; (5) to protect the body against infection; (6) to provide mechanisms to seal a broken blood vessel (clotting); and (7) to maintain fluid and electrolytic balance in the body.

Plasma

Blood is composed of plasma (a liquid), formed elements, and blood cells suspended in the plasma. Plasma makes up more than half the total volume of blood and is the carrier for blood cells, carbon dioxide, dissolved wastes, hormones, antibodies, nutrients, and fibrinogen (a plasma protein that helps blood clotting).

Serum

When blood clots, the liquid portion remaining is *serum*. Blood serum contains no blood cells. The major cellular elements in the blood are red cells (erythrocytes), white cells (leukocytes), and blood platelets (thrombocytes).

Demands

Red blood cells are formed in the adult in red bone marrow. Millions of old red cells are destroyed daily, either in the liver, the spleen, the lymph nodes, or in the vascular system itself. In a healthy person, the rate of destruction equals the rate of production so that a red cell count of about 5,000,000 per cubic millimeter remains constant. Red blood cells have an average life span of about 90 to 120 days before becoming obsolete.

Hemoglobin

A pigment, hemoglobin (Hgb), gives red cells their color. It has the power to combine with oxygen, carrying it from the lungs to tissue cells. Hgb also helps in transporting carbon dioxide from the cells to the lungs. This transportation of gases to and from cells is the principal function of red cells.

Its oxygen content gives arterial blood its bright red color. In order to carry oxygen, Hgb needs the mineral iron, which is ordinarily available in a nutritionally adequate diet. The condition known as *anemia* is due to a reduction in number of red cells or a reduction in the Hgb content of red cells.

Leukocytes

White cells vary in size and shape and are larger and fewer than red cells. The average number in an adult is 5,000 to 10,000 in 1 mm^3 of blood. Their function is primarily one of protection (soldiers). They can destroy foreign particles (eg, bacteria, fungi) in blood and tissues. This function is called *phagocytosis*, and the white cells performing it are *phagocytes*.

White cells are capable of ameboid movement and thus can pass through the walls of capillaries into surrounding tissues. This ability to enter tissue makes them useful in fighting tissue infection. An area of infection is characterized by a great increase of white cells that gather about the site to destroy bacteria. An example of this is seen in an ordinary boil (furuncle). The pus contained in the boil is made up largely of white cells, plus bacteria and dissolved tissue. Many white cells are killed in their struggle with invading bacteria. The battle is constant whether we are aware of it or not.

There are several types of white cells. In various diseases, the number of white cells in the blood may increase considerably, especially in acute infections. This increase, *leukocytosis*, is an important body defense response. Certain potent drugs interfere with the formation of these valuable cells, and the condition *agranulocytosis* (absence of granulocytes) develops. Neutrophils, the most numerous type of white cells, are produced by the red bone marrow. Monocytes, the largest type of white cells, are produced in lymphoid tissue.

Platelets

Blood platelets, which are smaller than red blood cells, are thought to be fragments of cells formed in bone marrow. Platelets number about 300,000 per mm^3 of blood. Their main function is to aid in the coagulation of blood at the site of a wound. When injured, platelets release a substance to hasten the formation of a blood clot.

Empiric Systems

There are also "functional" systems that have not been isolated anatomically but have been mapped clinically. One may find mention of these systems in professional papers as (1) the neurolymphatic system, which courses with the lymphatics; (2) the system connecting trigger points and referral zones; and (3) the neurovascular system, which courses with the arterioles. The Oriental meridian system associated with acupuncture is another member of this category. Specialized photography shows a distinct aura-like electromagnetic field surrounding the body, which some refer to as a system. These systems are, collectively, called the "subtle energy" systems of the body. Some of the largest universities today are conducting research of these empiric "systems."

THE RESPIRATORY SYSTEM

The cells of the body require a constant supply of oxygen to conduct the chemical processes necessary for life. Because of these processes, a waste product, carbon dioxide, is formed that must be removed from the body. Oxygen and carbon dioxide are thus continually being exchanged both within the body and between the body and the atmosphere by a process known as *respiration*. The organs performing this exchange of gases compose the *respiratory system.*

The respiratory system consists of the lungs and a series of air passages connecting the lungs to the outside atmosphere. The organs serving as air passages are the nose, pharynx, larynx, trachea, and bronchi. They carry air into the depths of the lungs and end there in thin alveoli where carbon dioxide is exchanged for oxygen.

The Nose

The nose has two major portions, one external and the other internal (nasal cavity). The external nose is a triangular framework of bone and cartilage covered by skin. On its under surface are the nostrils: the two external openings of the nasal cavity. The nasal cavity is divided by the nasal septum and separated from the mouth by the palate. Inhaled air is warmed, moistened, and filtered in the nasal cavity.

Cilia

Air filtering is done by the cilia of the mucous membrane lining the nasal passages. Cilia are numerous long microscopic processes that beat or wave to cause movement of materials across the surface and from the area. Ciliary movement is important in maintaining sinus drainage.

The Air Sinuses

Air spaces in several bones of the face and head open into the nasal cavity. They serve as resonance chambers in the production of speech and help decrease the weight of the skull. These air sinuses take the name of the bone in which they are found. Sinuses are lined with mucous membrane continuous with that lining the nasal cavity.

The Pharynx

The pharynx (throat) connects the nose and mouth with the lower air passages and esophagus. It is divided into three major parts: the nasopharynx, oropharynx, and laryngopharynx. Both air and food pass through the pharynx, carrying air from the nose to the larynx and food from the mouth to the esophagus. The walls of the pharynx contain masses of lymphatic tissue called *adenoids* and *tonsils.*

The Larynx

The larynx (voice box) connects the pharynx with the trachea. See Figure 5.21. The larynx is in the upper anterior part of the neck and is shaped like a triangular box. It is made of nine cartilages joined by ligaments and controlled by skeletal muscle. The thyroid cartilage is the largest. It forms the landmark in the neck called "Adam's apple."

Two membranous bands in the wall of the larynx form the *vocal cords.* The cricoid cartilage, located just below the prominent thyroid cartilage, is joined to the thyroid cartilage by a membrane. The emergency procedure of cricothyroidotomy to produce a

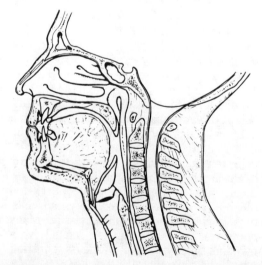

Figure 5.21. Schematic midsection of the face and neck.

patent airway is performed by puncturing this membrane.

The Epiglottis

Another important cartilage in this area is the epiglottis. During swallowing, the epiglottis closes the larynx, the soft palate closes the nasal cavity, and the lips close the mouth. Thus food is forced into the only remaining opening, the esophagus. This prevents food from entering the lungs. Except during swallowing or when the throat is voluntarily closed, the air passages are open and air is free to pass from the mouth and nose into the lungs.

The Trachea

The trachea (windpipe) is a firm tube of cartilaginous rings. It carries air from the larynx to the bronchi. Refer to Figure 5.21. The trachea is lined with cilia and mucous glands whose secretions provide a sticky film to keep dust and dirt out of the lungs.

The Bronchi

The trachea divides to form the two bronchi, which lead to the lungs. One bronchus enters each lung and there divides into many small air passages called *bronchioles* or *bronchial tubes*, which lead air into the final air spaces within the lungs.

The Lungs

The lungs are the soft air-filled essential organs of respiration. See Figure 5.22. They are elastic structures, almost filling the left and right sections of the thoracic cavity. The upper margin of each lung (apex) extends above the clavicle. The lower border (base) rests on the dome-shaped surface of the diaphragm. Between the two lungs centrally is the *mediastinum*. This central cavity contains the heart, great blood vessels, esophagus, and lower trachea.

Alveoli

The right lung has three lobes; the left, two. Within each lobe are separate branches of the main bronchus, and the lobes themselves are divided into segments. The last subdivisions of the air passages to the lungs are *alveoli*, which are closely surrounded by a network of capillaries. Alveoli are air chambers.

Pleurae

Each lung is enclosed by a membranous sac formed by two layers of serous membrane folded upon itself called *pleura*. The outer part lines the chest cavity (parietal pleura). When air enters a pleura, the sac expands to form a large cavity and the lung collapses. This condition of air in the chest outside the lungs is called *pneumothorax*.

The Physiologic Processes of Respiration

The walls of the alveoli are very thin, and it is here that oxygen passes into the blood stream and carbon dioxide is taken from it. This exchange of oxygen and carbon dioxide in the lungs is called *external respiration*. The oxygen entering the blood is carried by the red blood cells in chemical combination with hemoglobin. The blood, oxygenated in the lungs, returns to the heart and is then pumped through the arteries to the capillaries. Oxygen from the capillaries passes to tissue cells, and carbon dioxide from the cells passes into the venules to be carried back to the heart by veins. The exchange of gases between capillary blood and tissue cells is called *internal respiration*.

The Mechanical Processes of Respiration

Breathing (the cycle of inspiration and expiration) is normally repeated about 16 to 20 times per minute in an adult at rest. Breathing is regulated primarily by a respiratory center in the lower brain. This nerve center

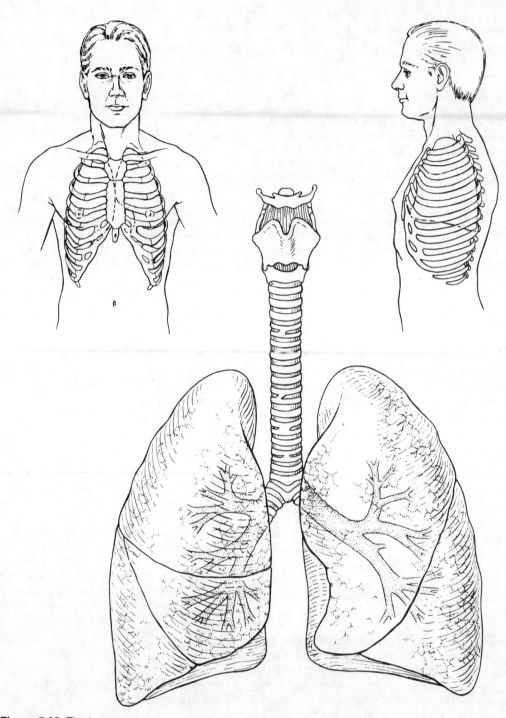

Figure 5.22. The lungs.

is sensitive to change in blood composition, temperature, and pressure, and adjusts breathing according to body needs.

Inhalation

Inspiration is an active movement. The diaphragm, the large muscle forming the floor of the thoracic cavity, contracts, flattening its domed upper surface and increasing the size of the cavity. About the same time, the muscles attached to the ribs (intercostals) contract to elevate and spread the ribs. This further increases the size of the cavity. Air rushes into the lungs and they expand, filling the enlarged cavity.

Exhalation

At rest during quiet breathing, expiration is a passive movement. As it relaxes, the diaphragm is forced upward by intra-abdominal pressure. Muscles attached to the ribs relax, permitting the chest to flatten. These actions reduce the size of the thoracic cavity to allow the elastic recoil of the stretched lungs to expel the air. More air can be exhaled from the lungs by forced expiration. This is done by contraction of the abdominal muscles (forcing the diaphragm upward) and of the muscles attached to the ribs (flattening the chest to compress the lungs and expel the air). When breathing becomes forced, as with exercise, expiration also becomes active.

Sounds caused by air moving in the lungs change with some diseases. These changes, heard with a stethoscope, assist in the diagnosis of diseases of the lungs such as pneumonia or tuberculosis.

THE DIGESTIVE SYSTEM

The digestive system is composed of the alimentary tract (food passageway) and the accessory organs of digestion. See Figure 5.23. Its main functions are to ingest, transport, digest, and absorb food so that assimilation can occur, and to eliminate unused material and the by-products of digestion. The products of the accessory organs help

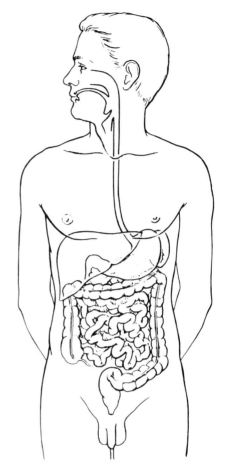

Figure 5.23. Schematic of the alimentary tract.

to prepare food for its absorption and use (metabolism) by tissues of the body.

Digestion consists of two major processes: one mechanical, the other chemical. The mechanical part of digestion includes chewing, swallowing, peristalsis, and defecation. The chemical part consists of breaking foodstuffs into simple components that can be absorbed and used by the body. In this process, foodstuffs are broken down by enzymes or digestive juices formed by digestive glands. Carbohydrates are broken into simple sugar (glucose), fats are changed into fatty acids, and proteins are converted to amino acids.

The Alimentary Canal and Accessory Organs

Anatomically, the alimentary canal is about 28 feet long, extending from the lips to the anus, and is divided as follows: mouth cavity (teeth, tongue), pharynx, esophagus, stomach, small intestine, large intestine (colon), rectum, and anus. The accessory organs aiding the process of digestion are the salivary glands, pancreas, liver, gallbladder, and intestinal glands.

The Teeth

The primary function of teeth is to chew (masticate) food. Secondarily, teeth help to modify sounds produced by the larynx and are used in forming words in association with the tongue.

A person develops two sets of teeth during life: a deciduous (temporary) set and a permanent set. The 20 deciduous teeth erupt during the first 3 years of life and are replaced during the period between the 6th and 14th years by permanent teeth. There are 32 permanent teeth in the normal mouth: four incisors, two cuspids, four bicuspids, and six molars in each jaw. Each tooth has two main parts: (1) the crown, that part visible above the gums, and (2) the root, that part not visible which is embedded in the bony structure of the jaw. The crown of the tooth is protected by enamel.

Tooth decay progresses from the outside inward. Once the protective enamel is broken, microorganisms attack the less resistant parts of the tooth.

The Salivary Glands

These three pairs of glands are the first accessory organs of digestion. They secrete saliva into the mouth through small ducts. One pair, the *parotid glands,* is at the sides of the face below and in front of the ears. The second pair, the *submandibular glands,* lies on either side of the mandible. The third pair, the *sublingual glands,* lies just below the mucous membrane in the floor of the mouth under the tip of the relaxed tongue.

Salivation

The flow of saliva is begun in several ways. Placing food in the mouth affects the nerve endings there. These nerves stimulate the glands to excrete a small amount of thick fluid. The sight, thought, or smell of food also activates the brain and induces a large flow of saliva. About 1,500 mL of saliva are secreted daily. Saliva moistens food in the mouth, which makes chewing easier. It also lubricates the food mass to aid swallowing. Saliva contains two *enzymes:* chemical ferments that change foods into simpler elements. These enzymes act on starches and break them down into sugars.

The Tongue

The tongue, a muscular organ, is attached at the back of the mouth and projects upward into the oral cavity. Refer to Figure 5.21. It is involved in taste, speech, mastication, salivation, and swallowing. After food has been masticated, the tongue propels it from the mouth into the pharynx. This is the first phase of swallowing. Mucous secreted by glands in the tongue lubricates food like saliva to make swallowing easier.

Taste buds located in the tongue make it the principal organ of the sense of taste. Stimulation of the nerve receptors of the taste buds causes secretion of gastric juices reflexively. This is necessary for the digestive process occurring in the stomach.

The Pharynx

The pharynx is a muscular canal that leads from the back of the nose and mouth to the esophagus. The passage of food from the pharynx into the esophagus is the second stage of swallowing. When food is swallowed, the larynx closes off from the pharynx to keep food from entering the respiratory tract.

The Esophagus

The esophagus is a muscular tube, about 10 inches long, lined with mucous membrane. It leads from the pharynx through the chest to the upper end of the stomach. Refer to Figure 5.23. Its function is to complete the act of swallowing. The involuntary movement of material down the esophagus is carried out by the process known as *peristalsis*, which is a wavelike action produced by contraction of the muscular wall. This "muscular wave" is the method by which food is moved through the entire alimentary canal.

The Stomach

The stomach is an elongated pouch-like structure lying just below the diaphragm, with most of its mass to the left of the midline (Fig. 5.24). It has three divisions: (1) the fundus, the enlarged portion to the left and above the entrance of the esophagus; (2) the body, the central portion; and (3) the pylorus, the lower portion. Circular sphincter muscles acting as valves guard the openings of the stomach above and below. The cardiac sphincter is at the esophageal opening, and the pyloric sphincter is at the junction of the stomach and the duodenum (the first portion of the small intestine). The cardiac sphincter prevents stomach contents from re-entering the esophagus unless vomiting occurs.

The functions of the stomach are both mechanical and chemical. The stomach acts as a storehouse for food, receiving fairly large amounts, churning it, and breaking it down further for mixing with digestive juices. Semiliquid food is released in small amounts by the pyloric valve into the duodenum, the first portion of the small intestine.

Gastric Juices

Glands of the stomach lining produce gastric juices (which contain enzymes) and hydrochloric acid. The enzymes in gastric juice start the digestion of protein foods, milk, and fats. The hydrochloric acid produced aids enzyme action. The mucous membrane lining the stomach protects the stomach itself from being digested by the strong acid and enzymes.

The Small Intestine

The small intestine is a mass of tubing about 22 feet long that is attached to the margin of a thin band of tissue called *mesentery*. The small intestine is divided for study into three continuous parts: the *duodenum, jejunum,* and *ileum.* Refer to Figure 5.23. It receives digestive juices from three accessory organs of digestion: the pancreas, liver, and gallbladder.

Mesentery

Mesentery is a portion of the peritoneum, the serous membrane lining the abdominal cavity. It supports the intestine, and the vessels carrying blood to and from the intestine lie within this membrane. The outer edge of mesentery is drawn together like a fan; the gathered margin is attached to the posterior wall of the abdomen. This arrangement permits folding and coiling of the intestine so that this long organ can be packed into a relatively small space.

The Pancreas

The pancreas is a long tapering organ lying behind the stomach. The head of the gland rests in a curve of the small intestine near the pyloric valve. The body of the pancreas extends to the left toward the spleen.

The pancreas secretes a juice that acts on all types of food. Two enzymes in pancreatic juice act on proteins. Other enzymes change starches into sugars. Another enzyme changes fats into their simplest forms. A portion of the pancreas has a special function: the production of insulin.

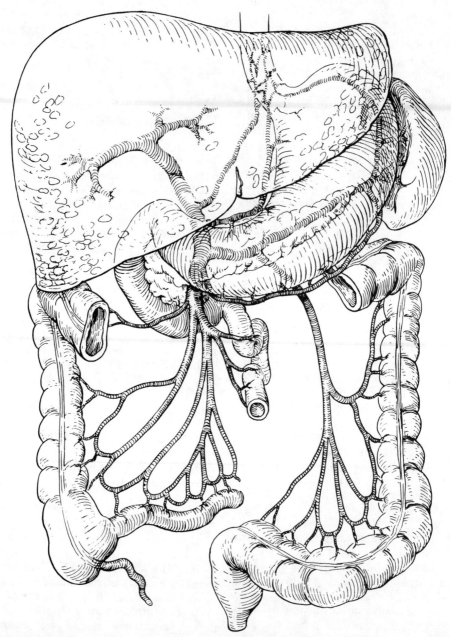

Figure 5.24. Schematic of the liver, stomach, and ascending and descending colon.

The Liver

The liver is the largest organ in the body other than the skin. Refer to Figure 5.24. It is located in the upper part of the abdomen with its larger (right) lobe to the right of the midline. It sits just under the diaphragm and above the lower end of the stomach.

The liver has several important functions. One is the secretion of bile, which is stored in the gallbladder and discharged into the small intestine when digestion is in process.

Bile contains no enzymes, but it breaks up fat particles so that enzymes can act faster. The liver is also a storehouse for body sugar (glycogen) and for iron and Vitamin B. It plays a part in the destruction of bacteria, toxins, and worn red blood cells. Many chemicals such as certain poisons or medicines are detoxified by the liver; others are excreted by the liver through bile ducts. The liver also manufactures part of the proteins of blood plasma.

Blood returning from the spleen, stomach, intestines, and pancreas is detoured through the liver by the portal vein. Refer to Figure 5.15. Blood drains from the liver by hepatic veins that join the inferior vena cava.

The Gallbladder

The gallbladder is a dark green sac, shaped like a blackjack and lodged in a hollow on the underside of the liver. Its ducts join with the duct of the liver to conduct bile to the upper end of the small intestine. The primary function of the gallbladder is the storage and concentration of bile when needed for digestion.

The Ileum

Most absorption of food takes place in the ileum. The walls of the ileum are covered with extremely small finger-like structures called villi that provide a large surface for absorption. After food has been digested, it is absorbed into the capillaries of the villi. Then it is carried to all parts of the body by blood and lymph.

The Large Intestine (Colon)

The large intestine is about 5 feet long. The *cecum*, located on the lower right side of the abdomen, is the first portion of the large intestine into which food is emptied from the small intestine. Refer to Figure 5.24. The *appendix* extends from the lower portion of the cecum in a blind sac. Although the ap-

pendix usually is found lying just below the cecum, by virtue of its free end it can extend in several different directions, depending on its mobility and length. The colon extends along the right side of the abdomen from the cecum up to the region of the liver (ascending colon). There the colon bends (hepatic flexure) and is continued across the upper portion of the abdomen (transverse colon) to the area of the spleen. The colon then bends again (splenic flexure) and extends down the left side of the abdomen (descending colon). The last portion makes an S-curve (sigmoid portion) toward the midline posterior area of the abdomen and ends at the rectum.

The main function of the large intestine is the recovery of water from the mass of undigested food received from the small intestine. As this mass passes through the colon, water is absorbed. Waste materials (feces) become more solid as they are pushed along by peristalsis. *Constipation* is caused by a delay in movement of intestinal contents and/or removal of too much water from them. *Diarrhea* results when movement of the intestinal contents is so rapid that not enough water is removed.

The Rectum and Anus

At the terminal end of the large intestine, the 5-inch-long rectum follows the curve of the sacrum and coccyx until it bends backward into the short anal canal. The *anus* is the external opening at the lower end of the digestive system. It is kept closed by a strong sphincter muscle. The rectum receives feces and periodically expels this material through the anus.

Digestion Time, Absorption, and Defecation

Within a few minutes after a meal reaches the stomach, it begins to pass through the lower valve of the stomach (pyloric). After the first hour, the stomach is half empty; and at the end of the 6th hour, none of the meal is present in the stomach. The meal passes through the small intestine, and the first part of it reaches the cecum from 20 minutes to 2 hours. After the 6th hour, most of it should have passed into the colon; in 12 hours, all of it should be in the colon. Twenty-four hours from the time food is eaten, the meal should reach the rectum. However, part of a meal may be defecated at one time and the remainder at another.

There is little absorption in the stomach. Most absorption takes places in the small intestine. The final nutrient products of digestion pass through the mucous membrane lining of the gastrointestinal (GI) tract and are carried to the liver and from there to the rest of the body. There is marked absorption of water in the large intestine. The residue is concentrated and expelled as feces.

Defecation is normally begun voluntarily by contraction of the abdominal muscles. Simultaneously, the sphincter muscles of the anus relax and there is a peristaltic contraction wave of the colon and rectum. Feces are expelled (defecated) because of these actions.

Feces consist of undigested food residue, secretions from the digestive glands, bile, mucous, and millions of bacteria. Mucous is derived from the many glands that pour secretions into the intestine. Bacteria are especially numerous in the large intestine. They act on food material to cause putrefaction of proteins and fermentation of carbohydrates. Although bacteria normally in the large intestine serve a useful purpose internally, they are contaminants outside the intestine.

THE URINARY SYSTEM

The urinary system, which filters and excretes waste materials from the blood, consists of two kidneys, two ureters (tubes carrying urine from the kidneys to the bladder), one urinary bladder, and one urethra (tube carrying urine from the bladder to the outside). See Figure 5.25. The urinary system helps the body maintain its delicate balance of water and certain chemicals in proportions necessary for health and survival. During the process of urine formation, waste

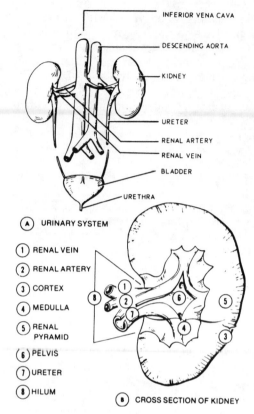

Figure 5.25. Schematic of the urinary system and cross section of a kidney.

products are removed from circulating blood for elimination and useful products are returned to the blood.

The Kidneys

The kidneys are bean-shaped organs about 4½ inches long, 2 inches wide, and 1 inch thick. They lie on each side of the spinal column against the posterior wall of the abdominal cavity near the level of the last thoracic and the first lumbar vertebrae. The right kidney is usually positioned slightly lower than the left.

Near the center of the medial side of each kidney is the central notch (hilum) where blood vessels and nerves enter and leave and the ureter is attached. The kidney is composed of an outer shell (cortex) and an inner layer (medulla). The cortex is made of firm reddish-brown tissue containing millions of microscopic "filtration" plants called *nephrons*. Channels called *collecting tubules* form larger tubes to deliver urine to the pelvis of the kidney.

Nephrons

Each nephron is a urine-forming unit. Nephron units receive and filter the body's total blood about once every 12 minutes. During this period, they draw off and filter the liquid portion of the blood, remove liquid wastes (urine), and return the usable portion to the circulation to maintain the body's fluid balance. The integrity of nephrons is essential for the complex filtration, reabsorption, and excretion process.

The Ureters

The pelvis of each kidney is drained by a ureter: a muscular tube extending from the hilus to the posterior portion of the urinary bladder. Ureters are smooth muscle structures, and urine is passed through each ureter by peristalsis. Drop by drop, urine passes into the bladder. Ureters are about 15 to 18 inches in length and about ⅛th inch in diameter.

The Urinary Bladder

The bladder, a muscular sac located in the lowest part of the abdominal cavity, stores urine. It normally holds from 300 to 500 mL of urine. The bladder is emptied by relaxation of the muscular value between the bladder and urethra and contraction of the muscles in the walls of the bladder that forces urine through the urethra.

The Urethra

The urethra is the tube that carries urine from the urinary bladder to the external opening (the urinary meatus). In the male, it is divided into three areas: the *prostatic portion*, which passes through the prostate gland; the *membranous portion*, which lies

beneath the prostate; and the anterior *penile portion*, which passes through the penis. The female urethra extends from the bladder to the meatus located just inside the superior aspect of the vaginal opening.

Urination

Urination (micturition) is the discharge or voiding of urine. It is done by contraction of the bladder and relaxation of the sphincters. The act of voiding in the adult, though dependent on involuntary reflexes, is partly under voluntary control. Voluntary contraction of abdominal muscles usually accompanies and aids urination.

The average quantity of urine excreted by a normal adult in 24 hours ranges from 1,500 to 2,000 mL—depending on fluid intake, amount of perspiration, and other factors. Urine contains protein wastes (urea), salts in solution, hormones, and pigments. Normal urine should not contain blood, albumin, sugar, or pus cells.

THE NERVOUS SYSTEM

The nervous system regulates, coordinates, and integrates all body systems. Its two major functions are communication and control. It enables a person to be aware of and react to the environment. It coordinates the body's responses to stimuli and keeps body systems working together harmoniously. The constant changes in environment require continuous adjustment of body activity.

Overview

The nervous system consists of nerve centers and nerves that branch off from them which lead to tissues and organs. Most nerve centers are in the brain and spinal cord. Nerves carry impulses from tissues and organs to nerve centers, and from these centers to tissues and organs. The neurons that carry impulses from the skin and other sense organs to the central nervous system

(CNS) are called *sensory nerves*. They make the body *aware* of its environment. Nerves carrying impulses from the CNS to muscles and glands are called *motor nerves*. They cause the body to *react* to its environment.

For study, major parts of the nervous system may be considered separately as (1) the central nervous system, which consists of the brain and spinal cord; (2) the peripheral nervous system, where the nerves are located outside the brain and spinal cord; and (3) the autonomic nervous system, which controls the activities of involuntary muscle and gland tissue.

Nerves, which appear as whitish cords, are bundles of nerve fibers bound together by a connective tissue sheath.

Neurons

The basic unit of the nervous system is the *neuron*, a cell specialized to respond to stimuli by transmitting impulses. Neurons differ in shape and function from all other body cells. Each neuron has three parts: a cell body and two types of processes extending from it. See Figure 5.26(D). Branched processes (dendrites) conduct impulses away from the cell body. *Impulses* are the neuroelectric messages carried by the processes. All communication between nerve cells is carried out through the dendrites and axons at the region of contact (synapse) between the processes of two adjacent neurons.

Neuron processes, whether dendrite or axon, are called *fibers*. Nerve fibers are often wrapped in an insulating material called the *myelin sheath*. Besides the myelin sheath, nerve fibers extending outside the brain and spinal cord (peripheral nerves) have a wrapping called *neurilemma*. The integrity of the neurilemma and nerve cell is essential for nerve regeneration following injury. In time, if the nerve cell body has not been destroyed, a peripheral fiber can regenerate.

Neuroglia

Nerve cell bodies and processes are bound together and supported by special connective tissue cells called *neuroglia*. Neuroglia literally means nerve glue. Several different types of neuroglia cells help form nerve tissue.

The Central Nervous System

As described previously, the CNS consists of the brain and spinal cord. These delicate structures are protected by two major coverings: bones and special membranes. The brain is encased by the bones of the skull that form the cranium; the spinal cord, by the vertebrae. The membranes enclosing both brain and spinal cord are the *meninges*.

The Meninges

Three layers of protective membranes (meninges) surround the brain and spinal cord. The outer layer of strong fibrous tissue is the *dura mater*. The middle layer of delicate cobweb-like tissue is the *arachnoid*. The innermost layer, which adheres to the outer surface of the brain and spinal cord, is the *pia mater*. Between the dura mater and arachnoid is the subdural space; between the arachnoid and pia mater is the subarachnoid space. Both spaces contain fluid.

Cerebrospinal Fluid

Besides protective bones and membranes, nature provides a cushion of fluid around and within the subarachnoid space, in the spaces within the brain called the *ventricles*, and in the central canal of the spinal cord. Cerebrospinal fluid (CSF), which is similar to lymph, filters from networks of capillaries in the ventricles. It is formed constantly, circulated constantly, and part of it is reabsorbed constantly into the venous blood of the brain. At any one time, an adult has about 135 mL of this fluid circulating, although over 500 mL is produced daily. If anything interferes with its circulation or reabsorption, the fluid accumulates. An abnormal accumulation of CSF in the cranium is called *hydrocephalus* (water on the brain).

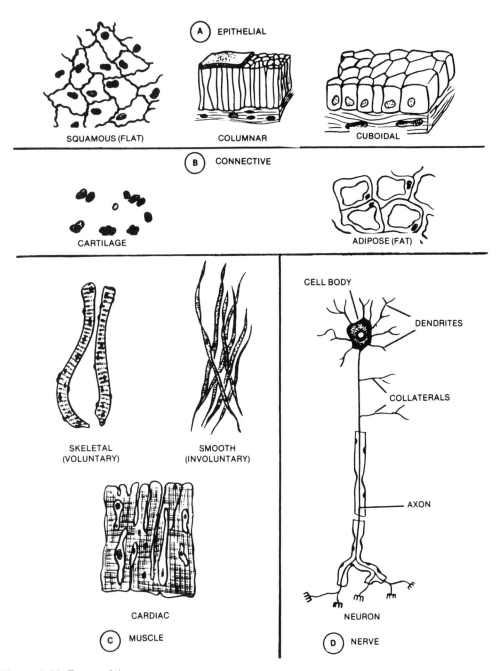

Figure 5.26. Types of tissue.

The Brain as a Whole

The brain, a mass of nerve tissues, is the highest level of the nervous system. It coordinates activities of the entire body; carries on the learning, thinking, and reasoning pro- cesses; and directs voluntary movements of the body. The brain may be divided into three parts: the *cerebrum, cerebellum,* and *brain stem.* The brain stem consists of the *midbrain, pons,* and *medulla.* The mid- brain serves as a connecting pathway between the right and left halves of the cerebrum and cerebellum and the remainder of the brain. See Figure 5.27.

The Cerebrum

The cerebrum resembles many small sausages bound tightly together. It is the largest part of the brain and is divided (but not completely) into right and left hemispheres. Each hemisphere has five lobes. The outer surface (cortex) of the brain is made up of gray matter, which is composed of nerve cells. The white matter within the brain is composed of nerve fibers, which lead to and from cell bodies in the gray matter.

Certain areas of the cerebrum are localized for specific functions, but it is believed that no one area functions independently. In the frontal lobe is the motor area that controls voluntary movements, the speech center, and writing ability. In the parietal lobe is the general sensory area that perceives sensations of heat, cold, touch, pain, pressure, and position. In the temporal lobe are the centers for hearing and smelling. The occipital lobe contains the visual center.

The Cerebellum

The cerebellum lies below the posterior part of the cerebrum. It coordinates muscular activity at an unconscious level. It also coordinates with the cerebrum to guide skilled movements. The cerebellum helps in the control of postural balance and to maintain equilibrium. If the cerebellum is injured

or diseased, movements are jerky and trembly.

The Pons

The pons is a bridge-like structure forming that part of the brain stem above the medulla. Nerve pathways between the spinal cord and other parts of the brain pass through the pons.

The Medulla Oblongata

This bulb-like structure attaching the brain to the spinal cord contains vital centers controlling heart action, blood vessel diameter (thus blood pressure), and respiration. Mechanisms controlling nonvital functions such as sneezing, hiccoughing, and vomiting are also in the medulla. Nerve fibers cross from one side to the other in the medulla, one fact explaining why one side of the brain is said to control the opposite side of the body.

The Spinal Cord

The spinal cord, protected by meninges and vertebrae, is about 18 inches in length. The cord is continuous with the medulla of the brain and terminates at a level between the 1st and 2nd lumbar vertebrae. Refer to Figure 5.2. The meninges enclosing the cord continue below the termination of the cord and are anchored at the sacrum and coccyx.

The spinal cord has two major functions: conduction and connection. Many nerves enter and leave the spinal cord at different levels. These nerves connect with nerve centers located within the spinal cord or with nerve centers in the brain. Nerve centers within the cord make up the *gray matter* of the cord's inner core. Surrounding the gray matter are columns of nerve fibers forming the *white matter.*

Nerve fiber columns in the spinal cord are called tracts. These tracts connect different levels of the nervous system. Tracts that transmit upward (ascending tracts) are sensory nerve fibers. Tracts that transmit impulses downward (descending tracts) are motor nerve fibers, controlling both volun-

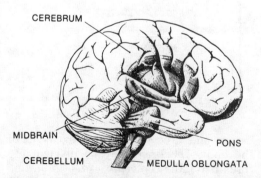

CEREBRUM

MIDBRAIN

CEREBELLUM

PONS

MEDULLA OBLONGATA

Figure 5.27. Schematic sagittal section of the brain.

tary and involuntary muscles. When the spinal cord is injured, the extent of disability depends on which nerve centers or tracts are damaged.

Careful and knowledgeable moving and transporting of patients suspected of having spinal injury is essential to minimize injury to the spinal cord. If the cord is severed or if many cord tracts have been damaged, patients lose feeling because sensory impulses cannot reach the brain. They are paralyzed because motor impulses from the brain can no longer reach muscles below the injury. Damage to the cord in the cervical area is particularly disabling because all cord tracts below the injury may be involved. Disease, injury, or chemicals (drugs) can cause loss of function by interrupting the conduction and connection pathways.

Reflex Centers

All sensory impulses entering the cord do not have to travel all the way to the brain to get a motor reaction. The gray matter in the spinal cord contains many reflex centers: places where incoming sensory impulses are shunted as outgoing motor impulses. There are reflex centers in both the brain and the spinal cord.

The knee jerk is an example of a spinal cord reflex. When the doctor taps the patellar tendon, the sensation is transmitted to a segment of the spinal cord at the lumbar level and a motor impulse causes extension of the knee. This type of reflex is an involuntary response. If lumbar segments of the cord are damaged, the knee jerk is absent. The doctor tests different reflexes during a neurologic examination because in certain diseases they deviate from normal.

The Peripheral Nervous System

The peripheral nervous system is composed of nerves located outside the brain and spinal cord. Cranial nerves and their branches stem from the brain; spinal nerves and their branches arise from the spinal cord.

Cranial Nerves

The 12 pairs of cranial nerves arise from the undersurface of the brain and pass through openings in the skull to their destinations. These nerves are numbered by Roman numerals. The vagus nerve, the Xth (10th) cranial nerve, contains both sensory and motor fibers distributed to organs in the thorax and abdomen. Other cranial nerves supply organs of special sense such as the eye, nose, ears, tongue, and their associated muscles. They also control muscles of the face, neck, thorax, and abdomen. See Table 5.1.

Spinal Nerves

The 31 pairs of spinal nerves arise from the spinal cord and pass through lateral openings (IVFs) between the vertebrae. Spinal nerves are numbered according to the level of the spinal column at which they emerge. The lumbar, sacral, and coccygeal nerves descend from the terminal end of the spinal cord and emerge in sequence from their respective vertebrae. These lower spinal nerves form the *cauda equina* (horse's tail) within the spinal cavity. Spinal nerves branch and subdivide into many smaller nerves after emerging from the spinal cavity.

Most spinal nerves carry both sensory and motor nerve fibers. Some fibers supply skeletal muscles and others supply visceral (smooth) muscle. Spinal nerves are two-way conductors, and if anything harmful happens to them, there can be both anesthesia (loss of sensation) and paralysis (loss of motion).

Plexuses

A nerve plexus is a network of spinal nerve subdivisions that appear as tangled masses in areas outside the spinal cord. The *brachial plexus*, for example, extends from the lower cervical spine to the shoulder region. Nerves emerging from this tangle supply the shoulder, arm, forearm, and hand. Pressure and/or stretching of the brachial plexus can cause paralysis in the upper extremity.

In a similar manner, the *sacral plexus* supplies nerves to the lower extremity. The

Table 5.1. The Twelve Cranial Nerves

Number/Name	Type	Origin	Distribution	Basic Function
I. Olfactory	Sensory	Nasal chamber	Nasal mucous membrane	Sense of smell and flavors except salty, sweet, bitter, and acid
II. Optic	Sensory	Retina	Retina	Sense of sight
III. Oculomotor	Motor	Midbrain	All ocular muscles except lateral rectus and superior oblique	Major down and out eye motion, pupil constriction
IV. Trochlear	Motor	Midbrain	Superior oblique muscles of eye	Major down and in eye motion
V. Trigeminal	Mixed	Pons and midbrain	Skin of upper face, ear, jaw, tongue, gums; teeth; muscles of mastication	Motor and chief sensory nerve of the face
VI. Abducens	Motor	Pons	Lateral rectus muscle of the eye	Major abduction motion of eye
VII. Facial	Mixed	Pons	Facial muscles, middle ear, anterior ⅔rds taste buds; lacrimal, nasal, sublingual, submaxillary glands	Muscles of expression, taste, salivation
VIII. Auditory	Sensory	Pons	Middle and internal ear	Sense of hearing and balance
IX. Glossopharyngeal	Mixed	Medulla	Posterior 3rd taste buds, pharynx, parotid gland, ear	Ear pain, swallowing, parotid parasympathetics, pharyngeal reflex
X. Vagus	Mixed	Medulla	Pharynx, larynx, heart, lungs, esophagus, stomach, abdominal viscera	Swallowing, hunger, speech, epiglottal taste, breathing, heart rate, ear and throat pain, alimentary tract pain, peristalsis, digestive juices
XI. Spinal accessory	Motor	Medulla and cord	Sternomastoid and trapezius muscles	Neck and shoulder girdle motion
XII. Hypoglossal	Motor	Medulla	Intrinsic muscles of tongue	Speech, eating

largest nerve in the body, the sciatic nerve, emerges from the sacral plexus. From the buttocks, the sciatic nerve runs down the thigh. Its branches supply posterior thigh muscles, the leg, and the foot.

The Autonomic Nervous System

The autonomic nervous system is that part of the nervous system which sends nerve fibers from nerve centers to smooth muscle, cardiac muscle, and gland tissue. Autonomic fibers supply impulses to body structures thought of as operating outside conscious control. The organs supplied are the heart, blood vessels, iris and ciliary muscles of the eye, bronchial tubes, parts of the esophagus, and abdominal and pelvic organs. See Figure 5.27A.

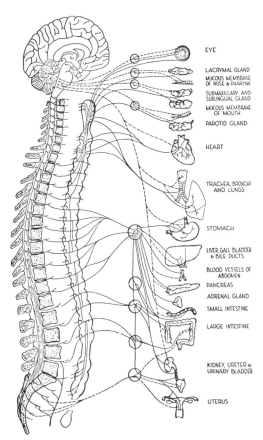

Figure 5.27A. Diagram of the distribution of the autonomic nervous system.

The autonomic nervous system is a part of both the central and peripheral nervous systems. It is not separate and independent. It has two divisions, sympathetic and parasympathetic. These two divisions receive impulses from the CNS by way of ganglia.

Ganglia

Ganglia are the relay stations of the autonomic nervous system. Neurons originating in the cord or brain conduct impulses to one or more autonomic ganglia. Other neurons conduct impulses from a ganglion to specific tissues or organs. Ganglia of the sympathetic division lie in a chain formation, like a string of beads, one chain on each side of the spinal column. Ganglia of the parasympathetic division are in or near the organs to which they send impulses.

Sympathetic and Parasympathetic Function

The sympathetic division of the autonomic nervous system regulates activities to prepare the body for maximum effort as a response to hazardous conditions. Sympathetic stimulation and response to stress go together. The parasympathetic division primarily regulates activities to conserve energy and to promote digestion and elimination. Generally, but not exclusively, sympathetic and parasympathetic impulses can be thought of as antagonists—like accelerators and brakes; ie, constricting or relaxing blood vessels, sphincters, and glands. See Table 5.2.

THE SPECIAL SENSES

Sensations of smell, taste, sight, hearing, and equilibrium are often called the *special senses* because special sensations are received by specialized sensory receptors that are sensitive to specific types of stimuli. Other important sensations such as touch, pressure, pain, heat, and cold are received through receptors widely distributed in the skin and underlying tissue, joints, and sometimes in viscera.

Table 5.2. Sympathetic and Parasympathetic Activation

Structure	Sympathetic Division Supply	Sympathetic Division Effect of Stimulation	Parasympathetic Division Supply	Parasympathetic Division Effect of Stimulation
Thyroid	T1	Increases secretion	X	Decreases secretion
Mucous membranes of head	T1–2	Vasoconstriction	VII	Vasodilation
Salivary glands	T1–2	Increases organic substances	IX	Increases watery substances
Pupils	T1–2	Dilation	III	Constriction
Lacrimal glands	T1–3	Vasoconstriction	VII	Secretion
Heart	T1–5	Increases rate and force of contraction, dilates coronary arteries	X	Decreases rate and force of contraction, constricts coronary arteries
Upper limbs	T1–6	Vasoconstriction, sweating, piloerection		
Bronchi and lungs	T1–7	Dilation, vasoconstriction	X	Constriction, vasodilation
Sphincter of Oddi	T4–8	Constricts	X	Relaxes
Gallbladder	T4–8	Relaxes muscle, constricts sphincter	X	Constricts muscle, relaxes sphincter
Stomach	T5–9	Decreases secretion and motility	X	Increases secretion and motility
Spleen	T6–8	Contracts smooth muscle	X	Relaxes smooth muscle
Pancreas	T6–9	Decreases secretion	X	Increases secretion
Liver	T8–10	Increases glycogen to glucose, increases protein metabolism, vasoconstriction	X	Opposite
Pyloric sphincter	T9	Increased tone, contraction	X	Relaxation
Adrenals	T9–10	Increases secretion	X	? (unknown)
Small intestine	T9–L1	Slightly decreases peristalsis and secretions, vasoconstriction	X	Increases peristalsis and secretions, relaxes sphincters
Kidneys	T10–L1	Vasoconstriction, inhibits	X	? (unknown)
Prostate	T10–L1	Contracts muscle and spermatic vein	S2–4	Increases secretion
Fallopian tubes	T10–L1	Contracts muscle		? (unknown)
Urinary bladder	T12–L2	Constricts sphincter, relaxes wall	S2–4	Relaxes sphincter, constricts wall
Lower limbs	T12–L2	Vasoconstriction, sweating, piloerection		
Uterus	L1	Contracts body	S2–4	Relaxes body, contracts cervix
Ileocecal valve	L1	Contracts	S2–4	Relaxes
Penis, clitoris	L1–2	Duct contraction, ejaculation	S2–4	Erection
Colon and rectum	L1–3	Decreased peristalsis	S3–5	Increased peristalsis
Anal sphincter	L3	Contracts	S3–5	Relaxes

Impulses from receptors for both special and other senses are carried by sensory nerve pathways to the cerebrum. There the impulses are converted into sensations and perceptions (awareness or consciousness of sensation). The parts of the sensory mechanism are (1) the sense organ or receptor, (2) the pathway by which the impulses are conducted to the CNS, and (3) the sensory center in the cerebrum. The sensory mechanisms of the special senses are summarized as follows.

Smell. Cells designed to perceive odors are in the olfactory membrane of the nose. The olfactory membrane is in the uppermost part of the nose, in the area above the upper turbinates. Impulses from the receptors are transmitted by the olfactory nerve to the temporal lobe of the brain. Although olfactory receptor cells are quite sensitive, they also can become fatigued. Odors that at first may be very noticeable may be less so on continued exposure. Smell is considered a primitive sense, and the detection of odors is more highly developed in animals than in man.

Taste. The sense organs for taste are taste buds, located in the surface of the tongue. The primary taste sensations are sweet, sour, salty, and bitter. The actual sensation of taste, particularly for distinctive flavors, is influenced by the sense of smell. Taste sensation is usually dulled when nasal membranes are congested or when the nostrils are pinched shut while eating. Impulses from taste receptors are transmitted by nerve fibers from two cranial nerves, the facial and glossopharyngeal, to the temporal lobe.

Sight. Cells in the retina of the eye are stimulated by light rays entering the eye (Fig. 5.28). These stimuli create impulses that are carried by the optic nerve to the visual center of the occipital lobe of the brain.

Hearing. Cells in the cochlea of the inner ear are stimulated by vibration of sound waves (Fig. 5.29). These stimuli create impulses that are carried by the *cochlear branch* of the acoustic (auditory) nerve to the auditory center of the temporal lobe.

Equilibrium. Beside having receptors for hearing, the internal ear contains three semicircular canals that regulate the sense

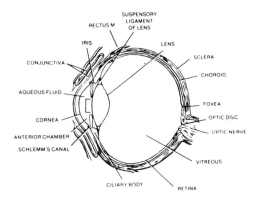

Figure 5.28. Schematic sagittal section of the eye.

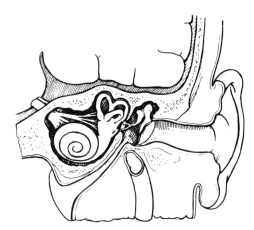

Figure 5.29. Schematic sagittal section of the ear: external, middle, and internal portions.

of equilibrium. Change in position of the head causes movement of fluid within the canals. This motion stimulates delicate nerve endings in the walls of the canals that sends impulses to the brain via the *vestibular branch* of the auditory nerve.

THE EYE

The eye is specialized for the reception of light. Each eye rests in a bony socket or cavity called the orbit, which is formed by several bones in the skull. The orbit provides protection, support, and attachment for the eyeball and its muscles, nerves, and vessels.

The Eyeball

The interior of the eye is divided into an anterior cavity (anterior to the lens) and a posterior cavity (behind the lens). Refer to Figure 5.28. A clear watery solution (aqueous fluid) is formed and circulated in the anterior cavity. A transparent semifluid material (vitreous fluid) is contained in the posterior cavity. The globular form and firmness of the eyeball is maintained by its fluid content, which also functions in the transmission of light.

The eyeball (globe) has an outer coat, a middle coat, and an inner coat. The outer coat consists of an invisible or transparent anterior portion (cornea) and a white fibrous nontransparent portion (sclera) that is directly continuous with the cornea. The middle coat holds the choroid, iris, and ciliary body. The inner coat is the retina, which coats the interior of the eye except toward its anterior surface.

The Lens

The lens is a small transparent disc-shaped structure situated immediately behind the iris and in front of the vitreous cavity. The lens is suspended in a capsule within the globe by a circular ligament (the suspensory ligament of the lens). This ligament attaches to the ciliary body. Muscle actions of the ciliary body affect the suspensory ligament and the consequent focus of the lens. The condition of cataract means that some portion of the lens has lost its transparency and has become cloudy or opaque.

Aqueous Fluid

The aqueous fluid is formed by a portion of the ciliary body and fills the two divisions of the anterior cavity of the eye (the anterior and posterior chambers). Aqueous fluid flows from the posterior chamber to the anterior chamber and drains via a series of channels into venous blood. Interference with the normal formation and flow of aqueous fluid can lead to development of

excessively high intraocular pressure (glaucoma).

The External Eye and Accessory Structures

The anterior surface of the eye and some of its accessory structures such as eyebrows, lids, lashes, and conjuctiva are readily visible. See Figure 5.30. An additional essential accessory structure, the lacrimal (tear) apparatus is shown in this figure. The eyelashes help to protect the entrance of foreign objects into the eyes. On the margin of the eyelids near the attachment of the eyelashes are the openings of a number of glands. Infection of these glands is commonly called a sty.

Specific muscles control the eyelids. The tarsal plate and the obicularis oculi muscle hold the eyelids in proper position against the eye. A levator (lifting) muscle opens the upper lid by pulling upward into the orbit, and the circular obicularis oculi muscle closes the eyelids.

A delicate mucous membrane (conjunctiva) coats the inside of the eyelids and the front surface of the eyeball. Acute bacterial infection of the conjunctiva is commonly called "pinkeye."

The function of the lacrimal apparatus is the secretion and drainage of tears. Normal blinking of the eyelids helps to spread the fluid evenly to provide a moist protective lubricating film over the exposed surface of the cornea. The formation and drainage of

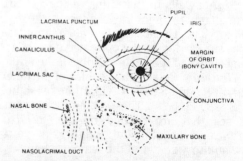

Figure 5.30. Frontal exterior diagram view of the eye and lacrimal apparatus.

tears are the natural ways in which the surface of the eye is kept clean and moist.

The Extraocular Muscles

Besides the levator muscles of the eyelids and the obicularis oculi, there are six sets of muscles located outside the eyeball. These muscles raise, lower, or rotate the globe within its socket. The muscles of the two eyes normally function in coordination so that both eyes move simultaneously and are aimed in the same direction. When coordination is impaired (eg, a nerve lesion), divergence or crossing of the eyes occurs (strabismus).

THE EAR

The ear, the organ of hearing, consists of three parts: the external ear, the middle ear, and the internal ear. These divisions provide for the reception and conduction of sound. The inner ear also contains the major mechanism for equilibrium. The structures of the ear, except that portion protruding from the head, are in the temporal bone of the skull.

The External Ear

The external ear consists of (1) the shell-shaped portion called the *auricle* or *pinna*, which projects from the side of the head, and (2) the external acoustic meatus, which is the canal leading toward the middle ear (Fig. 5.31). Near the entrance of the external canal, the skin contains wax-producing glands and hair follicles. This wax (cerumen) helps to prevent the entry of foreign objects into the ear.

The lobule (lobe) of the ear contains no cartilage, is composed of fatty tissue and of connective tissue, and lacks the firmness of the remainder of the auricle.

The principal function of the external ear is the collection and conduction of sound waves to the middle ear. The auricle is composed of cartilage covered with membrane

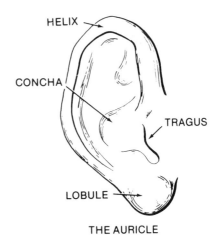

THE AURICLE

Figure 5.31. Diagram of the external ear.

(perichondrium) and skin. The prominent folded rim of the ear is the *helix*. A deep cavity (the concha) leads to the external auditory canal. In front of the concha and projecting backward over the entrance of the external auditory canal is a small triangular eminence of cartilage called the *tragus* whose undersurface is usually covered with soft hairs that help prevent insects and other foreign objects from entering the ear. The cartilage of the auricle is continuous with that forming the outer portion of the exterior canal.

The exterior auditory canal has two parts: an outer cartilaginous part and an inner bony portion formed by a passage in the temporal bone. The canal extends about 1¼ inches from its entrance at the bottom of the concha to the tympanic membrane (eardrum), which closes the inner end of the exterior canal. The tympanic membrane separates the inner end of the canal from the middle ear. The doctor uses a lighted instrument (otoscope) to examine the external canal and eardrum.

The Middle Ear

The middle ear (tympanic cavity) is an irregular space in the temporal bone filled with air and containing the three ossicles of the ear: *malleus* (hammer), *incus* (anvil), and *stapes* (stirrup). These small bones conduct vibrations from sound waves from the eardrum to the internal ear.

The *eustachian tube*, which connects the middle ear with the nasopharynx, has an opening into the pharynx that remains closed except during the act of yawning or swallowing. It then opens to admit air into the middle ear, thus performing its principal function of keeping air pressure equal on both sides of the eardrum. This tube is also an avenue of infection by which disease spreads from the throat to the middle ear.

The bony plate serving as the roof of the middle ear is quite susceptible to fracture during head injury and to the spread of infection from the middle ear (otitis media), either of which can result in intracranial disease.

The Inner Ear

The internal ear contains receptors for hearing and equilibrium. Refer to Figure 5.29. The receptor for hearing, the *organ of Corti*, lies in a structure called the *cochlea*, which is coiled and resembles the shell of a snail. Nerve impulses travel through the acoustic nerve from the organ of Corti to the auditory center of the cerebral cortex.

The internal ear also contains three semicircular canals that control equilibrium. Change of position resulting in fluid movements within the canals stimulate receptors in nerve endings that transmit impulses along the acoustic nerve to the cerebellum.

THE ENDOCRINE SYSTEM

The endocrine system is composed of glands of internal secretion (ductless glands). See Figure 5.32. These glands secrete hormones directly into circulating blood so that they can reach every part of the body and affect the function of specific tissues, thus influencing the activities of the body as a whole. Small in quantity but powerful in action, hormones are part of the body's chemical coordinating and regulating system.

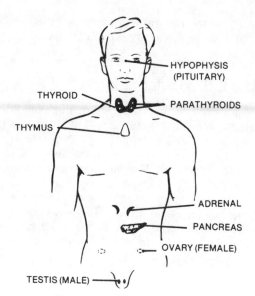

Figure 5.32. The endocrine glands.

The nervous system and endocrine system have almost identical roles. The difference is that the nervous system offers a quick response to changing environmental conditions; the endocrine system, a longer, more sustained effect.

There are six recognized endocrine glands: the thyroid, parathyroid, adrenals, isles of the pancreas, pituitary (hypophysis), and testes of the male and ovaries of the female.

The Thyroid

The thyroid gland, located in the front of the neck, has two lobes: one on each side of the larynx. The hormone produced by the thyroid is *thyroxin*. This hormone is associated with metabolism, regulating heat and energy production in body cells. Thyroid gland cells need the mineral *iodine* to manufacture thyroxin. Disorders of thyroid function include *hyperthyroidism*, which when severe causes a dangerous increase in the body's metabolic rate; and *hypothyroidism*, an opposite condition, which produces physical and mental sluggishness. An enlargement of the thyroid gland is called a *goiter*. When the enlargement is a nodular tumor, it is called an *adenoma*.

The Parathyroids

The parathyroid glands, usually four in number, are located on the posterior surfaces of the lobes of the thyroid gland. These glands produce the hormone *parathormone*, which helps to regulate the amount of calcium in the blood. Calcium, normally stored in bones, is released into the blood as required for normal nerve and muscle tissue function. When there is too little calcium in the blood, involuntary muscle twitching or spasm (tetany) develops.

The Adrenals

The two adrenal glands (suprarenals) are located above each kidney. Each adrenal functions as two separate glands having different functions: the *medulla* (core) and *cortex* (shell).

The medulla or inner part of the adrenal gland produces *epinephrine*. This is sometimes called the "flight or flight" hormone, and called *adrenaline* by the British. The medulla is stimulated to produce epinephrine by the sympathetic branch of the autonomic nervous system to give the body the extra push it needs in responding to emergencies.

The cortex, the outer part of the adrenal glands, produces a series of *adrenocortical hormones*, which include hydrocortisone. The adrenocortical hormones influence the salt and water balance of the body, the metabolism of food, and the ability of the body to handle stress. It is also an anti-inflammatory agent but tends to produce GI bleeding when administered artificially. External application does not produce this adverse effect. The cortex of the adrenal glands requires stimulation by a pituitary hormone (ACTH) for prolonged action.

The Pituitary

The pituitary gland, located within the skull, is also called the *hypophysis*. This small gland has two lobes, each producing distinctive hormones.

The anterior lobe hormone stimulates other endocrine glands to produce their distinctive secretions. For this reason, the pituitary gland is called *the master gland* of the endocrine system. The four hormones produced by the anterior lobe of the pituitary have names with the suffix "trophic," which means nourishing: *Somatotrophic hormone* (STH) means body nourishing. This hormone influences skeletal and soft-tissue growth. *Adrenocorticotrophic hormone* (ACTH) stimulates the cortex of the adrenals to produce its cortisone-like hormones. *Gonadotrophic hormone* stimulates the normal development of the gonads (the testes or ovaries) and controls the development of the male and female reproductive systems. *Thyrotrophic hormone* stimulates the thyroid gland to produce its hormone.

The posterior lobe of the pituitary gland produces a hormone that stimulates the contraction of the smooth muscles of the uterus, so it is important in childbirth. Another posterior lobe hormone, which helps prevent excessive water excretion from the kidneys, is called the *antidiuretic hormone*.

The Pancreas

Part of the pancreas functions as an accessory organ of the digestive system and a portion functions as an endocrine gland. Its endocrine gland function is carried out by groups of pancreas cells, called the *islands of Langerhans*, that produce the hormone *insulin*. This hormone is necessary for the normal use of sugar by body cells.

If insulin is not produced in sufficient amounts, sugar in the blood cannot be properly used by body cells, and the disease *diabetes mellitus* develops. A patient with diabetes mellitus requires continuous treatment—a combination of diet modification, education in modified living habits, correction of structural/functional disorders, and sometimes medication (insulin).

The Testes and Ovaries (Gonads)

The male testes are located in the scrotum; the female ovaries, in the lower abdominal cavity. Hormones produced by these glands stimulate the development of sexual characteristics that normally appear at *puberty* (onset of sexual maturity). They are responsible for the appearance of the secondary sexual characteristics; eg, pubic and axillary hair, changing of the voice, the beard in the male, and breast development in the female. These hormones also help maintain the reproductive organs in their adult state.

THE GENITAL SYSTEM

The male and female reproductive systems have their respective specialized internal and external organs, passageways, and supportive structures. The parts and functions of these systems are designed to make the process of fertilization possible. The female cell (ovum) must be fertilized by the male cell (spermatozoon). The normal result of fertilization is conception and reproduction.

The Male Reproductive System

The major parts of the male reproductive system are the scrotum, testes, epididymis, ductus deferens (vas deferens or seminal duct), seminal vesicles, ejaculatory ducts, prostate gland, urethra, and penis. The penis, testes, and scrotum are called the *external male genitalia* (Fig. 5.33).

The Scrotum, Testes, and Epididymis

There are two testes, one on each side of the septum of the scrotum. A testis (testicle) is an oval-shaped gland, about 1½ to 2 inches in length, which produces the male germ cells (spermatozoa or sperm) and the male hormone *testosterone.* Sperm are produced in great numbers, starting at puberty. Microscopic in size, each sperm has a head containing the cell nucleus and an elongated tail for movement. Sperm travel from the testes to a tightly coiled tube (the epididymis).

The Ductus Deferens

The *ductus deferens* is a continuation of the epididymis. The duct carries sperm from the

scrotum to the pelvic cavity. As the duct leaves the scrotum, it passes through the inguinal canal into the pelvic cavity as part of the spermatic cord. Spermatic cords, one on each side of the groin, are supporting structures. Each ductus deferens curves around the bladder and delivers sperm to one of two storage pouches called *seminal vesicles.*

The Seminal Vesicles and Ejaculatory Ducts

The seminal vesicles are located behind the bladder. During the storage of sperm in these vesicles, secretions are added to keep them alive and motile. The secretions and sperm form the seminal fluid (semen). Ejaculatory ducts carry seminal fluid from the seminal vesicles through the prostate gland to the urethra.

The Prostate Gland

The prostate almost surrounds the urethra at the neck of the bladder. Prostatic secretions are added to seminal fluid to protect sperm from potentially adverse urethral secretions. When the prostate gland becomes enlarged (hypertrophied) or swollen by inflammation or a tumor, it can seriously constrict the urethra. The size and consistency of the prostate gland is determined by the doctor via rectal examination.

The Urethra and Penis

The urethra, a passageway for seminal fluid and urine, has its longest segment in the penis. Several glands add secretions to the urethra: the largest being two bulbourethral (Cowper's) glands. Refer to Figure 5.33. The external opening of the urethra is in the glans penis (terminal portion), which is surrounded by a retractable fold of skin (foreskin or prepuce). The penis has an abundance of spongy tissue that becomes distended when the blood supply is increased (eg, erection during sexual arousal).

Surgical removal of the foreskin is *circumcision,* which is performed to reduce the possibility of an abnormal constriction of the glans (phimosis) or to reduce the pos-

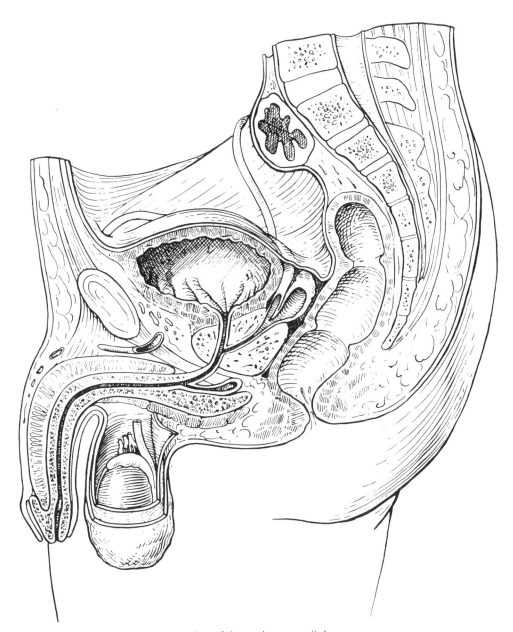

Figure 5.33. Schematic sagittal section of the male urogenital organs.

sibility of irritation from secretions that accumulate under the foreskin.

The Female Reproductive System

The major parts of the female reproductive system are the ovaries, fallopian tubes, uterus, vagina, and external genitalia

(vulva). The supportive structures for the internal reproductive organs are provided by a complicated arrangement of pelvic ligaments formed in part from folds of peritoneum lining the abdominopelvic cavity (Fig. 5.34).

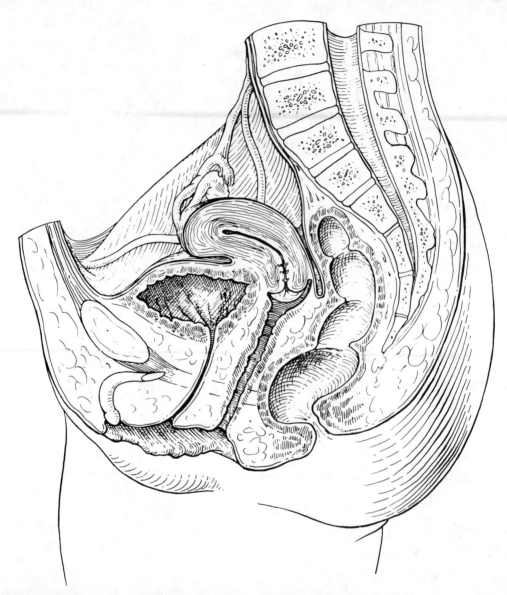

Figure 5.34. Schematic sagittal section of the female urogenital organs.

The Ovaries

The ovaries are two almond-shaped glands, one on each side of the abdominopelvic cavity. They produce female germ cells (ova) and the female hormones *estrogen* and *progesterone*. These hormones maintain the normal menstrual cycle. An ovum is expelled from the surface of an ovary in a process called *ovulation*, which occurs about halfway between each menstrual period.

The Fallopian Tubes

There are two fallopian tubes (oviducts), each curving outward from the upper part of the uterus. About 4 inches in length, each tube has a free end that cups near but is not attached to an ovary. The fringed surface of the free end of the fallopian tube carries an expelled ovum into the tube, and the ovum moves slowly on its way to the uterus. If fertilization takes place, it normally occurs as the ovum moves through a tube. The male germ cell must therefore travel up the fallopian tube to unite with the female germ cell.

An ovum expelled from an ovary is picked up by the free end of a fallopian tube for transportation to the uterus. Because there is no direct connection between an ovary and the corresponding fallopian tube, there is an interval where the ovum is "floating" within the abdominal pelvic cavity. For this reason, pregnancy might occur even when the right ovary and left fallopian tube (or vice versa) have been surgically removed.

The Uterus

The uterus, shaped somewhat like a large pear, is suspended in the pelvic cavity and supported between the bladder and the rectum by its system of eight ligaments. The normal position of the body of the uterus is *anteflexion* (bent forward over the bladder). Refer to Figure 5.34.

The uterus is about 3 inches long and 3 inches thick at its widest part. It has a thick wall of smooth muscle and a relatively small inner cavity. During pregnancy, it can stretch to about 20 times in size. The upper dome-shaped portion of the uterus is the *fundus*, the main part is the *body*. The lower neck portion is the *cervix*. The cervix serves as the canal opening into the vagina.

Menstruation

The inner lining of the uterus (endometrium) undergoes periodic changes during the menstrual cycle to prepare the uterus to receive a fertilized ovum. In preparing to receive the ovum, the mucous lining (mucosa) of the uterus becomes soft and swollen and uterine blood vessels dilate. If the ovum is not fertilized, the unneeded blood and mucosa are expelled from the uterus through the vagina. The process of menstruation begins at puberty and is repeated, unless interrupted by disease or pregnancy, about every 28 days until the age of 40 to 50 years.

The Vagina

This muscular canal extends from the cervix of the uterus to the vaginal opening in the vestibule of the vulva. The vaginal canal is capable of stretching widely to serve as the birth canal. Part of the cervix protrudes into the uppermost portion of the vagina.

A part of a female pelvic examination is the physical examination of the visible surface of the cervix and vagina, plus a laboratory examination of cervical and vaginal secretions. A Pap (Papanicolaou) smear is made to obtain these secretions for laboratory examination.

The Vulva

The several structures that make up the female external genitalia form the vulva. These are the *mons pubis, labia, clitoris,* and *vestibule*. The labia are two parallel sets of lip-like tissues: the *labia majora*, the larger outer folds of tissue; and the *labia minora*, the smaller inner folds. The *clitoris* is at the upper meeting point of the labia majora and labia minora. Between the labia minora is the *vestibule*, a shallow depression into which the urethra and the vagina open. The urethral opening is at the anterior roof of the vaginal opening. A series of glands, which may become infected, open into the vestibule. The largest of these glands are the *Bartholin glands* at the vaginal opening.

THE BUILDING BLOCKS OF THE SYSTEMS

Cells form tissues, tissues form organs, and organs form the various systems of the body. They are the building blocks of the body.

Cells

The cell is the basic functioning unit in the composition of the human body, as well as in all other living organisms. The human body is composed of billions of cells that vary in shape and size. Cells are microscopic in size. The largest is only about 1/1000 of an inch. Because of this, a special unit of measurement, the micron, is used in recording cell dimensions. One micron equals 1/1000 millimeter or about 1/25,000 of an inch. A group of the same cells is called a tissue and performs a particular function. The human body is composed of many groups of cells performing a variety of functions.

Cells constantly reproduce to replace worn out cells, build new tissues, and bring about the growth of the body as a whole. Cells reproduce themselves; ie, increase by dividing, maturing, and dividing again. This process is known as *growth by division*. It results in a mass of apparently identical cells. However, as cell division continues, differences begin to appear in various groups of cells as they develop the characteristics necessary to perform their roles in the development and functions of the body. This development of special characteristics is called *cell differentiation*.

Cells are composed of a substance called protoplasm. A typical animal cell is made up of a cell membrane and two main parts: the *nucleus* and *cytoplasm*, which are types of protoplasm. The nucleus controls all activities of the cell, including growth and reproduction. Cytoplasm is the matter surrounding the nucleus and is responsible for most of the work done by the cell.

Cell membrane encloses the protoplasm and allows the passage of fluid into and out of the cell. This permeable cell membrane is an important structural feature of the cell. It is through the cell membrane that all materials essential to metabolism are received and all products of metabolism are disposed of. The bloodstream and tissue fluid that constantly circulate around the cell transport materials to and from cells. The common chicken egg is a classic example.

Metabolism is the ability to conduct the chemical activities required for cell function. It includes using food and oxygen, producing and eliminating wastes, and manufacturing new materials for growth, repair, and use by other cells.

Tissues

A tissue is a part of the body composed of similar specialized cells that work together to perform particular functions. There are four main types of tissues, each of which has a particular function. Refer to Figure 5.26.

Epithelial Tissue

Epithelial tissue forms the outer layer of skin for the protection of the body. It is also a lining tissue. As *mucous membrane*, it lines the nasal cavity, mouth, larynx, pharynx, trachea, stomach, and intestines. As *serous membrane*, it lines the abdominal, chest, and heart cavities. As *endothelium*, it lines the heart and blood vessels. It lines respiratory and digestive organs for the functions of protection and absorption. It helps form organs concerned with the excretion of body wastes, some glands, and certain sensory organs for the reception of stimuli.

Squamous (flat) epithelial cells in a single layer compose such structures as the microscopic air sacs of the lungs. In other places such as the skin, squamous epithelium is in several layers or stratified. Columnar epithelium cells are more important in the formation of ducts.

Tissue Fluid

Tissue fluid is the body fluid that lies outside blood vessels and cells and is therefore also called *extravascular* (outside blood vessels) or *extracellular* (outside cells) fluid. Living body cells contain large amounts of water and must be bathed continuously in a watery solution to survive and carry on their functions. This colorless and slightly salty (saline) tissue fluid is derived from circulating blood.

Nerve Tissue

Nerve tissue is composed of cells highly specialized to receive and transmit impulses (electrochemical messages). As previously explained, nerve cells (neurons) are bound together by a special structure called neuroglia.

Connective Tissue

Connective tissue is distributed throughout the body to form the supporting framework of the body and to bind together and· support other tissues. It binds organs to other organs, muscles to bones, and bones to other bones. There are six types of connective tissue:

1. *Areolar tissue* is a fibrous connective tissue that forms the layer of tissue under the outer skin. It fills many of the small spaces on the body and helps hold organs in place.

2. *Adipose tissue* is a fatty connective tissue found under the skin and in many other regions of the body. It serves as padding around and between organs. It also insulates the body (reducing heat loss) and serves as a food reserve.

3. *Reticular tissue* is a fibrous connective tissue that forms the supporting framework of lymph glands, the liver, the spleen, bone marrow, and the lungs.

4. *Elastic tissue* is a fibrous connective tissue composed of springy fibers. It is found in the walls of blood vessels, in the lungs, and in many ligaments.

5. *Cartilage* is a tough resilient connective tissue found at the ends of the bones, between bones, and in the nose, throat, and ears.

6. *Muscle tissue* is composed of long slender cells held together by connective tissue. There are three types of muscle tissue: striated, smooth, and cardiac (heart muscle). Muscle tissue has the ability to contract (shorten) and by so doing to produce movement.

Striated muscle has fibers divided by transverse bands. Because most striated muscle attaches to bones, it is often called *skeletal muscle.* Skeletal muscle contraction is stimulated by impulses from nerves and, in theory, the nerve impulses can be controlled by voluntary (conscious) effort. Skeletal muscle tissue is therefore referred to as *striated voluntary muscle tissue.*

Smooth muscle lacks striations. It is found in the walls of internal organs (vis-

cera), blood vessels, and internal passages. Contraction of smooth muscle helps propel the contents of internal structures (eg, blood, intestinal contents). Smooth muscle contractions are stimulated by nerve impulses not usually under conscious control. Smooth muscle is therefore called *nonstriated involuntary muscle tissue.*

Cardiac muscle is found only in the walls of the heart; ie, myocardium is heart muscle.

Organs

An organ is a group of tissues that has combined to perform a specific function. The body is composed of many organs, each with its own specialized function. The heart, lungs, stomach, liver, and pancreas are commonly recognized as organs, but the skin is also an organ. The spinal column meets the definition of an organ but is not usually thought of as such.

CHIROPRACTIC'S HOLISTIC APPROACH TO HEALTH

The relationship between human structure and function has always been a concern of chiropractic. While it is common knowledge that a diseased organ may cause symptoms to appear in distant parts of the body, chiropractic has demonstrated clinically throughout the years that neurologic insults at the spinal column and other areas may cause symptoms to appear in remote organs and tissues. Likewise, as emotional disorders may lead to changes in structure, structural disorders may lead to emotional symptoms. The body is a total being: a whole even if its study is divided into systems and organs.

Structure/Function Relationship

Our skeletal structure is more than an osseous cage to hold vital organs or a bony hat rack on which nature has hung our muscles. The human body is a carefully integrated unit, not just the sum of its parts. The unifying and coordinating and controlling forces within the body are essentially the nervous, hormonal, and circulatory systems. There is no organ, tissue, or cell of the body that is not influenced directly or indirectly by these systems. Any dysfunction of one system may have extensive affects on other systems; eg, any dysfunction of structure may have an affect upon the nervous system because of the inherent relationship.

Balance and harmony among body systems results in normal functional tone. *Holism* is the theory that the determining factors in nature as a whole are irreducible to the sum of their parts. A human being is still a mystery even after we add up all the tissues, organs, and systems in the laboratory. Chiropractic recognizes this in its approach to health care.

As structure cannot be separated from function in the human being, neither should health care fail to recognize the human body's unification. Our bones are more than supports, our muscles more than pulleys, our nerves more than wiring, and our vessels more than fluid conduits. Chiropractic health care embraces this structure/function viewpoint, not only in its gross aspects but also at its cellular and molecular levels.

Healing Forces

The recognition that the human body has inherent healing powers is common to all ages and cannot be separated from considering the body as a total unit. These principles are ancient in origin. What is new to this century is chiropractic's re-emphasis of the doctrines of Hippocrates. Just as life is defined as the ability to respond to a stimulus, health must be considered the ability to adapt to internal and external stress. To neglect natural healing forces is to shun natural recovery manpower reserves. For these reasons, the relationship of biomechanics to biodynamics has been emphasized by the chiropractic profession.

Chapter 6

Human Relations in Health Care

Human relations as explained in this chapter involves the understanding of and empathy for the human needs of the sick and disabled. Its importance often runs parallel with the need for technical and professional services.

The chiropractic assistant is not removed from the doctor-patient relationship. She is an integral part of it. To the patient, doctor and assistant are a team. The doctor is judged by his choice of associates as much as he is as an individual. Because of this, this chapter describes many ways in which an assistant may develop her effectiveness in building patient rapport, respect, and admiration. Yet all explanation has one common denominator: Treat each patient at all times like you would like to be treated under similar circumstances.

Ever since the earliest civilizations, businessmen have realized that the success of business depends much on maintaining the good will of their clientele and customers. Even the healing arts realized that skills could be neutralized to a large degree if patient respect and admiration were not nourished. Thus, it is not a new thought that the foundation for human relations in health care is the doctor-patient and staff-patient relationships.

Faith is an unseen ally in any healing process, despite what discipline is used. For centuries, the family doctor was one of the most admired and respected people in the community. The doctor's reputation was based as much on his "bedside manner" as it was on his technical knowledge and skill. Unfortunately, with the rapid advance in technology and the increasing complexity in procedures and prescriptions, the medical profession lost much of this respect and admiration when the doctor-patient relationship became more impersonal, cold, mechanically administered. Fortunately, however, this has not been true of chiropractors. Doctors of chiropractic are keenly aware of the importance of positive human relations. They subscribe to a holistic and humanized form of health care.

Few big things but many small things result in positive human relations. The practice must be conducted skillfully, be fair to everyone, and be able to administer counsel, therapy, and fees wisely and justly. Staff must be practical, courteous, and decent. They must know when to be serious and when to have a sense of humor. They must be confidant, adviser, and educator—and frequently much more.

A patient needs and desires sincerity, gentleness, understanding, and affection from his doctor and assistants. The patient senses sincerity in voice, gentleness of touch, an understanding manner, and concerned responses. The doctor of chiropractic recognizes that the sick person resents being treated indifferently: as a nonbeing, case number, or disease entity. Wise healthcare providers recognize that they must be scientifically objective yet subjectively empathetic to those who seek care.

Almost every patient that enters the office is fearful to some extent. This fear must be reversed to faith, and it is reversed when the office staff is aware of the necessity of building positive human relations and by being sure that patients' questions are satisfactorily answered in nontechnical language. Most fear is fear of the unknown; questions unanswered are answers unknown.

ETIQUETTE IN THE PROFESSIONAL OFFICE

Office etiquette means observing common courtesies with fellow workers, your doctor-employer, patients, and the public. Etiquette, like ethics, can be summed up in one rule: Treat others in the way you would like them to treat you if the roles were reversed. When in doubt about proper office etiquette, watch the doctor for his example.

Rules of professional etiquette are just as important to know as the rules of professional ethics. For instance, the doctor should always be notified of the visit of another doctor even if an appointment has not been made. The same is true of telephone calls from another doctor.

Two of the most important expressions in our language are *please* and *thank you.* They are not and should not be unconscious utterances. Let them come from your heart rather than from habit. Most people crave recognition and appreciation.

Introductions. Learn to introduce people to each other easily. Despite know-ing the formal rules, your attitude and interest in people is the most important factor. In general, (1) honor a woman by introducing a man to her; (2) present a young person to an older person; and (3) introduce a patient to the doctor. When it's necessary to introduce yourself, say something like, "I'm Betty Smith, Dr. Brown's assistant. May I help you?"

Communication. Use the doctor's proper title. Never call the doctor by his first name unless you have been requested to do so. Do not call him "Dr. Jim" in front of patients, fellow staff members, or the public. Also, avoid use of the pronoun "he." Use "Dr. Brown will be with you soon" rather than "'He'll be right out." Use of the pronoun gives the impression of a casual or careless attitude.

The doctor's fees are also an area of sensitive human relations. The wise assistant will always discuss fees and arrangements at the earliest opportunity and arrive at a mutually satisfactory arrangement. Delinquent accounts must be handled with tact and common courtesy.

Respect. Respect the personal property of others; eg, respect office supplies and furnishings and the property of patients. Especially respect people's feelings. Never be too busy to answer a question with a smile and pleasant response. When help or cooperation is necessary, place your needs in the manner of a request, not an order.

Office etiquette between the assistant and the doctor-employer should be one of mutual respect. Abruptness and impatience is always mirrored back. As the doctor is frequently weighted with many responsibilities and anxieties, not burdened on the assistant, a good assistant will avoid adding further burden by being understanding, efficient, loyal, and trustworthy.

In the humanized practice, all patients are treated with respect. Instructions are explained friendly, manner, correspondence is issued promptly, delays are tactfully explained, every patient is offered personalized care and attention, and patients should feel admired and respected as special people. If not, how would the doctor and assistant build admiration and respect for themselves.

Guard Doctor-Patient Privacy. A patient deserves privacy. Health care is an intimate relationship. Phone conversations, discussions about fees, and case histories must be private and not within the range of others. Voices should not carry from consultation, examination, or therapy rooms. Dressing areas and preparation areas should be private, comfortable, and adequately supplied with clothes hangers and mirrors.

When the doctor is in consultation with a patient, screen calls and keep visitors occupied until he is available. Take notes of all calls for the doctor so that they may be returned later. The important subject of telephone etiquette will be covered in a following chapter.

Privileged Information. Gossip with patients and coworkers is unmannerly if not unethical. It may be uncomfortable for both you and the inquirer when you must decline to furnish information of a private nature, but confidentiality must be maintained. The law mandates it if a patient is involved.

Discretion. Human relationships should be friendly but not familiar. A health-care office requires close relationships among staff and patients. The subjects discussed, your tone of voice, and your general attitude help in drawing the line between friendliness and familiarity. A respectful and considerate attitude is always in good taste. Flippancy encourages insolence. Professionalism is reflected in quiet good taste, sincere empathy, and a businesslike decorum that is hospitable, gracious, and well mannered.

Positive human relations is the result of concern for both impersonal and personal impressions. On the personal side, the chiropractic assistant is cheerful, friendly, and warm. The office is no place to express personal moods. Nor is the office a good meeting place for friends and relatives or a place to receive personal mail. Keep your personal life separate from office matters. An assistant is hired to help solve the doctor's problems. He is not there to help solve assistants' nonhealth problems. Also, never offer to help the doctor on personal matters before he asks you.

The thoughtful assistant treats each patient fairly, with courtesy and without prejudice, regardless of the patient's social or financial standing in the community. She respects the patient's privacy, and she respects the doctor's privacy. Above all, the assistant has a keen desire to serve. She likes people. She has a deep desire to help the sick, the disabled, the aged, the immature. She accepts complaints as suggestions and patient irritability with understanding.

FIRST IMPRESSIONS

As explained, respect and admiration are difficult to develop if the doctor and assistant do not act the way the patient believes a doctor and assistant should act. In many silent ways, both doctor and assistant tell patients about their attitudes by the office and its impressions.

The Physical Office

Neatness and cleanliness are good examples of silent communication. Clean uniforms, clean furnishings and floors, neatly kept magazines, uncluttered desks, spotless equipment, and like concerns for housekeeping communicate to the patient as much as gestures, mannerisms, and tone of voice.

The office environment by itself can do much to add to or subtract from positive human relations. A clean, comfortable, attractive, well-organized office in many ways can do much to communicate *We care!*

Furnishings. Office furnishings should be cheerful and bright, avoiding the "hospital" appearance. This requires carefully selected drapes, carpeting, pictures, planters, and accessories. Good ventilation, air conditioning, comfortable armchairs, adequate lighting, soft music, uncramped space, concern for patient movement from room to room, and well-marked entrances and exits help to establish an environment reflecting concern for people's needs.

Flowers. Cut flowers will brighten a gloomy winter day. Patients will appreciate the cheerful sight of a bouquet, and the pleasant scent brings smiles to almost everyone's face. When cut flowers are placed in the office, use a sharp knife to remove an inch from each stem before putting the flowers in water. Do not pinch the stems with your fingers or use scissors. The container should be roomy enough for sufficient water but small enough to provide support for the stems. Be careful to remove all leaves below the water line to prevent rot. Change the water and trim the stems every other day. Cut flowers will fare best if they are in a cool but not drafty spot.

Administration

The alert assistant realizes that every factor within the office environment has a human relations aspect—even routine records. Patients become irritated when records are not neatly maintained and accurate, when financial information is not readily at hand, when statements are confusing, or when reports are delayed.

The concerned assistant realizes that an efficient appointment system is not just for the advantage of the doctor, staff, and practice. It is also a means to respect the patient's time. It reduces waiting time to a minimum, anticipates emergencies so not to disrupt the entire schedule, allows for different times for different procedures, and is efficient. Yet, it is humanized.

Helping the Doctor During New Employee Indoctrination

As human relations involves staff and patients, it also involves the relationship of staff among itself. This is especially true when new employees are added to the staff. Breaking-in a new member of the staff is not a task that should be treated without advance thought by all concerned. Once a person has been selected for employment, the training period is very important so that a humanized approach will be incorporated in training. The new person should be imbued with the idea that people learn by doing, not by endless listening, talking, and demon-

strating. It is one thing to tell the person how to perform a given task; it is another to have the trainee successfully demonstrate that she can do the job assigned.

Training a new person at one job at a time is another good rule. A new employee may be "snowed" if a variety of tasks is thrown at her in too short a time. Also make it a point during training to reserve some time after each training session to review and clarify any problem situations that are bound to arise.

Helping the Doctor During New Patient Indoctrination

When the doctor answers a patient's questions concerning the patient's condition, he not only relieves fear, he builds faith in the patient that he knows what is wrong (diagnosis), what to do about it (treatment), and creates added respect and admiration when he tells that patient how he or she can prevent recurrence and maintain maximum resistance.

The doctor is aware that the typical patient initially has six basic questions that must be answered: (1) What is wrong with me? (2) What caused it? (3) What can you do to help? (4) What can I do to help? (5) How long will it take to get better? (6) How much will it cost? The doctor's consultation and examination will be aimed at finding the answers to these questions. When the doctor answers these and associated questions, the patient has faith that the doctor knows what he is doing, and the patient places his health care in the doctor's hands with confidence. If these questions are not satisfactorily answered, the patient's fear will motivate him to seek the answers elsewhere. Thus, CAs should be alert to a patient's comment that one or more of these questions has not been answered to the patient's satisfaction. If recognized, bring this immediately to the attention of the doctor so that he can offer appropriate answers.

Direct consultation is but one medium the humanized practice uses to communicate to the patient. Patient information booklets, health tracts, reception room literature, written patient instructions that re-emphasize verbal instructions, printed office policies, as well as charts and illustrations and audiovisual programs are also effective auxiliary means toward patient education and motivation.

BASIC PSYCHODYNAMICS IN PROFESSIONAL HUMAN RELATIONS

The patient who is sick is under stress. One role of the assistant is to be sure she does nothing to add to this stress. The sick person needs a friend, an understanding friend. A friend who is cheerful, polite, well mannered, and poised. A friend who is efficient, calm in emergencies, devoted to her work, and soft spoken. A friend who is sympathetic, understanding, helpful, alert, and utterly dependable. Patients will love such an assistant and be devoted to her as she will be to them. This is one reason the career as a chiropractic assistant is so rewarding.

As human beings, we are all impelled by desires, fears, hopes, doubts, and emotional highs and lows, as well as selfish and self-centered thoughts. Recognizing such thoughts and motives early helps us control their intensity, duration, and expression when with patients. Nobody is perfect. All humans have potential contradictory emotions: some are constructive, helpful, and cheerful; others are unhappy, hostile, and revengeful. It is not unusual to have these tendencies conflict with one another, but wisdom helps us recognize them and make appropriate restraints because patients in discomfort are not interested in our feelings. They are only interested in their own feelings. The role of the professional in the office is to serve the needs of the patients.

Applied Psychology

The doctor's image and reputation are affected each time an assistant contacts a visitor to the office. By her attitude, the assistant can build the practice or diminish its effectiveness. In her hands, she has the ability to build human relations by creating an atmosphere of good will and efficiency or create negative relations by being nervous, overtalkative, aggressive, snobbish, or boorish. The chiropractic assistant is the doctor's ambassador of good will, his primary public-relations representative.

When you stub your toe, you suffer a musculoskeletal injury. But it is more than this. You hurt all over. The injury has its effects throughout your total being, physically and mentally. Because of the pain, all systems will be affected. Even your digestion may be affected. You undoubtedly will feel anger, which may affect your entire nervous, endocrine, and other systems. More is involved than just a stubbed toe.

A patient who is sick, disabled, or worried must be handled with special understanding of the nature and scope of illness or disability. When health is lost, security is threatened. We need sympathetic attention. When our security is threatened, we automatically become hypersensitive. Normal lighting may bother our eyes, normal odors may become offensive, and normal sounds may seem to be loud noises. Nothing tastes good. It is not unusual to develop hypochondriac symptoms and acquire new phobias. When we become sick, our entire being is affected, not just an isolated part.

Sick people have many fears. Fears of prolonged pain or disability, fears for the family's security, fears of income loss and of doctor bills. The chiropractic assistant must be empathetic with these feelings and understand why patients are sometimes irritable and grouchy. For some obscure reason, a patient may hide these symptoms from the doctor, yet openly vent them to or on an assistant.

When a patient is sick, he recognizes only one sick person in the world. Himself. He seeks personal attention, unhurried attention, immediate attention. Although he may be pessimistic, he expects all around him to be optimistic. While he may be hypersensitive, he will expect others to be insensitive to curt remarks, rude manners, and complaints. After all, he believes, he is sick and has the right to let the world know it. The wise chiropractic assistant will understand this.

Every practice will have a few problem patients, and every practice will have many patients with a few problems. Some patients will be habitually late yet complain on having to wait. Some patients will repeatedly disobey the doctor's instructions and complain of the slowness of their recovery. Most of these complaints will be to the assistant and sometimes in front of other patients. In such instances, the assistant's tact and grasp of psychology will be measured. Turning patients' complaints to renewed confidence, good will, and friendship is an art that develops with experience, a basic understanding of human nature, and a firm service philosophy.

Body Language

Body language is essentially nonverbal communication as expressed in body movements, gestures, and mannerisms. Behavior of the hands, fingers, arms, legs, feet, and head offer frequent signs that reflect a patient's inner feelings. Facial expressions, eye movements, voice tone, and inflection, as well as standing, sitting, and walking postures offer other signs.

Conscious or unconscious behavior in motion is an outward expression of inner attitude. Observation informs us that there is often an incongruity between verbal language and body language, between what a patient's words reveal and what his subtle actions are really communicating.

Body language offers both positive and negative signals to the careful observer. When an assistant sees negative groups of signs, it's her clue to try to remedy the situation. The patient is unconsciously trying to communicate something felt but for some reason cannot be put into words. For instance, if you say something that evokes a sign of confusion or doubt, it is your clue to offer more clarity or evidence.

When an assistant sees positive groups of signs, this tells her that the relationship is positive. If you make a statement that brings out a sign of acceptance and agreement, it is

your clue that your words are not meeting indifference or rejection.

Gestures reflect subconscious thoughts and feelings seeking expression. Gestures also influence thoughts and feelings in the observer. Body language is usually an unconscious reflex that expresses a feeling that has not been allowed vocal expression. However, some "actors" (eg, malingerers) may consciously apply body language in a few learned pantomimes to portray a feeling associated with a role.

Just as a doctor does not make a diagnosis based on just one symptom, so the interpreter of body language should be cautious in arriving at a judgment based on one or two attitude signs. Where one or two signs may be ploys to distract the observer, several signs expressed consistently serve as indicators to the experienced observer. The important thing is to weigh all evidence before arriving at a firm conclusion.

Other Forms of Nonverbal Communication

Self-fulfilling prophecies are communicated as much through nonverbal means as they are through direct words. Psychologists have long known that something as simple as a friendly smile offered when test sheets are passed out can raise the subjects' score. Students respond to their teacher's wordless expectations communicated through subtle facial gestures and voice tones as employees do to the nonverbal communications from their supervisors. Nonverbal communications serve as a medium in which one person's feelings and ideas are transmitted to another quite readily. The influence of such interpersonal expectation appears to vary with individuals in its clarity and effectiveness, however. These signals are mixed and contain subtle sequences and rhythms between voice tones, facial expressions, and bodily gestures.

An individual signal need not exceed a fraction of a second in duration to be interpreted. This draws attention to why action often speaks louder than words and why it is difficult to deceive the trained observer solely with verbal persuasion.

Eye Blink Rate

Hidden cameras used to record the eye-blink rate have shown that how fast a person blinks his eyelids is a good index of his state of inner tension. The normal rate of about 32 times per minute decreases during deep relaxation and hypnotic-like states, and increases rapidly during anxiety. Tests also have shown that when a person is not telling the truth, the rate of blinking rapidly increases from normal even if the person consciously tries to inhibit the reaction.

Pupil Reactions

Research has shown that the pupils of your eyes will reveal that you may be lying as well as indicate some of your innermost feelings. Some researchers believe that pupil size is a more accurate lie detector than the polygraph. Studies show that pupils distinctively dilate (become larger) when a person likes what he sees or is interested in it. Conversely, pupils contract (become smaller) when the subject is presented with an object or situation he dislikes or finds dull.

Handling the Emotionally Disturbed Patient

Positive human relations, dispensed by both doctor and assistant, is in itself a therapeutic agent of utmost value. Its effect has proved beneficial in almost all ailments that beset mankind. It may be curative solely by its own presence, or it may require assistance from other persons or therapies. It should frequently be combined with other forms of treatment.

Psychotherapy can be loosely defined as anything one person can do to improve the mental or emotional state of another person. Thus, it is anything that helps an individual cope with his feelings, motivations, behavior, or performance more effectively.

Words are not the only tools available. Doctors and assistants can influence others by their acts, manner, and attitudes possibly more than they can by words. It would be rare to talk a person out of an advanced mental disorder, soothe him with platitudes, pacify his concerns, or resolve his problems strictly by your prescriptions. Psychotherapy essentially is listening, giving and receiving feedback uncritically, helping a person develop his own solutions, helping the person develop confidence, and letting him talk things out and release bottled-up feelings.

The doctor's use of basic principles of psychotherapy involves a thorough history that is constantly updated, arriving at a differential diagnosis, creating formulations, and selecting a clinical approach specially designed for the individual patient. A positive doctor-patient relationship is probably the most important therapeutic measure available to any patient.

Listening attentively, being yourself, and showing personalized interest in the patient are powerful therapeutic measures available to the chiropractic assistant. The essential key to good care for the patient is in *caring* for the patient. This should be the entire staff's basic motivation.

The Underestimated Value of Applied Psychology

As a therapy in itself, positive human relations serves to function as a cure sometimes, a relief often, and a comfort always. In its superior form, it helps to prevent sickness. In its mediocre form, it attends to impending sickness. In its inferior form, it "treats" the symptoms of sickness.

The therapeutic effects of positive human relations are witnessed through a variety of methods; eg, listening, analyzing, and counseling. Besides its therapeutic value, it also has a diagnostic potential. It functions in diagnosis by alert observation, listening, responding, contacting, touching, testing, and interpreting. It serves as a contrast medium to emphasize the normal from the abnormal and subnormal, the real versus the unreal.

This "miracle" therapy of positive human relations is indicated in almost every conceivable physical and emotional ailment that besets mankind. It should be applied freely in all structural, functional, and traumatic disorders, and is particularly helpful in psychologic problems. It has proved its value in neurosis, career problems, marriage problems, and sexual problems—whether occurring singularly or coexisting with a disease process. It should be used liberally since it has little benefit when diluted.

Dependency

Therapeutic psychodynamics should not be used as a substitute for handling a problem that the patient is capable at the time to handle himself. Thus, it should not be used as a crutch. As any therapy, positive human relations can have an adverse reaction. Because of its potency and capability for relieving stress, a patient may become dependent on it and even addicted to it. Too frequent requests for office visits and telephone counsel are symptomatic of dependency. Severe anxiety and depression may result during withdrawal of the therapy. Disappointment may result in despair, anger, or resentment.

While an overdose of this powerful therapy may occur, underutilization is much more common.

The Application of Psychiatric Principles

One survey revealed that approximately 12% of problems presented by patients in a typical outpatient practice were clearly psychiatric in nature and that psychiatric problems were the second most frequently presented complaints. From 20%–80% of general practice will require some use of psychiatric principles. Every successful practitioner, regardless of discipline, is aware of this necessity.

Here are some assumptions regarding the management of psychiatric problems:

1. Psychiatric treatment and the use of psychologic principles in everyday practice represent a necessary and desirable dimension of competency for both doctor and assistants.

2. The primary-care physician should obtain and maintain astute awareness of the psychologic factors present in all illnesses whether these illnesses present as physical or psychiatric problems.

3. The primary physician should obtain and maintain a considerable degree of skill not only in recognizing psychiatric problems but also in managing these problems on a continuing basis.

4. Primary physicians should have a familiarity with the body of knowledge available regarding human growth, development, and behavior throughout the life cycle and at each stage of the cycle. This is regarded as core-content knowledge.

5. Core-content knowledge is not enough. Physicians (and assistants to a limited degree) should also develop core-content skill in putting this knowledge to use in the practice just as any doctor must develop and refine his clinical skills. These skills, once developed, can be lost due to "disuse atrophy" or lack of feedback. Education in this field must be continual to keep alert to the current state of the art.

6. Some of these core-content skills involve the following:

- Handling doctor-patient and assistant-patient relationships
- Good counseling and interviewing techniques
- Awareness of the role of the illness in the patient's psychic and social economy by the doctor
- Self-awareness
- The appropriate administration of somatopsychiatric therapies.
- Attributes of consideration, compassion, acceptance, empathy, responsibility, and flexibility
- Problem helpfulness and resolution ability
- Use of family members in the treatment process
- Psychiatric illnesses have two common characteristics. They take time, and they deserve more than common sense advice. As some patients require specialized services, the doctor should have knowledge of community resources for handling emotional and psychiatric problems. The doctor also should have a friendly professional relationship with local counselors, a psychologist, and a psychiatrist with whom he can discuss and refer patients when necessary.

7. Every family physician is exposed to the entire range of psychiatric problems (from mild to severe). Thus, he must be able to recognize and manage them on either a continuing or emergency basis according to his skill, desire, and the patient's needs and consent.

All patients presenting with psychiatric problems do not require the specialized care of a psychologist or psychiatrist, and only the most severe cases require hospitalization. The clinical judgment of when or how to refer a patient to a specialist is one of the core-content skills of the doctor. Often, the primary physician can treat the illness effectively.

The assistant must be aware that patients with major or minor mental or emotional illnesses are human beings who are suffering. They are seeking help to cope with the problems of life. Like a patient with a purely structural disorder, they have a right to be treated with dignity and concern. They are not malingering. A patient suffering a psychiatric illness has a right to be in the doctor's office and receive the best chiropractic care possible. Such patients are never "taking the doctor's time" without cause.

The experienced doctor will be alert to treat the patient as well as the complaint. The nature of recommended therapy should be based on the individual needs of the patient involved. Some patients require only simple advice while others need in-depth counseling or possible referral. All patients require understanding.

The Assistant's Role in Case Management

While the doctor understands that patients with psychiatric illnesses require special considerations, he may fail to offer all assistants specific instructions regarding what to do or not do. Here are some basic recommendations that he will likely expect an assistant to understand:

• Be empathetic, not sympathetic. With empathy you place yourself in the other person's position so you can appreciate his experience. With sympathy, you *feel* with the patient and most likely will take on the patient's feelings of hopelessness and fear.

• Do not give pep talks, preach, threaten, bribe, or moralize. Don't do anything that implies that the patient *could* change if he *would* change. Will power by itself is rarely the answer. Since there is a difference between sin and sickness, and a patient's behavior and values may be different from yours, do not attempt to set or enforce your morals. Never advise a patient to "have faith," "keep your chin up," or "try a little harder." Patients will feel rejected by such vague generalities and trite comments. Likewise, do not advise patients to "straighten up" or "pull yourself together." If they *could*, they *would*. Most likely they have tried and failed repeatedly. They need professional help.

• Be *reality oriented*. Separate fact from opinion. Be professional and poised, and do not let yourself be emotionally drawn into the patient's problems. Be helpful whenever possible, but recognize that the patient's troubles are those of the patient and not yours. Treat the patient as an adult who you may be able to help, not some child you should lecture.

• Do not hold the belief that a patient's problems will automatically disappear with a new job, a new hobby, a new spouse, a vacation, or some other change in environment. Changes in scenery only result in old problems in new places. The problem must be assumed to be with and within the patient; ie, the problem moves with the patient until it is resolved.

AN OVERVIEW OF PSYCHIATRIC DISORDERS

Some psychiatric problems can be roughly compared to the severity of a common cold. Some are like mild pneumonia, others like moderate emphysema, but only a few are considered malignant. Psychiatric illnesses, as most health disorders, rarely have a sudden onset. They develop slowly, and symptoms may only appear in the later stages. The dynamic symptoms are but the tip of the iceberg. It must be recognized that as pain and fever fulfill a specific and helpful purpose in the survival process, so do psychiatric symptoms. The doctor must be concerned with what *caused* the symptoms plus what is maintaining them now.

It must be assumed that the patient has had his successes and failures, has learned to relate to other people, and has learned to work and live and survive in a relatively suitable manner. A new problem arose, the patient tried to cope with it according to his experience, and efforts have failed. Why have previously successful methods of coping failed this time? Is the reason the patient or the situation? Can the problem be resolved or must the patient learn to adapt?

Coping Mechanisms

All behavior is purposeful, even neurotic behavior. Behavior is never random or capricious. It is goal oriented. People attempt to adapt to their environment as they perceive it. Behind every action lies a reason related to the life history of the individual and associated with an emotional or physical need. Ahead of every action is a goal, a purpose, a promise of need gratification. Thus, all behavior is some type of coping mechanism, and all that psychotherapy can do is attempt to improve an individual's coping skills. In psychiatric illness, every symptom can be considered an action—an action that has a need behind and a purpose ahead.

As a coping organism, an individual lives a life beset by three basic types of problems and influences: (1) problems rising from the external environment, (2) stressful inner feelings resulting from memories of past actions or refusal to act when capable (guilt), and (3) impulses within arising from sanctions and prohibitions of a moral or ethical conditioning acquired since childhood (conscience).

A coping individual must defend against these attacking forces by warding off attack by some shielding mechanism (eg, flight, rationalization) or by acquiring a weapon to attack or alter internal and external negative environments (eg, fight). In other words, he can (1) *attack*, change the environment or act to alter it; (2) *retreat*, run

away to avoid the stress of the environment, get out of the situation, surrender; or (3) *coexist*, adjust to the problems in the environment, change the environment or the self a little, tolerate an undesirable situation if a better one cannot be developed. These are rational alternatives, but they are rarely accepted as such by involved patients. The typical patient suffering a psychiatric illness seeks a magic wand, frequently going from doctor to doctor in quest of an easy solution to a difficult problem.

While physical impairment can be readily measured, psychologic impairment is difficult. How sick is sick? If a patient is in pain, we know he is sick, but we do not know how severe or widespread the sickness is. The same is true of psychiatric distress. The degree of psychiatric illness can be determined only by the methods the patient uses to cope with the stress. Whenever a person is confronted with a problem, he calls on his coping mechanisms to help re-establish the status quo before the stress occurred.

If the stress is more severe than the patient can handle, the individual is forced to resort to more pathologic coping mechanisms that are classified into five levels:

1. *Alarm and mobilization*, characterized by anxiety, inefficient hyperactivity, frustration, withdrawal and depression, and sympathetic nervous system responses in preparation for fight or flight.

2. *Partial detachment and attempted compensation*, characterized by neurotic symptom formation and behavior, less obvious anxiety, erratic and nonproductive behavior, and the development of phobias, obsessions, compulsions, intoxications, addictions, or somatizations.

3. *Transitory ego rupture with prompt restoration*, characterized by severe neurotic and brief psychotic episodes such as panic attacks, catastrophic and demoralizing feelings, irrational excitement, violent behavior (homicidal, suicidal, sexual, or convulsive) of a temporary episodic nature.

4. *Persistent ego rupture or exhaustion with marked detachment*, characterized by varying degrees of erratic excitement, dis-

organized behavior, withdrawal, apathy to the point of inactivity and unresponsiveness or even mutism, hallucinations, delusions of persecution or grandiosity, confusion, bewilderment, forgetfulness, and disorientation. Most patients at this stage require institutional care.

5. *Complete ego failure*, characterized by continuous uncontrolled violence or retarded depression ending ultimately in death unless controlled. Most primary physicians will treat patients using first- and some second-order coping devices. Specialists are necessary for the treatment of severe levels in a restricted environment.

As explained, if a doctor is to treat a psychiatric illness adequately, he must determine how the patient got sick and what keeps the sickness going. Remember that psychiatric illness does not "just happen" any more than pneumonia or a slipped disc just happens. Illness (physical, functional, or psychiatric) develops for one or more reasons. The development of a neurosis has seven aspects: (1) a predisposing personality, (2) a current conflict, (3) an external precipitating stress, (4) the development of anxiety, (5) a primary gain (symptom-forming factor), (6) the symptom complex, and (7) the secondary gain (symptom-fixing factor).

The Person Behind the Illness

A person with a pure personality problem will rarely appear in the doctor's office consciously seeking help for the problem. Almost always, he comes because of some physical or functional symptom or disability. Thus, it is important to keep in mind that behind the problem presented is the patient's basic personality. He has always had this personality and will always have this personality (modified only according to profound conditioning). He is a unique individual. There is no one else like him. He has his own way of handling stress, and he will try in the future to handle new stresses in like manner. In this sense, behavior becomes quite predictable.

Psychoanalytic theory holds that an adult neurosis develops from the roots of a childhood neurosis. While we can assume that some degree of childhood neurosis existed, that memory is often forgotten. Still, adult symptoms often mimic those occurring in childhood. As the personality develops from childhood to adulthood, habitual behavior becomes more rigid and presents with a somewhat fixed behavioral pattern. Thus, in adult neurosis, we often see an adult reacting to stress as if he were immature.

A psychiatric illness is usually associated with a current conflict or problem that is perceived by the patient as a threat. Conflicts, such as marriage problems and career dissatisfaction, involve the person's self-image and superimposed on and related to the predisposing personality. During the course of treatment, the patient may reveal this current conflict to the doctor, he may conceal it, it may be repressed from conscious awareness, or the patient may fail to see its relationship with his symptoms.

It is understandable that a patient with a predisposing personality and a current conflict is waiting for something to happen. Based on past experiences, he seeks solutions to his problems. Neurosis resulting from chronic stress in ineffective problem solving is usually precipitated by some external situation. This explains why the illness manifested when it did, but this external precipitating stress should not be confused with the current conflict. If a person is having a current conflict in his marriage and attempts suicide, some specific external stress must occur to precipitate the act. For example, chronic feelings of insecurity (current conflict) might have been augmented by learning of his spouse's infidelity (external precipitating stress).

Tolerable or intolerable anxiety occurs in stress when the individual doubts his capabilities of successfully applying fight or flight mechanisms. Thus, we have the quality and quantity of anxiety and its manifestations superimposed on (1) the predisposing personality, (2) the current conflict, and (3) an external precipitating stress. Now, if the stress becomes long standing or very severe and the anxiety becomes overwhelming, secondary defense processes are forced to manifest themselves.

Psychiatric Symptom Formation

When an individual can control anxiety by applying healthy defense mechanisms, illness does not result. However, when unhealthy defense mechanisms are applied, illness invariably results. The strength of the personality determines its ability to tolerate stress. Whether by healthy or unhealthy means, the primary gain in the illness process is the relief of anxiety. These means or mechanisms themselves are often witnessed as symptoms such as forgetting recent events or conversations. Such symptoms are therefore the result of the patient's attempt to control anxiety. The symptoms manifest in a wide variety such as development of an aversion, a phobia, a compulsion, an obsession, a temperament change, a psychosomatic syndrome, or some schizophrenic world of fantasy.

Unfortunately, these symptoms are accompanied by increased anxiety and/or depression that tells us the symptom was not totally successful in relieving the anxiety. Thus, a cause must be found behind the symptom. The paradox is that the symptom, as the most dynamic factor, tends to conceal and reveal. The symptom also creates the secondary gain or symptom-fixing factor.

Even if the cause behind the symptom is known, what keeps it going? The concept of secondary gain is the most recognized answer to this question. The symptom is not easily given up by the individual because he has learned that it offers certain advantages in relieving some anxiety. To give up the symptom means to confront the basic anxiety again, and the patient wishes to avoid this at all costs if possible.

Besides the emotional rewards, there also may be another reward in not giving up the symptom. For instance, the man having marital difficulties who develops a heart condition from "overwork" may unconsciously recognize that his continuing disability will help prevent his wife from leaving him. In fact, he may unconsciously do things that will discourage healing. Likewise, a woman with a "back problem" may recognize that her continuing disability will help her receive more attention and help from her husband. Thus, she may unconsciously do things to delay recovery (eg, heavy lifting, falling). If this is done consciously, the patient is malingering. But secondary gain efforts, being unconscious, are definitely not cases of malingering. To complicate the matter, the patient may consciously or unconsciously become aware later in the process that there is a financial reward for the presence of an illness, disorder, or symptom in the development of secondary gain. This is commonly seen when the possibilities of financial settlement for an industrial or automobile accident become apparent. This might be observed in the patient progressing on schedule who suddenly has a "relapse."

The aim of a psychiatric symptom is to distract attention from the real problem. Unfortunately, while it tends to relieve anxiety in one area, it tends to cause anxiety in another. A symptom should be viewed as the outward sign of an inward problem. That is, while the individual tries to hide unacceptable feelings and create a symptom designed to control the anxiety, attempts become outwardly apparent to the keen observer. Thus, the attempt to conceal can actually reveal.

The psychiatric symptom (psychologic defense mechanism) manifests as pathologic behavior expressed in thought and action. It is characterized by irrational behavior beyond conscious control; thus, it is involuntary. If it were under conscious control, the symptom would be viewed as normal problem solving, and adaptive, purposeful behavior. Besides being involuntary, the psychiatric symptom is never really successful even if it is purposeful but it does help to relieve part of the basic anxiety. Because of this, the individual is afraid to give it up.

During therapy, the doctor must determine why the symptom manifested when it did, under what circumstances it occurs, and why it occurs under some situations and not others. Why does it occur at night but not in the morning? Why does it occur at home but not at work? What purpose does the symptom fulfill for this individual at a particular time?

As the doctor studies the psychiatric symptom, he must consider its four aspects: (1) as a coping device; (2) as an attempt at adapting, with the risk that maladaptation may lead to personality scarring; (3) as a purposeful defense mechanism designed to shield against or avoid anxiety; and (4) as a tactic to survive within interpersonal relationships.

The personality changes with development of the symptom as the old personality and new symptom unite. As the symptom is now part of the individual's coping technique, it can be used for secondary gain to obtain something previously perceived denied or defend a possession previously felt to be in jeopardy. Thus, the illness may unconsciously be used to maintain a disintegrating marriage, gain financial compensation, avoid unpleasant career situations, manipulate people, express hostility, or satisfy thwarted needs or have them fulfilled by someone else. Thus, the individual unconsciously tends to view the symptom as a definite asset—but not completely because there is a conflict.

The symptom that is an expression of a wish, usually a forbidden wish, expresses itself along with denial of the wish. It is as if one part of the personality is saying "go" while another part is saying "stop." Dreams also can express a forbidden wish and a denial of that wish, and this is the basis of dream analysis according to Freud.

When a doctor analyzes the psychiatric symptom, he can perceive the adaptive and defensive mechanisms used by the patient. Armed with this knowledge, the doctor can then analyze other symptoms and coping methods used to face life. Again, coping patterns tend to result in repetitive behavior that is fairly well predictable.

Authorities define symptom characteristics slightly different. Neurotic behavior was viewed by Eric Berne as game type behavior in *transactional analysis*. He taught that there is always an ulterior motive with a pay-off, the act is unconscious, and it involves another person. Jay Haley stated that it is the result of some extreme influence, the behavior is beyond conscious control, and it involves another person. Freud's position was that the behavior was unconscious, was an expression of both a wish and a denial of a wish, was designed to solve a problem but is unsuccessful, is related to childhood neurosis, and usually involves another person or persons. These authorities view neurotic behavior as coping behavior, unconscious and involuntary, repetitive, reflecting a conflict within oneself or about someone else, and indicates the general coping behavior of the person.

Understanding Anxiety and Depression

Anxiety

Anxiety is an unpleasant feeling or apprehension of danger often characterized physically by rapid heart beat, shortness of breath, palpitation, pupil dilation, extremity paresthesia, nausea, and/or anorexia. It may be strictly of mental origin or be a symptom of physical illness as in acute heart attack, alkalosis, hyperventilation, or a reaction to or a complication of a wide range of physical dysfunctions. It can defend against, substitute for, or precipitate depression. In schizophrenia, it may be a symptom of dammed-up psychologic tension. Regardless, it is viewed as the essential element in the development of mental illness whenever noted.

Anxiety occurs when an individual feels that something will happen and the subject lacks control. As all behavior is purposeful, anxiety has an aim—an attempt at protection from internal and external dangers. It alerts the personality to a threat, it prepares the body physically for a "flight or fight" response, and it alerts the individual's defenses. In many instances, an anxiety response is healthy. It is maladaptive when the anxiety is so severe that the threat is not realistic to the response.

Differentiation

Anxiety is referenced to the future; depression is oriented to the past. With anxiety, a person is afraid of what *might* happen. In depression, a person feels hopelessness because of something that *did* happen. Anxiety is linked with *fear;* depression, with *guilt.* An individual expresses anxiety when he perceives a threat and feels *helpless.* A person expresses depression when he perceives a loss and feels *hopeless.* Thus, an individual may express both anxiety and depression if he perceives a threat and has feelings of hopelessness. Frustration is the result when a person perceives a wish or a need and simultaneously feels helpless in acquiring the wish or need.

Depression

When we hear the word *depression,* we usually think of an individual being blue, sad, sorrowful, melancholy, or in very low spirits. However, depression as a clinical syndrome is more broadly defined. Psychologically, depression is a response to a loss, especially a loss of self-esteem. As anxiety, it can be a symptom of physical disease as well as be of mental origin. It is frequently associated with cancer and viral infections because of the illnesses and their restrictions. It also may be the result of a loss of income, a loss of somebody close such as in death or divorce, or used as a defense against or a surrender to anxiety. Depression can be viewed as *anger turned inward:* repressed hostility showing distinct biochemical changes within the body.

The five cardinal symptoms of depression are (1) the patient looks tired (fatigue) and acts tired (psychomotor retardation); (2) self-neglect in attire, personal sanitation, grooming, etc; (3) feelings of dejection, sadness, guilt and sorrow; (4) loss of social interest with a tendency toward withdrawal from people, things, food, sex; and (5) characteristic insomnia: the individual falls to sleep rapidly but awakens in the middle of the night and has difficulty returning to sleep.

Depression is greatest in the morning, but eases as the day progresses. Other characteristics include dependency, guilt, dire hopelessness, loss of self-esteem, distorted thought processes, indecisiveness, narcissism, mixed feelings of love and hate (am-

bivalence), and the physical symptoms of fatigue.

Organ Language and Psychosemantics

The study of psychosomatic illness reminds us that the control of body functions makes a lasting imprint on the mind and becomes part of mental processes. As we learn to control our bodies and their biologic functions, we build our psychic structure. The mind is not created independently of the body. It is very definitely linked with it.

Many authorities suggest that the most satisfactory way to deal with tension is by *action*, the least satisfactory is by *thought*, and in between is *speech*.

Neurotic Symbolism

A person suffering from psychosomatic illness can be compared to a heated tea kettle. If steam cannot escape from the spout, the lid blows off. In a similar way, people accumulate tension that is almost certain to explode in symptom formation. The point is that tension (energy) should be used in productive work or speech. Short-circuited energy can disturb body function. If people cannot express tension by acts, thoughts, or words, if they cannot express what is disturbing them, then one or more of his organs will try to say it for them. Thus, the person with nausea, who lacks evidence of organic disease, may be indicating that he cannot "stomach" situations. The person with an itch often "lets things get under his skin." Careful observation finds that body language expresses in many symbolic formulas.

The function of the mind is to promote the control of ourselves and our relations to other people. Remember that when feelings and thoughts exist that cannot be expressed by words, thoughts, or actions, they may find expression through some organ or system. The result is a "language of the organs" that can express itself in illness if the personality is not sufficiently developed to solve its problems through other channels. The organ that "speaks" is most likely the organ whose function was in ascendancy when environmental conditions were threatening and produced pain (anxiety). But constitutional predisposition, identification with an authority (eg, boss, parent, teacher), or other factors may also determine the "choice of organ."

In the context just described, it can be recognized that physical symptoms are often symbolic of neurosis. A feeling of oppression in the chest accompanied by sighing respirations in the absence of organic findings may suggest that the person has a "load on his chest" which he would like to get rid of by talking about his problems. The person who has lost his appetite and consequently becomes severely undernourished is often emotionally starved as well as physically starved. The common symptom of fatigue may be due to an emotional conflict using so much energy that little is left for other purposes. Emotional tension of unconscious origin frequently expresses itself as muscle tension giving rise to aches and pains, and sometimes these are represented by sharp pains such as seen in neuralgia. An ache in the arm may suggest that the person would like to strike someone but is prevented from doing so by the affliction. Itching can represent dissatisfaction with the environment in which the individual takes out on himself; martyr-like, he scratches himself (shows aggression) instead of someone else. "Weak legs" and vertigo are common physical expressions of anxiety. The digestive tract is, above all other systems, the pathway through which emotions are often expressed.

Alert Listening

Casual remarks can offer important diagnostic clues. Be aware of the importance of side remarks and apparent irrelevancies because important clues are often obtained in this way. Considerable anxiety may also be hidden behind laughter and jokes. The middle-aged man who with a laugh "guesses that he's cracking up" is often referring to his anxiety regarding his potency and future usefulness. The middle-aged woman with her half-expressed anxiety regarding the imminence of menopause may be anticipating

the end of her femininity. Both expectations are, of course, based on false beliefs that may require discreet clarification by the doctor.

An interesting analysis of the semantics of organ language shows that expressions concerning organ function exist as close parallels in many languages. The analysis done several ways in which words for organs and their functions are employed to indicate some degree of psychosomatic influence.

1. Some expressions imply a conscious awareness of the autonomic concomitants of emotional reactions. For example, "to be scared spitless" or "it makes my flesh creep."

2. There are expressions in which the word for an organ is employed as a substitute for an emotional attitude—for example, "soft-hearted" or "have guts." Some of these expressions have a shade of concrete physiologic meaning. For example, "spineless" or "no backbone," referring to the loss of muscle tone associated with a lack of initiative.

3. One group of expressions has implications proved accurate on psychoanalytic methods. For example, "I can't stomach him" or "I'll just have to swallow the consequences of that decision."

4. Another group of expressions indicates a long-standing awareness of psychosomatic relationships. For example, "Just the thought of that gives me a headache."

GENERAL EDUCATIONAL OBLIGATIONS

Although the typical patient may be in the office for a considerable time, the doctor will not have the opportunity to spend a great deal of time with each patient. The majority of total office time will likely be spent in contact with one or more assistants. Thus, while the doctor has a relatively brief time to develop the doctor-patient relationship, assistants have a greater opportunity to enhance this relationship.

Developing Levels of Consciousness

Each doctor and assistant has the professional obligation to develop three distinct stages of consciousness within each patient. These are (1) health consciousness, (2) chiropractic consciousness, and (3) Dr. X consciousness. From the viewpoint of an individual practice, consciousness of the individual doctor is the most important in regard to practice stability. If the patient is just health conscious, he may hold the opinion that he can treat himself adequately and thus be vulnerable to the dangers of over-the-counter patent medicines and home remedies. While chiropractic consciousness is a higher level than health consciousness, it does not ensure the security of the practice. However, if the patient is Dr. X conscious, he is at the same time both chiropractic conscious and health conscious.

Office Literature

Because of time limitations, the doctor's influence cannot rest on the office visit alone. Patient instruction sheets help to extend the doctor's influence. The use of printed guides and instructions also offers constant reminders of the doctor's services. Their use helps to minimize errors in communication, they save time in repeating oral instructions by the doctor and assistant, they impress patients with the office's thoroughness and efficiency and make patients more receptive to recommendations, and they indicate special consideration for the patient's welfare by not depending on the patient's memory.

The alert doctor and assistant will be aware that typical patients are not interested in the technical aspects of their condition. The patient is interested in the removal of pain, discomfort, and how the condition affects their lifestyle. Therefore, it is important that patient's everyday activities, hobbies, work, and personal habits be considered along with the clinical aspects of the condition.

The practice has a moral obligation and responsibility for the patient's health. Thus, the doctor should anticipate possible patient stress by questioning the patient about common activities. If the patient is left with the impression that the doctor is only interested in people when they are in the office, the patient will question the doctor's motives. Confidence in the doctor will diminish. The doctor can enhance confidence by showing the patient how to avoid overstress during the holidays, while on vacation, and during spring cleaning, sports, or recreational activities. Helpful tips on eating and sleeping habits are often appreciated. Special instructions during the prenatal and postnatal period are welcomed. This will show that the doctor and assistant care about the patient's welfare.

Many commonly used patient instruction sheets, diet forms, exercise routines, and safety measures while lifting or on vacation are available from the American Chiropractic Association.

HUMAN RELATIONS IN PATIENT CONTROL

Patients initially believe that they will receive competent service when they enter a doctor's office. They receive service, pay for it, and leave with the conclusion that they received what was expected. Patients are under no obligation to refer others to the practice. They paid for what they received. Yet without constant patient referrals, a practice cannot grow. New patients must be available to replace those who are dismissed, die, or move from the community.

Building Good Will

The question arises: What motivates patients to refer others? The answer is found in the answer to another question: Why does one technically competent doctor have a highly successful practice while another technically competent doctor has difficulty in maintaining his practice? The answer is that the successful practitioner and his staff place emphasis on building positive human relations.

Almost invariably, the successful practice will be characterized by patients receiving VIP treatment. Alert staff members are hosts and hostesses to every patient in the office. They recognize that the average person is hungry for attention, and attention is freely served. Patients are thanked. Patients are appreciated. Patients are complimented. The watchword is *hospitality*. Patients are allowed to talk, to express themselves, and to question. Good assistants are good listeners.

The successful practice has a staff that likes to brighten the day for patients with a kind word, a friendly gesture, a compliment. A patient's positive acts are praised. Promptness in appointments is praised. Prompt payment of bills is praised. Prompt recovery is praised. Cooperation is praised. Such praise is not idle flattery; it is sincere recognition.

The staff of a successful practice is considerate, thoughtful, and sympathetic. Patients' birthdays and anniversaries are remembered. The staff is aware when a patient's daughter graduates from college or a son enters a new business. Alert offices make a point of knowing such things and sending a thoughtful card or offering a considerate comment. The considerate staff knows that while few patients may avail themselves of office coffee, tea, or fruit juice, all patients appreciate the gesture. A few raincoats or umbrellas available for loan to help the patient caught in an unexpected shower are a sign of special consideration. Yes, patients will talk more about such extra kindnesses than they will about excellent technical service that is expected. It is doing more than the expected that counts.

The staff of a successful practice never argues with patients. The staff agrees, and refers to the constraints of "office policy." Yet, flexibility is always offered when possible. Patients are allowed to express their point of view, and their suggestions are always given sincere consideration. If you win an argument with a patient, you lose the patient. Without patients, there is no practice.

Without positive human relations, there is no practice growth. Any assistant or doctor who becomes irritated by eccentric patients or becomes arrogant or too impressed by his or her own dignity is their worse enemy.

As explained previously, patients who are sick or disabled are worried and fearful. The staff of a successful practice recognizes this and offers assurance within ethical bounds. Constant reassurance, encouragement, and inspiration help the patient continue with the recommended treatment plan. Doubt, discouragement, and apathy result in patient "drop-outs." Continual explanation results in reassurance. Even slight results offer encouragement, for results are facts. When results become more evident, the patient is inspired. During inspiration, when the mind is in a high state of expectation and belief, it is highly receptive to suggestion.

Successful human relations is giving patients what they don't expect or more than they expect. It's a warm smile, attention to a new hairstyle, the availability of a lending library, a "smile" button on dismissal, a sense of humor, a concern for the personal touch, an "I care" attitude, a small bowl of mints in the reception room, or a list of "health and safety tips" for patients planning a trip. Is it so unusual that patients will be motivated to do "something extra" for the office that does something extra for them?

Every human being has certain preferences, beliefs, theories, convictions, and habits—some good, some bad. Doctors and their assistants are no exception. However, it is very detrimental to positive human relations when a doctor or assistant attempts to persuade patients to accept his or her ideas as gospel. A patient's smoking habits, eating habits, or sexual habits are none of the staff's business unless there is a direct proved connection of the habit and the patient's condition. If smoking bothers you or other patients, it is good policy to improve the ventilation or provide a special area. If you prefer a vegetarian diet, keep the fact to yourself. If you are a "born again" Christian, that's your personal business. If you like to have a cocktail before dinner or are a total abstainer, the average patient could not care less and resents your attempting to impose your ideas.

Patients are human, and humans are not perfect. They prefer not to be. They enjoy many habits of which you might not approve that they feel are none of your business (and they are probably right). They come to the office for a health service, not a lecture or a sermon. When you accept patients as they are (a combination of strengths and weaknesses), they will accept you. You have your hang-ups, patients have theirs. Accept this, and go on to provide what patients want in a manner better than their expectations.

Preventing Patient Drop-Outs

While clinical chiropractic is science oriented, the practice of chiropractic must be patient oriented if it is to achieve its potential for success. Patients are human. They are people struggling with their health problems, family problems, financial problems, career problems, and a multitude of other concerns.

Remember that the successful practice is a humanized practice, one that recognizes patients as they are, not as you might wish them to be. The staff that builds a successful practice is not one that lives in a pseudo-technical-scientific ivory tower—ordering patients about, talking to them in professional jargon, subjugating them with airs of superiority, or deducing patients' ignorance in health habits. The successful staff is one that offers the public an opportunity to share its knowledge, experience, services, and facilities upon request.

Meeting Patient Needs

The successful office recognizes that patients present both physical and emotional needs and tries to the best of its ability to fulfill these needs within a professional atmosphere. This takes identification with and a willingness to relate to human beings, especially sick human beings. In the same manner, patients must relate to the doctor

and his assistants. This takes encouragement and rapport conditioned by agreement, faith, and inspiration.

We are living in what some have called the "Computer Age" or the "Space Age." It is true that science and technology are evolving faster in a few months than they did in several decades a generation ago. We live in an era of rapid change: changing environment, changing values, changing morals, and so forth. With such change, we witness more emphasis being placed on "image" than "substance," more interest in masks than the faces behind the masks. The "professional image" of the health practitioner so often portrayed today is one of an efficiently programmed, never wrong, scientific superbeing. It should be remembered that the friendly, homespun, often bumbling but always human doctor of years past had little worry of a malpractice suit.

The word *personality* comes from the Greek word meaning *mask*. Patients wear masks, doctors wear masks, and their assistants wear masks. We all try to hide our real selves from the world. In humanizing the office environment, we must learn to drop our masks: to be caring, open, honest, and kind. We are not dealing with "patient Smith," "the 3:15 appointment," or "the patient with tennis elbow." We are dealing with friend Mary Smith, Pastor Brown, or Jimmy Burns.

We should learn to look through the masks of patients to see the real person. This is how we harmonize with feelings, and feelings are always the precursors of actions. Such rapport is not always easy to develop, but it's the *magic* of human relations. Armies follow generals who have this magic, often to the ends of the earth and their own destruction. Employees burn the midnight oil, great attorneys mystify juries, zealots are created in causes, and patients become referral centers when caught up in the magic.

It is strange that some staffs forget that people do not like being sick. They are not in a doctor's office by choice. They are bitter and resentful of being forced into a painful situation against their will. The chiropractic assistant should not become intimidated by this situation. Do not, in fear of saying the wrong thing, draw yourself inward like a turtle and say nothing under the excuse of being shy. Shed your shell by not seeing a "patient" before you but a potential friend. Be understanding, be concerned; show empathy and kindness, but be natural. Let your warmth express naturally to turn a stranger into a friend, a welcomed guest.

Avoid Self-Prophesies

Be careful of your expectations. People have a way of fulfilling your prophesies. Assistants who expect patients to be cordial, cooperative, prompt, and friendly will find that patients reflect this attitude. In contrast, the assistant who expects patients to be irritable, uncooperative, or even hostile will find her predictions come true. *When effects are not to your liking, change the cause.* You will find by experience that you have the power to determine the attitudes and actions of others by your attitudes and actions.

Advantages of the Humanized Practice

While every practice has its share of drop-outs, the successful office keeps the number to a minimum. Although every patient may not need intensive health care, everybody needs some form of health maintenance or preventive program. Patients do not become drop-outs because their needs were fulfilled; they drop out because their needs were not being fulfilled. They were forced to seek fulfillment elsewhere. When a patient abruptly switches from one practitioner to another, it is because the motive to switch became greater than the motivation to stay.

When a practice is humanized, a few happy patients lead to more happy patients. The reverse is also true: when a practice becomes dehumanized, a few drop-outs lead to many more. Both positive human relations and negative human relations are contagious. Some practices may exist by advertising volume alone with a large turnover, but they will never be successful in the true sense of the term—nor will such offices be happy places in which to work.

A bruised ego often prevents one from realizing the cause of drop-outs. Symptoms preceded the act, but they were not recognized: dissatisfaction, unappreciativeness, uncooperativeness; chronic late, missed, or changed appointments; collection problems; no referrals. When these symptoms are noticed, they indicate a breakdown in human relations, a breakdown in communications, a breakdown in motivation.

What the Doctor Expects

While your doctor-employer will expect you to sincerely try to please everyone, he knows that it is impossible to please everyone every time. Some people are difficult to reach. The realist is aware that 5% of the patients will cause 95% of your problems. But you cannot spend 95% of your time coping with 5% of the patients. You must serve all. Each practice has its personalities, procedures, services, and facilities that will appeal to many but not everybody. If you or the doctor spend too much effort in trying to satisfy the eccentricities of a small minority, you may dissatisfy the majority. This would be self-defeating.

We are living in a very mobile society. The typical family moves on the average of every 5 years: six or seven times in a lifetime. Moving or being transferred from the community is a cause of unavoidable drop-outs, but new referrals must replace these patients. For this and other reasons, most doctors will maintain statistics to arrive at a drop-out versus referral ratio. When drop-outs exceed referrals, the practice is in trouble. When referrals exceed drop-outs, the practice is healthy and growing. Changes in trends of these figures serve as signals.

When a patient is dropped from the practice for whatever reason, be sure to make and keep copies of all pertinent records before passing them on to whoever takes over the case. Court records show that this type patient is more likely to file a malpractice action than any other patient the office may have treated. A special place in your files should be reserved for such case files.

Use "Address Correction Requested" on the outside of envelopes to ensure patients are at the addresses you have in the records. Even if your letter is forwarded, you'll never know that the patient has moved unless you use this "ACR" notification on your envelopes.

Handling Complaints and Criticisms

Healing Reactions. During the course of case management, it is not unusual for a few patients to experience new or exaggerated symptoms for a time. These symptoms are often the result of various structural and functional changes occurring during the normalizing process. While the doctor understands this, some patients may feel that the treatment is doing more harm than good. If a patient should mention such a "reaction," report this to the doctor immediately as the patient may fail to do so. The doctor will then explain to the patient what is happening and put the patient's fears at ease.

Slow Healing. Sometimes a patient with a chronic condition or long-standing disease process will complain about the slowness of recovery. It must be remembered that a disorder of long duration has been well established and may be characterized by various degenerative processes. Such conditions are often slow in recovery under the best treatment possible. When you become aware of patient discouragement, mention this to the doctor so he may counsel the patient accordingly. Patient discouragement and impatience are traits of the sick that are not difficult to understand. Complaints must be handled with poise, assurance, and empathy. Never treat them lightly.

Family Worries. While family criticisms are rare, they do arise occasionally. This especially occurs when a family member is severely ill or in distress. These criticisms usually come by way of the telephone, and most doctors will want to talk with these people. Some people, however, will impose on the doctor's time unnecessarily, and it is the CA's job to use her talents to reassure them without putting them through to the doctor immediately. Remember your feelings when a loved one is critically ill or in pain. Be considerate, but never enter a discussion regarding the patient's condition and the management of the case.

Symptom-Free vs Optimal Health. The typical patient's primary concern is to be free of symptoms and undertake a normal lifestyle. The doctor's primary concern is this too, but he is also interested in developing the patient's state of health to one of maximum resistance to recurrence of the condition. Sometimes the outward symptoms fade rapidly, while a true return to normal or maximum potential may take a much longer period. If the patient has not been educated to the need for extended care, he will have a tendency to quit the outlined program before maximum benefits have been achieved. If you recognize such anxiety within a patient, report this to the doctor so he may explain the facts and possible consequences of premature dismissal.

Whenever you are confronted with a complaint or criticism, be polite, stay calm, keep your voice soft and slow, and maintain a professional poise that is sympathetic with the patient's viewpoint. Let the patient express himself. Listen carefully; he may be right that a mistake has been made. Listen so you can obtain the facts. Listen between the words to seek a motive or unexpressed concern. Don't argue. When the patient has expressed himself, tactfully review the facts and separate facts from opinions. If you cannot handle the problem, tell the patient you will report the situation to the doctor to see how the problem can be resolved.

Coping with Negative Personalities

While it seems fundamental that the assistant must know how to cope with all types of people and to be helpful, courteous, kind, and considerate, these attributes are often taxed by the grumpy patient. Although most patients are enjoyable to meet, there is always a minority that appear irritable, unreasonable, and sometimes quite rude. Even in such a situation, the assistant must keep her control and composure, and maintain a friendly professional attitude.

Unreasonable Patients

The assistant must realize that the average irritable patient is not being personal. The patient is likely venting his spleen at the person available. Fear, discouragement, pain, fatigue, and anxiety are just a few factors contributing to such a patient's frame of mind. However, the experienced assistant knows that her cheerful and understanding attitude can do much to calm patients' fears and enhance a more positive attitude.

The typical reception room has people with varied needs and temperament. While most patients will be easy to relate to, you will occasionally have to cope with the ill-tempered complaining person who will upset the reception area atmosphere. When you see signs of impatience such as fidgeting, fussing, and grouching, be pleasant and reassuring. Always offer a courteous reason the doctor is late if the time is past the appointment schedule. Cranky and whiny children can often be placated with a coloring book or toy.

Irritability and stubbornness are often expressed as the result of fatigue, nervous tension, impatience with a chronic disorder, or worry. The patient may be openly contradictory. However, a CA's patience, understanding, and soothing personality will do much to calm and reassure the situation. The inconsiderate "troublemaker" who fumes and fusses, is argumentative and often misrepresents the facts can be handled without argument with poise, patience, and politeness.

Inconsiderate Patients

Inconsiderate "smart alec" patients will tax the assistant's poise. The "smart alec" is characterized by impatience, intolerance, egotistic and cocksure attitude of self-importance, and difficulty in responding to suggestions. Again, patience, understanding, and a positive sense of humor should be your response.

Indecisive Patients

Both deliberate and indecisive patients require special handling. The slow-moving, indecisive, slow-thinking, and overly careful patient should be talked with in a slow, deliberate, and clear manner. Instructions must be carefully made point by point, and then reviewed point by point. "Reasons why" must be offered to make instructions logical.

Timid Patients

The timid patient, like the indecisive patient, has difficulty in making up his mind—especially when alternatives are presented. When you talk with this type of patient, offer facts and features and place emphasis on the personal benefits involved. Offer messages confidently, clearly, and enthusiastically.

Suspicious Patients

Every office has its share of suspicious patients that measure your understanding of human nature. The suspicious patient will doubt the doctor's judgment, doubt your sincerity, and be cynical of his future. Handle the situation by instilling hope through logical, clear explanations.

Snobbish Patients

Snobs are recognized by their constant attempt to "put down" you, the doctor, the profession, or all healing arts in general. Their slighting remarks and airs of superiority require a rigid professional attitude, firm politeness, and understanding that the snobbish are frequently overcompensating for strong feelings of inferiority within themselves.

Chattering Patients

The patient who babbles endlessly usually does so in sentences without meaning or direction. The habit is, essentially, just a means to release inner tension through self-expression. Be tactful and tolerant, and try to guide the conversation to a meaningful subject by courteously directing and closing conversations. Beware of becoming involved in gossip or rumors. They are favorite subjects of a chattering patient.

Lessons from the World of Business

The doctor is not a businessman, yet the businessman can tell the doctor much about human relations. As the customer is the most important person to the businessman, the patient is the most important person to a doctor. The patient is the purpose of all activity of the practice. Remember that the doctor and his assistants are more dependent on the patient than the patient is on the practice. The patient can go elsewhere and achieve comparable services. The practice is being favored by offering the staff an opportunity to serve. Misguided physicians and assistants sometimes have this truth reversed.

Yes, the business world recognizes the value of its customers. Elaborate systems are maintained to keep in frequent contact with customers, enhance good will, and maintain customer and product loyalty. Business constantly studies the wants and needs of its customers. Business seeks answers to why customers buy or stop buying. Everything possible is done to develop this most valuable asset of any business—the customer.

Control of the Situation

The typical patient entering a doctor's office seeks help. To help the patient, the doctor must have control in the doctor-patient relationship. This control is founded on a desire to serve the best interests of the patient at all times. All physical and personality characteristics of the staff should reflect this attitude. If the doctor and his assistants do not understand the desires and needs of a patient, the patient will not be inclined to follow instructions or might be motivated to seek fulfillment elsewhere. The practice not only loses face, it loses an opportunity to serve and ultimately suffers an economic loss. Thus, control is necessary to maintain positive patient relations and safeguard the financial stability of the practice.

CHILDREN IN THE OFFICE

Any chiropractic practice adopting the philosophy of preventive therapy should emphasize the treatment of children, for childhood presents the golden age of prevention. Care during childhood can often foresee serious consequences of apparently slight abnormalities, thus offering the best time to take preventive measures.

The Child Visitor

Besides the child patient, a parent may visit the doctor accompanied by one or more children. Caring for these children when the patient is attended is often the responsibility of an assistant.

The Child Patient

From a human relations viewpoint, children within a practice offer a stabilizing factor. The child patient of today is the adult patient of tomorrow. If cared for intelligently, a child will become a worthy patient. Children complain little, are unobservant of minor inefficiencies, do not worry about fees, and are unaware of trifling inconveniences often irritating to adults. In cases where the child is the patient, it is the parent who is more often a problem than the child.

The child is preoccupied with self. Cooperation is ensured if the child is understood at his level and gentleness, kindness, and patience are offered. The child who likes the doctor and his assistants becomes an automatic booster for the practice. He will tell of his experiences to his immediate family, relatives, school chums, neighbors, and teachers. This is always beneficial to the practice: positive public relations.

The Frightened or Timid Child

The assistant may have to cope with the frightened or timid child. The correct approach to use is determined by the child's age and temperament. The technique is to put yourself in the child's place and communicate with the patient in a manner the child understands at the particular age and temperament presented. With any child, you must (1) win confidence, (2) arouse interest, and (3) gain cooperation. Any child, as any adult, is a distinct personality that must be approached according to that person's nature.

The doctor's office may arouse fear within the child. The surroundings are new and strange; the people are new and strange; the equipment may be new and strange. The child's previous experience in a doctor's office may have resulted in a painful experience or a morbid fear of injections is associated with any doctor's office. Such fears should never be responded to by glib remarks of reassurance, laughter, or labeling the child a "sissy." On the other hand, both mother and child should be told what a good patient the child is when the child is cooperative.

The unexpected is as frightening to the typical child as a painful experience. When children are old enough to comprehend that a procedure may cause some discomfort, they should be told beforehand and an appeal made to their braveness and "grown-up" courage. If you tell a child a procedure will not hurt and it does, confidence will be lost and you will have a difficult time being believed again. Tell the truth, and emphasize how much better the child will feel when he gets better.

Never underestimate the intelligence of the child patient. Children are keen observers, are more intelligent, and absorb much more than adults suspect. This is also true when you are speaking with a parent and you do not think the child is listening. Likewise, don't feel that the child fully understands just because he nods his head up and down in agreement.

The frightened or timid younger child is witnessed by the patient clinging to the parent's hand and being "dragged" reluctantly from room to room. Such a child, however, is usually quite intelligent and observant of every movement of you and the doctor. Under extreme suspense during examina-

tion and therapy, the frightened child will be tense and rigid. Thus, it is necessary at first to spend time to acquaint him with each procedure, explain what will be done and how, tell about the use of instruments to be employed, and win confidence beforehand.

The Bashful Child

The bashful child usually acts in a manner similar to the frightened child except for not expressing abnormal tenseness. He often holds his mother's hand in a relaxed manner, expressing a sense of freedom and curiosity while he nuzzles the parent and uses his thumb or a finger as a pacifier. Such children usually adapt to discomfort well when handled kindly and tend to hold back tears if their tolerance is not exceeded. The jovial attitude of others can do much to bring the bashful child out of his "shell."

The Moody Child

A moody child may fluctuate from cooperativeness at one moment to hostility at another. Such moods usually reflect some casual remark made by some adult, or they may be a method to control the parent by extending or withholding cooperation. The doctor may wish to treat such a child without the presence of a parent or to ignore the situation and proceed as usual without comment.

The Hysterical Child

The assistant usually will not have the training to handle a truly hysterical child. This takes professional training that may require a stern measure. Hysteria may be an effect of fear or used as a psychologic weapon. Parents of a hysterical child should not be permitted in the treatment room.

The Unmanageable or Temperamental Child

The apparent unmanageable or temperamental child is rarely as bad as he may seem on the surface. The attitude usually reflects fears from experiences based more on the child's imagination than reality. These cases can be handled with gentleness, patience in explanations, and assurance that the patient will not be tricked in some manner. The development of confidence in you and the doctor is primary. This type of child should be treated alone, not in the presence of a parent, where the "chip on the shoulder" has little impression. Children of this nature respond exceptionally well to staff once they are convinced that you mean to do what you have to do and there is no alternative.

Significance of Age Groups

Infant Care

A newborn child presents the least difficulty. If crying cannot be pacified and adult patients appear irritated, the parent should be asked to take the child to a private room until the doctor can see the patient.

During examination and therapy, your assistance may be necessary to support a small baby to prevent the child from squirming from the doctor's grasp. If the examination or treatment room is drafty or chilly, it may be necessary to wrap the baby in a blanket, exposing only that part necessary for examination or treatment.

Childhood

When the assistant makes appointments for several children on the same day, many doctors feel that the appointments should be grouped if possible. Children appear more cooperative when they are together and not left entirely in an environment of strange adults. However, siblings of the same sex are often jealous of attention, competitive, and restless.

Childhood, which extends from infancy to adolescence, evolves the child from a state of biologic helplessness to that of mature self-dependence. Between these extremes, many changes are witnessed (some normal and some abnormal) in the child's structural, functional, and emotional development.

About the age of 2 years, the average child begins to understand simple instructions and can often be coaxed into cooperation. Between the ages of 2 and 6, the child's attention span is short, the body is restless, the mind resists discipline, and contrary acts of will are obvious. Equipment must be guarded as the urge to destroy is common. This period between 2 and 6 years is the most difficult age group to deal with, not only because of the child but because a reprimand may bring resentment from a parent.

After the age of 6, reason can be appealed to according to the child's intelligence level. During the period between 6 and 12 years, the child develops reasoning and independence that is not so easily placated by a toy or cute comment. Self-interest evolves to a greater interest in the world about him, and curiosity arouses to a greater degree. By communicating with such a child in a serious manner, avoiding deflating attitudes, and handling him in a somewhat adult manner, security, relaxation, and cooperation of the patient are achieved. Bright children have a tendency to throw tantrums because they are alert to the effectiveness of the weapon. Such a tantrum is not true hysteria; it is an act that requires the doctor's management.

With the onset of the teen years, both boys and girls often resent having a parent present during consultation, examination, and therapy. The assistant must use great diplomacy in separating child from parent.

Both doctor and assistant must express constant enthusiasm toward the child patient, striving to make the event of the visit a happy occasion rather than a chore. All ethical means should be used to impress the child favorably that he is more than a little person in an adult world. The child must be impressed that you are interested in him as an individual and concerned about his welfare.

Practices handling many children are the least altered by economic trends. The reason for this is that parents want to give their children every possible advantage, even if it takes financial hardship and personal sacrifice. Despite family budget, anything that benefits the child's welfare is a justifiable expense.

Managing the Child-Patient's Parents

Parents are important aspects to consider in the care of children. Not only is a parent part of the situation in the office, the parent is involved in the child's case management, home treatment, and possibly as a factor in the condition under treatment.

Although both parents may accompany a child patient on a visit to the office, it is usually the mother. Either parent can be a great help to the doctor in the child's case management or the mother or father may be possessive, unreasonable, or blinded to the actual situation at hand. Sometimes a child is easily managed in the presence of a parent, sometimes not, and at other times it may be better to allow the child to decide.

The Intruding Parent

When a child is asked to do something, a child's reaction time between suggestion and action is longer than in the adult even when the child is willing. Sometimes a parent feels she is helping the doctor when she constantly repeats every directive of the doctor to the child. The parent's constant intrusion at this point of seemingly delayed reaction tends to confuse the child-patient and hinders the doctor-patient relationship. The parent's repetition intimates that the child is retarded or has a hearing problem. The same is true in the assistant-patient relationship. If you ask the child to "step on the scale to be weighed," the parent may follow with, "Billy, step up on the scale." When you ask, "Bill, turn around and face me," the parent repeats instantly, "Turn around, dear, and face the lady." In such instances, a tactful, "I believe Billy understands" will usually suffice.

The Overly Sympathetic Parent

The too sympathetic parent can be a problem at times. Such a parent constantly reminds the child that she knows just how much the child is hurting or feeling. The result is magnification of the condition in the child's mind. Without such reinforcement,

the child might be more cooperative. It is easy for a child to become unmanageable when subjected to this constant excessively sympathetic routine. One must be tactful and firm in requesting the parent not to talk to the patient while the child is being examined or treated unless it's absolutely necessary.

Parent Consultation

The first time a parent calls to make an appointment for a child is the best time for the assistant to state the office's policy regarding child care. The doctor may first want to see the parent alone on the first visit unless there is an emergency or the child is in pain. If an assistant is not available to tend to the child during the doctor-parent consultation, the parent should be asked to bring another adult with her during the visit.

By interviewing the parent alone, considerable information can be obtained about the child, and the doctor has an opportunity to explain the reasons behind office policy in child care. This tends to relax the parent, condition the parent of what to expect, and gain cooperation from the parent from the beginning.

Parental Communication During Treatment

When children are under treatment, the assistant should be prepared to handle an increased number of telephone calls. Most of these calls can be handled by the assistant once she becomes acquainted with the parents, child's condition, and treatment plan. It is important for the assistant to discuss this policy with the doctor-employer to determine what questions she should respond and which questions should be referred to the doctor. Frequently, the doctor will prepare a list of questions from which she will question the parent; eg, temperature, pain or distress, breathing difficulty, vomiting, diarrhea, and last meal?

Mothers often like to discuss with the assistant home treatment prescribed by the doctor. They may feel that another woman's viewpoint will help to clear their understanding. If the assistant is familiar with the instructions, she should offer an explanation in nontechnical terms and/or provide printed instructions approved by the doctor.

History Taking and Its Rationale

If it is the duty of the assistant to take a portion of the history, details should be listed regarding the child-patient's eating habits (including the amount of sweets and soft drinks), sleeping habits, recreation and exercise habits, and general behavior and temperament. Avoid vague and generalized answers.

In recording a child's history, data concerning development and past illnesses and disorders are important. Those conditions having adversely affected normal growth and development constitute the developmental history. Severe vitamin deficiencies (eg, rickets), endocrine disorders (eg, hypo- or hyper-thyroidism), and metabolic disorders may have an effect on skeletal growth and muscular function. The age of occurrence of such disorders is important to record. The age of walking and teething also should be noted.

A record of the child's present and past health status represents the *medical history*. The parent should be questioned regarding the child's birth, the pregnancy in general, labor abnormalities, and whether instruments were used during delivery. Such childhood diseases as diphtheria, scarlet fever, measles, rheumatic fever, rickets, typhoid, allergies, etc, should be recorded accurately and in detail, along with unusual weight gain or loss. Special concern should be given to any spinal condition, past or present. Questions concerning abnormal shoe wear, irritability, manner of walking, frequency of headaches, general behavior, and "growing pains" are also significant.

Mensuration

Most growth normally occurs in three cycles classified as the infantile period (*in utero* to 2 years), the juvenile period (from 8 to 11 years), and the adolescent period (from 13 to 17 years). Normal growth within any of these periods may be influenced by under- or over-nutrition, disease, or trauma.

Structural growth, usually measured by standing height and limb measurements, does not occur in an uninterrupted, smooth, even, bilateral manner. Both the body as a whole and its individual parts go through periods characterized by acceleration and retardation.

The doctor may ask the assistant to take several measurements of the child-patient. In general, the length of the extremities from the sole of the foot to the pubis should be approximately ⅜ of total body length during normal infancy. This relationship gradually changes with age until the pubis is approximately at the midpoint of the total length of the body. Structural measurements should always be taken bilaterally when extremities are measured. The information gathered is important in disorders of the extremities, especially those involving the epiphyses.

The Initial Examination

After the doctor reviews and enhances the history taken by the assistant, an examination will be scheduled. The examination of a child and that of an adult is similar except for age factors. The doctor's observation faculties must be much greater, however, as the child has more difficulty in expressing subjective feelings or describing an accurate picture of a complaint.

Office Rules and Procedures

Special rules and procedures must be established within the practice if child care is to be emphasized and made pleasant, efficient, and profitable. Several aids are explained below.

Special Hours. Special hours on certain days can be reserved for the treatment of children. They will feel more at home in the presence of other children. From a public relations standpoint, the grouping also educates other parents of the need for chiropractic care for all children of all ages. As children appear to be more cooperative in the morning, the best hours for scheduling younger children are from 9:30 to 11:30 am. Printed excuses can be used to schedule high school students during school hours.

Special Attitude. A special attitude is necessary in the care of children from the moment the child enters the reception room to the time of dismissal. The behavior of both assistant and doctor is largely reflected in the child's attitude. Every impression instilled during points of contact is important. Each procedure offered must be carefully limited to the capacity of the child's tolerance.

While everybody appreciates and remembers kindness and friendliness, children tend to do so more than adults. Children in the office are little strangers, afraid of a world they never made. By nature, they are apprehensive of changes in routine procedures, thus consistency is important. At the same time, children will usually take to new procedures more rapidly than adults if a change is explained and care is taken to develop their enthusiasm. As with adults, the most important factor before beginning any procedure is to get the patient relaxed and in a receptive frame of mind. Any professional method that attains patient relaxation is well worth the effort.

Preconditioning. It is often a good policy to have the assistant spend some time with the child-patient prior to entrance of the doctor. An understanding assistant can do much to ease the child's fear and develop confidence in the doctor to enhance an excellent doctor-patient relationship. If an assistant asks the child about his hobbies, interests, and likes and dislikes, answers questions about equipment and procedures, and reassures the child that there is nothing to fear, the child is conditioned to accept the whole procedure as a pleasant experience and will be receptive to the doctor when introduced. Such attention flatters the child's ego and makes him feel a VIP. He will be more relaxed, more suggestible, and more responsive to the doctor's presence. Confidence and cooperation will be almost assured.

Testing. Certain tests must be given to children just as they are to adults. The need for imagination when dealing with children is obvious. As children have a tendency to get excited, it is important to calm them before testing. For this reason, basal metabolism tests on youngsters under 6 years of age are rarely accurate. It is helpful with young children to divert their attention and calm them by telling them a story or make a game of the procedure. The mouthpiece of a basal metabolic rate (BMR) instrument, for example, can be likened to the oxygen mask of a space ship.

Home Safety Instruction. It is important that the assistant help the doctor in teaching safety measures when a parent is in the office. All parents should be warned to keep medicine out of the reach of children, flush old medicines down the toilet, and practice good safety habits in the home. Young children should be taught to avoid matches, gas stoves, electric appliances, cleaning fluids, poisons and pesticides, slippery surfaces, and climbing on ladders and trees. The safe use of sharp instruments such as scissors and knives should be taught. Once older children are taught the proper use of such things, they no longer need be hidden.

Office Safety. The assistant must be constantly aware of safety measures so that accident prevention is primary. Cautionary vigilance is imperative. Children should never be left in a room alone. Their imagination can become so overactive that it results in mischief. The doctor should summon the assistant if a child must be left in a room and a parent is not present. One should not be surprised when a child, who is not sufficiently matured, reacts to animal instincts. When an unsupervised child gives vent to inherited traits, such actions must be understood by the assistant and reacted to with calmness and understanding. With small tots, toys are often important. Avoid toys with sharp edges, small objects that may be swallowed, things that might break easily, or toys that require running or jumping. Building blocks, coloring books, rubber or clean stuffed animals, and animated picture books are common choices.

Scheduling Control. The doctor of chiropractic may accept many cases of behavior disorders such as retardation, hyperkinesia, severe nervousness, or temper tantrums or tics. Thus it is important that waiting time be held at a minimum. This requires alert scheduling. If the patient is late, time from the appointment reservation must be deducted so that the next appointment can be taken on time with a minimum of waiting. Waiting adds to tension. Kindness, special consideration, and efficiency are essential in such case management. To reduce waiting time to a minimum, try to have everything possible in readiness beforehand. If waiting is unavoidable, children love to hear stories. Learn to be a good story teller.

Periodic Check-Ups. In most practices, children will be scheduled for check-ups before vacations, camps, and supervised sports, and before school opens. Because these appointments will likely be made in June and August, the assistant in charge of scheduling must anticipate time for these children.

Confidential Information. The law also protects clinical data of a minor from all but a parent or guardian. Overdoting relatives may telephone and inquire about a child's health. Never release any information without the consent of the parent or guardian. Refer all inquiries to the parent or guardian.

Third-Party Forms. Schools and camps may require certain forms to be completed. The assistant will usually fill these forms out for the doctor's signature. If a vaccination history is required, this must be reported by the parent to an MD or DO.

Building Positive Relationships with Children

When a child's enthusiasm is properly cultivated and stimulated, the child can do much to the indirect education of parents, friends, relatives, and acquaintances to the value of chiropractic services. To develop this state of mind, several factors should be considered. Following are some thoughts to enlist in developing better cooperation of both child patient and parent.

Self-Image Development

Children love flattery regardless of their age. Boys like to hear that they are brave, have good bodies, and have the ability to be an athletic champion if they work at it. Girls like to be complimented on their beauty, form, dress, and potential ability to become wonderful dancers, ballerinas, and attractive to boys. Flattery helps to solidify the office-patient relationship.

Remember that better results are obtained and a closer relationship can be established in many instances if parents of an older child patient are excluded from the examining and treatment rooms. Nothing will yield better dividends in health care than gaining the patient's confidence and satisfaction by minimizing fears and anxieties.

Communication

A child should be spoken with at his level of understanding and recognized as a unique individual. Speak to the child as much as possible in an adult manner so that his consciousness will be raised rather than relating to him as a "mere child." At the same time, never exceed the child's level too much. Stoop when you speak so that you are at the same head level, eliminating the image of a very large and overpowering person.

When special instructions are given to the child to execute outside the office, instructions should be given directly to the child (if he can comprehend) in the presence of a parent. This flatters the ego of the child who then feels important and responsible. The presence of the parent offers third party assistance if recall is necessary.

Avoid giving a direct command to a child or using a paternal attitude. It may arouse opposition as the child gets enough of this at home and school. By putting your instructions in the form of a request or suggestion the child will more happily comply with what you desire.

Both doctor and assistant should choose their words carefully in communicating to children who do not quite understand their meaning. Words such as manipulation, regulate, disciplines, and other technical jargon often stir the imagination to fearful anticipations. Never discuss details of techniques or procedures in front of the child-patient. The doctor will only discuss a child's unfavorable prognosis with a parent in private. Any child's questions should be answered honestly in terms the child can comprehend. While unpleasant details can be minimized, a good relationship will be broken if the child learns he has been lied to or tricked.

High-quality educational material geared to the child's level should be in the reception room, just as it should be for the adult level. The ACA has an excellent coloring book and several pieces of child-oriented literature available.

Special Attention Pays Dividends in Human Relations

Most doctors will not treat a child-patient with a chronic condition on the first visit or will only offer a simple prophylactic therapy. This allows the child time to evaluate the office, staff, and surroundings and arrive at the conclusion there is nothing to worry about. Much can be accomplished during the first visit if nothing more is done but to wean the child from his worries, fears, tensions, and apprehensions. Winning of confidence is the goal. When the child leaves the office smiling, a good relationship is ensured.

Special recognition is deeply appreciated by a child. It is good office policy to record birth dates and send a card in remembrance. Send children a special valentine from the doctor and staff. Offer companionship to the older child-patient showing you appreciate the patient's intelligence and maturity by, within reason, liking things he likes and not liking things he doesn't like. Show interest in the child's skills and hobbies, and note these in the patient's records as a reminder.

It is policy in many offices that every new young child-patient be given some sort of gift when he leaves the office for the first time; eg, a balloon, set of crayons, coloring book, rubber ball, or ice cream cone certificate. This special attention endears the child to the office and increases the desire to return. It is not so much the value of the gift as it is the instilling in the child that you feel he is someone special.

When children are frequent visitors to the office, various gadgets are helpful. For instance, lollipops have proved to be standard equipment in many offices as excellent tranquilizers of younger children. If an assortment is available, let the child choose the flavor. It adds to the pleasure and feeling of self-importance. However, never use such a device as a bribe for good conduct. Rather, use it as a reward for good conduct.

Children take their play very seriously, but sometimes you may have to take the time to point out certain possibilities. Give the child only one toy at a time. Once he tires of it, give him another. A "kiddie korner" equipped with a small table and chairs can be adapted within a 4-foot by 4-foot space in most reception rooms if many children are cared for in the practice. Such a space makes small children feel at home, minimizes disciplinary problems, and alerts the casual adult patient that the practice is concerned with the health care of children.

While relationships with child-patients should be cordial and friendly, they should not become *too* familiar. A respectful distance must be maintained or it will stymie respect and require discipline. Be friendly in a reserved manner. Children are not adults, thus they must always be understood and handled as children.

THE ELDERLY IN THE OFFICE

Because of the high incidence of degenerative musculoskeletal diseases, elderly patients are seen in chiropractic offices far more than children. As with the very young, the very old require more time, patience, assistance, and closer attention.

Age Considerations

The process of aging begins at birth and stops only with death. It is a gradual process. Changes occur in a fairly predictable pattern, but the rate of change varies from one individual to another. Old age is a period often marked by mental confusion and vagueness, and this must be considered in extending aid. Chronological age, however, does not make a person young or old. Some people are young in spirit and alert mentally at 90 years and others are old at 25 years. The chronological age of 65, however, is arbitrarily considered the dividing line point between middle age and old age.

Special Human Relations Considerations

As a group, the elderly tend to be talkative yet secretive, and sometimes hostile, rude, and childish, but their remarks should not be taken personally. Most of their hostility comes just from the resentment of the effects of growing old.

Assistant Maturity. Attendants should be nonjudgmental, stable, and even-tempered—attributes known as maturity. A mature assistant will possess self-respect and pass this respect to others through kindness, tolerance, and patience for the elderly. Sincere interest and gentleness is deeply appreciated. However, old people detest and are quick to recognize insincerity. Communicate slowly and distinctively without appearing patronizing.

Schedule Logically. An elderly patient usually will take more time than a young adult. The appointment assistant should be aware of this and schedule accordingly. Do not rush elderly patients. As mentioned, it will injure their self-esteem.

Develop Empathy. Probably the most important attribute necessary in caring for the elderly is empathy. This takes a projection of one's personality into the problems and personality of another person. It takes imagination. For example, imagine that you are a person who has lost your job, lost most of your friends, lost a part of your hearing and vision, lost many of your teeth, lost your ability to speak fluently and decide quickly, and lost much of your health and pride. Then replace these losses with new pains, stiff joints, a slumped posture, circulatory deficiencies, constipation, and the embar-

rassment of being unable to do simple tasks and remember a recent conversation. If you can imagine this and appreciate the feelings involved, you will have empathy for the elderly. It is no wonder that their insecurity is often expressed as hostility.

Preserve Pride. It will often seem easier and quicker to do something for the elderly patient rather than let him do it for himself because it takes him so long. However, oversolicitousness will force him into a dependent role—a role he does not want and one that is incompatible with a healthy outlook on life. Avoid the temptation to "take over." The aim of proper assistance is to permit the patient to do as much for himself as he can, with only a minimum of assistance. His small accomplishments will mean much to him. Help patients to help themselves, and always ask if assistance would be helpful before giving it. Most elderly people guard their independence. Respect this.

Special Considerations of Trauma

Age is often a distinct factor in many musculoskeletal injuries. As a group, older people are susceptible to fractures. Their vision and hearing may be impaired, increasing the possibilities of accidents. Atrophy of bone and connective tissue occurring as part of the aging process may also increase susceptibility to fracture, sprain, and strain. Additionally, the elderly may be poorly nourished, poorly coordinated, have a decline in postural stability, and have difficulty walking. With advanced aging, one's level of proficiency progressively deteriorates.

Senior citizens may have disorders predisposing to a variety of complicating disorders; eg, cerebral ischemia, osteoporosis, arthritis, postural hypotension, weakness, and neurologic disorders that affect locomotion. While such disorders predispose a person of any age to injury, the elderly are particularly at risk because of concomitant factors that accompany advanced age.

Musculoskeletal injuries of the elderly range in severity from relatively minor soft-tissue injuries to severe crushing fractures.

Older females are especially prone to fractures. Males, as a group, most commonly sustain fractures in their younger years, up to the age of 45.

ADDING THE PERSONAL TOUCH

It has been emphasized throughout this chapter that any individual who is sick, in pain, or worried must be dealt with in an atmosphere of understanding and consideration. When health is lost, a sense of security is lost, and that person is operating on the motivation level of self-preservation and threatened personal safety.

A Review of Fundamentals

While the doctor's diagnostic and therapeutic skills help to restore confidence and relieve some patient stress, a strictly scientific approach is not enough. The patient's emotions and frame of mind also must be considered. The patient looks to the doctor and staff for friendship, understanding, and recognition as a special human being rather than a *case*. The state of rapport between patient and office staff can be as important as the technical service.

Office staff should at every opportunity be kind and empathetic to every patient. Sincere interest in the patient and the patient's problems should be expressed. Remember that the apprehensive new patient to the office enters new surroundings, experiences odors from antiseptics, sees strange equipment, and confronts new personalities with which to cope. There are many fears and anxieties about fees, what the doctor may do or recommend, debts, and loss of income from services. Without proper understanding, an assistant may view such patients as "difficult," yet it is not abnormal if a patient should appear nervous and irritable.

While a patient's feelings may be held from the doctor's view, they are often openly expressed to an assistant. The assistant, however, should never take this personal.

The patient is only "letting off steam" from an internal "boiler" the best way he can at the moment. By establishing a pleasant relationship from the start, by obtaining friendly cooperation, by being patient without condescension, and by avoiding anything that would contribute to increased patient tension, the assistant is far ahead in establishing positive patient relations.

A competent physician, a spotless office, and shiny equipment are not substitutes for kindness, friendliness, and personal interest from the doctor and his staff. To the patient, there is just one patient that counts despite the volume of patients that must be seen. Sometimes all that is needed is a smile and friendly remark and a feeling that he is not being hurried in one door and out the other.

Patients appreciate the personal touch. As the doctor rarely has the time, a telephone call from an assistant to discuss progress is always appreciated, but it must have the doctor's permission. Good scheduling avoiding prolonged waiting time is also appreciated for it shows respect for the patient's time. Thus, delays should be explained with regret.

As unfortunate patients may visit the doctor, the assistant should be careful not to display revulsion, antagonism, or condescending airs to those who are disfigured, maimed, scarred, or handicapped; those with tic, spastic tremors, parkinsonian movements; or those with ugly skin conditions. Nor should these afflictions be ignored. The patient knows his condition, and so do you. Don't make believe that the patient isn't what he is. This is unrealistic and not appreciated. Hold a positive attitude, radiate confidence, build good cheer, be optimistic, and the patient will too.

This positive attitude does not erase the fact that there will be problem patients. Some will be chronically late or tardy, some uncooperative, some fail to follow instructions, some will use crude language, and some will unfairly criticize the practice and its procedures and policies. Remain professionally firm and tactful in such instances. Despite experiences, each patient should be greeted with a smile on entering and leaving the office. The patient should leave with the feeling that the visit was important, he or she is important, and the scheduled return visit is important.

Patients appreciate "extra" services beyond expected technical services. Service organizations go to great lengths to offer their clientele extra but highly important auxiliary services. In the personalized chiropractic office, these extra services may be home-therapy equipment such as braces available for loan, a lending library, bus schedules, travel tips, a simple beverage while waiting, placing a call for a taxi, or some other "extra" service.

The Role of Office Records

All offices should maintain accurate and comprehensive clinical and financial records. The need for this will be explained in future chapters. As all patients are different and present different variations in disorders, such records serve to provide better health service. But if we wish to serve the *total* person, there is a need to custom-design technical services to be harmonious with patient's emotional needs.

When office records also incorporate personal data about each patient such as special interests, hobbies, likes and dislikes, aspirations, etc, doctor and assistant are more able to speak "in the patient's language." The power of persuasion will be increased many fold when you know how to explain office procedures and policies in terms of patient interests.

Personal Public Relations

As a representative of the office, every contact between you and a patient within the office and every contact between you and a person outside the office subtly affects the doctor's reputation. Negative attitudes on your part discourage patients from returning and discourage others from entering the practice. The assistant who constantly creates good will wherever she goes is a distinct practice builder. Everyone likes the friendly, sympathetic, pleasant assistant who is truly interested in people as individuals. This interest is shown by remembering people by name; by being interested in their children, work, and hobbies; and by being a good listener.

The Art of Communication

The more you know about a patient without appearing inquisitive, the more effectively you can communicate with that person. The person's home address, clothing, posture, car, gestures and other body language, occupation, hobbies, and educational background can tell you much. By listening carefully to what the patient talks about, you can become alert to his likes, dislikes, worries, self-image, pride, and aspirations. You can soon learn how the person arrives at a decision, how he reacts to a motivational block, and what "special interests" he reveals only to those whom he feels close. Knowing such things allows "personalization" of the approach. You will then be able to explain complicated subjects by using analogies meaningful to the patient. You can draw parallels that ease tensions and develop inspiration.

If you listen carefully to the patient, you will be able to use the patient's key words in feedback to convey you understand what the patient feels and means to say. By paraphrasing the patient's words, you also will be able to instruct the patient in terms he will understand. This act serves to reinforce rapport, enhance the patient's ego in that you "talk the same language," and invite the patient to drop some communication defenses because you have proved you were closely paying attention and are interested.

This is not a new technique: it has long been used by successful salesmen, marketing experts, and others. In the June 1965 issue of *Reader's Digest*, within an article titled "The Delicate Art of Asking Questions," John K. Langemann states:

There is a powerful tool that many professional counselors—clinical psychologists, doctor, ministers—have learned to use in getting to the bottom of personal problems that people bring to them. Instead of trying to reassemble the facts (who said or did what to whom) or to give specific advice, they listen for and encourage all expressions of *feeling*, however faint or fleeting. In statements that begin "I feel," "I wish," or "I don't care if. . . ," the interviewer acknowledges, perhaps by repeating their content. Or he may just note, "You feel very strongly about that, don't you?" or "Is that so?" Having feelings recognized without judgment or criticism often has an almost magical effect in making a person open up. The truth comes out, and with it, often self-insight.

Appealing to a Patient's Inner Needs

Positive relations based on a sound understanding of human nature has both clinical and economic benefits. It has been proven that a patient with a positive attitude will heal quicker than one with a negative attitude. On the other hand, a positive mental attitude in the doctor and assistant enhances the effect of professional skill. From a practice standpoint, it keeps established patients associated with the practice and encourages referrals that attract new patients to the practice.

Because there undoubtedly will be equally competent and equipped offices in your area, it will be human relations factors that differentiate your office from another. It will be human relations factors that determine which practice patients enter, remain, and boost. Competent health service can be found somewhere; special humanized service is more difficult to find. People will go where their thirst for personalized attention can be satisfied to some degree when other factors are equal. Many doctors and assistants literally force some patients out of the practice simply by failing to nourish emotional hungers.

We are living in a highly technologic-oriented society. We are classified by codes and numbers, and our lives appear to be manipulated by computers and indifferent "red tape." Yet our inner needs for individuality often go begging for recognition and attention. The average person today is not looking for professional competency, sophisticated technology, or efficient case administration. These factors are expected—taken

for granted. The quest is for warmth, reassurance, appreciation, and personal recognition.

Just as a business having an abundance of excellent technology can operate in the red, so can a health practice. On the other hand, it is not unusual for a business or a health practice to double its income in a few years once it recognizes the importance of serving people's inner as well as outer needs.

During the initial interview, you may learn that a patient has been switching from one practice to another for the same condition. This is a clue that emotional needs went begging. The reasons offered will be endless, but rarely will they be the true reason for changing from doctor to doctor. Here are some thoughts that probably enter the patient's mind many times:

- "I was kept waiting for long periods. My time was considered unimportant."
- "I was treated like a child."
- "I was hurried here and there, and nobody had the time to listen to me."
- "I was just another case to them."
- "I was criticized when I suggested a second opinion from a specialist."
- "I couldn't understand what they were doing or why they wanted to do it. They talked in highly technical language."
- "My complaints were belittled and made light of."
- "I wasn't a human being to them. I was the 2 o'clock insurance whiplash."
- "They played favorites, and I found this insulting."

If we analyze these complaints carefully, we come to one conclusion. All the reasons listed involve insults to the patient's ego. They all said in unspoken words, "You don't count" or "You're not important."

Several years ago, before the Conference of TransCanada Medical Plans, Dr. Ernest Dichter reported on the conclusions of his motivational studies in business and the professions. One of his statements is pertinent to this topic:

Summarizing our findings, what had happened was that while the world was changing very rapidly; while the patient in this world was changing at least at the same pace; while all the medical equipment, medical knowledge and drugs were developing at an ever-increasing rate, the human aspect in the doctor-patient relationship had fallen behind. A psychological lag had taken place....

Fortunately, the chiropractic profession did not fall into this psychologic lag as has the allopathic profession. This is probably because the "human touch" is an integral part of chiropractic therapy and chiropractic has emphasized concern for the total individual.

Chiropractic physicians and their assistants have learned the importance of applying scientific know-how with positive human relations. They take the time to establish a personal rapport with each patient before giving impersonal instructions. The patient is given concentrated, undivided attention. People are truly listened to and professionally "catered." Patients are escorted in their choices rather than directed. The humanized chiropractic practice offers an abundance of "special" services and "extra" favors. The doctor directly makes referral appointments with specialists showing personalized concern. A patient's complaint or question is never made light of or belittled. Even if an assistant may be responsible for the administration of a procedure or therapy on a particular visit, the patient should never leave the office without visiting with the doctor.

Printed instructions should be preceded by oral explanation. Literature should be considered "reminders," not "recipes." If time permits, personalized typewritten instructions are better for they signal, "This is especially for you." In this regard, Robert Levoy in *The Successful Professional Practice* refers to Les Giblins' remark that "No girl likes to receive a carbon copied love letter."

Resolving and Preventing Complaints

A pessimist will react to a complaint as a personal put-down, while an optimist will react to a complaint as an opportunity for self-analysis. Some doctors and assistants think they live in a type of ivory tower because of their specialized training. Complaints are considered insults because they believe that patients do not have the *right* to complain. Yet these same professionals will take their car to a garage and tell the mechanic to "Change the oil, check the plugs and points, and repair the flat in the trunk." Most people would become highly indignant if the mechanic answered, "Don't tell me how to do my job. I know more about automobiles than you do. I was certified as a top mechanic in one of the best trade schools and have been working in this field for 25 years." Would not these professionals think, "But it's my car!"

When a person seeks service, even health service, he takes for granted that the agency has personnel that are competent and qualified. This does not mean that customers or patients do not have the right to ask questions, complain when they think service is below standard, or believe an oversight or error has been made. In fact, questions begging answers mean a person is interested. Disinterest is shown by the person who stops talking, becomes withdrawn. Thus, complaints and questions should not be reacted to as affronts to ability. When your reactions are negative, more complaints, questions, and objections are created.

There are many reasons why a patient may object, question, or complain. It is important that both the doctor and his assistants be prepared to respond in a professional, human, personalized manner. Here are a few examples:

1. *People need facts to support their position.* Chiropractic is a minority profession. It is probably the least understood healing art of the three major health provider groups. Because of this, a patient's neighbors, friends, relatives, or coworkers may not think the patient is doing the right thing by entering the practice. When a patient is exposed to negative comments and doubts, the patient needs answers to questions and concerns eased to defend his position against those who do not understand.

2. *People need to know what is being done and why it is being done.* Many chiro-

practic procedures are new to the patient. Apprehension is not unusual when a person is placed in a situation that is strange. Fear of the unknown is one of our greatest fears. Because we are unfamiliar, we fear making errors spotlighting our ignorance that would subject us to ridicule. Thus, it's normal that a person exposed to new ideas and "different" procedures will ask questions to gain a clear understanding of who, what, when, where, and why. Thus, avoid becoming irritated when you are asked even simple instructions to be repeated.

3. *People need conflicting thoughts resolved.* When conflict is not solved, anxiety results. Patient questions indicate a strong need for reassurance. They need reassurance that the x-ray films recommended are not dangerous as an article stated in some magazine. They need reassurance that a remark made by another doctor many years ago to the effect that "Chiropractic treatments may be harmful" is not true. They need reassurance that "deep heat" will not cause pain. Many patients realize that the doctor has gone to a great deal of trouble in consultation and examination to arrive at a differential diagnosis and recommend a treatment plan. The more "well read" the patient is, the more there is need to clarify misunderstandings, hearsay, and half-truths. A patient with conflicting thoughts is not usually seeking an alternative to the doctor's recommendations. He is seeking answers to why his generalized beliefs are not true in his particular case.

4. *People need adequate justification for their acts.* Gestalt psychology emphasizes that people really don't know why they act the way they do. Although we make a choice consciously, this conscious selection is based on many deeply subconscious beliefs (some rational, some not), conditioned reflexes, programmed responses, and fixed behavioral patterns of which we are unaware on the intellectual level of consciousness. While we may be aware how we feel, we are unable to know exactly *why* we feel this way. Thus, we must rationalize actions. When we want a new car or a new dress or suit, we buy it. We rationalize our actions in terms of "good quality," "will last a long time," "a good investment," "cheaper than repairing the old one," and other conscious justifications. Subconscious urges for status, selfishness, self-indulgence, ego gratification, etc, are repressed from conscious awareness for they would surely result in painful guilt and prevent us from having what we *want*. Therefore, when a diagnostic or therapeutic procedure is recommended or a treatment plan is prescribed, the patient's investment in time, money, and effort must be justified in harmony with personally accepted criteria. Quality health care "eases pain and discomfort," "safeguards against income loss," "enhances personal performance," "improves resistance," and so forth.

5. *People need their priorities put in proper perspective.* Most people have fixed sources of income, and their wants often exceed their means. We want a nice car, a comfortable home, attractive clothes, a swimming pool, exotic vacations, good education for our children, and the other good things in life. But these things are meaningless if we don't have our health. Thus, patients must be shown and convinced that health care is the priority consideration. They must be persuaded at times that professional services should not be postponed until "the patio is completed," "until the Christmas bonus comes in," or "the new business gets off the ground." Such excuses may seem highly irrelevant to those of us who work in health care, but they are not to the average patient. The patient must be continually educated, persuaded, and convinced of the value and benefits of professional services. This takes explanation, illustration, demonstration, and a large degree of "salesmanship" sometimes so the patient will want health care more than anything else. To nurture this frame of mind, the patient must be shown that the doctor's professional services are a means to achieve and appreciate other wants, goals, and needs. Health care is not an alternative to or an obstacle in the path of a patient's personal goal attainment.

6. *People need their self-concept reinforced.* It is often said that the profession of chiropractic reached its present status solely because it achieved results in cases

where traditional health-care methods failed. There is much truth in this, as the average person, habitually programmed by social forces, will risk deviating from the established pattern only when all conventional avenues have become exhausted and desperation forces considered of the irregular. Thus, many patients new to chiropractic health care are apprehensive. This tension can be relieved by showing patients that their selection was the right one. It can be brought out that great sports figures like quarter-miler Ken Randle, discus-thrower Mac Williams, and high-jumper Dwight Stones attribute much of their success to chiropractic. You may mention that Rocky Marciano and Muhammad Ali called for chiropractic care frequently, as have several professional golfers such as Arnold Palmer, many professional baseball players (including Babe Ruth), and four-time bowler of the year, Earl Anthony. John D. Rockefeller, Sr. and Hubert Humphrey were chiropractic supporters. Many famous past and present actors and actresses such as John Wayne, Bob Cummings, Jane Fonda, Carol Lawrence, Robert Goulet, to name a few, have been chiropractic patients. These famous personalities could afford the best, and they chose chiropractic care.

7. *People need to disguise their unfulfilled emotional needs.* Chronic complainers will not openly admit that the doctor or assistant is not fulfilling their needs for friendship, warmth, or reassurance to the degree expected. No, they disguise their disappointment by faultfinding, irritability, uncooperativeness, ignoring statements, and other methods "to get back at you." The patient who complains about almost everything is really trying to express dissatisfaction with the interpersonal relationship. Look for the reason such a patient feels insulted, ignored, belittled, or angered. Patient irritability, sulking, pouting, and other behavioral changes are signals that there has been some breakdown in positive human relations that needs immediate repair.

Throughout your career, review these seven points frequently. You will find them not only helpful in your relationships with patients, but also in your relationship with any person who complains about something with which you are associated. Naturally, some complaints from the patient's viewpoint have a logical rather than an emotional basis such as an error in a bill or exceedingly long waiting periods. Most complaints, however, will reflect other motives. In summary:

• People need facts to support their positions.
• People need to know what is being done and why it is being done.
• People need conflicting thoughts resolved.
• People need adequate justification for their acts.
• People need their priorities put in proper prospective.
• People need their self-concept reinforced.
• People need to disguise their unfulfilled emotional needs.

The public is becoming more critical of health-care practitioners each year, but this is not a new phenomenon. It has been growing for several years but only recognized by the most alert health-care personnel. The criticism is not technology oriented, it is human-relations oriented. As far back as December 1955, E. L. Koos, PhD, brought this out in an article titled "Metropolis, What City People Think of Their Medical Services," which was published in the *American Journal of Public Health* and copyrighted by the American Public Health Association, Inc. The article told of a study of 1,000 families selected at random in a city of 350,000. Dr. Koos reported:

1. There was almost no criticism of technical competence.
2. Only 19% thought health care cost too much.
3. As many as 47% criticized the physician's handling of his practice.
4. The greatest criticism involved the doctor-patient relationship.

Sixty-four percent of the replies indicated that modern, technic-centered medical practice lacked the human warmth of the old-time general practitioner (who possibly knew less about medicine, but more about his patients). Those who are defensive regarding criticisms of modern medical care have been known to charge that this attitude exists only among the older age groups who view the passing of the family doctor with nostalgia. Our data do not bear this out, for the respondents in the families with husbands under 40 years of age were even more definite in this criticism than were those in the older age group.... We can probably best sum up the position of the people of "Metropolis" regarding their medical care in these words: they tend to be *satisfied* with what they get and to accept its cost, but they *dislike the way it is provided.*

An assistant who has little knowledge of human nature tends to turn a deaf ear to complaints, while the trained assistant knows how to turn a complaint into an affirmation. The experienced assistant knows that a questioning patient is an interested patient, a participating patient, a person seeking answers who wants to be a good patient but needs help.

The Art of Gentle Persuasion

A good salesman will tell you that it is almost impossible to sell a person who says, "I agree with everything you say, but I don't want it." On the other hand, the average person will put up various specific reasons for not purchasing (objections, complaints, excuses). The good salesman will have a ready answer for each objection, knowing that when all objections are answered, the person is in a position where he must buy because his reasons for not buying have been erased through explanation, illustration, demonstration, and agreement with advantages of features and benefits. To understand this is to understand the gentle art of tough-minded persuasion.

Whenever the alert salesman is presented with a new objection for which he does not have a ready answer, he writes it down and later thinks of a good reply in case the objection should ever again be raised. Health-care personnel can learn a lesson from this

practice as most complaints are universal in the health-care field. When the same complaint becomes common, it is an indication that the subject matter has not been properly covered within the patient's orientation to the practice's procedures and policies.

There are several methods by which the assistant can be taught or learn from experience to cope with general patient complaints and turn dissatisfaction into inspiration. A few are listed below:

1. *If a patient asks a question that is difficult to answer, rephrase the question into one you can answer.* If a patient should ask, for example, "Why are the doctor's fees so high." you could respond, "If I understand you correctly, Mrs. Brown, you're asking if the doctor's fees are unusual for these types of services. I can assure you that Dr. Smith is very careful in seeing to it that his fees are based on those usual and customary throughout the community for identical services." Such a response to a patient's inquiry tells the patient that you were listening attentively, showed friendly respect in answering the question, but had to put the inquiry into proper perspective.

2. *Inexperienced assistants have a tendency to anticipate a complaint and attempt to answer it before it is fully given.* This is an error, for a patient may feel the interruption is a "brush off." It may be interpreted as "I don't want to hear you. I know what's best for you." When you refuse to listen attentively, you are telling patients you don't care, are not concerned, and have more important things to do than bother with them.

3. *Third-party testimony avoids being placed between a patient and his goal or a conflict in personalities.* This is done by prefacing your answer with such phrases as "According to national statistics," "Health-care surveys indicate that ... ," or "The latest figures state that...." For instance, if a patient should criticize the fact that the practice does not have evening hours, you might reply, "According to a recent national survey, most patients prefer daytime hours so they can spend evenings with their families and friends." By so doing, you divert the

patient's complaint to the statistics and benefits rather than office policy. Never try to prove that *you* are right. Let figures and statistics do that. It's always better to say, "It has been found that . . . ," rather than, "Our policy is. . . ."

4. *Avoid answering a direct question with a curt "yes" or "no."* Remember that more is at stake from a human-relations standpoint than an answer to a question. If a patient should ask, "Isn't it true that . . . ?," offer a "yes—but" reply. In other words, agree and then disagree. For example, "I felt that way once until I learned that . . . ," "Many people think that, but the majority feel . . . ," "What you say is certainly true sometimes, however . . . ," "I can understand your viewpoint, but recent evidence indicates. . . ." The patient must be handled as an intelligent person who has some slight misunderstanding. His complaint or question should be accepted as a logical occurrence from the individual's viewpoint. If he is in error, it's not his fault that his information was incomplete or inaccurate.

By being aware of reasons a patient may object, question, or complain, the assistant is in a better position to resolve and prevent poor human relations. Once the assistant masters the art of coping with complaints in a friendly manner, dissatisfaction can be converted into inspiration. The basic key to successful problem solving in the office is to be on the patient's side. Never appear to be an antagonist or a block to a patient's goal. This would be a "no-win" position.

Filling the Communications Gap

Self-preservation is one of our most basic urges. When we feel our health is threatened, we call on all our energies to return us to as normal as possible. Anyone who will help us has our respect. Any information that will help is appreciated. However, while the typical patient will crave for the whys and wherefores of his illness and treatment, he is also often timid in asking for answers to his worries and fears. On one hand the patient wants to know the facts, and on the other hand, he may be afraid to hear the truth. "No news is good news" is not the solution as the related anxiety still burns.

Answering Silent Concerns

When John Smith is ill, he wants to know why he is sick, what can be done to return his health, and how he can prevent the disorder from returning once it has been seemingly corrected. After being examined, he wants to know the details of what is wrong and what is right; what he must do and not do to speed recovery; how long it will take and how much it will cost; and answers to many other associated questions. He begs for answers even if he does not ask questions. He wants to understand. He wants a simple explanation, not Latin or Greek mumbo-jumbo. He wants his confidence built up, not his intelligence put down.

The patient needs and deserves an explanation. When a procedure is recommended, he wants to know "why?" When an abnormal condition is found, he wants to know what it means. When a certain therapy is applied, he wants to know why it will help. He wants to be informed before anything is performed, and he wants the explanation in a simple step-by-step manner that he can understand. He wants you and the doctor to explain what you are doing and why you are doing it before you do it. He wants you to vocalize the features and benefits of each of your actions. Always remember that many routine things you do are not routine to the patient. What may be obvious to you may be confusing or fearful to the patient.

Health care is a learning situation. Time and again it can be shown that the best-informed patient is the most motivated patient; the least-informed patient, the most uncooperative. We should be alert, however, to recognize that effective communication does not depend on how much is explained to the patient but on how the patient interprets what is said. A doctor or assistant may offer a "technically correct" explanation that is completely misinterpreted by a patient. Patient feedback is the best method to determine proper interpretation. Misinterpretation results when we take for granted the patient understands.

Leverage Through Illustrations

Offering a simple verbal explanation does not guarantee learning. While we learn through our senses, behavioral scientists tell us we learn only about 10% by what we *hear*, a large 85% by what we *see*, and about 5% through the senses of taste, touch, and smell. Thus, telling is far inferior to showing. Comprehension and recall are greatly enhanced when we use visual aids; eg, models, charts, pictures, graphs, drawings, demonstrations, and dramatizations.

This shows the advantage quality patient literature has on enhancing patient education. It reinforces what has been said and shown in the office. Take-home literature tells patients "We care" by helping them prevent trouble, by helping them understand health problems and office policies, and by assuring them that important points were not accidentally omitted in the office explanations. Such literature can also add authority to what has been explained.

While most patients want to learn, they have difficulty in learning because they have been conditioned to poor learning habits. Because we are all exposed to so many unimportant words and commercials, we often develop a conditioned response to "turn off." We don't hear the important because we don't listen. We don't see the important because we don't really look. Realizing this, we must use as many of the patient's physical senses in teaching as we can and as often as we can to make a firm impression. We must re-emphasize, paraphrase, repeat, and review. We must build mental pictures through analogies and frequent varied examples and comparisons.

Teaching helps the patient, and it helps the practice. Patients want to understand and appreciate the features and benefits of the health services offered. Patients want to learn and be informed. Motivation to learn and appreciate must not be taken for granted; it must be constantly stimulated through repetition of benefits (personal value). Each patient must be shown the personal value for each consultation, examination, therapy, teaching, and policy. If they are not convinced of the value, they will only think in terms of time, price, effort, and immediate results.

External Communications

Patient education within the office is only one method of filling the communications gap. In the office, the patient is a captive audience. Communications outside the office for both assistant and doctor take more assertive action. External communications of this nature mean arranging for the practice to get noticed, remembered, and known throughout the community.

The practice also receives recognition when it bestows recognition. Local newspapers offer an abundance of announcements by which the office can recognize the achievements and advancements of others. Congratulatory letters are welcomed and remembered. The office that "doesn't have the time" to get involved with the community is all too often the office that the community doesn't get involved with to any great extent. Think and talk good about people, and they will think and talk good about you.

Remember that it is the extra and the unusual that impress people the most. It's usual to send greeting cards at Christmas; it's unusual to send cards at Thanksgiving. It's usual to have black-and-white letterheads; it's unusual to have blue or brown letterheads with a matching typewriter ribbon. There is nothing unprofessional about being unusual if it is done in good taste.

Health practice begins with a desire to serve others. It is not a gimmick. Therefore, when you join community clubs and organizations, it should never be a gimmick to gain personal attention. You can expect only to receive in the same spirit in which you give. If you give sincerely and freely of your time to community affairs, the community will return in kind. Dedicated community service is a medium to further your professional image and that of the practice you serve.

Enthusiasm Is Contagious

The more successful the practice, the better setting for the CA to have opportunity for career development and advancement. Thus, besides loyalty and efficient job performance, the assistant has a strong personal motive to assist in practice development.

Enthusiasm is contagious if it is natural. Enthusiasm is not something that can be learned in the classroom. It is something that is the effect of working each day in a practice, witnessing the results first hand, and becoming absorbed in the professional atmosphere and its contribution to the community. As one performing an important job in an important field, you have a right to be enthusiastic about your occupation and the people with whom you are associated.

Effective salesmen are enthusiastic salesmen because people like enthusiastic people, and, of course, you are a salesman for your office, your doctor, and the profession of chiropractic. By being affirmative, cheerful, and confident about your position and work, you help people like yourself more because your project interest through your enthusiastic attitude. Because enthusiasm is contagious, the best way for you to encourage people to have greater interest in you and confidence in your employer is to display such confidence.

At parties, club meetings, showers, and other social affairs, you will inevitably be asked about the job you hold. When you reply that you are employed in a chiropractic office, the next question will likely be, "How do you like it?" If you enjoy your work, you can win friends for the office by saying enthusiastically that you enjoy it. If you don't enjoy it, it's a sure sign you are in the wrong occupation. If you respect and admire the doctor and what he does, say so from the heart. If you don't, you should certainly look for other employment. People who have no opportunity of learning about chiropractic in general or your doctor-employer in particular can learn about chiropractic through you.

The enthusiastic assistant doesn't lock her job in a desk at night. When she leaves the office, she takes the excitement and challenge of chiropractic with her. She discusses it with her friends. She explains what it is, what it does, and the health services provided. It would be a rare person you meet that would not benefit from the services of a chiropractor at some period in life. Most people need chiropractic health care periodically. You do a distinct favor for your friends, your doctor, yourself, and your community when you help them to select a chiropractic physician whose professional skill, concern, and integrity are acknowledged.

Chapter 7

Responsibilities of an Administrative Assistant

Proper scheduling and planning help any office function smoothly with less possibility of omitting necessary actions. The doctor in charge will identify each assistant's duties and functions and discuss her responsibility for the performance of each assigned task. During her initial orientation and training, these functions may be subdivided into procedural steps necessary.

Task plans and work schedules eliminate the confusion of who should perform a specific duty. It eliminates the question, "What do I do next?" Work schedules based on good planning eliminate the need to work beyond expected hours, except for rare emergency situations. Keep in mind, however, that a plan is not a permanent thing. As conditions change, the doctor must revise schedules, duties, and responsibilities to reflect changes. Flexibility is a necessary qualification for a chiropractic assistant.

Patient handling and patient control are the two major factors determining the success or failure of any practice. As professional competence should be taken for granted, patient satisfaction makes the difference in success or failure. This one factor determines a high or low patient return and a high or low referral rate.

This chapter describes common duties of an administrative assistant. In both the professional and business world, however, specific job descriptions vary to meet the needs of management.

OVERVIEW

It is frequently stated that the doctor should not be required to do anything in his office that an assistant can do as well or better. Valuable clinical time would be wasted if the doctor had to answer routine telephone calls, make appointments, supervise patient flow, send out notices and reminders, type letters, make billings, file records, and attend to the various other duties necessary to administer and manage the business side of a practice. To be efficient in his profession, the doctor must delegate much authority and responsibility for many office details to his assistant(s) so that his time will be used optimally in doing that which he has been specially prepared—helping the sick to get well and helping the healthy stay well.

The extent of delegated administrative responsibility depends largely on the nature of the practice itself, the assistant's experience and training, and the size of the administrative staff. In a small solo practice with one assistant, the assistant will be required to assume several small roles. In a large office with several assistants, the number of duties will be reduced, but their scope will be expanded for each assistant.

An assistant with knowledge in basic administrative procedures, office equipment, secretarial methods, and bookkeeping systems will find little difficulty learning to become a capable administrative assistant within a chiropractic office. Major tasks usually performed by one or more administrative assistants include directing the flow of patients, reception area supervision, filing and record keeping, appointment and scheduling control, billings, telephone responsibilities, typing letters, general office management, inventory control, computing patients' fees, instructing patients about office policies, and record filing among other tasks. These duties usually concern the reception, business, dismissal, and communications areas of the practice. See Figure 7.1.

A solo assistant will undoubtedly be involved in technical duties and responsibilities as well as administrative duties and responsibilities. These technical duties involve certain routine data recording, measurements, laboratory tests, x-ray procedures, administration of certain therapies and rehabilitation procedures, and other clinical aid. The extent of clinical assistance also depends on the nature of the practice itself, the assistant's experience and training, the size of the staff, and pertinent state laws and regulations. The typical role of technical assistants is described in Chapters 13 and 14.

General Office Philosophy

As described in the previous chapter, health practice is a very human environment. With most patients, the initial office contact is by the telephone. Know proper telephone etiquette, be cheerful but not familiar, and sincerely want to help the caller. After the telephone contact, the next is with the patient in the reception area. This contact also

---

TYPICAL ADMINISTRATIVE ASSISTANT
DUTIES

Patient Relations

- Opens office
- Reception room supervision
- Directs the flow of patients
- Orients patients to office policies
- Answers general questions about fees and procedures
- Appointment and scheduling control
- Telephone responsibilities
- Sends appointment reminders or makes telephone calls
- Supervises the patient recall system
- Sends congratulatory and referral thank-you notes
- Sends birthday and anniversary cards to patients
- Attends to special needs of children and elderly
- Checks office heating, cooling, and ventilation quality
- Incidental housekeeping
- Maintains office laundry control
- Implements office public relations programs

Secretarial and Business Administration

- Routine stenography and typing
- Contacts with doctor's telephone answering service
- Pulls and files records
- Computes patient fees
- Processes incoming and outgoing mail
- Receives payments
- Credit arrangements and control
- Routine billing procedures
- Prepares and mails statements
- Accounts receivable records
- Payroll and accounts payable records
- Daily and periodic bookkeeping and balancing
- Reconciles bank statements
- Maintains office petty cash account
- Prepares referral letters, forms, and reports
- Invoice checking
- Nonclinical inventory control
- Assists patients in completing office forms
- General business office management
- Closes office

Figure 7.1. Some typical responsibilities of an administrative assistant.

helps to establish the success or failure in patient satisfaction. In both physical appearance and mental attitude, assure that the office has a reception room and not a waiting room. A waiting room is the result of poor appointment scheduling.

The patient new to the practice entering the reception area should be properly greeted, and the initial registration should be completed. The doctor may wish you to take some preliminary case history using a standardized form. If the patient is asked to record information, a clipboard and pen should be provided. Conversation with the patient should be professional and cheerful. A sincerely interested, reasonably relaxed, politely inquiring attitude will elicit more information in less time than a hurried, tense questioning period.

Keep your personal and office problems to yourself. The patient is there to bring his or her problems to the office. Patients do not want to listen to the problems of others.

Showing interest in a patient's well being, family, and outside interests is a good practice builder. Another key to successful administration of a practice is personal warmth that recognizes each patient as an individual. Such an attitude can produce more confidence, increase patient referrals, and reduce office fee complaints than any other personal attribute.

Before the doctor sees the patient, the doctor should be given a few moments to review the patient's case records. When the doctor is ready, the patient should be introduced, "Doctor, this is Mr. Jones." The continuing patient can be introduced, "Doctor, Mrs. Smith is ready."

After the initial consultation, the doctor may wish you to help in the examination procedure or perform some basic tests and measurements. After the information is gathered, the doctor usually asks the patient to schedule an appointment for an evaluation of his findings. This evaluation is usually given verbally, but some doctors may also give the patient a written summary report for the benefit of an absent spouse or parent.

During the initial consultation, the doctor explains the need for suggested examination procedures. During the evaluation ap-pointment, the doctor discusses his findings from the examination and his prognosis under a specified treatment program. This procedure is called obtaining *informed consent*. It means the doctor will describe the procedures necessary and receive the patient's consent prior to any recommended examination or therapy. The patient will be informed of likely consequences, dangers, and other factors so that the patient's consent is given with knowledge of inherent dangers or risks, if any, to which the patient will be exposed.

Aiding Professional Service

Definite office policies and carefully planned procedures are the prerequisites for running a smooth, efficient practice. Keep in mind, however, that a *definite* policy does not necessarily mean a *fixed* policy. Periodic staff meetings are regularly used to analyze the different phases and procedures involved in the professional services offered, seek areas of improvement, and voice doctor and assistant expectations. Quality communications require understanding another person's viewpoint and expectations. See Figure 7.2.

Office policies and procedures are generally designed to support the doctor's three major services: (1) consultation, (2) examination, and (3) treatment. *Consultation* and history are required to help the doctor determine the type of examination necessary to isolate the cause(s) of the patient's complaint. They are also necessary to counsel the patient against harmful acts and toward healthy behavior. *Examination* is necessary to profile the patient's structural and functional status to arrive at a diagnosis and prognosis under the recommended therapies. *Treatment* is designed to help the patient return to as near a state of health and resistance to disease or normal stress as possible.

The typical office will offer five different forms of health care depending on the case involved at any particular time: (1) emergency, (2) acute, (3) chronic, (4) rehabilitative, and (5) prophylactic care. *Emergency care* is that minimal care necessary to aid

---

BASIC EXPECTATIONS

Basic Employee Expectations	Basic Employer Expectations
Proper instruction	Advice to be followed
Clear lines of authority	Standard production
Nonconflicting rules and regulations	Flexibility to change
Impartial treatment	Good attendance
Personal respect	Responsible behavior
Reasonable production standards	Loyalty
Appreciation of complex problems	Good morale
Good working conditions	A team spirit
Opportunity to achieve personal goals	Support to achieve practice goals

Figure 7.2. Basic expectations of employees and employers. Priorities vary according to the individuals involved.

---

the patient until an appointment can be scheduled for more detailed consultation, examination, and therapy. *Acute care* usually concerns unanticipated situations such as accidents, strains, and sprains that, although painful, leave little permanent damage or predisposition to recurrence if properly treated. *Chronic conditions* are usually those that are long standing and therapy is used more to check progress of the condition rather than reversal of the stubborn disease process. *Rehabilitative conditions* are those of either an acute or chronic nature where the disorder has been checked and therapy is directed to return the patient to that state of health enjoyed before the onset of the disorder. *Prophylactic care* is preventive in nature, striving to maintain optimal health and resistance of the patient.

Remember that all office policies and procedures are designed and administered to aid the practice's services and the types of cases seen. From the time patients enter the office until they leave, every procedure should be planned to support the best interests of each patient. By so doing, the best interests of the practice will be served. Patient handling, case management, and practice control are just different aspects of professional health care. Each aspect must run smoothly and efficiently in a well-organized manner.

Office policies, procedures, records, forms, systems, supplies, equipment, and furnishings are but vehicles to reach the goal of professional health care. They should never be considered an end in themselves. The assistant should be alert that systems originally designed to aid the practice, in time and habitual use, have a tendency to dictate to the creators of the systems. The patient is always more important than any procedure.

OPENING THE OFFICE

Acting in the capacity of office manager, the administrative assistant should be the first person to arrive at the office each morning. She should immediately follow a daily routine of getting the office in order. Here are some basic duties:

1. Assure that all rooms are clean and neat.

2. Check temperature. Set thermostat so that temperatures range between 70° and 75° Fahrenheit.

3. Make certain there is proper ventilation and adequate fresh air circulation so that it is a pleasant and refreshing place to work.

4. Develop a list of the day's appointments that gives each patient's name, time of appointment, and reason for visit. Using this list, pull established patient record cards from the files and prepare one for each patient new to the practice. This will help to ease pressure and maintain efficient patient flow throughout the day.

5. Open and organize the daily mail. Do not open personal letters addressed to the doctor or staff.

6. Complete tasks left over from the previous day.

7. Double check the office environment, and attend to as many preparation details as possible before patients arrive.

GREETING PATIENTS

In review, the patient received the first impression of the office by the telephone and the second impression by the physical appearance of the office's exterior and receiving area. Now the patient is ready for the third impression. This is the point of contact when the patient is personally "approached" by an assistant. Depending on the quality of this approach, either positive or negative impressions will be made.

Importance of a Positive Approach

In marketing a product, authorities rate the "approach" as high as 80% in importance to all sales. As a health practice is not a business but a profession, the word "salesmanship" is a poor term to use. On the other hand, it is difficult to completely differentiate salesmanship, public relations, and common sense in human relations. Obviously, the approach in a chiropractic office to either a new or continuing patient is important to practice success. When poorly handled, through a thoughtless act or a tactless word, impression of the doctor's skills and professional service standards may be sharply minimized in the mind of the patient.

An assistant should greet the entering patient with a smile and cheerful welcome as if she were the hostess in her home, being gracious and pleasant to make the patient feel welcomed and at ease. The rules of courtesy, appearance, decorum, hospitality, and tact apply. A kindly smile (never forced) will do much to tell the patient in distress that he or she will be served with consideration. Your words, voice tones, facial expressions, gestures, grooming, posture, and carriage are important parts of making a positive approach.

First words as first impressions are important. Phrases such as "Good morning," "Good afternoon," or "May I help you?" are warm opening remarks. Avoid stern expressions such as "What can I do for you?" or "What seems wrong?" These openings often frighten the timid patient. It is good policy always to use the name of the patient in the opening statement if it is known, but do not ask, "How are you today, Mrs. Smith?" This may invite a problem.

After the patient is made comfortable in the reception room, inform the patient, "Dr. Jones will be with you directly, Mrs. Smith." This is better than "Dr. Jones will be with you in a few moments" because the latter implies uncertainty. The word "directly" in the first statement implies a short wait, yet it is noncommittal.

If a patient enters the receiving area while you are on the telephone, acknowledge the patient with a smile and friendly nod. If you are busy at the desk, stop momentarily to greet the patient and exchange a few words. Suggest a magazine if you will be a few moments. Always be friendly and interested, but avoid excessive socializing even if you know the patient well. Avoid selective favoritism to any patient.

It is a rare patient who enjoys a long wait in a reception room. To many, it's annoying. All patients deserve a courteous explanation of why a long delay is necessary. When a patient has been waiting a considerable time beyond the scheduled appointment, the assistant should re-enter the room and graciously apologize for the delay: "We're sorry, but an unforeseen situation arose that delayed our schedule a little." Never let the patient remain in the reception room well past the appointment time without an explanation. It is discourteous and unprofessional behavior. Nothing less than good social conduct should be the guideline of a hostess.

Proper atmosphere and patient contact are two major points in a proper approach. The assistant holds the responsibility for developing a receptive patient attitude before the patient meets with the doctor. In its simplest terms, the goal is to have the patient like you, the doctor, and the professional services. Your initial smile and friendly greeting are much more than a rule to be memorized. They set the stage for all that follows.

When a patient new to the practice is greeted for the first time, show where coats can be hung, and then obtain the basic office information. Be sure to offer extra special assistance with clothing of the elderly, physically handicapped, or painfully distressed.

When patients enter the practice, basic information must be obtained such as patient's name, home address, residence telephone number, occupation, business address, employer if not self-employed, business telephone, marital status, how the patient was referred to the office, health insurance information, and how the patient wishes to pay for the doctor's services. If the patient is a woman, further information about the number and ages of children should be recorded. This basic information is often recorded on an index card and kept on file for administrative reference. In many offices, the doctor also desires the assistant to take some basic case history data such as childhood diseases, surgical history, accident history, disorders under treatment by another doctor, and other facts. A standardized form is usually provided.

If the doctor desires, record the pre-examination history for the patient new to the practice. Prepare a folder for the patient, insert history and other data obtained, and then prepare an office visit slip (Fig. 7.3), and attach it to the folder. Mention the doctor's time schedule (on time or delayed). When the doctor is ready, escort the patient to the consultation room and introduce the patient to the doctor.

Types of New Patients

While there are exceptions to all generalizations, there are four general types of new patients to a practice. We will describe them briefly so you will be in a better position to handle the type of appointment necessary.

1. *The Referred Patient with a Positive Attitude.* One type of patient will be characterized by being referred by a satisfied patient and, because of the referring patient, will have a high regard for the profession and positive expectations for relief of the disorder. Such a patient will respect office policies, value the doctor's professional opinion, and have been somewhat indoctrinated to office procedures beforehand. This type of patient is usually interested in a complete rehabilitation program, and appointment schedules can be established accordingly depending on the clinical judgment of the doctor.

2. *The Positive Patient with Scheduling Problems.* Another type of patient is one who presents with a history calling for a complete rehabilitation program but for one reason or another such a schedule is not possible at this time. Reasons may be financial, an occupation requiring out-of-town traveling, baby-sitting problems, or another factor that would prevent keeping scheduled appointments or present great difficulty in so doing. Such a patient has a high regard for the doctor and the profession, realizes the necessity of complete rehabilitation but is compelled not to engage in it at the present. The only alternative is to place the patient on some type of temporary program that would allow the patient the maximum amount of comfort possible within a schedule that would allow for the patient's current situation.

3. *The "Tough-Minded" Skeptic.* This type of patient does not have a high regard for the profession. Usually, such a patient has been filled with years of negative propaganda, but previous care for a disorder has

JAMES R. PIERCE, D.C.
Chiropractic Physician
86543 Center Street
Anytown, Oklahoma 12345

No. 2984   Date _____

Patient's Name _____

Address _____

Services Rendered	X	Fee
Consultation		
Complete Examination		
Limited Examination		
Roentgenography		
Thermography		
Electrocardiography		
Electrodiagnosis		
Electromyography		
Laboratory Test(s)		
Spinal Adjustment		
Cryotherapy		
Galvanic Therapy		
Hydrocollator		
High-Volt Therapy		
Interferential		
Iontophoresis		
MENS		
Meridian Therapy		
Microwave Diathermy		
Shortwave Diathermy		
Spondylotherapy		
Taping/Bandaging		
Traction		
Ultrasound Diathermy		
Ultraviolet		
Supplements		
TENS		
Support/Brace		

DB   NC   WC   MC   MA   WF   Total

Next Appointment on _____ near _____

Please Give to Receptionist
Before You Leave

Figure 7.3. Sample visit slip. Unless fees change frequently, nonvariables (eg, films, supplements) may be printed in the right column to show standardization.

not been beneficial. He has called your office on the advice of a friend but is highly skeptical. While such a patient will often manifest clinical indications for comprehensive examination procedures, he is usually not psychologically prepared for such a recommendation. He enters the office expecting either a limited service or a "miracle," to pay a fee, and then to return whenever "he has a mind to."

For the doctor to try to alter such deeply entrenched opinions on one visit would be folly. The patient would likely nod his head up and down during a detailed presentation, but on returning home and exposed to negative friends and the return of established negative thinking patterns, he would feel that he was the victim of some type of "high-pressure salesmanship." A definite future appointment is rarely scheduled for this type of patient unless something occurs to change his attitude.

Although the patient is left to his volition, the doctor of chiropractic will plant the seeds of what should be done from a rational standpoint. This is the doctor's moral and professional obligation though he feels that his constructive suggestions may be going in one ear of the patient and out the other. The patient should realize that only first-aid service has been provided and a more comprehensive service is available when the patient is ready. By enlightening the patient of the need for a comprehensive program, the DC fulfills his obligation. The responsibility for further action is placed squarely on the patient. He is free either to ignore the advice or later think about it and take positive action.

If the patient chooses to ignore the doctor's advice, he assumes responsibility for progression of the disorder and any complications arising from lack of proper care. In any event, the patient is not in a rational position to criticize the doctor, the profession, or the practice for any reason. He can only speak affirmatively since his fate is in his hands. He cannot say that the doctor took advantage of him. He can only say that the doctor pointed out the folly of continuing without treatment and suggested a constructive program regarding his condition that should be considered. The patient has

been educated that chiropractic health care is not only interested in relieving pain and discomfort, it is also obliged to prevent health disorders from recurring or progressing if possible.

4. There is another type of patient who on the surface appears to be the skeptical type just described. It is important that both assistant and doctor make proper differentiation. This fourth type of patient has become discouraged with the superficial first-aid treatment received in the past even if it was all that he would allow. He has recently been informed of the comprehensive services of your office and is now prepared to have a full diagnostic workup and a comprehensive rehabilitative plan outlined. This is his sole purpose for calling for an appointment. Thus, this patient is more akin to the first type of patient discussed than the third type. If this type of patient is suspected on the telephone, enough time in the appointment schedule should be allotted for proper orientation.

GREETING VISITORS

Every office, be it business or professional, has a regular stream of salesmen and solicitors calling. Many are important to the operation of the office. Others are unproductive or unnecessary time-consuming callers. The handling of nonpatient visitors is a matter that you and your employer should discuss early in your association. Together, you can set a firm policy in dealing with them. Many professionals and/or their assistants designate specific hours or days solely for meeting with solicitors and salesmen.

In handling these callers, it is important to remember that your office may need the service or product offered. You must have good equipment, supplies, and service to run an office efficiently and profitably. Therefore, do not be abrupt with salesmen. Give them the attention and courtesies deserved. Do not discriminate against them provided they follow established office policies. Salesmen are not only your best source of information, they are also carriers of good will or ill will. Besides, salesmen and their families need chiropractic care too. Avoid the attitude that all callers other than patients are nuisances.

If a salesperson should call at the office without an appointment, request a card and the purpose of his visit. Tactfully find out if the subject is important enough to be called to the doctor's immediate attention. After talking to the salesman, you may decide that he has something of interest for your office. It is then up to you to schedule an appointment with the doctor when the salesman can present full information on his product or service. These people will often leave some literature for the doctor to review.

Although most doctors do not want to be pestered with insignificant decisions and details, they do want to make major decisions. The extent of your ordering and purchasing will depend on your experience, the policy characteristics of your office, and the specific faith and authority given to you by your employer.

If the visitor is another doctor, bypass all waiting patients and escort him to an inner room. Then notify the doctor. Such visits are usually for a specific purpose and can be handled quickly.

TELEPHONE DUTIES

Attitude

The ring of the telephone should spur your sincere interest, helpfulness, and empathy. Your tone of voice should reflect a friendly, professional attitude. No matter how busy you may be at the moment, take a slow deep breath, put a smile on your face, and let the caller know you "care." The caller must be convinced through your tone that the office has people who are courteous, efficient, concerned, and eager to help.

Technique

Telephone technique is expressed in voice quality, volume, pitch, clear pronunciation, and rapidity of speech. A good telephone voice reflects sincerity, warmth, friendliness, professionalism, graciousness, and understanding. Volume need be no different from that of an in-person conversation. Don't yell; don't mumble. While callers cannot see your hand gestures and head nods, they will "feel" your smile. A pleasant well-modulated voice shows your response is free from strain and tension. Voice quality alone may calm or reassure a nervous patient.

Because the telephone is a low-fidelity instrument, many overtones and undertones witnessed in personal conversation are lost. Therefore, it's often helpful to pitch the voice slightly lower than normal. If you have a high-pitched voice, speak slower and lower. Transmission is best when the mouthpiece is held about one inch directly in front of the lips. Here are some simple rules in developing good telephone technique:

• Smile, greet the caller pleasantly, and listen attentively. Visualize the caller. The caller will form an image of you through your voice and manners.

• Answer promptly, on the first ring if possible, but once you pick up the phone, assume an unhurried manner. Before you speak, clear your mind of previous tasks.

• Hold the mouthpiece about one inch from your lips and speak softly and clearly, avoiding monotones. Don't use slang, "mod talk," or professional jargon. Keep personal chatting to a minimum.

• Record name (and often telephone number) immediately. Take notes, request necessary spelling and use phonetic spelling if necessary. Don't put the caller on hold if you expect a long delay. If you put the caller on hold, quickly return to the person and explain any delay.

Words Reveal

Words come from the mind, but the way they are spoken reveals your heart. When you meet someone face to face, you can express your cordiality by a smile, a nod, or a wave of your hand. But over the telephone you must find other ways of transmitting your feeling of friendship. Over the telephone, the smile, the nod, the wave of the hand, can only be shown by what you say and how you say it. You can sound uncertain, abrupt, bored, or irritated. Or you can be confident, courteous, sparkling and friendly. You can make yourself a real person instead of "just a voice."

All appreciate a person who speaks over the telephone clearly and pleasantly, not too fast or too slow, neither too loud nor too soft, with a careful enunciation of each word and syllable. A pleasant voice is an asset—not only on the job but in everyday life. It saves time and avoids confusion. It makes friends and wins promotions, and it dissolves resentment and reveals culture. It invites opportunity and secures a cordial relationship.

The way your voice rises and falls, the way you show what is important by proper emphasis, the way shades of feeling appear in your voice—these give vocal color and help make it pleasing and convincing. For example, the way you say the words you use in answering a call is important. Suppose they are, "Dr. Smith's office." In these words you can accomplish much. By a pleasing tone, you seem to ask, "Is this the office you are calling?" By the helpful expression in your manner, you ask, "What may I do for you?" You imply that you are pleased to receive the call. All that—in just three words!

Pronunciation Enhances Understanding

To be easily and accurately understood, it is necessary, of course, to speak clearly and distinctly. Pronounce carefully, giving proper form to each sound in every word. Try this: Open your mouth slightly and while hardly moving your jaw or tongue, speak a few sentences. You have heard people speak that way and probably had trouble in understanding them. They are suffering from stiff jaws, lazy lips, or sleepy tongues. It's no wonder their words sound mumbled, shut in, or "swallowed" instead of being nicely formed and directed. It should be obvious that chewing gum or eating should be avoided while using the telephone since they interfere with distinctiveness.

It's more important to speak unhurriedly and distinctly over the telephone than when face to face. That is because the listener cannot see the changing expressions of your face. Without distinctiveness, other good voice qualities will be lost. You can frequently tell whether your voice is easily understood by noticing the number of times others ask you to repeat what you have said. Experiment until you have reduced these requests to a minimum.

If you cannot hear the caller clearly, use extra tact and courtesy. Never say, "I cannot hear you," or "I can't understand you." Rather, say that it seems you have a bad connection and ask the caller to speak a little louder or slower.

Monitor Your Rate of Speech

A moderate rate of speech is important. Sometimes you may be tempted to talk too fast over the phone because you are busy and believe you are saving time. If you speak too rapidly, however, the chances are you won't be nearly as well understood and you must use valuable time repeating. It pays to take time for courtesy, too. Telephone conversation should neither be too fast nor too slow. If too fast, words are jumbled and parts of words are lost to the ear. If too slow, words seem disconnected and lose meaning and interest. Ordinarily, the very act of speaking clearly will tend to prevent talking too fast.

Voice Tone

Be as sincere and natural to everyone over the telephone as you are face to face. If your voice loses its natural tone, try to determine why. Is it due to a monotone or mechanical way of speaking? If so, put more expression in your tone by varying phrases. Perhaps you are speaking too loud or not loud enough. Ask a friend whether your telephone voice resembles your natural voice.

Care in using correct mouth action for any sound will assure that the sound is formed rightly and clearly. You'll be astonished at the variety and importance of mouth action required to form different sounds.

To sound any particular note on a musical instrument requires a special position or action such as pressing a violin string at exactly the right point and drawing the bow correctly. So too there is a special position or action of the lips, tongue, or jaw for every sound used in speech. The lips sometimes close or take a slightly parted or rounded shape; the jaw moves up and down; the tongue moves to certain positions. For a pleasing tone, drop your jaw so that there will be sufficient space between the teeth.

Answering the Telephone

In review: Try to answer each call as promptly as possible. If other lines are used, politely ask the caller to hold for a moment while you respond to the other call and return as soon as possible. Offer to return the call if you feel the delay will be longer than one minute. If the party on hold is there longer than anticipated, take their name and number and have the call returned rather than leaving them "dangling" on the phone.

Most doctors will have set policies for handling routine and emergency calls. For instance:

Rapidly identify the office. For example, "Good morning! Suburban Chiropractic Clinic. This is Miss Anderson speaking. How may I help you?" Never just say, "Hello," "555-5834," or "The doctor is busy!"

Quickly determine the reason for the call. If in doubt, ask a tactful question. For example: "Yes, Mr. Brown?" This infers that you are ready to hear why he called. Visualize the caller while speaking and listening.

Accurately gather the facts of the call. Obtain the caller's full name with correct spelling and phonetic breakdown, reason for the call, and final disposition. Recap this information to the caller to verify the facts before you hang up.

Be friendly. If you are acquainted with the caller, let him know that he is recognized. For example, "Hi, Mr. Peterson. It's good to hear from you." To be sure of the name of the caller, repeat it during the conversation. People like to hear the sound of their name.

Although most calls will be for an appointment, many new patients will ask to speak to the doctor directly. Your "How may I help you?" will usually resolve this problem. Or you may say, "If you wish to make an appointment (or reserve time for consultation), I can help you as I have the appointment book here at my desk."

Avoid direct answers to specific questions regarding the doctor's fees or professional procedures. Give a polite general answer to the effect that the doctor's fees and procedures are usual and customary in the area and that a personal visit with the doctor would be necessary to discuss specifics as each patient requires individualized attention.

The caller may ask, "Do I have to be x-rayed?" Respond that all patients do not require films but the necessity must be discussed with the doctor in the light of each patient's individual needs.

Calls the Assistant Can Resolve

Don't feel that your function is to "screen" calls for the doctor. Such an attitude appears to separate the doctor from his patients. Your function is to handle those calls you can so the doctor's clinical time will not be reduced. An able assistant can manage calls about appointments, take messages, answer questions about third-party claims, receive a favorable progress report, answer requests for general information, take requests for a housecall, answer complaints or misunderstandings about a bill, answer calls from salespeople, and manage nuisance calls.

Sometimes a caller refuses to identify himself. This may be because the caller is a "skeptic," has been recently mistreated by another practitioner, or is "shopping around." Most people with legitimate motives will identify themselves and their suspicions. If a mystery caller demands to speak directly with the doctor, ask for his name and number so the call may be returned or suggest that a letter be forwarded. Be polite, even in the most demanding situations.

Sometimes a relative or neighbor of a patient will call seeking information. Unless you are sure the caller is a parent of a minor, remember that all information is *privileged information* and that a release form is necessary before any information can be communicated—even to the point that the person in question is a patient of the doctor. Speak in a way that others nearby will not hear the conversation, especially other patients. Never discuss a call with other patients or they will suspect that you do the same about their calls and conversations.

Following are two common examples of routine questions:

• Is Dr. Smith a good back doctor? Answer: Yes, Dr. Smith is an excellent chiropractic physician. He offers professional health-care service.

• How much does he charge? Answer: How long have you had this problem? After further discussion of the patient's complaint and without mention of fees, state: "Dr. Smith will be happy to discuss fees with you. If you would like to arrange a private consultation before a regular appointment, he can see you either next Monday at 10:15 in the morning or Wednesday at 3:45 in the afternoon. Which is the best for you?"

Calls the Doctor Must Resolve

While the assistant should give the impression that the doctor is always readily available, she should not put calls through to the doctor unless she feels it is totally necessary. If in doubt, place the caller on hold and brief the doctor of the problem. It's important not to interrupt a doctor's rapport or procedure with a patient being treated unless it's vital or an emergency. Most calls that must be handled by the doctor can be noted by you so the doctor may return the call between patients or after the last patient of the session has left.

If you have a question, message, or special caller on the phone, there are ways to inform the doctor. You may use some predetermined buzzer or light signal indicating the doctor is wanted, in which case he could excuse himself from the patient for a moment. Another procedure sometimes used is

to write a note (Fig. 7.4) and personally take it to the doctor. Place it so the doctor can see it at a glance without it being visible to the patient. He can then do whatever is necessary without the patient being aware of the delay or annoyed by the interruption.

Always knock before entering a private office or examination room. Be careful not to walk in on a patient unannounced while he is unclothed or in an otherwise potentially embarrassing situation.

If the doctor is available but speaking on another line, inform the caller that the doctor is speaking on another line. Ask if the caller would rather wait or have the doctor return the call. If the doctor's current conversation is extended, return to the line and

TELEPHONE MESSAGE

For ___

Date ___ ☐ Patient
Time ___ ☐ Prospective Patient
Recd by ___ ☐ Nonpatient

☐ ON HOLD ☐ Please Call Back at ___
☐ URGENT ☐ Will Call Again at ___

Name ___

Telephone Number ( ) ___

Message: ___

Remarks: ___

Backup Attached: ☐ Clinical file
☐ Ledger
☐ Other ___

Figure 7.4. Sample telephone message slip.

explain the situation: "Dr. Jones is still on the telephone. I'm sorry. Would you prefer to hold or may I ask him to call you back?" Never say, "The doctor is still talking" or "I'll have him return your call." Rather, say, "Dr. Jones is still in conversation" and "May I ask Dr. Jones to return your call?"

When the doctor is busy but wishes to speak immediately to certain callers, be sure you know the names of such callers. In such situations, say, "Dr. Jones is expecting your call. Please hold, and I'll see if I can get Dr. Jones on the line for you, Mrs. Peters."

If the doctor is out of the office, be tactful and factual. If he is out of town attending an educational program, say, "Dr. Jones is attending a special seminar (doing some graduate work) in Cincinnati this week." Offering such information informs the caller that the doctor keeps abreast of the times. Avoid use of the word "Convention," as it has negative connotations to many people. If the doctor is in town but out of the office, simply say, "Dr. Jones is out of the office and is scheduled to be back by 2 o'clock this afternoon." Avoid statements that may be embarrassing to the doctor such as "He isn't in yet!" (why not), "I don't know where he is!" (golf), "He hasn't come in yet!" (tardy), or "He's out for coffee" (no patients).

Call Records

A memorandum should be made immediately of every telephone call that needs the attention. This memo should contain date, time of call, name of person who called, telephone number of caller in case he is to be called back, the main points of the conversation, what the assistant did about the call, and, if necessary, some comments about the conversation. Refer to Figure 7.4.

Follow-up Calls

The assistant has many more duties besides the actual handling of patients face-to-face. An important function is the telephoning of patients for periodic spinal examinations or appointments that have been long standing.

The doctor may also wish you to check the status of certain patients during the early stages of treatment. Figure 7.5 shows a typical log sheet for this purpose.

Patients often forget how long it has been between spinal examinations, or an appointment made several weeks ago may have been forgotten. Because people tend to forget and because "no shows" waste everyone's time, a few minutes on the telephone confirming the next day's appointments will keep office time productive. Thus, it's helpful when recording a patient's appointment that you also include the patient's telephone number. When you do call, never "call to remind" the patient. This tends to insult a patient's memory. Call to "confirm" or "verify" the appointment.

Outgoing Calls

If you must make several outgoing calls such as for appointment verification, allow about 5 minutes between each call to give a person who is trying to reach the office a chance to make connection. A constant "busy" signal may discourage a patient and cause him to call another doctor.

For frequently dialed outgoing calls, have a list of the numbers handy to your desk and keep it updated. It will save valuable time.

Answering Services

Many offices use some type of answering service or device when the office is closed. It is usually the responsibility of an administrative assistant to obtain the messages from the service—passing on urgent messages to the doctor, and responding to unessential requests personally. Often the assistant will feel she is too busy to respond to some calls, feeling that the service has told the caller when office hours begin and that the patient will call back. This is an error. Keep in mind that when callers receive an answering service, they already have suffered a "let down" in reaching the coolness of the service when in need of help. It creates a warm impression when the assistant replies to the call instead of requiring the

Patient's Name	Phone No.	File No.	Major Complaint	Present Status		Remarks
				Improved	Unim-proved	
				☐	☐	
				☐	☐	
				☐	☐	
				☐	☐	
				☐	☐	
				☐	☐	
				☐	☐	
				☐	☐	
				☐	☐	
				☐	☐	
				☐	☐	

ACUTE CASE FOLLOW-UP LIST   DATE _____

Figure 7.5. Sample acute case follow-up list.

patient to make a second effort to reach the office.

When an answering device is used, the assistant plays back the tape, notes the caller's name, phone number, and a brief summary of the message. Calls are then returned to those who left messages.

Pressure Shows Your Personality

One test of a good assistant is the way she handles calls when under pressure and the last thing she needs is for the telephone to ring. A good assistant will be calm and courteous, doesn't panic, and will not "take it out" on the innocent party on the line. You never know who that will be. It could be an important community leader, a colleague of the doctor, a patient in distress, or the doctor's wife.

Summary of Highlights

While doctors of chiropractic rightly believe that clinical skills and services are the major factors in developing a successful practice, an assistant should realize that the psychologic impressions made on patients in their association with the office are equally important. Positive initial impressions and continuing impressions are an integral part of developing and maintaining a successful practice.

A patient is more than a sick body; he or

she is also a sensitive psyche. Each contact with the doctor or any member of the office team, no matter how minute, has one of two reactions. It either builds patients' confidence, creates greater respect, and develops further appreciation for the doctor and what he represents, or it builds patients' doubts and resistance, and lowers respect and appreciation for the doctor and what he represents. This action is not a sometime thing. It is constant. It begins with the first contact.

Visualize the new patient. Before a new patient calls the office, it may be often assumed that the person is in trouble. He probably has had difficulty for a long time, even if "off and on." He probably has run the gamut of self-medication and home remedies. He probably has been to one or more MDs or DOs with unsatisfactory relief. He has tried to follow the advice of well-meaning friends and neighbors with unfavorable results. It is even possible that he has been to another DC. Someone whose advice he respects has now suggested he try your office. He is skeptical but groping for relief. He has hope or he wouldn't make the call. His optimism or skepticism will be enhanced by the first person he speaks to from your office and the continuing impressions he receives from the doctor and staff. The patient's first impression of the office is usually by telephone. The second impression is usually his reception at the office. Both are likely under the control of a CA.

In closing a call, review the details. Remember your "Thank you's" and "I'm sorry's." Hang up gently; you can spoil a pleasant good-by by jarring the ears of the person on the other end of the line. It's usually a good idea to allow the caller to disconnect first.

Keep personal calls brief. Visualize the plight of the mother with a sick child who cannot contact the office because the line is busy. Frustrating! Limit personal calls during office hours to emergencies, and make such calls as brief as possible.

MANAGING THE RECEPTION ROOM

First impressions are the strongest because they are the longest lasting. First impressions may be modified, but this takes a much longer time. *Well begun is half done.*

The receiving area is the second point of patient contact with the doctor's practice. The call to set the appointment was the first point of contact. The patient's susceptibility to impression continues in the receiving area. It is an important area as this is the first tangible evidence of the environment of the practice and possibly of the services to be received. Even before the patient has personal contact with an assistant in the receiving area, the external appearance of the office building and the receiving area itself has made an impression—adding to or subtracting from the impression created on the telephone.

From a clinical viewpoint, the reception room is a nonproductive area. Yet it is one of the most important rooms in the office. It is here that the new patient receives his first close impression of the doctor's neatness, taste, consideration for detail, cleanliness, and patient comfort. It is here that the returning patient gathers his thoughts before he sees the doctor. The reception room can either enhance or deflate the doctor's image and that of his services.

Overseeing the Receiving Area

The reception, dismissing, and business areas of the office are the chief domain of the administrative assistant. Before the first patient arrives, and throughout the day, observe these areas as if you were a patient. Periodically, check neatness of magazines, wastebaskets, lighting, ventilation, room temperature, general cleanliness, and tidiness. If the condition of the furniture, condition of wood and paint, color scheme, and furniture arrangement is not the best, feel free to call this to the attention of the doctor discreetly.

The reception area need not be large, but it should be comfortable, hospitable, and sunny if possible. Furnishings should be in good taste, coordinated, and chairs should have arms so patients with low-back disorders may arise without excessive strain.

Sound Control

Rarely should the actual reception room contain a desk. Conversations with entering and leaving patients are private and should not be within the range of other patients. One exception to this pertains to the group practice of several doctors who share a common receptionist whose duties are solely those of a receptionist. When an assistant is seated within the reception room, conversations are not private, and much time can be lost in idle conversation.

Listen as you would if you were a patient. Are there annoying interoffice sounds from equipment, intercoms, voices? Are there extra-office sounds from street noise? Remember, once you become used to a certain environment, you automatically become unaware of visual and audio impressions witnessed by a patient new to the environment. Soft background music is often used to induce relaxation and cover voices from adjacent rooms.

Clocks, radios, and television sets have no place in a professional office. Clocks constantly remind the patient how much the doctor may be behind schedule and add to the irritation. Avoid radios and TVs because it is difficult to select a program that would not irritate somebody. Prized antlers or bear rugs should be avoided because many people are not interested in the doctor's prowess as an animal killer, and they frequently frighten children. Care should also be taken in selecting pictures. What appeals to one may offend another. Seek to establish a pleasant atmosphere.

Several means can be used to reduce irritating noises. For interoffice noise, ceilings acoustically tiled, deep pile carpeting, snugly fitting doors, soft background music, conversations kept low, and especially noisy equipment placed in special sound-proofed rooms will be a great help. It is sometimes helpful to lower the ring of the telephone bell or use a phone chime in the business office. Street noise can be reduced by closing windows, providing windows with double-paned glass, covering windows with heavy drapery, and placing large shrubs near the windows. When appropriate, such suggestions will be appreciated by the doctor.

Policy Announcements

Sometimes it is necessary to post notices within the reception area that aid patients and procedures. Such signs should always be of professional appearance. If the sign is paper, place it under glass within a picture frame and mount. Never "thumb tack" it to the wall. Signs, usually of bakelite or plastic, announcing "Please Register" assure the assistant that no one patient in the reception area has not been properly greeted. Embarrassing situations regarding fee policy, payments for service, or check cashing can often be prevented by a small professional announcement near the business desk that describes office policies.

Reception Room Literature

Reading materials should be neatly placed in a magazine rack. Topics should have a varied interest to meet the needs of patients with different preferences. The material should be patient oriented rather than office oriented. One exception to this is the office of the new practitioner who wishes to educate as many people as quickly as possible to the benefits of chiropractic health care. He may restrict literature to that of "chiropractic" and "natural health" publications. Professional journals and newsletters, however, should not be placed in the reception area. Health literature designed specially for lay people are welcomed in most reception rooms.

For some reason, many patients associate the progressiveness of the doctor with the type and date of reception room literature. For this reason, monthly publications should be removed when they are 2 months old; weekly publications when they are 2 weeks old.

Educational Literature

Either in the reception room or preparation rooms or both, an adequate supply of modern chiropractic educational literature should be on hand. When tactfully suggested by the doctor or an assistant, patients enjoy reading chiropractic literature. If they had little interest, they would not be in the office. If a patient casually mentions a friend or relative that has a health disorder and is not a chiropractic patient, you may suggest a specific piece of literature that the patient may wish to forward. Chiropractic educational material prepares the mind of a patient or prospective patient for further information.

The American Chiropractic Association has a variety of quality educational literature and supplies. An array of titles is available for general health education, children and classrooms, back injuries, safety, insurance, and career opportunities within chiropractic.

Reception Area Supervision

In most practices, an administrative assistant takes responsibility for housekeeping control. A schedule should be established for daily, weekly, semimonthly, monthly, and less frequent responsibilities for each assistant, cleaning help, landlord, and others involved.

A messy office and dusty equipment can do more to discourage goodwill than things you or the doctor can say. Usually it will be the role of a technical assistant to supervise spotlessness of examination and therapeutic equipment. An administrative assistant should supervise business equipment such as typewriters, duplicating machines, dictaphone equipment, files, etc.

Because it is one of the first impressions on the patient, the reception area requires constant attention. Its appearance reflects the personality and character of the practice. Because of constant patient flow, frequent attention must be given to scattered magazines, gum wrappers, arranging supplies, straightening files, and emptying wastebaskets. Any wastebasket that may receive food particles, moisture or liquids, discarded adhesive tape, etc., should be lined with a plastic bag. Daily dusting and sweeping is usually necessary, and special attention should be given to the tidiness and cleanliness of rest rooms. Heavy cleaning such as vacuuming, floor maintenance, window cleaning, and washing woodwork is typically performed by an outside cleaning service.

Check throughout the day to see that all rooms are well ventilated. Check heating and aircooling levels, spray with air freshener when necessary, check lighting, pick up clutter, straighten furniture and magazines, restock literature displays, and oversee the neatness of all rooms. The bright, cheerful, well-organized reception area reflects a bright, cheerful, well-organized assistant.

Vinyl or wood floors should be cared for daily. Wood furniture should be dusted, leather or plastic furniture should be cleaned with a damp cloth and saddle soap, and upholstered furniture should be brushed and fluffed. Dust and fingerprints should be wiped from desks and table tops. Lamps should be dusted and bulbs replaced as necessary. The magazine rack should be clean and well organized; discard old issues. Window shades should be adjusted and draperies straightened. Empty wastebaskets and replace liners. Check rest room soap, towels, and toilet paper.

Wipe dust from plant leaves and use leaf spray. Plants will require moisture and nutrition. Dead leaves should be removed, and the plants should be rotated for sunlight.

Periodically see that upholstered furniture is dry cleaned or shampooed, that lamp shades are cleaned, that desks and tables are washed and polished, and that the frames of pictures or paintings are polished. See that draperies are professionally cleaned annually. Upholstered furniture should be vacuumed weekly. Dust paintings with a soft dry cloth as necessary.

SUCCESSFULLY MANAGING A PROFESSIONAL APPOINTMENT SYSTEM

The most frequent complaints from patients do not concern fees, health services, or house calls but rather the time wasted in waiting in the reception room when the doctor is behind schedule. Waiting complaints are heard twice as much as complaints about fees. It is natural for patients to become irritated when they have established a specific appointment time and are kept waiting a half hour or longer. Yet this is what happens in offices that are not run efficiently. This is poor management, poor human relations.

The doctor's reputation and the practice's image must be developed on an appointment system that is truly *a system* which does not deteriorate into a "catch the doctor when you can" procedure. Patients are people whose time and appointments are just as important to them as they are to the practice. Poor appointment management results in businessmen missing important dates, employees being "docked," and the development of animosity rather than good will.

Many practitioners feel strongly that no patient should leave the office without an appointment. Such an appointment may be the next day, as with an acute situation, or several months ahead, as for a periodic examination.

Handling and Making Appointments

General community economics has little to do with the success of a practice. Some practices thrive in poor times; others flounder in good times. One imperative for a successful practice is a controlled appointment system. Such a system considers the best interests of the patient and the practice. It is important then to allow enough time for each patient and his or her needs. Allowance also must be given to the examination or treatment that takes a little longer than

anticipated. This takes experience by the assistant: knowledge of the doctor's habits and knowledge of his patients. With experience, the alert assistant will judge fairly well what type of consultation, examination, or treatment will be necessary and how long such a procedure usually takes. Proper calculation of the time necessary for a patient's appointment greatly reduces reception room waiting, improves the quality of care, and contributes to positive public relations. A free period (about 20 minutes) scheduled midmorning and midafternoon allows for catch-up or to enter an unexpected emergency case.

To the doctor of chiropractic, the appointment book is his diary and record of activities. On it, he schedules his time. Thus, handling and making appointments must be done accurately and intelligently. Three basic points should be remembered:

1. Assure that names, addresses, phone numbers, time of appointments, and spellings are correct before you enter them into the book. Repeat them to the patient for verification. There is no room for overlooked appointments or misunderstandings in a well-run office. Open times in the appointment book are unproductive nonincome-earning periods. Crowded or duplicated periods in the appointment book are sources of dissatisfaction.

2. If in doubt about an appointment, verify it. This will avoid an error and will aid you when you fear the patient might have overlooked the appointment.

3. A record should be kept of canceled appointments made by phone or in person. This information is important when reviewing the work done that day and the work to be done in the future. The record also serves as a reference for charges and may have medicolegal implications.

People are human, and humans make mistakes. When the patient enters, the appointment book should be checked to assure that the patient is not too early, not too late, coming at the right hour, or even arriving on the right day.

Even the best appointment schedules can be disrupted. First, tardy patients do happen. A very late patient should be asked to reschedule the appointment or wait until there is time in the schedule for him. This explanation must be tactful, never sharp or paternal. Second, sometimes it is difficult for the doctor to dismiss a talkative patient. When the assistant suspects this, it is not inappropriate for her to remind the doctor that the next patient is waiting. Third, occasionally a person may drop in without an appointment. If it's not an emergency, schedule an appointment for the next day if possible. And fourth, emergencies happen that cannot be avoided.

Patients in severe pain take precedence over others with less priority. Most patients waiting will realize that they may be in the same condition sometime and will require immediate attention. Explain the occurrence in general terms to waiting patients so that they will understand.

Types of Appointment Books

The appointment book is a prerequisite of a good appointment system, and there are many types designed to fit a variety of needs. Some doctors with special needs have sheets printed to their specifications.

Most books have a line for every 15 minutes and offer two columns: One for the patient's name and the other for the services to be rendered. Some books allow one page for each day, while others show Monday through Saturday on two opposing pages, three days to a page. Most doctors and assistants prefer a large appointment book revealing the weekly schedule at a glance. Appointment books come either bound or loose leaf, and choice is a matter of personal preference.

While the 15-minute-line appointment book is the most common, many offices find this division impractical and prefer 5-minute or 10-minute intervals. This offers better accommodation for different types of consultations, examinations, and therapies. It is also more flexible for practices that require seeing more than four patients per hour on typical visits. Appointments must be scheduled according to services rendered.

Appointment Responsibilities and Techniques

The doctor schedules appointments by day, but it is an assistant who is responsible for arriving at an agreeable time of day for the patient. Because this assistant has this responsibility, she must have the authority to control the scheduling.

Some doctors like to schedule all severe cases at one period during the day and check-up visits during another. Likewise, some doctors like to schedule all extensive examinations during one part of the day (mornings or afternoons), while others prefer them interspersed between regular appointments. This is a matter of policy determined by the doctor's preferences.

In a busy office, it is rarely possible to give a caller an appointment at the exact time desired unless the appointment is being made far in advance. The assistant, however, should always let the patient know that the doctor is available and will see him as soon as possible. If a distressed caller is put off for several days, he undoubtedly will turn to another doctor who is more accommodating. Usually, a continuing patient not in distress or a new patient with a chronic condition will not mind if an appointment cannot be arranged for several days. Even in these situations, however, a 5-day wait is about maximum to suggest.

Appointments made by telephone are rarely forgotten by the patient as the patient has taken the initiative. However, appointments made in the office are apt to be forgotten, especially when the patient's condition begins to improve and distress is not a constant reminder. For this reason, most doctors will have printed appointment cards as a reminder. If the appointment is for a period over a week away, a telephone call on the day before the appointment is advisable to verify the appointment. Such a procedure helps to avoid "holes" within the appointment schedule because of forgotten appointments.

On the other hand, some doctors have the policy that an appointment should never be confirmed by telephone. Their reasoning is that calling patients to remind them of their time reservation often acts as an invitation to cancel or change the appointment. A patient may respond, "Glad you called. I was just going to phone you. It's not convenient for me to come in tomorrow. I'll let you know when I can make another appointment." Thus, it is felt that the office should not be the stimulus for a cancellation or appointment change. As health processes may be involved that are unknown to the patient, nothing should be done to encourage development of a tentative health-care plan. As shown, there are many strong points on both sides. The final decision whether to verify appointments or not must be decided by the doctor.

Managing the Appointment Schedule

Each new patient should be informed of the office's appointment policies when they are about to complete their first visit. This is usually at the dismissal desk. At this time, the assistant learns the most convenient time of day and days of the week for each patient and then tries to accommodate the patient's desires as close as possible when making appointments. It is helpful to note such desires on the patient's record for reference.

If the health-service program agreed to requires several visits a week for several weeks, the assistant should suggest blanketing a series of appointments for specific times during specific days in advance. This shows consideration for the patient's desires, eliminates further conversation about appointments in the near future, and serves also to act as a commitment between office and patient.

Most doctors prefer appointments be scheduled at regular intervals if possible. When it is necessary for a patient to be seen three times a week for several weeks, schedule the patient Monday, Wednesday, and Friday or Tuesday, Thursday, and Saturday. Patients to be seen twice a week could be scheduled Monday and Thursday, Tuesday and Friday, or Wednesday and Saturday. Patients to be seen once a week or less

frequent can be scheduled any time available.

Appointment Reminders

As previously described, some doctors prefer patient appointments verified by telephone and others do not. Most practitioners, however, do prefer the use of mailed reminders when appointments are made far in advance. Thus, if an appointment is greater than 3 weeks in the future, notify the patient through the mail so that it arrives about 4 days prior to the appointment. Many offices use a fill-in printed type of appointment reminder for this. Such printed cards have spaces for the patient's name and the date and time of the appointment reserved. If the appointment is made when the patient is in the office and not by telephone, the appointment is recorded in the appointment book in the presence of the patient and a note is made in a small tickler file to mail the appointment reminder.

It's good psychology to offer a patient a choice of two different appointment times. This gives the patient an "either—or" choice and a sense of being in control rather than being dictated to by the assistant. On the other hand, rarely give more than two choices as this contributes to the difficulty of a decision and wastes time at the appointment desk. By learning time preferences of various patients and recording this information within their records, you can conserve your time as well as that of the patients.

Return Appointments

Many practitioners prefer that every patient leaving the office has a definite appointment and that the name be entered in the appointment book in the patient's presence. Some doctors believe that a patient without a specific appointment will feel "discharged" if symptoms disappear and left to an unstable health-maintenance program. This would be an injustice to a comprehensive health-care service. Another reason is that if the doctor tells some patients to return in 2 weeks, they will often appear 2 weeks later when you do not have an opening. Thus, give the patient a specific day and time for the next appointment even if the appointment is 6 months in the future. If you are aware that the doctor has told the patient, "We'll do another progress examination in 3 months," note this in the appointment book so that adequate time will be allotted. Note any procedure you can anticipate if more time will be required than for a routine visit.

Future-Appointment Refusals

The doctor assumes responsibility for proper case management, but he cannot do this if the patient does not grant the authority to direct and schedule necessary appointments for care and evaluation of progress. In fairness to both doctor and patient, this policy must be maintained. A patient who refuses to accept a future appointment should understand that the doctor cannot be responsible for the consequences. When a patient refuses to accept a specific appointment, he assumes responsibility for the effects.

If a patient refuses to accept a future appointment after your tactful explanation, make a memorandum of the future appointment together with the patient's refusal. Post the memo within the patient's file. An accurate detailed record may relieve the doctor from responsibility for the patient's condition if the patient suffers a relapse because of lack of treatment.

Completing Incomplete Appointment Schedules

A tactful administrative assistant can efficiently control the appointment schedule by manipulating appointment times to suit practice needs and individual patient demands without disrupting the cordial doctor-patient relationship so necessary in health care. It is her responsibility to see that the appointment schedule is as complete for every practice day as possible.

After a practice has been operating for several years, it is possible to have the appointment schedule productive in advance 95% of the time. This is achieved by referring to the periodic examination list and developing a *recall list* (Fig. 7.6). If, for example, today is Friday and you note three openings for next Monday, check the appointment book for patients scheduled to come in later next week for a periodic examination. Call these people, and ask if they would mind coming Monday rather than the previously scheduled Wednesday, for example. Most patients who have not been to the office for several weeks or months usually do not mind such a slight appointment change. If this procedure fails, call "once a month" patients who are scheduled later in the week and attempt to move them to Monday. "New patient" calls and emergency calls will usually fill openings created by changes necessary to complete Monday's schedule. Monday is probably not the best day to use as an example because patients have a tendency to overextend themselves on the weekend, and the telephone is usually quite busy early Monday morning.

Patients who admire the doctor and respect the services readily cooperate with tactful requests. The objective is to see that each practice day represents a minimum of lost production time. When using a system to complete incomplete appointment schedules, note each patient's cooperativeness in their record file. Avoid requesting the same patient to change his time reservation on consecutive occasions, and avoid asking patients to change their time reservation if previously they appeared uncooperative or annoyed during the request.

In newly established practices, it is difficult if not impossible to maintain a completely full schedule for the simple reason that patient volume has not been developed to that point. In such situations, group appointments as close as possible to each other. Rather than allowing four 15-minute openings in an afternoon, it is better for the doctor to have an open hour at the beginning or end of the afternoon for correspondence, reading, case study, or personal business.

New Patient Referral Follow-up

It is important when making an appointment for a patient new to the practice to ask

Patient's Name	Phone No.	File No.	Last Major Complaint	Present Status	Appt. Made	Appt. Not Made

RECALL LIST   DATE _____

Figure 7.6. Sample recall list.

who referred him to the doctor. If it was another doctor, record this fact as it is customary that a report of your doctor-employer's findings and recommendations be sent immediately to the referring doctor. If you learn this on the telephone, try to arrange an appointment for the patient at the earliest opportunity as a professional courtesy.

Obtain the patient's name (correct spelling), address, telephone number, the condition for which he is being referred, and possibly the length and type of treatment he has received. This will help you prepare initial records, offer the doctor an overview of the situation, and save time for all involved. If the referred patient lives many miles away, consider travel time and possibly lodging arrangements.

If it is found that the entering patient was referred by a patient of your office, the referring patient should be sent a "Thank you" note or letter. Some doctors use a printed fill-in-type card. However, most doctors believe that a printed card is too impersonal and prefer an individually typed letter be forwarded. Many offices have on file several numbered "form letters" of this nature that can be personalized. Several are necessary as patients who refer usually develop a history of referring several people to the office. When numbered "form letters" are used, note in the referring patient's file the letter's number so the same letter is not sent twice to the same patient. If it is, the personal touch will be lost and feelings may be injured.

Appointment Book Responsibility and Authority

As one assistant should have the responsibility for appointment scheduling and control, the book must be considered her personal domain. Most doctors will respect this assistant's authority. She alone should make and change all appointments. It is also her responsibility to write clearly and accurately so that others can easily read her entries and notations.

If one assistant has the responsibility for the smooth functioning of the appointment schedule, she must have absolute authority to control it. There are two major reasons for this. First, the doctor who makes an appointment for a patient without informing the assistant is committing a definite breach of professional taste. Second, appointment book problems are multiplied in the two or more doctor office that has several staff assistants. Everyone is tempted to make appointments. If various doctors and assistants make appointments, disorganization and chaos follow.

On the surface it may appear that anyone can look at the book, see an opening, and insert a name for the time reservation. Such a policy does not consider the problems involved. For example, the assistant supposedly in charge of the appointment book has just spoken with Mrs. Anderson and told her that next Monday at 3 pm would be open for her daughter Mary. Mrs. Anderson says that's fine but she must check with the school to see if Mary can be excused early that day, and that she will call back in 20 minutes. Meanwhile, when the assistant is away from her desk for a moment, the telephone rings and is answered by a doctor or another assistant who schedules a patient in the apparently open 3:00 post. A few minutes later, Mrs. Anderson calls to confirm the 3:00 appointment. Tempers flare that could have been avoided if the caller who telephoned while the assistant was away from her desk was informed that the assistant in charge of appointments would return her call shortly.

Necessary Information for Making Advance Appointments

Put as much information as possible in a small space in your appointment book. For example, if a patient is scheduled for an extensive examination, noting this allows for proper time estimation as well as alerting the staff of necessary preparation. Most offices code standard procedures; eg, diathermy (D), x-ray (X), traction (T), spinal manipulation (M), physical examination (P), ultrasound (US), urinalysis (UR), and so forth. With experience, you can judge how long each procedure usually takes and schedule the appointment accordingly.

Obviously, a patient requiring several procedures will need a longer time reservation than a patient requiring one or two procedures. An entering patient requiring extensive examination will need a longer time reservation than a patient for a routine progress evaluation. A patient suffering a severely painful disorder probably will require more time than a patient suffering a minor acute disorder. Different procedures and different situations require different time requirements. Even age is a factor. A senior citizen will usually require a longer time reservation than a teenager suffering the same complaint. If the assistant must control patient flow with maximum efficiency and minimal effort, she must be able to see at a glance why the patient is scheduled.

When setting advance appointments, mark holidays observed by the office. Also cross out all days when you know the doctor will not be in the office for such reasons as seminars, conventions, vacations, and other predictable absences. This prevents errors requiring many telephone calls and apologies to change scheduled appointments.

Your employer may be an examiner or a consultant for an insurance company. If an examiner, the company will refer applicants for life insurance to your office for examination prior to approving the policy requested. When this happens, be sure to obtain the name of the insurance company since it will be they who are responsible for the bill. If the company requires certain laboratory tests, note this in the appointment book. The doctor will inform you how long an average insurance examination will take. Note this for reference.

If your employer is a consultant for an insurance company, one of his roles will be that of reviewing claims. If the volume is extensive, he may wish you to allot several hours a week in the appointment book to review claims.

Handling Difficult Appointment Requests

An administrative assistant frequently receives some unusual appointment requests. Mental and emotional balance is the key in handling such situations. First, remember that a health practice is a service operation. Its primary goal is to help people in need. Second, office policies must be guarded. If there are too many exceptions, satisfying the needs of a few patients may be detrimental to the needs of the majority. By keeping in mind the needs of individual patients and the needs of the practice as a whole, logical decisions can be achieved.

Telephone requests for a definite appointment time can be a problem. If the time requested is available, reserve that time for the patient. If the requested time is filled, offer two alternatives as near the request as possible and say something to the effect: "What is your second choice, Mr. Brown? I probably can be more helpful then, and, if there is any change in the schedule, I'll call you immediately." Intelligent patients will appreciate this consideration. Even if no change in the schedule occurs to satisfy the original request, telephone the patient and say, "Sorry, Mr. Brown, but there has been no change in our schedule so I'm verifying your second choice at 1 o'clock Wednesday. If a change does occur, and I'll do my best to help you, I'll call you immediately." This again reassures the patient of your personal interest and enhances office good will. Good will is the essence of practice security and growth.

Telephone requests for an immediate appointment are handled in the same way as requests for a definite time. We are not referring here to the emergency call,

rather the call for an immediate appointment because of impending travel or personal convenience. If the patient should call and request an appointment for later that day, make the appointment if an opening is available. When you do, say, "You're very fortunate, Mrs. Kingsley, it just so happens that we just had a schedule change." Never say, "We just had a cancellation." Patient attitude should be developed to the effect that a cancellation never occurs. Patients should be educated that cancellations are not permitted.

The continuing or entering patient who enters the office without an appointment and requests immediate service requires tact. Explain office procedures, yet comply with the request if the patient can be worked into the schedule without too much confusion. Here again, we are not referring to what would be called an *emergency.* Avoid the word "cancellation" and say, "Because of a recent change in our schedule, the doctor can see you soon." Then have the patient seated in the reception room and begin the entering patient process. These occurrences test the efficiency and tact of the assistant in charge of appointments. By being interested in patient's needs and without disrupting good practice management standards, everybody benefits. Such situations, however, should be rare for any one patient.

A patient who habitually enters the office without an appointment and requests immediate attention or the patient who frequently calls late for a time reservation must be discreetly educated to the necessity of adhering to office policy. It's only policy because it's in the best interests of all patients. Some patients feel that while the doctor prefers appointments, they are not absolutely necessary, at least not for them. An attitude as this soon grows to a lack of respect for the doctor because the assistant was not in control of the situation. Yes, some patients will bully assistants.

Tourists. Offering service to tourists is often a perplexing problem for the doctor. On one hand, he is faced with a person in need and it is his professional obligation to help. On the other hand, because he lacks experience with the patient, a thorough history and examination is necessary to provide competent care. Few tourists are willing to go such an expense when they know they will be leaving town soon. The doctor can suggest two things: Either perform the necessary examinations and tests, or telephone the patient's hometown doctor (at the patient's expense) and see what he suggests. The patient must decide what course of action he prefers. First aid is always extended on request, however.

A practice operating on office hours rather than an appointment system requires a different approach. Prior to World War II, most doctors treated patients during certain hours rather than giving each patient a specific appointment. The appointment system has since slowly gained in popularity and is now used by most practitioners. In the office-hours system, patients are seen in the order they arrive. It is important for the receptionist to record each patient's name in their order of arrival. This serves a threefold purpose: it avoids questions about who sees the doctor next, provides a record of patients the doctor has seen that day, and allows the assistant to gather in sequence patient files.

The major disadvantage of the office-hours system is that most patients tend to come about the same time. This means the office and doctor may be idle at some hours and then be forced to handle a large volume of patients at other times. This situation can be avoided, however. If, for example, office hours are from 2 till 6 o'clock, tell half the patients to come between 2 and 4, and the other half between 4 and 6. Experience will tell the alert assistant the best way to manage the particular practice philosophy of her employer.

Handling several progress reports or inquiries by telephone may dominate lines needed for appointments. If the practice manages many acute disorders, the doctor may ask patients to report their daily progress. Patients, on their volition, may call the doctor's office to report their progress or to ask questions regarding their condition. Such calls may be routine for the practice. Abuse of the telephone is seen in the patient attempting to obtain detailed professional counsel or a diagnosis over the telephone. These abuses are often called "nuisance" calls as they interrupt the doctor when he is in consultation with another patient. Many practitioners feel that legitimate progress reports and inquiries should be encouraged.

To avoid "plugging" lines during peak office hours or interfering with a doctor-patient relationship during care, practices having many of these calls can set aside a special time each day during which patients can reach the doctor by telephone. This special time, a "Telephone Hour," is sometimes printed on the office's stationery, sometimes it is posted in the dismissal area, or both. When a telephone hour is established, it is usually placed at the beginning of the day. If placed at the end of the day, conflict may arise because of an extended schedule accommodating drop-in patients or emergencies requiring an immediate appointment.

When a telephone hour is specified, office policy usually requires that telephone appointments will not be scheduled during the telephone hour nor will progress reports or inquiries be accepted at times other than the telephone hour. As always, controlling policy requires tact by the assistant so that no patient will feel that they are being "victimized" by an office policy. And, of course, there will always be justifiable exceptions.

Problems arise in house calls that are different from those of office visits. Out-of-office visits are usually made for one of two reasons. Either the patient is bedridden because of an acute condition and the doctor must afford enough relief so the patient can come to the office for thorough care, or the patient is bedridden because of some chronic degenerative condition. For whatever reason the doctor makes house calls, the assistant should schedule them to the mutual convenience of the doctor and patient in the most efficient manner.

Because of unforeseen delays resulting from case management, traffic conditions, or climate, it will be impossible to give the patient anything more than an approximate time for the doctor's arrival. When scheduling the appointment by telephone, ask what major streets or landmarks are near the residence and note this for the doctor. Check the address in your city directory, and see to it that the doctor's bag contains a city map. If the doctor makes a regular round of house visits, prepare a *routing list* so he need not crisscross the town after each visit. The list should be prepared considering both the location of the patient's residence and the urgency of the visit. A copy of the list should be at the office so if the doctor needs to be contacted you will have an approximate idea where he will be at any time.

A record of out-of-office visits can be handled several ways. For example:

1. When the doctor returns, the assistant can note on her copy of the routing list the services provided, the fee involved, whether the fee was paid or charged, and other points the doctor wishes recorded. These points are then transferred to the patient's record in the office file.

2. The doctor may carry a pad of printed house call slips that he fills out at each residence visited. When he returns to the office, he gives these to the assistant for processing.

3. The doctor may keep a small pocket notebook using two facing pages for each day's entries. Patient names, addresses, and approximate appointment times are entered on the left-hand page. Notes about services provided, patient's condition, charges made, and payments received are recorded on the right-hand page directly across from the patient's name. Such a ledger is usually kept at the appointment desk so that the assistant can schedule the out-of-office visits efficiently. The doctor picks up the ledger as he leaves the office and returns it to the assistant when he completes the calls. Data from the ledger are transferred to permanent patient records in the office.

Appointment Planning Influence on Case Management

The efficiency of almost the entire office can be aided greatly through a well-planned appointment schedule. Good planning maintains an even patient flow through the office

and avoids idle time. As time means money, planning affects practice economy. Orderly scheduling prevents overcrowding and allows patients to be cared for in an unhurried manner. Thus, good planning has a direct relationship to both the clinical and psychologic atmosphere of the practice.

Only in slipshod helter-skelter offices will appointments be considered just names in the appointment book. The assistant should never enter an appointment unless there is reasonable assurance that the appointment will be kept. Each patient must be educated to the importance and seriousness of the time reservation with the doctor. When the assistant recognizes the seriousness of efficient appointment planning and respects the authority and responsibility the doctor has given her, patients will reflect this attitude. On the other hand, if the assistant assumes a lackadaisical attitude in appointment planning and is unimpressed with the importance of efficient scheduling, patients will reflect this attitude. This would be detrimental to a good doctor-patient relationship.

Good planning means to live in reality—to face situations of the practice as they are and not as we wish them to be. Office policies are not laws; common sense and good judgment are needed to know when it is logical to bend the rules and when it is not. We must have administrative mechanics, but people are not machines that can be operated with simple push-button controls. Living in reality, the wise assistant anticipates some appointment changes, tardy patients, broken appointments, last minute cancellations, times when the doctor will be late, and sensitive, irritable, and demanding patients.

Besides the concerns described, patient relations can suffer if the following situations are not well planned in patient scheduling.

Patients Who Commute

A patient may live several months in Arizona during the winter, reside in Minnesota during the summer, and vacation on the coast. The doctor recommending a comprehensive health plan must adapt the ideal to anticipating many appointment irregularities in routine. Either the ideal must be amended or the doctor must restrict his care to prophylactic care until the patient can be convinced it will be necessary to reside in the doctor's community for a longer period than originally planned. While several doctors in different areas who practice closely alike may cooperate on a case of a commuting patient, it is difficult. In any event, it is important that the assistant ask how long the patient expects to be in the area when planning appointments.

Shift Workers

Employees working in factories requiring a rotating shift pose a problem in maintaining a regular appointment schedule. Entertainers presenting both matinee and evening performances also have difficulty. Before accepting a patient under these conditions, the doctor must educate the patient on the importance of following the case plan, and the doctor and patient must agree on ways to correct irregularities to the recommended schedule. It would be folly to embark on a comprehensive program for a serious condition if it is felt that adherence to a schedule could not be made. If ways to correct expected irregularities can be found and agreed to, this information should be passed on to the appointment assistant and recorded in the patient's chart. If the doctor and patient cannot agree on a logical method to establish an effective appointment routine, it would be better to postpone the recommended service until a satisfactory schedule can be maintained. Policemen, firemen, nurses, and others on rotating shifts present similar problems.

Unstable Personalities

The more unstable the patient's personality, the more important it is that the patient be educated and periodically reminded of appointment policy. Skeptical, high strung, overemotional, flighty, severely neurotic, or unstable patients need constant guidance and reinforcement. If such patients fail to profit by the advice, the doctor may be forced to postpone further service until full

cooperation can be obtained. If the recommended case program cannot be followed, the patient is wasting money and the doctor is wasting time that could be better spent with more cooperative patients.

Adverse Traveling Conditions

Patients living many miles from the office may be subjected to bad driving conditions, inclement weather, undependable transportation systems, and other unpredictable problems that place a severe hardship in maintaining appointment regularity. Here too, attempts must be made to find a logical solution.

Sales and Service People

Some types of sales or service positions and truck drivers require extensive traveling to meet customer needs. This may involve a multicounty route or unpredictable service calls to remote areas from the home community of the doctor and patient. It is important that anticipated irregularities in the recommended appointment schedule be explained to the patient and means sought to protect regularity.

The doctor can examine a patient to determine the cause of a health disorder. He can recommend to the patient a plan felt to be the best method to correct the disorder in the shortest possible time, if it is possible. When the patient accepts the program, he can expect that the doctor will do everything possible to see that the plan is carried out. Likewise, the doctor must expect the patient to cooperate to the fullest in following recommendations. But the doctor cannot do it alone.

Returning a sick or disabled person to health is a difficult enough task without adding to it the negative influences of broken appointments, changed appointments, cancellations, and other irregularities to the recommended schedule. Barriers to offering the best professional service possible must be identified as early as possible, and attempts must be made to eliminate them. To do less would be an injustice to both the patient and the doctor.

Handling Broken, Changed, or Late Appointments

Patients who cancel or change appointments without due notice or justification must be tactfully reminded of office policy else the assistant contributes to the patient's delinquency and helps to establish a negative habit pattern. The patient should be made to feel, in a polite way, that the doctor's treatment plan has been greatly inconvenienced by the schedule being disrupted. The assistant might say, "Mr. Jones, you realize that a time reservation has been personally set aside for you. When so many people want time to see the doctor, it really isn't fair to the doctor or your health. I know you will see that it won't happen again." When a patient did not have the courtesy to call to change or cancel an appointment, a letter can be sent to the patient who does not have a telephone.

Unworthy Patients

If the patient habitually misses, cancels, or changes appointments without justification, he must be considered an unworthy patient. If the case program is being affected, the doctor must have a heart-to-heart talk with the patient on the importance of regularity. If this fails, steps must be taken to postpone further service until cooperation can be given. This may not be possible in the newly established practice where every patient is important to the practice's economic stability. Nevertheless, a practice cannot be controlled or a professional health service provided if it is based on uncooperative patients who are unworthy to both the practice and their health needs.

"No Shows"

Chronic "no shows" must be handled in the same manner as that for patients who habitually cancel appointments without due notice or justification. Such unworthiness suggests a profound lack of appreciation of the doctor and his services. This lack of respect may be the result of the patient's personality, negative environmental factors, or negative conditioning.

The cause also may be within the doctor's office. Was the first telephone contact handled effectively? Were first impressions of the office positive? Did the assistant who first greeted the patient present a warm and professional approach? Were the history taking, examination, and case presentation conducted professionally? Does the staff maintain the highest professional standards, and do their attitudes reflect sincere concern for the patient's welfare? Was the patient adequately educated to office policies, and were appointment policies stressed? An objective analysis of the important phases of patient contact will often spotlight weaknesses in the office system.

Time Reservation Charges

If a patient cancels at the last moment or fails to notify the doctor that he's not coming in, some doctors feel the time reserved should be charged. This, of course, is strictly up to the doctor. Doctors who charge a fee usually do not like to charge a patient for the first offense. For the patient who habitually cancels, the charge serves to motivate regularity. Some doctors post an announcement in the reception area that appointments not rescheduled within 24 hours of the time reserved will be charged a fee for the time reserved (eg, $15).

While a charge for a broken appointment is legal in most states, many doctors feel that the procedure is psychologically unsound except in special situations. The basic problem requiring correction is education of the patient to the need for regularity.

Several canceled appointments will severely affect office economics. Most doctors base their fees on anticipated patient volume and projected expenses. To the practice with a tight schedule, cancellations and "no shows" represent a drastic influence on practice stability. If the office is open 200 days a year and if the doctor charges $20 for a standard office visit, one broken appointment daily represents a $4,000 annual loss; three broken appointments a day, a $12,000 deficit.

Resolution Techniques

Several methods in handling canceled appointments are used. One common method applied when a patient calls to cancel an appointment is to suggest another time immediately. If time allows, the CA can then call a patient who desired an earlier appointment but was unable to obtain one.

With a "no show," the assistant should initial the notation of the missed appointment. With the patient's file folder on her desk for reference, the assistant can telephone the patient and say: "Hello, Mr. Smith, this is Dr. Godfrey's office calling. Dr. Godfrey was sorry you missed your time reservation this morning and asked me to phone and arrange a visit this evening—or would tomorrow morning be better?" Calls to "no shows" should be made approximately a half hour after the patient was due. The goal is to arrange another appointment as soon as possible so the patient's schedule will not be too upset.

There are three main reasons for a "no show": (1) the patient forgot the appointment; (2) the patient feels so good that he feels future appointments are unnecessary, or (3) the patient feels worse and is discouraged in continuing treatment. These reasons deserve further explanation:

1. If the patient simply forgot the appointment, there usually is no difficulty in quickly arranging another.

2. If the patient says he feels so good that he doesn't feel an immediate appointment is necessary, the assistant should respond to the effect: "It's wonderful you are feeling so much better, Mr. Smith. Dr. Burton will be glad to hear that because that is what he has been working toward. Let's arrange an appointment for Thursday or Friday so that you can discuss this with Dr. Burton and avoid any recurrence of the problem. Which would be better, Thursday at 10 am or Friday at 3:15 pm." If the patient still refuses your suggestion for an appointment, let him know that you will give the doctor his message and that the doctor may want to call him. Depending on the circumstances of the case and your report of the conversation, the doctor may wish to call the patient to

explain the difference between the relief of outward symptoms and achieving as much of a permanent correction as possible.

3. If the patient says he feels worse, is discouraged, and doesn't wish to continue treatment now, the assistant can comment: "Mr. Smith, it's only human to get discouraged when response isn't as fast as desired. However, the fact that you haven't responded suggests further treatment is necessary to get you well. Dr. Burton would not have asked me to call if he was not thoroughly convinced that further therapy is necessary. Let me arrange an appointment for you Thursday morning at 10:30 or Friday afternoon at 2:15. Which would be better for you?" If the patient still refuses an appointment, let him know that you will pass on his message to the doctor. Again, depending on the circumstances, the doctor may wish to call the patient to attempt to re-establish rapport.

In essence, the effectiveness of any appointment control system (or any office system for that matter) depends primarily on the doctor. If the practitioner is lackadaisical, deficient in professional deportment and authority, does not take time to adequately train his assistants or supervise their performance, he will find that patients reflect this attitude in their attitudes toward the recommended appointment schedule. If either the doctor or assistant hesitates to tactfully discuss appointment irregularities with lax or uncooperative patients, they cannot expect to maintain control of the appointment schedule. Poor consequences are inevitable.

Tardy Patients

Patients late for appointments cause another type of problem. Because people meet unsuspected problems, occasional tardiness must be accepted as part of life. On the first offense, the late patient only needs to be reminded that he is late and that the doctor will see him when possible. Whether the patient will receive the total service scheduled will depend on the type of service specified and how tight the appointment schedule is. The habitual late patient is a more serious problem. With tact and sympathy for the patient's excuse for being late, the assistant should arrange a new appointment if the schedule would not easily allow him to be worked in. Patients with undependable appointment habits must be educated to the importance of their time reservations. This is only logical, however, if the doctor and the staff are punctual.

Delayed Doctor

Patient irregularities are not the only reason schedules get disrupted. The doctor may be late in arriving at the office. If patients are waiting, the assistant should inform the patients the reason for the delay. If the doctor is extremely delayed, new appointments should be made for those patients who do not wish to wait.

Sometimes situations arise when the doctor must cancel one or more appointments. Bad weather, emergency professional meetings, and other unforeseen situations may require several appointments or even the entire day's appointments be changed. When this happens, patients should be notified immediately by telephone, telegram, or mail—whichever is the more appropriate. When the schedule is changed, another appointment should be offered at the same time.

When changing a patient's appointment, the assistant should tactfully offer a reasonable explanation why the appointment must be changed. Avoid such abruptness as: "Mr. Jones, this is Dr. Carey's office. We must cancel your appointment for next Wednesday. Could you come in Friday?" Such a cold approach would be received by most patients as an indication of little concern for patients' interests and personal problems. A better approach would be something like this: "Mr. Jones, this is Dr. Carey's office. Dr. Carey must attend a special meeting in Capitol City at your appointment time. He asked me to call and extend his apologies and asks if we can arrange a convenient time for you—like next Monday or Tuesday?" In this instance, you have used tact, appreciated the inconvenience to the patient, and offered the patient a choice in selecting the new appointment.

Handling Emergency Situations

While emergency situations are not everyday happenings, it is important that you know what to do. There are two basic types of emergencies: those that happen when the doctor is in the office and those that occur when he is not.

When the doctor is in the office, any emergency should be brought to his attention immediately. If he is out of the office such as at his residence, at a meeting, or out socially, you should know where to reach him. Your employer will have a personal calendar that lists his engagements. If the doctor is out of town or unavailable for emergency needs, he will have arranged with another doctor to cover patient needs. Be sure you know who this substitute is and where he can be located during your employer's absence.

If a telephone call reports an emergency, keep calm and in control. Be careful to write clearly and accurately the necessary information of who, what, when, and where. Most emergency situations can be handled quickly and efficiently if you are calm, cool, and collected. After noting the important information, retrieve the patient's file and bring both the file and your notes to the doctor. If you are communicating with a substitute doctor by telephone, relate from the patient's file the patient's history, working diagnosis, and other points questioned.

The following usually indicate emergency situations:

- Severe pain
- Unusual swelling, edema
- Difficult breathing
- Inability to move, paralysis
- Dizziness, vertigo
- High fever
- Fainting, unconsciousness
- Sudden visual disturbances
- Anuresis
- Hemorrhage of any type
- Severe vomiting
- Cyanosis, jaundice, pallor
- Convulsions, seizures

Legitimate telephone requests for emergency attention of an established patient must be given priority appointment time even in a full schedule. Specific procedures for coping with these situations depend solely on the doctor's practice philosophy and state legal requirements. Time must be borrowed from other patients—usually prophylactic or unworthy patients.

Experience shows that the emergency patient should only receive services solely of an emergency nature. If an emergency patient new to the practice is accepted and extensive examination and therapy are provided during a full schedule, a poor precedent is established with that patient. In addition, it is unfair to those patients scheduled who were inconvenienced by the emergency.

Maintaining Appointment Continuity and Control

Continuity

Log patients on regular appointment schedules at the same hour whenever possible. It helps to establish a habit pattern. Likewise, when the schedule is known for several weeks in advance, blanket these appointments in advance. On the other hand, if a patient is accustomed to a specific time and day for his appointment and cannot be allotted that time, inform the patient immediately.

Control

Appointment schedules should be arranged as far ahead as possible to suit the patient's convenience. However, the patient should not be allowed to determine the interval between appointments. This is a clinical judgment. When the patient makes such a decision, the doctor is no longer in authority of the case. If the doctor is to be responsible for case management, he must have the authority to direct the quantity and quality of service.

While the assistant should be specific in the patient's appointment day and time, she should not mention the specific length of time reserved for the patient. Never say, "We've scheduled you for a 15-minute reservation next Friday, Mr. Johnson." When the day of the appointment arrives, different patient conditions and situations may develop that require a shorter or longer visit than originally anticipated. Some CAs handle this by scheduling three or four patients simultaneously followed by a break. This allows flexibility needed for patient care, makes fullest use of examining and treatment rooms, avoids delays for the doctor while patients are being prepared for examination or treatment, and helps handle the problem of the tardy patient.

The office appointment book must be considered restricted property and its schedule confidential information. Never allow a patient to view the appointment schedule. The volume of patients scheduled for any one day or the openings present are the business of the appointment assistant and the doctor; no one else.

Policy should be explained in detail at the dismissal desk following the first visit. A good explanation here will do much to minimize the possibility of future changed or canceled appointments. Also, the assistant is in a prime position to reinforce the doctor's concern for "case control" and the value of regularly scheduled check-ups in preventing relapse. A doctor's staff can do much to create an impression of punctuality, concern, efficiency, and cooperation in the minds of patients by rigidly setting a positive example.

The Control Sheet

A practice in control operates efficiently without unnecessary open time in the appointment book, without rush periods, and without seasonal trends. This takes patient education to the value of health services, preventive measures, and the value of health maintenance. However, before anyone can be educated, there must be a desire to learn. Desire is based on need, admiration, and respect: human relations.

The efficient office has a minimum of unproductive time. This requires few broken appointments, changed appointments, and tardy patients else the practice is not in control. A *control sheet* is helpful in analyzing problem areas. It is a sheet on which each patient scheduled for the day is listed followed by several columns to indicate the patient's next appointment, a broken appointment, a canceled appointment, a changed appointment, or if the patient was a new referral.

The exact scheduling of the patient's next appointment is important to patient control. No practice can be considered under control when patients are allowed to arrange their next appointment on their volition. For all practical purposes, a patient without a scheduled appointment must be considered lost to the practice because it cannot be assumed that the patient will return.

From both a human relations and an economic viewpoint, it is important to record the number of cancellations and the reasons for the cancellation. From a clinical viewpoint, the doctor is interested in cancellations and appointments changed to a later date as such changes may affect his prognosis. It is also an indication that the patient is assuming responsibility of the case and is directing his appointment schedule. When a patient assumes such control, there is a breakdown in the doctor-patient relationship allowing the patient to question the doctor's authority and sincerity. A *control sheet* allows the doctor to analyze the quantity of these occurrences. When the number of new referrals does not exceed the number of patients lost to the practice, the practice is not growing; it is diminishing.

There is nothing unprofessional about an assistant calling a patient to determine the reason for not meeting a scheduled appointment. If the appointment was scheduled for the patient's welfare, no inquiry suggests lack of the doctor's interest. The reason may be a simple oversight, or it could mean a breakdown in communications. Obviously, if the practice does not show interest and concern for the patient's welfare, the patient will lose interest and concern for the doctor's services. If a patient becomes discouraged or has a complaint, the doctor must know this to analyze it and keep similar situations from recurring. For his sake and the patient's, the doctor is obliged to determine the reason behind cancellations.

A cancellation may be the result of a death in the family. If so, the doctor will have an opportunity to forward an appropriate sympathy card. Whatever the reason, communications must be maintained so that positive action can take place. Professional conduct should never be less than good social conduct. Communication of sympathy, congratulations, and the like cannot be expressed if the facts are not known. This takes follow-up. Intelligent patients appreciate this consideration.

Obviously, all legitimate reasons for cancellation are excusable. Yet even with justifiable excuses, the patient must be impressed with the necessity of maintaining the treatment schedule. If appointment changes are not justifiable, office policy must be reaffirmed to the patient through education and motivation. The results of these conversations should be noted in the patient's record. It cannot be overemphasized that the office's concern with cancellations and changed appointments reaffirms in the patient's mind the importance of office policy and the staff's interest and concern in the welfare of the patient. When the patient is thoroughly impressed with the seriousness and importance of the appointment, there is greater desire by the patient to see that there are few appointment irregularities.

Appointment Scheduling

The appointment book is the place of battle against time. The entry system must be unified and informative. Entries should be made in pencil so that changes, cross-outs, and erasures can be made neatly.

During late afternoon or early evening before the day in question, many offices telephone to confirm appointments for the next day. This may be in addition to reminder cards that were given to the patient when he was last in the office or those mailed several days before for a time reservation made by telephone.

Patients sometimes make appointments for friends and family members—in person or by telephone. Determine if the appointment is for a patient new to the practice or an established patient. Record as many important data as possible such as the full name, complete address, telephone number at home and at work with extension, and family name when different from patient's name (eg, married daughter). Try to determine why the appointment is being made, and ask the age of the prospective patient. Is there an urgency to the appointment? Try to find the needs of the patient, how long the disorder has existed, or if the patient has been to another doctor for the condition or is under care of another doctor for another reason. Determine what specific instructions the person might need (eg, forms to be prepared prior to the visit).

You can measure your success at the art of scheduling two ways: (1) when patients come to the office confident that they will see the doctor without unreasonable delay, and (2) when the doctor and staff are productively occupied with neither too few nor too many patients.

If the doctor has recommended a future appointment but the patient fails to make arrangements, the reason should be noted in the patient's record. A "Will Call" must be considered the same as a cancellation and treated with appropriate follow through.

As referrals are the life-blood of the practice, human relations factors must be considered. The foundation for most entering patients will be referral from current patients. Surveys conclude that most patients new to the practice will be referred by active patients. No practice can survive or grow if it depends on referral by location, the yellow pages, or other external influences. When one realizes that 94% of new patients are the result of direct patient referral, note the importance of recognizing and thanking each patient for each referral. Printed "fill-in" cards are not recommended as they lack the human, personal touch. Human relations cannot be mechanical.

Human relations and patient control are analyzed by noting factors such as patient load, the number of patients with a definite future appointment, why some patients do not have a future appointment, and the quantity of cancellations and the reasons offered. The number of changed appointments, the quantity of new patients admitted, the services rendered, collection difficulties, and other facts offer helpful "trouble-shooter" information.

When the appointment book shows an in-sufficient number of patients scheduled to maintain full production capabilities, a system of recalls should be considered. In this procedure, the doctor reviews his files and selects several patients that do not have scheduled appointments, are considered worthy patients, and have not been to the office for several months. Such patients have not been educated by the doctor on the importance of preventive or maintenance care. Statistics show that for every eight patients telephoned, five of eight will accept an appointment. Patients are contacted each day until the appointment schedule is filled to a desirable degree, allowing for new patients and emergencies. Never attempt to "pressure" a patient into a return visit.

Handling the "Demand" for an Appointment

An assistant's judgment must decide whether a patient's urgent request for an appointment is a true emergency or not. If in doubt, ask the doctor. Frequently, however, answers to tactful questions provide the information necessary to arrive at a competent judgment whether the patient should be "squeezed" into a full schedule or put off until the next opening.

In asking questions about a patient's symptoms, never "play down" the patient's problem. His complaint is very real to him, while you are looking at the situation from an objective viewpoint. The patient should feel you are genuinely interested, as you are, and allow him an opportunity to air how he feels and what is happening. Most patients will be more receptive to suggestions after they have expressed themselves than when you first answer the phone.

If the patient persists that an immediate appointment is necessary, politely explain that the schedule is full and the doctor is running late. If he feels he cannot wait until tomorrow, say that you will be happy to work him in. Remind him that the doctor could only take a quick look at his condition today, and you would rather give him an appointment tomorrow when the doctor will have more time to thoroughly investigate the problem. As few patients want a hurried visit when not necessary or enjoy waiting a long period only to be rushed in and out, most patients, after discussing the problem with you, will ask what time the doctor can see them the next day. However, never refuse an established patient emergency care when requested—it could constitute malpractice.

IT'S NOT ALWAYS WHAT YOU SAY, BUT HOW YOU SAY IT

A CA should never let a patient browbeat her (eg, for the sake of economy or expediency) to do anything that would not be ultimately in the patient's best interests. Actions should be designed to enhance the doctor-patient relationship and support the doctor's authority in case management.

Semantics and Case Management

During the course of treatment, never ask a patient, "How do you feel?" If the patient does feel better, fine; if he does not, you invite a complaint. It is better to greet returning patients with a positive question such as, "What improvement have you noticed so far?" This suggests to the patient that it takes time for the healing process but improvement is expected. However, if you can see obvious improvement, there is nothing wrong in mentioning it to the patient. In fact, it is positive reinforcement.

Patients rarely leave a practice because they have a complaint. They leave when people involved do not listen. See Figure 7.7. Any patient complaint, no matter how seemingly casual or trivial, should be taken seriously. Evaluate every comment, and follow with appropriate comment or action. During acute illness, complaints may come from family members who are apprehensive about a loved one. Do your best to ease their fears or they may be passed on to the patient, but never infer a "promise" that could be mistaken as a guarantee.

You will occasionally be exposed to a sensitive human-relations situation in which a patient mentions that another doctor or a member of the immediate family disagrees with your doctor-employer's opinion. When this happens, maintain professional poise, be courteous, and disagree friendly. Indicate that while you respect the other person's opinion, your employer has a fine reputation for having excellent judgment in such matters. Build the doctor without tearing down another person.

Help the patient recognize that the doctor is not a magician. The patient must assume a share of responsibility in the healing process such as following the doctor's advice and recommendations. The doctor's role includes teaching the patient certain preventive practices, explaining methods to enhance the healing process, educating the patient in certain dietary habits and therapeutic exercises, or recommending acts such as more rest, staying home from work, and activity changes. A patient's recovery depends a great deal on active participation in the health program. The chiropractic assistant serves the patient's and the doctor's best interests when she encourages the patient to become actively involved in the health plan.

Only a fraction of lost customers can be attributed to death, moving, unadjusted complaints, lower prices, or better services in the business world. The majority of customers lose interest because of personnel indifference or disinterest. A breakdown in human relations is the major cause of clientele loss. There is no reason to think this is not also true in health practice. Patients who are responding well and those who are not will remain in the practice if they feel the doctor and assistant are competent and interested in them as individuals. They leave the practice when interest is not continually reinforced. This interest is maintained by having singleminded focus on the patient, his condition, and his problem.

Both doctor and assistant should leave all thoughts of family problems, organizational interests, and other personal concerns aside during office hours. Energies must be concentrated on and directed to the most important aspect of the practice—the patient.

SOME VERBAL MESSAGES AND THEIR HIDDEN MEANINGS

Message	Meaning
I need your advice on something.	I'm really confused.
No, I'm not upset!	I don't want to talk about it because you never listen to my viewpoint.
I know, I know.	Stop bugging me. You've said this all before, but I have my own reasons for doing it this way.
Forget it. It doesn't matter.	I don't want to talk about it any more.
I was afraid this was going to happen.	I told you so. I tried to warn you, but you just wouldn't listen.
Let's think about it for awhile?	I'm not sold on it.
I agree, but . . .	You're dead wrong, and I'll show you where.
It doesn't matter!	My feelings don't count, do they?
That's a ridiculous deadline.	What's in it for me for the extra effort?
Sorry, it's office policy.	My opinion is fixed.
Whatever you say.	You're an exasperating tyrant.
Some people think that . . .	I think that . . .
I was only trying to help.	Judge my intentions, not my actions.
It was an accident.	Will you forgive me?
He's that way with everybody.	He's that way with me too!
You've got to be kidding.	I've about reached my limits.
What I'm trying to say is. . .	Would you PLEASE listen?

Figure 7.7. Some innocuous phrases and their frequently hidden meanings. Strong messages can often be stated softly, but the feelings behind them can be loud and clear to an attentive ear.

Every thought or act that is not patient oriented distracts from the quality of the practice. If thoughts of the staff are filled with patient concern, the practice will maintain positive momentum.

Periodic tests and examinations, comparative studies, and progress reports indicate to the patient the doctor's thoroughness and concern. The assistant must be aware of the purpose of these procedures so she can reinforce their need and benefit whenever the opportunity arises.

Semantics and Patient Relations

Many expressions mean different things to different people. The effects of semantics on good human relations are difficult to overemphasize. Technical words between doctor and assistant often become matter-of-fact among the staff, but we should remember that chiropractic terminology is often "over the head" of the average patient. When patients are exposed to confusing terms and do not understand them, they can feel "put down," uneducated, and alienated. When you see that "gazed, confused" look, respond with, "In other words, ..."

Look for signs of poor understanding or unfavorable connotation when explaining routine consultation, examination, evaluation, laboratory and therapeutic procedures, and fee arrangements. The list shown in Figure 7.8 shows some examples of common word use.

OFFICE RECORDS

The typical chiropractic office requires a variety of records. In this variety, there are two basic classifications: administrative records and clinical records.

Office Records and Functions

Administrative records aid scheduling, financial control, analyzing practice growth, and recording information for business and tax purposes. Examples include entering patient data forms, daily record sheets, permanent ledger, petty cash record, appointment book, and patient financial records. Examples of administrative support records are excuses, authorizations, form letters, collection systems, request forms, various types of memos, and other support records and forms.

Clinical records concern the health-care aspects of the practice. Examples include patient history forms, examination and case history forms, case progress records, and laboratory and radiographic records.

Entering patient data, patient history, and initial examination findings may be recorded on one comprehensive form. However, for ease in comprehension, we will describe them in this chapter as if they were separate records. Financial records will be explained in Chapter 8.

Any employee involved in the preparation, organization, or filing of records should fully understand how they are to be processed efficiently. Neatness, accuracy, and completeness are not only clinical and ad-

ministrative requirements, they may also be legal necessities. When assistants are delegated the responsibility of gathering information from a patient to be entered in case records, accuracy and completeness must be above criticism.

Typical Office Records and Communications

Good records protect the interests of both the doctor and patient. Accurate information helps the doctor provide quality services, helps in the continuity of patient care, and serves as a clinical and legal history of the relationship between doctor and patient.

Printed forms save preparation time as well as indicate a well-organized office system. The type of records and reports necessary depends on the nature of the practice and is determined by need. Yet, this is often a problem. Some burden time and result in poor control. Too many increase "red tape" in patient handling and practice control. The ideal would be an inventory of records and forms offering the least number of items in stock that would allow the simplest and most efficient method of practice management.

Necessary paperwork in health care is large. Figure 7.9 shows a list of major printed matter described in this book.

Common Record Flow

At this point, it is helpful to explain the flow of records within a typical office.

1. Initial telephone contact. An assistant puts basic information on a card at the time of appointment scheduling that is held in a "Future Appointments" file. It will be reconfirmed by the assistant on the patient's arrival, and additional information and case history will be added.

2. Established and new records are made ready for the day's patients. The doctor will likely want to quickly review each patient's file before he sees the patient.

COMMON EXPRESSIONS AND COMMON ALTERNATIVES

Avoid	Use
adjustment	correction
old patient	previous patient
waiting room	reception room
exam	examination
appointment	time reservation
pain	severe discomfort
spinal care	health care
good patient	conscientious patient
dressing room	preparation room
doctor is late	doctor has an interrupted schedule
treatment	therapy
cancellation	change in schedule
spine doctor	doctor of chiropractic
vitamins/minerals	recommended supplementation
diet	nutritional menu
doctor's charge	professional fee
take care of	pay for
doctor is busy	doctor is in consultation
routine spinal check	periodic spinal examination
cost	investment
down payment	initial payment
treatment reaction	healing sign
first aid	emergency care
business	practice
budget plan	extended payment plan
What do you mean?	Help me understand better.
price for	fee for
office girl, CA	assistant
Just a minute!	One moment, please!
cost of tests	fee for examinations
office help	technicians, staff
convention	conference
call to remind	call to confirm, verify
Sign here	Your signature goes here.
course	seminar
When will you pay?	You select a payment date next month!
for me, us, the office	for the doctor's records
muscle exercise	tissue rehabilitation
Do you understand?	Have I been clear?
brace, corset	support

Figure 7.8. Many words produce different reactions in different people. The above list compares some common words and phrases with alternatives that usually generate a more positive response.

Accounts payable system and office checkbook
Accounts receivable cards and file
Address book
Adhesives
Appointment book or system
Appointment cards
Appointment reminder cards
Area code book
Area map
Assistants' activity calendar
Assorted manila envelopes for large mailings
Authorization forms
Birthday file (patient) and cards
Business equipment inventory list
Business supplies inventory list
Carbon paper
Case history forms
Cash disbursement reminders
Clinical equipment inventory list
Clinical supplies inventory list
Control sheets
Correspondence "In" and "Out" trays
Daily charge slips
Desk trays
Dictionaries (standard and medical)
Dietary instruction sheets
Dispensed supplies and appliances inventory list
Doctor referral list
Doctor's activity calendar
Embossed label marker
Entering patient data forms
Equipment cleaner
Equipment data file (eg, operator instructions, warranties, etc)
Erasers and correction fluid
Exercise instruction sheets
File folder signals
Form letter file
Furnishings inventory list
Glass cleaner
House call forms
Insurance report forms
Laboratory request forms
Ledger sheets
Lending library record
Letter opener
Log and accounting books
Long-distance telephone memo slips

Mailing labels
Medicare receipt slips
Memo pads
Paper clips
Past-due stickers
Patient file folders and labels
Patient progress forms
Payroll records
Pencil sharpener
Pens and pencils
Personnel time cards
Postage scale
Professional stationery and cards
Radiology record forms
Recall file system
Receipt pads
Reception room literature
Reference catalogs
Referral cards or slips
Release forms
Reminder pads
Rubber bands
Rubber cement
Rubber stamp pad and ink
Rulers
Scissors
Sign-in sheets
Stamps
Staple remover
Stapler and staples
Statement stuffers
Statements and envelopes
String and twine
Tape dispenser
Tapes (transparent and mailing)
Telephone message pads
Telephone number list
Thank you notes
Three-hole paper punch
Thumb tacks
Tickler files
Travel expense record forms
Typing paper
Typing ribbons
Various rubber stamps and a holder
Work/school excuses
Worker's Compensation forms
Wrapping paper for package mailings
X-ray film filing envelopes/labels
X-ray film mailing tubes
Zip code book

Figure 7.9. A listing of typical business office supplies.

3. During the visit, the doctor will enter notations concerning case actions and progress, and note on the visit slip the services rendered. Refer to Figure 7.3.

4. When the doctor dismisses the patient, the patient presents the visit slip at the check-out desk. An assistant totals the slip, determines how fees will be paid, and enters the completed visit slip in the record. The patient's next appointment is scheduled.

5. Appropriate entries are made for recall, thank-you letters, etc, and entered either in the case record or another file. If laboratory work is necessary, an assistant makes necessary arrangements and offers the patient appropriate instructions. If vitamins or minerals are dispensed or if rehabilitative equipment has been loaned or rented, entries are made within the records. If the office has a lending library, books leaving the office should be noted.

6. When it is known that the patient is scheduled for x-ray on the next visit, note this in the record so that an identification marker may be prepared before the appointment.

The flow of records within an office is determined by office policy. The above list offers a general system that must be amended to fulfill the needs of a particular practice.

Emergency Telephone Numbers

Although dire emergencies are rare in a chiropractic office, they do happen and the entire staff must be prepared to act calmly and decisively. People can have strokes, heart attacks, and seizures in a chiropractor's office just as they can have them anywhere. This requires established policies, procedures, and training. A log of important telephone numbers will save time and eliminate confusion. See Figure 7.10.

Closing the Communications Gap

Even in a small practice, a communications gap can exist between doctor and assistant.

EMERGENCY TELEPHONE NUMBERS	
Service	Telephone Number
Paramedic Squad	_____
Ambulance Service	_____
Hospital	_____
Fire Department	_____
Police	_____
_____	_____
_____	_____
_____	_____

Figure 7.10. Sample format to list emergency telephone numbers.

The best preventive is to remember, "If it's worth remembering, it's worth a written notation." A written record eliminates guesswork and avoids the chance of forgetting instructions or patients' comments. Even the best of memories may fail at the most inopportune moment. In times of personal sickness or vacation, written records will carry on in your absence.

When patients telephone *progress reports*, note their comments in their records and date of the call. When information is passed verbally to the doctor or another assistant, record a reminder for reinforcement. Be brief, but be sure to include the necessary facts of who, what, when, where, and why, if known.

All correspondence should be copied. Memos given to patients are best made in duplicate so a copy can be placed in patient files.

In larger practice requiring several assistants and possibly more than one doctor, a *clinical routing slip* is helpful when several people are involved during a single patient visit. This routing slip enables each staff member to initial services as they are completed. This can avoid an oversight.

Purchase orders facilitate both record keeping and inventory control. The office copy of a purchase order will automatically file information about the name of the supplier, what was ordered, the quantity, the cost, and the order and expected delivery date. Standard forms can be obtained at an office supply store or from mail-order catalogs. The doctor's name and address can be imprinted on the POs or rubber stamped at the office. They can be obtained prenumbered if desired. A sample purchase order form is shown in Figure 7.11.

Standard Operating Procedures

An office run in a business-like manner should contain a procedure notebook or file incorporating office policies, standard procedures, and doctor-assistant relationships. The assistant should know what the doctor expects of her, and the doctor should discuss what the assistant can expect from the doctor. A procedural reference, often called the "Office Bible," should include statements regarding office regulations, employee duties and responsibilities, employee benefits, growth opportunities, and serve as a compilation of rules and systems that al-

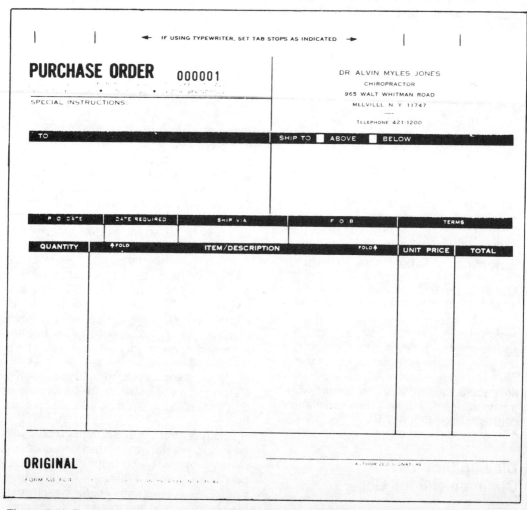

Figure 7.11. Typical purchase order form (reprinted by permission of Histacount, Inc)

low the practice to run smoothly. Whenever a policy is changed, a notation should be made within the notebook or file folder. This reference removes guesswork and helps in orienting new employees to office policies.

Entering Patient Data

When patients new to the practice enter the office, they are typically greeted, seated comfortably, handed a clipboard to which a card, slip, or sheet has been attached, and are requested to document some basic information (Fig. 7.12). Usually, the first entry is the patient's *name* and *address. Date of birth* is a more courteous request than *age*, and it provides information that can be transferred to a birthday record book if the office sends cards. A space will be provided in which the patient is asked to briefly describe the *chief complaint.* For legal and insurance reasons, it is good policy to have this description in the patient's handwriting. *Marital status* is commonly requested, as is the number and ages of *children*, if any. This offers the doctor an overview of the family environment. Date of marriage will be asked if the office sends out anniversary cards. *Employer* and *occupation* information is requested. This is necessary if the case is (or may be in the future) an industrial accident. Occupation data is necessary if the work activities of the patient must be controlled. If the patient has been *referred* by a patient or doctor, a space will be provided to enter this information. This is important so proper acknowledgment may be sent to the person referring the patient. Space also will be provided for the entering patient to list *health and accident insurance* data. The form usually concludes with a statement of office policy concerning payment for services rendered by the office such as "Payment is expected at the time of visit unless other arrangements have been made in advance." Whatever office policy is, the patient should be informed as soon as possible. After the patient completes the form, the assistant should check it to be sure all appropriate blanks are filled and that the writing is legible.

Entering patient data are often called pa-

tients' personal or statistical data. Besides the entries described above, this information should contain the parents' or guardians' names if the patient is a minor, the name of the person to be billed, the patient's home and business telephone numbers if applicable, and mailing address if different from that of the residence.

Patient History Form

After this initial information is obtained, the next data-gathering step is to obtain a record of the patient's health history. In many offices, either an administrative or technical assistant may be responsible for collecting some of this information. The history records why the patient is consulting the doctor, when present symptoms first appeared, how long the disorder has existed, what the patient has done about the condition, and other facts helpful to case evaluation by the doctor. The data gathered by an assistant are usually restricted to the patient's chief and minor complaints; the patient's medical, surgical, and obstetrical history; and family, social, and accident histories. This information serves the doctor as clues to a crime would serve a detective. Therefore, although an assistant may take some basic information, the doctor will review each point in greater detail with the patient.

Case history forms come in a variety of sizes, shapes, and styles. There are small cards, large cards, double cards, sheets and multiple sheet forms. The nature of some practices requires modest information while others need extensive information. Styles range anywhere from a 6 × 9-inch card to several 8½ × 11-inch sheets. Although professional printing houses have a large selection of case history cards and sheets to choose from, many doctors wish to personally design them to meet particular needs.

To save patient and office time, some doctors use a form requiring only a simple "Yes" or "No" answer that can be checked or encircled by the patient. These forms are usually designed so that a group of questions relates to a specific system of the body.

CONFIDENTIAL PATIENT INTRODUCTION

Date _____

Patient's Name _____ Phone No. _____

Mailing Address _____

Age _____ Date of Birth _____ Soc. Sec. No. _____

Occupation _____

Employer _____

Name of Wife or Husband _____ Phone No. _____

    Occupation _____

    Employer _____

Patient's Nearest Relative _____

    Address _____(not at patient's address)_____

Have you had previous chiropractic care? _____ When? _____

ARE YOU INSURED? _____   (PLEASE CHECK BELOW)

_____ Blue Cross/Blue Shield   _____ HMO

_____ Group Health and Accident Insurance   _____ Disability Insurance

_____ Union Health Benefit Plan   _____ Owner's Landlords & Tenants Insurance

_____ Accident & Health (Individual)   _____ State Workers' Compensation

_____ Medical & Surgical Service Plan   _____ Federal Workers' Compensation

_____ Medicare/Medicaid   _____ Federal Employee Health Benefit Plan/
                                                          CHAMPUS/Veteran's Administration
_____ Interscholastic Insurance
                                                    _____ Other

PAYMENT IS EXPECTED AT TIME OF VISIT

    Name of person responsible for payment _____

HEALTH AND ACCIDENT INSURANCE POLICIES ARE IN ARRANGEMENT BETWEEN THE CARRIER AND THE PATIENT WHICH ARE USUALLY DESIGNED TO OFFSET A LARGE PORTION OF THE TOTAL COST. THIS OFFICE WILL PREPARE ANY NECESSARY REPORTS AND FORMS TO ASSIST IN MAKING COLLECTIONS FROM THE INSURANCE COMPANY TO THE PATIENT. ANY AMOUNT AUTHORIZED TO BE PAID DIRECTLY TO THIS OFFICE WILL BE CREDITED TO THE PATIENT'S ACCOUNT. IT SHOULD BE UNDERSTOOD THAT ALL SERVICES FURNISHED ARE CHARGED DIRECTLY TO THE PATIENT WHO IS PERSONALLY RESPONSIBLE FOR PAYMENT, INCLUDING THE SMALL CHARGE FOR COMPLETING THE FORMS.

    Patient's Signature _____

                                                                        ACA Form 18

Figure 7.12. Confidential patient information form. This entering data form offers third-party information and states office policy regarding financial relationships. Available from the American Chiropractic Association.

Chief Complaint

The *chief complaint* data gathered here are an elaboration of those recorded on the entrance form. The chief complaint is the primary motive for the patient seeing the doctor—why the patient is seeking help. Although a patient may present several complaints, one will usually stand out as chief among the group. In cases of an acute and chronic complaint, the acute situation would usually be the chief complaint. If a patient complains of a chronic cough and of being overweight, the cough would be the chief complaint. The chief complaint will usually be the most painful, severe, potentially dangerous, or urgent complaint.

Past and Related Histories

The patient's *medical history* records serious past illnesses, operations, miscarriages, births, drug or food sensitivities, congenital difficulties, and past medical and chiropractic care and the results obtained. *Family history* concerns the health status of siblings and parents, which may offer clues regarding possible hereditary influences. The patient's *social history* relates to where the patient lives, marital status, number and ages of children, type of work, work environment, smoking and drinking habits, and similar activities. The *history of accidents* and their effects are also recorded. If present complaints appear to have resulted from an accident or work-related injury, details of how, when, where the accident occurred is important.

The patient's history, the doctor's diagnosis, the therapy recommended, and the patient's progress record form the patient's case record (chart). Without this record, few doctors could remember from one visit to another what was previously learned. Such records must be referred to (often for many years) whenever the patient visits the office.

If an assistant is responsible for recording some of the patient's history, absolute privacy must be granted the patient. Such confidential information is not for the ears of strangers, friends, or even relatives except for a minor patient in the presence of a par-

ent. If a patient appears to feel embarrassed to tell an assistant necessary information, the assistant should be tactful and memo this to the doctor. The matter should not be pressed.

Examination and Case History Form

The doctor's examination begins with the patient's history. During consultation, he will probe the information acquired and arrive at a judgment of what type of examination procedures would be best suited for the particular complaints involved. Where the assistant has left off, the doctor will explore deeper and conduct more intimate questioning if necessary. A comprehensive patient history can offer most information necessary to arrive at an accurate diagnosis.

At the completion of the consultation, the doctor proposes the type and scope of the examinations necessary. With patient agreement, the examination proceeds or another appointment will be scheduled for the necessary tests. After examination, the doctor records or dictates the results of his physical examination, orthopedic and neurologic tests, spinal analysis, x-ray findings, laboratory findings, and other data necessary to profile the patient's condition.

In a simple acute case, this whole procedure may be completed in a matter of minutes. In a severe chronic condition of an obscure nature, the process may take from several days to several weeks before a diagnosis and prognosis are determined. Regardless, after the examination and evaluation of the patient's history and examination findings, the doctor will meet with the patient to discuss the recommendations for treatment, risks involved, and options, or referral to another practitioner.

Some doctors do not like the restriction of a standardized format. They prefer to develop case histories in their own way for each case. Some doctors prefer to dictate case histories and have them later typed on plain white bond. Such typing should use headings so that review can be made easily. X-ray findings and laboratory reports also should be included in the case history along with the physical examination findings, results of the spinal analysis, and other test results.

Case Progress Records

Once a patient enters therapy at the office, each time the patient returns on subsequent visits or the doctor visits him at the patient's residence, the patient's condition is recorded, together with changes in treatment or changes to previously given instructions. Progress notations are a permanent record of what was done and offer a chronologic patient status. While the patient's history shows the patient's status at the time of the initial visit, progress records show the patient's state of health at subsequent points in time.

Once a therapeutic program is established for a patient, subsequent care should be handled smoothly in a well-organized manner. Only minimal verbal instruction among staff members is necessary if procedures are firmly established. Patient progress records should indicate the date of each visit, therapies offered (type, strength, distance, pressure, duration, special instructions, etc), type of service the patient is to receive on the next visit, necessary diet menus, supplements, exercises, supports or braces, home therapies, and new instructions and changes to previous instructions.

The doctor should initial all entries made by himself. The assistant should initial all entries made by herself. If the doctor dictates notations, the assistant's initials should precede the doctor's initials (entered after review and approval). This review guards against an inaccurate entry. It is especially important in offices where several staff members make entries on a patient's record. If the assistant is new to the office, it also differentiates her entries from those of her predecessor.

Brief, accurate, and neatly prepared case histories and progress reports help the doctor to help the patient. Such records can supply data for chiropractic clinical research, and they can be used as evidence in lawsuits. If the patient moves or changes

doctors, copies will likely be forwarded to the next attending physician. Thus, the need for accuracy and detail should be obvious.

Legal Considerations

Medicolegal considerations are subjects explained in Chapter 12. However, a few points will be summarized here as they pertain to the need for accurate comprehensive clinical records.

Medical histories, progress reports, and other patient records are "privileged communications" that always must be treated as highly confidential records. They are protected by law as such. Office records belong to the doctor and must never be copied or information from them disclosed without express authorization from the doctor *and* the patient. If these records are needed by others and authorization is not given, they must be subpoenaed. The doctor and chiropractic assistant are equally bound by this principle of secrecy.

Case histories and reports are legal documents that may have to be produced in court as evidence. This is especially true in accident cases involving suits for damages where the doctor's testimony would be required. This again underscores the necessity for accuracy, neatness, legibility of handwriting (if not typed), completeness, and dating and initialing of all entries. The quality of patient records may mean the difference of winning or losing a legal case.

Advice Restrictions

There are times when an assistant must discuss certain confidential information with a patient. At these times, the assistant must be alert that she does not transgress the Chiropractic Practice Act by directly or indirectly offering information that might be construed as recommending a type of treatment or making a diagnosis. These are the sole prerogatives of a licensed practitioner. For instance, if a patient asks whether to continue a certain type of home therapy recommended by the doctor although the treatment is increasing the patient's discomfort and the assistant is aware that such side effects are quite common, she would be in error to tell the patient either to stop or continue the procedure. To say, "It's okay, many people have such symptoms at the beginning of treatment" would be a serious medicolegal error. If the patient's condition becomes worse, the doctor might be liable and the assistant charged with practicing chiropractic without a license. Also, if a patient asks the assistant, "I have a 'slipped disc,' don't I?" and the assistant responds with a casual remark, "Well, it seems like it," she would be in an embarrassing position if the doctor arrives at a different diagnosis. The assistant also should be aware that a doctor's "working (tentative) diagnosis" may be different from his final diagnosis.

Required Reports

There are various instances, especially in communicable diseases, where the doctor is legally obligated to report to certain authorities. Usually, it is the local or state Department of Health. It's often the assistant's responsibility to complete forms from information given by the doctor and see that the doctor signs the report before it is mailed. Births and deaths are probably the two most important events that must be registered in every state. Only in a few states do doctors of chiropractic practice obstetrics. However, in a growing number of states, chiropractic physicians are authorized to sign death certificates. Other situations that may require reports to authorities are cases of criminal assault, venereal disease, drug addiction, child beating, abuse of the elderly, and blindness. In these instances, state laws vary considerably and the assistant must be alerted to legal requirements and informed of changes in requirements. According to local needs, the assistant should see that a proper amount of necessary forms is on hand in the office at all times and that such reports are processed promptly.

Consent and Release Forms

As the number of lawsuits for damages against doctors has increased in recent years, the use of consent and release forms has increased to protect the doctor from an unjustified malpractice claim. Pertinent forms are commercially available, or the doctor or doctor's attorney may design a form and have it printed locally. When a rarely used form is needed, the assistant may type it as needed or keep a few on file. A carbon copy should never be used as an original, however.

Referral List

Each doctor develops a list of particular specialists to whom he or she refers patients for specialized attention. See Figure 7.13.

Other Records and Forms

A variety of office forms and records were described in previous chapters, and several are explained in this chapter. In Chapter 8, regarding office economics, the functions of patient receipts, charge slips, daily work sheets, petty cash slips, financial arrangement forms, expense records, patient statements, collection systems, financial account records, permanent ledger sheets, financial authorization forms, daily control sheets, payroll records and time cards, and other subjects of this nature will be explained. In Chapter 14, concerned with the duties of a technical assistant, laboratory request slips, radiology record forms, x-ray ID cards, dietary instructions, corrective exercise forms, and patient instruction sheets will be described. Chapter 11, which concerns insurance and other third-party relationships, offers descriptions of health insurance claim forms and worker's compensation forms.

OFFICE FILING SYSTEMS

An efficient filing system should provide for at least three basic types of records: (1) patients' case histories and financial account records, (2) correspondence, reports, reprints, documents, etc, and (3) record books, inventory sheets, personal notes, etc.

Figure 7.13. Sample specialty referral list format.

Some records are designed to hold more than one set of information and others require new folders for the data. That is, some records are designed to incorporate history, examination findings, progress reports, laboratory reports, and similar data, while others require a separate document.

An office may use different filing systems for different categories of patients. Some offices use the same file, but folders are color coded to show the appropriate category. An increasing number of offices use color coding to provide subdivisions within a particular major category to differentiate cases; eg, Medicare, Medicaid, Worker's Compensation, Health Insurance, Accident Insurance, and other types.

Basic Filing Requirements

Most offices file strictly alphabetically by the patient's last name in clinical files or subject of the topic to be filed in nonclinical files. See Figure 7.14. In large volume practices where several patients may have the same name, patients' records are filed by case number and each patient's number is cross-indexed to an alphabetical list incor-porating the patients' addresses. It is not unusual in large practices to have several patients with the name Mary E. Smith or John J. Jones. Despite the system used, guides should be used to divide the file drawers into appropriate sections, and patient folders or pockets should be used to hold all records of a patient or topic.

It is necessary to refer to a patient's records on return visits, to complete insurance forms, to review case progress, and to supply a variety of information needed from time to time. Thus, prompt accurate filing is important. Besides patient record files, card files that can remind the assistant of important dates and matters to be taken up in the future reduce burdening memory with sundry details.

Pulling Files

The custom in organizing patients' files is to place the newest material (that with the latest date) at the front of the folder with records running in chronologically. When records are pulled for patients with appointments, they should be placed on the doctor's desk in the sequence that the patients are to

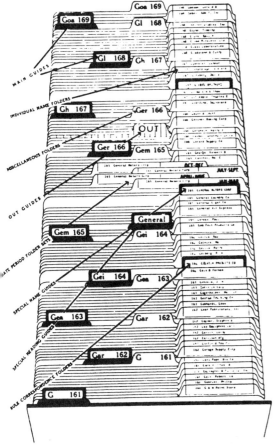

Figure 7.14. An alphabetical file arranged in four positions.

be seen. The best time for initial organization is usually at the end of the previous day or in the morning before the first patient arrives.

For follow-up visits where a new record is not necessary and the appointment has been made for several weeks, records can be pulled once each week when reminder notices are sent. For patients new to the practice, however, entering patient data and history data must be obtained after the patient arrives, thus the file cannot be given to the doctor until just before the patient is introduced.

Safety and Security Considerations

If a patient's record cannot be found, first look through the entire letter of the alphabet to see if it has been previously misfiled. Next, check the desks of other staff members where files are commonly placed when in transit.

Whenever any document is removed from a patient's file, an "Out Card" should be inserted that notes what was removed, who removed it, and the date it was removed. This card should be placed in the position of the document removed. Such a record will save much frustration in locating missing documents (Fig. 7.15).

Be cautious in keeping records out of sight of patients. Never leave them lying around or open on a desk. People are curious and can easily be frightened by what

OUT

DATE	MATERIAL	DATE REMOVED	TO BE RETURNED	CHARGE TO WHOM	REMARKS

Figure 7.15. A typical out card. Actual size is 8½ × 11 inches.

they read and misunderstand. All records developed at the office are records that belong to the doctor. You may have to tactfully explain this to patients. Use a release form, under the doctor's and patient's specific authorization, when there is need to send information to an insurance company, attorney, another doctor, or another third party.

Avoiding Space Waste

Several methods can be used in saving file space: (1) Loose papers take less space than those having bulky fasteners, clips, or staples. Of the three, staples are the best unless papers must be separated. (2) Transfer papers and records that cannot be destroyed, yet are rarely referred to, to other storage facilities. If the material is stored in boxes, label the contents of each box on the outside.

Federal and state statutes of limitations and the doctor's desires determine what should be destroyed and what should be stored in active or inactive files. The doctor will usually wish to keep all case, legal, and financial records despite the statutes of limitations involved. However, with the doctor's approval, grossly outdated correspondence, literature, and records no longer useful or pertinent can be destroyed periodically to save filing and storage space.

Filing Systems

Both efficiency and accuracy are the key words to remember in good filing. Avoid accumulating charts to be filed by setting a certain time each day for filing. Take care to file charts in their proper order, and be alert to any name or address changes to maintain accuracy. Although a patient has been in the office before, verify the address, phone number, occupation, and other basic data periodically.

There are two general filing systems popular in chiropractic offices: alphabetical indexing and numerical indexing. Numerical indexing became popular shortly after World War II. In recent years, however, this system has been replaced by the simpler alphabetical indexing method.

Alphabetical Indexing

The most simple alphabetical indexing method uses three units. Unit 1 is the last name, Unit 2 is the first name, and Unit 3 is the middle name or middle initial. There is little difficulty in assigning the correct alphabetical position in the file to each patient's record when indexing is done in the unit method.

Unit 1	Unit 2	Unit 3
Jones	John	J.
Jones	John	L.
Jones	Mary	P.
Jones	Mary	W.

A more detailed type of alphabetical indexing uses five units. Unit 1 is the last name in capitals, Unit 2 is the patient's title, Unit 3 is the first name, Unit 4 is the middle name or middle initial, and Unit 5 is the nickname or name by which the patient prefers to be called.

Unit 1	Unit 2	Unit 3	Unit 4	Unit 5
JONES	Mr.	John	J.	Johnny
JONES	Dr.	John	L.	Jack
JONES	Mrs.	Mary	P.	Mary
JONES	Miss	Mary	W.	Mary

Two difficulties sometimes arise within the three-unit system. First, family chart errors are difficult to avoid; and second, confusion results when patients have the same last, first, and middle initials. The five-unit system allows a married woman to use her formal name (eg, Mrs. John J. Jones), which would distinguish her from another Mary J. Jones. It also allows patient differentiation by title (Mr., Dr., Mrs., Miss), and shows the name by which the patient prefers to be called. This system greatly reduces the risk of having two files labeled identically.

It is often best to presort all charts to be filed before they are actually inserted into the filing cabinet. This organization saves time and effort by proper sequencing at your desk. Filing can be completed without going back and forth from drawer to drawer.

In alphabetical indexing, it is helpful to make a miscellaneous folder for each letter of the alphabet and place it behind the last name folder under the particular letter of the alphabet. File any material for which there is no separate name folder in this "Miscellaneous" folder. Filing should be done within this folder alphabetically rather than by date. Papers relating to a particular name or topic can be clipped together, and when they reach a logical number, a separate folder may be made.

Numerical Indexing

In this system, numbers are used on file folders that are arranged numerically (Fig. 7.16). The advantages of the system are those of fast and accurate refiling, the opportunity for indefinite expansion, and confidentiality.

Numerical indexing often is used in large practices conducted by several doctors and assistants. While numbers lead an illusion of being modern and concise, the system has several drawbacks. In the numerical indexing system, each patient is assigned a case number. The patient's folder is labeled first by case number, and this is followed by the three-unit alphabetical system (eg, 1423 Jones, John L). A small cross-index card is also prepared that contains the same information in reverse (eg, Jones, John L 1423). This card is filed alphabetically in a separate file, and the patient's case records are filed by number in the master file. Numerical indexing also requires a log book to be maintained that lists each number assigned so the same number will not be used twice. The extra steps involved in the cross-index card and the case-number log offer few advantages over the simpler alphabetical system.

Standards

Generally accepted rules of filing come from The Association of Records Managers and Administrators (ARMA), a recognized

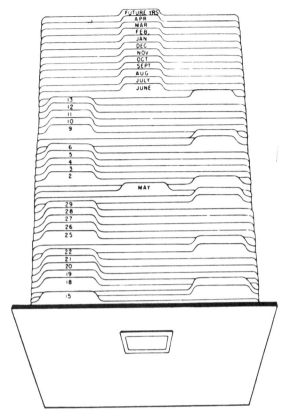

Figure 7.16. A current-patients file arranged numerically.

authority in the field of records management. ARMA guidelines have been developed over a 30-year period by committees of veteran records managers and file management professionals. For current guidelines, contact ARMA, 4200 Somerset Drive, Suite 215, Prairie Village, Kansas 66208.

Types of Files

It should be recognized at this point that several different types of files are used in chiropractic offices depending on the nature of the practice, its size, and the personal inclinations of the doctor(s) involved. Current case records, inactive case records, a subject file, a correspondence file, tickler files, a public relations file, financial record files, and x-ray and microfilm files may be separate or filed within the same cabinet.

Current, Active, and Inactive Case Record Files

Patients' records should be separated into at least active and inactive files. Every office should have some cut-off point (eg, 3 or 5 years). Thus, if a patient has not visited the office in at least 3 years, his or her records can be changed from the active to the inactive file. The cut-off point is a matter of the doctor's preference.

Many offices divide patients' records into three distinct categories: (1) *active patients* who are currently under care and patients who owe the office money whether they are under care or not, (2) *inactive patients* who are not currently under care and do not owe the office money but are likely to return, and (3) *former patients* who are not under care and do not owe the office money but are unlikely to return. The latter category is commonly used for patients who have not been heard from in 3 or more years, have moved from the community, or are deceased.

Active, inactive, and former patient files are usually placed in an alphabetic file where the folders are inserted behind alphabetic guides. When the files become crowded, they may be subdivided according to second letters (eg, Aa Al, Am Az). Subdividing enhances organization and rapid retrieval.

As the active patient file is under the greatest use, it should be placed in a convenient location as near to the pertinent CA's desk as possible. The file is first divided by month. Next, the current month is set according to the days of the week beginning with the present date and following through to the same day 4 weeks from the present. When a current patient is dismissed and receives the next scheduled appointment, the assistant files the patient's record in the appropriate divider for easy access.

Patients scheduled ahead for a longer interval have their folders placed in the monthly division. They will remain there until their specific date becomes current. For instance, if today is January 9, and the patient is scheduled for her next visit in 2 weeks, the file will be posted in the January 23 location. However, if the patient is scheduled to return in 2 months for a periodic examination, the file will be posted behind the March tab. About 4 weeks before the March appointment, the folder will be placed under the appropriate day tab. This system is essentially a *tickler file*. When the assistant is ready to arrange the next day's case records, they are already gathered and only need sequencing according to *time* of appointment.

Despite the system used, case records should be filed separately from other materials, preferably in a separate cabinet if not a separate drawer. If the patient's chart is not a self-contained folder, a manila folder should be labeled for each patient according to either an alphabetical or numerical color-coded system. This case record folder should contain all pertinent history, examination reports, laboratory reports, progress records, and correspondence about the patient. Financial information may be included here or in a separate file.

When active patients can be designated as *inactive* or *former*, their records should be moved. Sometimes deceased patients or patients who have moved from the neighborhood are placed in a "closed" file. For storage economy, inactive and closed files can be placed in a distant storage room so valuable office space is not burdened.

The 15 × 28-inch four-drawer letter-size filing cabinet is the conventional style. This type cabinet also comes in two-drawer and three-drawer models. They occupy considerable room depth but not too much width. Another design has long shelves on which the folders are placed on end, tabs are easily read, and processing is rapid.

Few doctors destroy records—and for good reason. Regardless of statutes of limitation, a patient may return after many years or a patient's children may benefit from knowledge within a parent's record. It is not unusual for a patient who has moved from the area to return many years later. When storage of inactive, former, and closed files become a problem, microfilming is one solution. Microfilm is being replaced with the increased use of office computers where data are stored on disks.

Subject File

When the subject is more important than the writer, the information is filed by *subject* in an alphabetical file. For instance if the doctor wishes to keep a technical paper on *diathermy*, it could be placed in a subject file rather than under the name of the author. Office nonpatient correspondence, however, should be filed alphabetically by author.

In a file arranged alphabetically by subject title, the basic file is arranged as follows: (1) a durable separator with the letter of the alphabet in the left position, (2) main subject guides with center tabs that can be labeled, and (3) subheading folders with tabs in the right position. Papers within a subject folder should be arranged by date, with the most current date in front.

In typing labels for subhead folders, it helps in filing if you type the label with the main heading in capitals and the subhead in initial capitals. The subhead is usually typed on the first line, and the main heading is typed on the second line. A sampling of subject titles is listed below:

    ASSOCIATIONS

    BILLS PAYABLE
    CONTRACTS
    EQUIPMENT
    EXPRESS MAIL ACCOUNT
    FORM LETTERS
    INSURANCE
    POSTGRADUATE EDUCATION
    SUPPLIES
    TAXES

Invoices for office expenses can be filed under "Bills Payable" and then transferred to the "Taxes" file after they are paid. Before transfer, the date and number of the check issued in payment should be noted on the invoice. "Equipment" subjects would include purchase orders, related correspondence, descriptive brochures, and price lists. These files can be divided into "Office Equipment," "Diagnostic Equipment," and "Therapeutic Equipment" when desired. Similar information may be filed under a "Supplies" tab that may be subdivided into "Office Supplies" and "Clinical Supplies" sections. A file also can be made for each

professional association of which the doctor belongs. And, if he is a member of certain committees or commissions, this file may be subdivided accordingly to accommodate this type information. Under the "Taxes" file, receipts for deductible expenses can be stored. An "Insurance" file can be subdivided to differentiate between "Office Insurance Policies" and the doctor's personal and family insurance policies. The "Postgraduate Education" file should hold records of the doctor's attendance.

It is advisable to maintain either an *alphabetical list* or a *card index* in subject filing to prevent filing material under a new heading when one already exists for the general subject. An alphabetical list is made by typing main headings in full capitals and the subheading in initial capitals. After each subheading, type in parentheses the main heading under which the subheading is classified. Sufficient space should be left between each item to allow for adding new subjects and to keep the list current. For example:

    INSURANCE

    INVESTMENTS

    Itineraries (Travel)

    Leases (Contracts)

    MEETINGS

    Minutes (Meetings)

    PERSONNEL

In a card index, a card is prepared for each subject heading and subheading. In subhead cards, the main heading is typed somewhere on the card for reference. A card index is usually preferred in extensive filing systems because it is easier to keep current. It also allows for cards that cross-reference subject headings, subheadings, and synonymous titles.

Correspondence File

As most correspondence within an office concerns patient's, copies of letters and reports about cases can be placed within a patient's case record folders. The general correspondence file refers to correspondence that does not specifically relate to a specific patient. This type of correspondence is filed alphabetically by the writer's name or the name of the company, institution, organization, or agency from which the letter was issued.

Some offices divide the correspondence file into two sections: (1) incoming correspondence and (2) outgoing correspondence. Most doctors, however, prefer to staple the incoming letter and its answer together and file it under the name of the incoming letter's author or company name. Generally, the assistant removes all letters at the end of the year that are over 3 years old. According to office policy, these are either destroyed or placed in storage.

Cross-Reference Sheets

Besides the cross-reference files needed for a numerical indexing system, other cross-reference files contribute to an efficient filing system. For instance, a letter received concerning several patients can be handled two ways. Either the letter can be copied and a copy placed in each pertinent file, or the letter can be filed in the records of the first patient named in the letter and a cross-reference sheet placed in the records of other patients with a note explaining where the original letter is and what it is about.

Whenever a document, letter, report, or form can be found under two or more names or subject titles, a cross-reference sheet or one or more copies should be made. Printed cross-reference sheets are available at most office supply stores. When they are printed on brightly colored paper, they are quickly noticed. See Figure 7.17.

Cross-reference sheets are also valuable within clinical subject files. For instance, a report on "The Use of Diathermy in Osteoarthritis of the Shoulder" may be filed under

---

CROSS-REFERENCE SHEET

NAME OR SUBJECT:

Robert, R. J.

REGARDING:

Recommendation, Dr. George M. Abernathy

DATE:

January 11, 1991

(see)

NAME OR SUBJECT:

Abernathy, Dr. George M.

Figure 7.17. Typical cross-reference sheet.

"Diathermy" and cross-referenced under "Osteoarthritis" and "Shoulder Disorders."

If you have only one main file that is set up by name and occasionally have material that should be filed by subject, or have only a subject file and have material that should be filed by name, you can combine such occasional folders in the main file. This is done by either (1) putting a cross-reference sheet under the name in the miscellaneous folder behind the alphabet letter that begins the name or (2) including a folder labeled with the person's name (last name first), which would be a subject in a subject file.

Patient Relations File

Some offices wish to keep close account on patient relations. In this type of file, canceled appointments, broken appointments, and other data relative to poor cooperation can be filed. On the positive side, the names of patients who have referred others to the practice can be recorded so that appropriate thanks can be forwarded systematically.

Financial Record Files

An alphabetically arranged credit file contains cards for patients who have been extended credit. When a charge is made or a payment is received, the transaction is recorded first on the daily control sheet and then on the patient's account card whose information is used in preparing statements. Colored tabs or small removable label signals are often used to distinguish delinquent account cards, with different colors identifying the stage of delinquency. Efficient financial record systems will be described in the next chapter.

X-Ray Files

X-ray films are probably the only patient clinical records that are not filed with the patient's case records. Because their size can be large (eg, 14 × 36 inches), films are filed in specially designed cabinets. The envelopes are usually filed alphabetically by patient name and sometimes cross-referenced by an x-ray film number.

Microfilm Files

Microfilm was once the popular answer when storage became a problem. Local companies as well as Remington Rand and Xerox outlets perform this service. Sources are listed in the yellow pages of the telephone directory. Besides clinical records, microfilm is helpful in storing books and clinical papers. For instance, an 869-page reference book can be reduced to ten 4 × 6-inch cards occupying only ⅛-inch file space. Many outdated technical papers are only available on microfilm.

With the increasing popularity of office computers, microfilming is being replaced by storing data on computer disks. Sheets are "scanned" by an instrument that sends a copy of the information to the computer. Some computer "hard disks" can store information in a quantity equivalent to over 100 books. See Chapter 10.

Tickler Files

The need for an orderly reminder system is necessary as every assistant has the responsibility of seeing that certain things are done at some time in the future.

A well-organized *tickler file* is helpful in keeping special notations and memoranda in order. This system is usually a small file containing a card for each day of the year. Each morning, the card for that particular day is removed and reviewed. The information listed usually has approaching due dates for insurance policy premiums, taxes, withholding reports, subscription expirations, and other reminders of what should be done that day. Some doctors like to be reminded of personal anniversaries, approaching birthdays of family members, pledged charitable contributions, and other dates of approaching events. Patients' birthdays and anniversaries may also be noted in a tickler file.

A small tickler file is helpful in preparing the doctor's calendar. In this file is a tab for each month and 31 subtabs for each day of the current month. Notations are made on file cards, and the cards are filed according to the date the matter requires attention. If an item is recurring (eg, board meetings), the card is moved from week to week, month to month, or as necessary. It is obvious, however, that a tickler file cannot replace an appointment calendar, but it can serve as a reminder for many events.

Reminder Calendars

Reminder calendars serve a similar function as a tickler file (Fig. 7.18). These calendars come in various sizes. Two common designs are the desk calendar and the portable type having a box by each date for recording events. The desk calendar and box calendar, however, limit the number of possible entries compared to a tickler file.

It is ideal when every member of the staff has a calendar of some type or a yearbook in which entries are made for important appointments, conferences, special dates, things to remember personally, and things to remind others about. Besides his regular calendar or yearbook, a doctor may carry a pocket memo book outside the office to jot down important items to be remembered and transferred to his calendar.

Follow-up Files

A *follow-up file* is a large type of tickler holding folders. It offers an excellent method to follow-up requests waiting an answer, matters that have been referred to others for action, orders for future delivery to receive or to place, items requiring periodic consideration, and promises made for future actions. The follow-up system can be handled in one of two ways: either the material itself is placed in the follow-up tickler file or a cross-reference sheet is placed in the tickler and the material is left in its normal file.

Filing Philosophy

No practice or business can be operated successfully unless its key people can retrieve information quickly. Good practice management and control mandate more

records and efficient filing of subjects than described so far. The number of new patients in a given period, the number of broken appointments in a given period, the number of x-ray and laboratory examinations in a given time, and other accounting are ways doctors have of objectively analyzing and controlling their practice. This is impossible without good assistance and adequate records.

Unfortunately, the average doctor is a poor businessman. He usually considers records and their maintenance a laborious chore and procrastinates and rationalizes at every opportunity in this area. Therefore, the importance of an assistant who is accurate, conscientious, and efficient in record and filing responsibilities cannot be overestimated. Studies show time and again that the doctor who has accurate and detailed records of important phases of the practice, and analyzes them carefully, is bound to be more successful than one who does not.

Accurate case records are as important to the patient as they are to the practice. Our legal system recognizes this. Judges may not accept verbal testimony if unsupported by documentation. On the human side, rare is the doctor who is thorough in record keeping who does not maintain strong doctor-patient relationships: a basic key of practice development.

The prime requisite of any good record system is accuracy, completeness, and immediate accessibility. No system is any better than the manner in which it is used. All systems require alert attention: no system will run itself. The major purpose of many records is to provide comparative information that is complete, accurate, and simple to file, pull, and analyze.

TYPICAL OFFICE EQUIPMENT

Many offices will have the following business equipment:

Calculator	Embossed label
Desk organizer	maker
Desk trays	Fax machine
Desktop computer	Filing cabinets

DOCTOR'S MEETING CALENDAR FOR 19__

Organization's Name	Meeting Place	Regular Meeting Date/Time

January	February	March
April	May	June
July	August	September
October	November	December

Figure 7.18. Sample meeting calendar.

Dictation recorder/   Modem
   player   Music system
Duplicating ma-   Office intercom
   chine   Paper punch
Electric letter   Pegboard system
   opener   Postage meter
Electric paper   Postage scale
   shredder   Printer (computer)
Electric pencil   Scanner
   sharpener   Spiral binding ma-
Electric stapler   chine
Electric typewriter   Tape dispensers
                         Telephones

The office will periodically receive mailed announcements of new equipment available. Although the office may not have need for such equipment at the time, it is often helpful to file these brochures for future reference when needs change. Whenever a new piece of equipment is considered, investigate different brands and types, and compare features, benefits, and costs. Maintenance and service considerations are just as important as initial purchase price. This research will help the doctor to arrive at a purchase decision.

Dictation Equipment

Some management consultants feel that, in the ideal situation, the office should have a central dictating machine with a microphone in each consultation, examination, and therapy room where the doctor might be. The person assigned typing duties should have a transcribing unit. Dictation immediately after consultation, examination, or therapy when recall is greatest is faster and more accurate for the doctor than writing reports long hand. Dictation equipment eases the chore of developing a referral letter, preparing a case report, creating general correspondence, entering reminders, making special notations within a patient's file, and storing other information that should be recorded or processed.

Duplication Equipment

It is a benefit to most offices to have some form of copy machine so that duplicates of records can be sent to the doctor's colleagues or a patient's attorney or insurance company when authorized. Copying capabilities also allow patient's financial records to be copied and used as an account statement at the end of the month.

PURCHASING AND INVENTORY MANAGEMENT

Typical Business Office Supplies

In any professional practice, ordering of supplies must consider both quality and economy. Poor economic procedures in purchasing can place a hardship on the practice that hinders financial growth. If an assistant is given the responsibility of selecting and ordering office supplies, she should shop as she would for a personal purchase, keeping both professional quality and economy in mind.

An office will require an inventory of basic supplies necessary to carry out functions. Refer to Figure 7.9.

Ordering Supplies

Quantity purchasing and comparative shopping offer distinct savings to the office. When buying supplies that are used frequently in the office, check for quantity discounts. If three or four units are used each month, determine the price break on a dozen units. A rule is to order a 6-month supply. Less than that is usually poor economy. If you buy too far ahead, you burden office capital. You also may find that an item needed today will not be in the future because of changing policies, procedures, or systems. The doctor would not want a large quantity of something in stock when a new and better product is introduced to the market. A supply purchasing control sheet is shown in Figure 7.19.

Many doctors will set up a system in which a specified assistant may order common supplies without his continued authorization up to a certain dollar amount of purchase (eg, reorders totaling under $100).

SUPPLY PURCHASING CONTROL SHEET

Item/Size	Date Ordered	Quantity Ordered	Cost	Date Rec'd	Supplier	Telephone

Figure 7.19. Typical supplies purchasing control sheet format. You may also wish to make columns for the name of the manufacturer, the reorder point, purchase order number, check number of payment, etc.

Checking Deliveries

Check ordered items on delivery. If something is delivered in an unsatisfactory condition or a mistake has been made, do not accept delivery. If damaged goods are not discovered until after delivery, call the supplier immediately and ask him to pick up the damaged goods when he makes delivery according to your specifications. Careful surveillance of ordering and receiving procedures will save the office time, money, and frustration.

The professional office is always quality conscious. Most doctors prefer quality bond letterheads, second sheets, envelopes, and statements that are coordinated. Cheap carbon paper will not give the clean copies desired or will it last as long as the higher quality grades. Because file folders are handled so frequently in the office, folders with reinforced tabs enhance durability. The better grades are of heavy material that adds greater life to the folder subjected to frequent use. Cheap typewriter ribbons, as carbon paper, are apt to be heavy and smudgy at the beginning of use but quickly result in faded copy. Silk or nylon ribbons are more expensive than cotton, but they give much longer wear. Carbon ribbons are the most expensive, have the shortest life, yet present the finest appearance.

Clinical Supplies

Unlike a commercial business office, the chiropractic office requires supplies over that necessary for the business side of the practice. Examination, therapy, laboratory, and x-ray facilities require basic supplies. Figure 7.20 shows a brief listing.

Representatives from vitamin/mineral companies and office supply houses may call on the doctor to keep him abreast of developments, leave pertinent literature, and

Absorbents	Nail cutters
Acupuncture needles (if utilized)	Orthopedic braces and supports
Adhesive felt	Paper cups
Adhesive spray	Protective padding
Artificial airway	Razor
Benzoin tincture	Regular and elastic bandages
Blades	Safety pins
Cervical collars	Shoe lifts
Chafing powder	Skin pencils
Contact lens suction cup	Slings
Cotton balls and tips	Spine board (emergency)
Deodorants	Splints
Disinfectants	Stockinetts
Eye patches	Styptics
Head rest paper/chest towels	Swabs
Heel cups	Tape scissors
Hydrocolator packs	Therapy creams (eg, ultrasound)
Ice packs	Therapy sprays (eg, Fluori-methane)
Jaw wedge	Tweezers
Magnifying glass	Various gauze pads and adhesive tapes
Massage lotions	

Figure 7.20. A listing of typical clinical supplies.

take orders. Be courteous to these sales-men, check with the doctor to see if he would desire to meet with them for a few minutes, and advise them of the best time to see the doctor.

Inventory and Storage Considerations

A running inventory of supplies is the best procedure to assure enough materials are always available. A simple record can be developed by listing on a sheet of paper every supply item in the office. Record the date of the last order for each and the quantity ordered. After each month or sooner, count the quantity on hand. If you are low on any one item (eg, less than a month's supply), reorder as indicated. This record will prevent running out of any one item and give you a good guide to quantity purchasing. See Figure 7.21.

A central storage facility is more efficient than several storage cabinets scattered throughout the office. A central facility re-

duces both inventory time and duplication of paperwork. All items should be stored neatly in an organized manner so you can tell at a glance the quantity of each item available. For items requiring considerable time between order and receipt, be sure to note this on your inventory record. It is often helpful to note the reorder point for each item stocked.

HANDLING MAIL AND CORRESPONDENCE

On or near each assistant's desk and the doctor's desk should be trays to receive incoming and outgoing forms, reports, and correspondence. Processing should be frequent, smooth, and alert to emergency situations. Filing, however, may be delegated to a certain period of each day, but carry-overs from day to day should be avoided.

Organization is the key to smooth function. The filing system should not only be one where you can retrieve material quickly,

INVENTORY CONTROL SHEET

Item/Size	Reorder Point	Date	Quantity on Hand	Date	Quantity on Hand

Figure 7.21. Sample inventory control sheet format.

it also should be a file where everyone in the office can retrieve information quickly.

Your work area should always be ready for "inspection." By taking pride in your work, your methods, and your responsibilities, you will be happy and productive in your career.

Policy and Procedures

Every office receives a large quantity of mail each day: some of it is very important, some of it is of casual interest, and some of it can be classified as "junk" mail. In many offices, it will be the responsibility of an assistant to sort the mail, slit the envelopes, and stack them in an orderly fashion. To do this, the doctor must inform the assistant what he considers junk mail that is not to be forwarded to him, what incoming mail he wants to see, what priorities should be given to certain types of mail, and how the mail should be sorted and organized. Incoming mail marked "personal" should not be opened.

When incoming mail arrives, sort it into three piles: (1) letters requiring the attention of someone outside the office, (2) letters needing the doctor's personal attention, and (3) letters requiring your or another CA's attention. When opening mail and you notice a letter referring to an enclosure that is not there, note its absence on an attached slip before forwarding it.

If you attend to part of a letter before sending it to someone for further action, mark the paragraph that has had attention. Write the date and "done" or "noted" in the margin and initial.

In opening mail, be sure to remove all contents from the envelope. Patients frequently insert small notes when paying bills. These can be easily overlooked and discarded if the envelope is not carefully inspected.

Although it is usually good policy to fold and insert approved letters in their addressed envelopes as they are prepared, do not seal the envelopes or attach the postage immediately. Wait to the time for mailing as you or the doctor may think of a necessary or helpful enclosure later in the day.

Daily Record

Keep a simple daily record of important mail sent *from* the office for action by another person. This is especially important in insurance records, reports, contracts, and other legal documents. Such a record serves as a check on the receipt and disposition of mail that gets misplaced and for follow-up if necessary.

Outgoing mail records are usually designed on three-hole drilled loose-leaf sheets for simple storage in a ring binder. Five vertical columns are titled "Date," "Description," "To Whom Sent," "Action To Be Taken," "Follow-up." If you keep the record with a pencil or pen rather than with a typewriter, the sheets should be ruled. If typewritten, double space between each entry. See Figure 7.22.

In the "Date" column, show the date the material was mailed. Under "Description," note the date of the communication, the name of the sender, and the subject matter. "To Whom Sent" refers to the person to whom you addressed the material. In the "Action to Be Taken" column, the action checked on the transmittal slip or mentioned in a cover letter is noted. Write the deadline for disposition in the "Follow-up" column if it is necessary to monitor that proper action is taken. When follow-up confirms that the necessary action was taken, write "did," the date, and your initial in the margin.

Transmittal Slips

Transmittal slips speed intra- and interoffice communications where there is no need for a journal record of the correspondence or for elaborate explanation. See Figure 7.23.

The Doctor's Correspondence

When giving letters to the doctor for his signature, separate those that he dictated from those that you or someone else wrote for his signature. Some doctors prefer that letters given to them for signature not be accompanied with the carbon copy or envelope.

	CORRESPONDENCE RECORD			
Date	Description	Sent to	Action to Be Taken	Follow-up

Figure 7.22. Sample daily correspondence log sheet.

John J. Jones, D.C.

2200 Main Street - Center City, Missouri 76543

☐ For your information   ☐ Please rush
☐ For your   ☐ For your action
   approval   ☐ In answer to your request
☐ For your file   ☐ To accompany
☐ For your comments
☐ For your signature   ☐ Returned as requested

☐ PLEASE RETURN

Figure 7.23. Typical transmittal slip format.

Enclosures should be paper clipped to the letter, but this is not necessary if the enclosures are bulky. In all cases, however, the letter should mention the enclosures as a postscript notation.

Preparing Enclosures

When enclosures are approximately the same size as the letter, fold the enclosures, then fold the letter and slip the enclosures inside the last fold of the letter so when the letter is removed from the envelope, the enclosures come out with it. If the enclosures are smaller than the letter, they can be stapled to the back of the letter in the upper left-hand corner. If two or more enclosures are sent, place the smaller one on top. If enclosures are larger than the letter, either put the unfolded letter and enclosures in a large first-class envelope or affix the letter's envelope to the face of a large envelope. An envelope with a letter (inserted or attached) must contain first-class postage. Large en-velopes can be marked third-class when de-livery speed is not urgent.

Organizing Incoming Mail

Doctors usually prefer their mail to be orga-nized when placed on their desk. Following is a common priority order, from top to bot-tom:

1. Telegrams
2. Special delivery letters
3. Express mail
4. First-class clinical mail
5. First-class business mail
6. Third-class mail
7. Journals
8. Newspapers
9. Magazines
10. Catalogs

An assistant properly trained in screening mail will save the doctor a large amount of valuable time. In most offices, an assistant will process payments received, appointment requests or changes, and bills to be paid, and have the authority to discard mail that the doctor has classified as junk mail. In offices not using a purchase-order system, the doctor may wish to approve (by initialing) bills to be paid. An assistant may also be authorized to complete insurance forms for the doctor's signature.

X-Ray Films

When your office receives x-ray films from another office, leave them in their mailing envelopes or tubes. You will then have the proper size envelope or tube if the films are to be returned. X-ray films (as patient files) are the property of the person or institution who makes them. When requested, return films to the sender when your doctor-employer has made his analysis. The longer they remain in your office, the more chance there is of being misplaced or damaged. This would reflect a poor image of your office.

Certified and Registered Mail

When certified or registered mail is sent requesting a return receipt, attach the returned receipt to the office copy of the mailing. This is proof that the letter was received by someone at the address (certified mail) or was personally received by the addressee (registered mail).

Letters Containing Checks or Money Orders

Letters containing checks need special attention. Examine each check carefully. Be sure it is signed and that the date is appropriate. Banks will not pay, as a rule, postdated checks. Many banks will reject a check that is dated too far in the past (eg, 6 months old). Also review each check to assure that the written amount and figures agree. Improperly prepared checks returned from your bank cause confusion in the office's bookkeeping system. When the check

is properly made out, enter necessary data within your daily record, and assure that no errors have been made in transferring information.

Patients are humans who make both intentional and unintentional errors. When noted, the assistant should tactfully call this to the patient's attention so a correction can be made. As some patients write checks with a minimum of funds in the bank, all checks processed in a day should be submitted to the office's bank the same day received. First come, first served.

If a check is received marked "In full settlement of account" or "Final payment on account" and the amount is below the account's balance, discuss it with the doctor. Acceptance of the check may make it impossible to collect the full balance due.

Document Routing Slips

If several people should see correspondence, a report, document, or publication, routing slips can be used effectively. The originator need only write the sequence of the routing. Each person then initials and dates his review before forwarding it to the next person on the list. See Figure 7.24.

ROUTING SLIP			
Route	Name	Initial	Date
	Dr. Jackson		
	Dr. Andrews		
	Betty		
	Alice		
	Donna		
	File		

Please initial, date, and forward

Figure 7.24. Typical routing slip format.

Handling Mail in the Doctor's Absence

If the doctor is scheduled to be out of the office for several days, the assistant should be informed of what mail she is authorized to respond to and what mail she should hold for the doctor's return. Any mail you are normally authorized to process would usually be done in the doctor's absence. However, there may be some correspondence that the doctor wishes you to acknowledge receipt with a note that he will reply on his return.

When the doctor is away from the office for an extended period and it is his habit to contact the office periodically, sort correspondence according to priority and note the essence of each letter so you can report to him quickly. Contact him immediately if his urgent attention is needed.

Holding File

Copies of correspondence requesting information that cannot be replied to immediately should be placed in a holding file. This file should contain a copy of the request until it can be fulfilled. A holding file is also a constant reminder of things to be done. Mail received during the doctor's absence that requires his immediate attention should be banded, marked "Urgent," and placed on his desk.

Postage Considerations

If most office outgoing mail is first-class, all you likely would need would be coils of stamps. Coils are better than sheets because they require less space, are easily stored, and are easier to tear apart at the perforations.

As first-class mail rates are determined by the ounce, multiples of the same stamp can be used for mailings of over one ounce. However, if the office is required to send considerable third-class mailings or parcel post packages, a postage meter would be of benefit.

Postage Meters

If a postage meter is available at your office, certain precautions should be observed. Be sure to change the date on the meter the first thing each day. Assure the meter is set for the correct amount for each new classification or each different weight of mail. Make daily entries in the meter record book showing ascending and descending totals. If these totals do not balance, the machine requires immediate servicing. When the meter is refilled at the post office, take the record book with you. Purchase an adequate amount of postage so that trips to the post office can be kept to a minimum. If any mistakes have been made while metering, take the unused meter stamps with you to the post office to obtain a refund. If unfamiliar with the operation of a postage meter, ask your doctor-employer for detailed instructions or request that a company representative demonstrate its use.

HOUSEKEEPING AND EQUIPMENT SERVICE

Cleaning Services

Heavy or specialized cleaning such as carpet cleaning, floor maintenance, window cleaning, furniture waxing, and wall and woodwork scrubbing are usually performed by a commercial cleaning service. When necessary, an outside service should dry-clean or shampoo upholstered furniture.

Equipment Service and Repair

Major equipment should have a maintenance checklist attached to assure that the manufacturers' recommendations are followed. Periodic dusting, cleaning, and oiling (if necessary) add to the service life of clinical and business office equipment.

Periodic Inspections

There are two common facility inspections that should be made periodically: that of the office's general appearance and that for its safety to patients, visitors, and staff.

Appearance Inspections

Patients tend to view professional offices with a critical eye. A carefully designed office with appropriately selected furnishings will not support the image or the impressions desired if the office becomes dusty, cluttered, or takes on an excessively worn look. Periodic office inspections, within and without, are required to see that the environment is maintained to the level of high standards. Even when cleanliness standards are high, negative impressions can result when leaves and papers accumulate in exterior shrubs or when wall hangings and lamp shades become crooked.

Safety Inspections

Be careful that accidental shocks, cuts, bruises, slips, and trips are avoided. Frayed electric cords, electric cords coursing in traffic areas, sharp edges, wobbly furniture, supply boxes stored on the floor, slippery floors, loose carpets, loose grab bars and railings, and icy exterior walkways in winter are the most common hazards.

Monthly safety inspections of the office are good insurance. A format for periodic safety checks is shown in Figure 7.25. The entire staff should have an emergency fire plan, and at least one good fire extinguisher should be centrally located.

POLICY AND PROCEDURAL CHANGES

A procedure is a plan, and a plan is not a permanent order because conditions change with time, personnel changes, and growth of the practice. Likewise, a definite policy does not necessarily mean a fixed policy. Once patient volume substantially increases, it is not difficult to get so involved in practice routines that where the practice is headed fails to be recognized. The alert doctor must revise schedules, duties, and responsibilities to reflect necessary

changes, as conditions evolve within the practice.

Office policies and procedures are the result of a series of developments and modifications over the life of the practice. If the practice is growing, it is not the same today as it was last year or will it be the same next year. Periodic staff meetings should be regularly used to analyze the different phases, procedures, and control points involved in the services offered and to seek areas of improvement. This forces the entire staff to think creatively and regain a perspective of the practice as a whole.

The doctor is in the best position to appreciate his practice's overall objectives; however, rational flexibility is essential because he is not directly involved in the detailed implementation of every item within the office's procedural manual. As assistants must work with and integrate specific policies and procedures each day, they often can provide constructive suggestions. A format for a recommended change in procedure is shown in Figure 7.26. This could be done verbally, but placing your ideas on paper encourages each suggestion to be thought through from various viewpoints.

BUSINESS AND PERSONAL DUTIES FOR THE DOCTOR

An assistant may have certain duties to fulfill for the doctor that do not specifically concern patient relations. Greeting nonpatient callers, making travel arrangements for the doctor, and helping the doctor in his organizational work are examples.

Nonpatient Callers

The assistant who serves as receptionist fulfills a responsibility to her employer first and visitors to the office second. Greeting patients of the office has been described. Here we shall explain how nonpatient callers can be handled efficiently.

While the doctor may instruct you how to treat specific nonpatient callers, many instances must be dealt with with a few spe-

OFFICE SAFETY CHECK

	Check		Corrective Action Necessary
	Date	Initial	
Exterior			
Entry			
Reception Room			
Consultation Room			
Preparation Rooms			
Examination Rooms			
Treatment Rooms			
X-Ray & Dark Room			
Business Office			
Storage Rooms			
Toilets			
Laundry			
Children's Area			
Personnel Lounge			
Other			

Figure 7.25. Sample format for a safety check sheet. A similar checklist can be used for appearance evaluations.

RECOMMENDED CHANGE IN PROCEDURE

Date: _____   Re: _____
                          _____
By: _____   _____
                          _____

Current Procedure   _____
                         _____
                         _____
                         _____
                         _____
                         _____
                         _____

Suggested Procedure   _____
                         _____
                         _____
                         _____
                         _____
                         _____
                         _____
                         _____

New Procedure Advantages _____
                         _____
                         _____
                         _____
                         _____

( ) Approved by _____   Effective Date: _____
                               ( ) Enter in Procedural Manual
                               ( ) Route to: _____
                                             _____
                                             _____

( ) Not Approved. Reason: _____
                         _____

Figure 7.26. Sample format for recommending a change in office procedure (reprinted by permission of Behavioral Research Foundation).

cific guidelines. Regardless, you will be expected to greet any caller with good manners, determine the name of the caller, his company affiliation, if any, and the purpose of the visit so you will know what to say and what not to say.

When you know the doctor's preferences, he may have you judge which callers he will meet during office hours, who he wishes to avoid, who should be seen by someone else in the organization, and who you should take care of yourself. You will be expected to tactfully explain to callers who the doctor will not see at a particular time.

Maintain the good will of the person by making his contact with the office both pleasant and helpful, while simultaneously controlling office routine. After you greet the caller, determine the purpose of the call, give the caller your prompt attention, display genuine interest, and express a helpful attitude. If the caller is to be introduced to the doctor, make the visitor comfortable during the waiting period.

Business calls with appointments produce few problems. However, there are certain instances that should be discussed with the doctor so you will be alerted to his policy. Here are a few examples:

- Callers soliciting a contribution
- Callers the doctor will see without an appointment
- Callers who are friends of the doctor
- Callers the doctor does not want to see
- Callers the doctor wants you to handle
- Callers to be referred to others in the practice

Organizational Aid

Many doctors of chiropractic are active in professional and civic organizations. Related duties frequently require assistance of the doctor's employees. For instance, he may ask an assistant to keep his calendar of meeting dates and a list of time/costs involved (Fig. 7.27), and to alert him before an important event. An assistant may be asked to assume responsibility for paying dues, typing organizational correspondence, or taking minutes of a committee meeting.

A doctor participating in research or developing a professional paper will usually use an assistant's services for typing a manuscript or report. She may be asked to help with editing and proofreading, and maintaining a list of individuals to whom original articles or reprints are sent. This subject will be described in Chapter 9.

You may find it helpful to keep a list that specifies:

- The name of each group
- The amount of dues and when payable
- The current office held by the doctor and date term expires
- Meeting dates
- How you can help (delegated tasks)

Doctors with heavy speaking schedules will usually assign an assistant the task of maintaining the calendar, seeing to it that speaking notes or slides are properly arranged, and handling correspondence related to public appearances. Many doctors keep a log of personal activities. See Figure 7.28.

Meeting and Travel Arrangements

You may be asked to book transportation or to make hotel reservations for the doctor. When this is requested, you will need to know what persons to contact (travel agents, airlines, railroads, rental car agencies, etc) and their addresses and telephone numbers. Each doctor will have a personal preference to what type of transportation he desires. He also might have personal preferences to specific hotel or motel accommodations. Keep a list of preferred hotels/motels in frequently visited cities, their addresses and telephone numbers, and the price range for types of accommodations available.

Most doctors will use credit cards while traveling so an account of expenses can be readily determined. Know what credit cards the doctor has and record the cards' numbers and the telephone number of the issuing company if a card is lost or stolen. See Figure 7.29. Before making reservations, assure which cards the transportation carrier

ORGANIZATIONAL ACTIVITIES

Date	Organization	Activity	Cost	Time Consumed
			$	
		Total		

Figure 7.27. Listing of organizational activities, recording costs and time contributed.

and the hotel/motel involved will accept. The same should be done for traveler's checks.

Personnel Data

Another helpful log is that for personnel in a multiperson practice. This should include each staff member's name, title, address, and telephone number in the event off-duty personnel must be contacted. Data concerning the doctor's attorney, accountant, banker, insurance agent, and travel agent also can be placed on this list for ready reference. See Figure 7.30.

Postgraduate Education Log

Most states have established specific continuing education requirements for annual relicensure. The number of hours required and the courses and seminars approved vary from state to state. Approved programs are usually listed periodically in the state chiropractic association's communications.

It is helpful to develop a continuing education log (Fig. 7.31), listing all educational programs attended by the doctor whether approved for relicensure or not. Programs not approved in one state may be approved in another in which the doctor holds a license. File and safeguard all certifications of attendance so that proper credit can be given.

DOCTOR'S PERSONAL WEEKLY ACTIVITY SCHEDULE

Month _____ Week of the _____

	MONDAY	TUESDAY	WEDNESDAY
8:00 AM			
8:30 AM			
9:00 AM			
9:30 AM			
10:00 AM			
10:30 AM			
11:00 AM			
11:30 AM			
Noon			
12:30 PM			
1:00 PM			
1:30 PM			
2:00 PM			
2:30 PM			
3:00 PM			
3:30 PM			
4:00 PM			
4:30 PM			
5:00 PM			
5:30 PM			
6:00 PM			
6:30 PM			
7:00 PM			

UNDERSTANDING PROFESSIONAL PUBLIC RELATIONS

It is a commonly held belief that doctors within the healing arts need better public relations. Perhaps this is because the scientific and technical aspects of practice are so emphasized in the educational environment. While doctors must to a certain degree be objectively detached in their clinical approach, the secret of building solid patient and public esteem lies in the individual physician living up to his concept of being a "good doctor."

Be it good or bad, everybody has public relations. Positive public relations is that attitude and course of action taken by any individual or group desiring to identify its actions and goals with the welfare of the people to gain widespread understanding and good will. Public relations is not merely the propagation of favorable publicity regardless of merit. It is not phony promotions and cheap publicity stunts designed to ma-

DOCTOR'S PERSONAL WEEKLY ACTIVITY SCHEDULE		
Month _____ Week of the _____		
THURSDAY	FRIDAY	SATURDAY
8:00 AM		
8:30 AM		
9:00 AM		
9:30 AM		
10:00 AM		
10:30 AM		
11:00 AM		
11:30 AM		
Noon		
12:30 PM		
1:00 PM		
1:30 PM		
2:00 PM		
2:30 PM		
3:00 PM		
3:30 PM		
4:00 PM		
4:30 PM		
5:00 PM		
5:30 PM		
6:00 PM		
6:30 PM		
7:00 PM		

Figure 7.28. Sample personal activity schedule for a week.

nipulate public opinion. Public relations is *identification* with the public welfare: education to mutual concerns, and operating in the public interest and communicating this performance. As the business world has learned that it can, and must, take a careful account of the attitudes and wishes of the public before it evolves its programs of action, so do health-care professions.

Public relations begins in the local community and takes shape through the contacts of individual people with one another.

In both the business world and the professions, a good reputation is founded on good works communicated truthfully and candidly. It must be recognized that the modern doctor of chiropractic is a combination of scientist and healer. As a scientist, his powers of analysis and integration have led to growth from fixed orthodoxy and illogical traditions. As a healer, however, he also must be aware of basic psychologic and human relations facts contributing to the "art" of his profession.

DOCTOR'S CREDIT CARD LOG

Issuing Company	Card Number	Expiration Date	Telephone No.

Figure 7.29. Sample credit card log sheet.

PERSONNEL/ADVISER LOG

Name	Title	Address	Telephone No.

Figure 7.30. Sample log-sheet format for personnel and advisers.

Doctors and their assistants should never become so preoccupied with the "case" to the neglect of the *person* involved. It is unfortunate that many patients neither look for nor evidently expect to find in their doctor the same qualities of compassion, sympathy, and reassurance that were once taken for granted in the healing arts. But this attitude is held with reluctance. Patients would prefer a doctor who is more important as an individual than all his scientific skills and instruments. Patients would prefer a doctor who, in turn, rates the patient more important as an individual than the disease or disorder presented.

Poor public relations, ill-will and resentment take place when either a doctor or assistant fails to put himself in the patient's place. Patients inevitably react negatively to a transaction in which they are expected to understand without knowing the facts as understood by the doctor and assistant. Thus, it's the doctor's and assistant's responsibility to explain the facts to patients and

DOCTOR'S CONTINUING EDUCATION LOG FOR 19 __					
Month	Program	Date	Place	Hours	Approved by
JAN					
FEB					
MAR					
APR					
MAY					
JUN					
JLY					
AUG					
SEP					
OCT					
NOV					
DEC					

Figure 7.31. Sample continuing education log sheet.

the public in words that can be understood.

Public relations in chiropractic can be approached from both an individual practice viewpoint and a professional viewpoint—these are overlapping and indivisible functions. Such programs are but practical devices by which the profession may and does prove its devotion to the community.

Ethics, a service-oriented attitude, and high-quality conduct are the basis on which any public relations program must be built. What is good public relations for the doctor is good public relations for the profession, and vice versa. However, a well-planned, high-quality national or local public relations program will profit the profession little if the individual practice is not completely imbued with the attitude of positive public relations and the development of safeguards making poor public relations impossible.

Interpersonal relations generally involve the four steps of attention, interest, desire, and action. The goals of mass public relations and community relations programs are to gain public attention and interest in public health in general and chiropractic health in particular. The development of patient desire and action is a function of the individual practice. Without patient interest and desire, there can be little practice growth.

Relating to the Public

The goals of chiropractic must be to strengthen weak spots in public belief. As early as 1910, Theodore N. Vail, then president of the American Telephone & Telegraph Company, said: "In all times, in all lands, public opinion has had control of the last word."

Our presidents recognized the power of public relations. In one of his debates with Stephen Douglas, Abraham Lincoln said: "Public sentiment is everything; without public sentiment, nothing can succeed. He who molds opinion is greater than he who enacts laws." And President Harry Truman once observed: "You hear people talk about the powers of the president. In the long run, his powers depend a good deal on his success in public relations."

Most practitioners agree that a chiropractor's public relations efforts must be directed toward obtaining favorable opinion. This is an educational process requiring a change in public attitudes, which comes about as the result of long-term exposure and influence.

Public opinion is but the concert of individual opinion. It is based on information and belief. If it is wrong, it is wrong because of wrong information and consequent erroneous belief. It is the obligation of everyone—those who meet the public—to see that the public has full and correct information, thus a positive image of chiropractic.

When each practitioner and his staff realize that the power of public opinion is the supreme arbiter in public affairs, when they accept the thesis that opinion is subject to change, and when they recognize the basis of success is involvement in organized public relations activities, then chiropractic public-relation, efforts of communication should and will follow.

Building Public Confidence

There is no doubt that public confidence is essential to public relations success. It is both cause and effect. Unfortunately, too often participants in a public relations program get overcome with the tools and tend to concentrate solely on the means rather than the end. Merely getting chiropractic's name in the paper or a chiropractic spokesman on TV or being invited to speak before a meeting is not good public relations. The positive results that may or may not come from that exposure is. Thus, the amount of public confidence built into a public relations program becomes the determining factor of the soundness and effectiveness of that program.

It is essential to understand that chiropractic does not merely want exposure. It needs positive exposure, well-timed exposure, and well-planned exposure that fulfills its role in a progress strategy. Exposure, any kind of exposure, therefore, is not the goal, as some would believe. Positive exposure that fits into the general plan and has a role in building public confidence is the key. It becomes necessary, therefore, that the techniques and approaches used in building public confidence should change from time to time and be influenced by current conditions. In this respect, a good public relations program builds on a foundation of previous campaigns but changes to meet new conditions, new opportunities, new challenges.

Public relations is not a cure-all nor should it be considered a one-treatment method for correcting a traumatic public opinion problem. In its most effective form, public relations is a preventive-health method of assuring public confidence. It requires defined objectives and consistency of purpose. In terms of involvement, it is a 12-month-a-year activity, year in and year out.

Like the health of an individual, public relations is in a state of constant flux. Therefore, it is foolhardy to assume that once a "healthy state" is achieved the job is done. Consistency is the only key to security. National, state, and local ongoing PR programs are essential if a positive image is to be achieved and maintained.

Media Action Projects

The American Chiropractic Association has available to the profession a comprehensive portfolio titled *Media Action Projects Kit* designed to help state and local chiropractic associations develop positive relations with radio, television, and newspaper personnel. The kit offers guidelines for strengthening media relations and improving public communication benefits. Projects concern radio and television public service time, press information, news releases, space announcements, health columns, techniques for dealing with controversy, and so forth. An abundance of how-to facts, proven dos and don'ts, and a plentiful supply of samples and forms are offered.

Community Action Projects

The ACA also has developed a portfolio titled *Community Action Projects Kit* designed to help state and local chiropractic associations develop positive community relations. The kit includes the implementation of health and professional literature, posters, speaking engagements for the doctor, health fairs and exhibits, bumper strips, industrial safety programs, films, youth programs, billboards, and community service awards, along with political and educational involvement at the local level.

Chapter 8

Professional Office Economics

A doctor's priority is to care for the health needs of his patients in the best manner possible. Besides the health care rendered patients, there are numerous economic matters that must be considered. Chiropractic is not a business, but there is a business side to practice. This aspect of practice is described in this chapter.

The objective of this chapter is to isolate the more troublesome and time-consuming problems of managing a chiropractic practice and offer proved solutions. Described are common systems, methods, and procedures designed to provide control over office financial records such as patient billing and collections, bookkeeping, and financial reports. Because the problems encountered in all practices are not the same, the fundamentals of each system are described. Each system represents a basic concept that can be customized to the needs of almost any practice.

The doctor's administrative assistant is very much involved for it is she who sends out the doctor's statements, collects his fees, keeps records of earnings, collections, and expenses. If the business aspect of practice is not well governed, funds will not be available to continue operation or for practice and staff development.

INITIAL CONSIDERATIONS

The doctor of chiropractic is a highly skilled physician dedicated to promoting the health of the people of his community. At the same time, he is the owner and operator of a facility who functions in the economic sense like the traditional entrepreneur who assumes the risk and management of a business. The doctor must invest a sizable amount of money in education, office space, furnishings, equipment, personnel, and consultants. In addition to his clinical expertise, he must supervise, manage, and lead other phases of practice.

Most doctors seek two principal rewards from the pursuit of their vocation: (1) the intellectual stimulation and personal satisfaction of exercising a special expertise in the service of their community and (2) the benefits available to their families, assistants, and themselves from the financial remuneration their profession commands. Both rewards are influenced by the efficiency of the business side of their professional practice. The less time spent on business affairs, the more time to achieve satisfaction in the pursuit of their chosen field and provide service to their patients. The more accurate and current their financial records and systems, the more they will collect in billings and the better they will know how much they have available for remuneration. In short, financial records and reports representing the business side of practice can either work for or against the goals of the practice depending on their quality.

There is nothing unprofessional about using sound business techniques in managing a practice or is there anything inhumanitarian with recognizing that a doctor must charge and collect for the services he renders. Because of the demands of our times, health practice has turned to business and industry for efficient management ideas and practices. Efficient and frequently automated systems are being used in health care to free the doctor and his staff from time-consuming business details so more time may be applied to direct patient care. These systems eliminate duplication of data in records, journals, and ledgers. The doctor can then supervise most business functions in a fraction of the time it took in the past and still have the advantage of records that are accurate and up to date.

UNDERSTANDING THE DOCTOR'S FEE

The doctor must establish a definite fee schedule to determine charges for his services. However, this schedule need not be rigid. One doctor may simply apply the usual and customary rate for various services in his area, while another may feel justified by special training and experience to charge slightly higher fees.

Regardless of the system used, proper handling of fees is essential. How fees are discussed with the patient by the doctor or assistant and the office's method of billing and collecting may either add to or subtract from the doctor's reputation in the commu-

nity and the economic success of the practice.

There are several methods by which the doctor may arrive at his fee. Increasingly, standardized fees are being adopted by the individual practitioner rather than charging according to the patient's ability to pay—which was a common practice in the past. One system is a *relative value system* where services are given a value relative to other services. Fees may be keyed to those usual, customary, and reasonable in a particular area, taking into account the professional time, knowledge, and responsibility required. An administrative assistant must be thoroughly familiar with the system if she is expected to explain the doctor's fees to patients. This is usually done at the first visit after entering data are recorded.

Standardized Fees

Most offices have a standard fee for routine office calls and a standard fee for the initial visit of a patient entering the practice that includes examination, history, and/or treatment. There also are charges for special tests, therapies, supplements, supplies, and other needs that would not be considered routine. The word *routine* used here refers to a procedure used with most all patients.

Professional fees charged by the doctor and paid by the patient are part of the doctor-patient relationship. Interference with this relationship or other contractual relationships of the respective parties is not condoned. Where third-party contracts call for reimbursement based on usual, customary, and reasonable fees, charges should be consistent with customary fees of the profession in a given geographical and/or socio-economic area.

Care-Basis Fees

Care-basis fees are not usual and customary in the chiropractic profession. The term refers to payment for the correction of one or more disorders, but there is no known currently acceptable statistical basis for computation of a "care-basis" fee for chiropractic services. DCs may assume unnecessary legal risks when participating in this type of contractual relationship as there may be an implied warranty despite contractual language disclaiming warranty. Third-party payers and/or patients are within their rights to require itemization of approved services.

Some doctors argue that care-basis fees offer the advantage of (1) establishing a climate where the patient will put a value on the health service rather than the individual components of the service, (2) establishing within the patient the expectancy of being under care for a specific length of time rather than for a certain number of visits, and (3) providing an incentive to the physician to deliver to the patient the maximum results with a minimum of office visits. However, the majority of the profession feel that these advantages do not outweigh the risks involved.

Unit-Basis Fees

Unit-basis fees are also not usual and customary in the chiropractic profession. Unit pricing calls for detailed justification of the medical necessity for each unit of care given.

Prepaid Fees

Fees based on a prepaid system are usually considered unprofessional today, although in years past the system had many supporters. In the early years of chiropractic, many patients suffered from chronic conditions for which they had seen numerous traditional physicians with little or no relief. The prepaid system (eg, prepayment for 90-days care) gave the doctor of chiropractic some assurance that the patient would be committed to a length of care necessary according to clinical judgment to witness relief. Thus, many doctors felt that prepayment would give them added control over the patient to offset periodic negative influences and patient discouragement during the recovery process. The prepayment system also allowed the recent graduate some

working capital when patient volume was at its lowest. However, an office functioning on a prepayment basis must be willing to render a financial adjustment quickly to the patient who prematurely terminates care. The same risks involved in care-basis fees must also be considered.

Most practitioners feel that patients should return to the office because they want to, not because they have to because of some prior financial commitment. The contention is that the doctor on an office call basis knows where he stands with the patient at all times. The continuing patient reflects signs of patient satisfaction, respect, and confidence. The doctor is always aware that the doctor-patient relationship is intact.

HMOs. Health Maintenance Organizations (HMOs) are essentially group practices operating on a prepayment system. They differ from individual practitioner prepayment plans in that they offer a broader scope of service to patients.

Discounted Services

Years ago when health practice was less complicated and more informal, doctors would find themselves reducing a fee for a friend, reducing a fee because a patient was about to finance a new home, and writing a "no charge" here and there for reasons appearing humanitarian at the time. The result was a low gross income and an even lower net income. Doctors were increasingly busy and increasingly losing money. The result was reduced practice development and increased discouragement.

The public today feels that it is not necessary for a professional to offer discounts. If fees are priced fairly, there is no room for a discount. There are, however, some exceptions. When a patient is seen more than once during a single day for the same illness, many physicians will make a reduction for the subsequent visits. When several patients from the same family are seen in the office at the same time, many physicians will charge the initial office visit fee for the first patient seen and follow-up visit fee for the second patient. Likewise, when two patients in one family are seen at the same time during a house call, many physicians will charge the regular scheduled rate for the first patient seen and a reduced fee for the second patient. These practices are usually limited to the doctor offering a family type of health service.

Professional Courtesy

Each doctor is faced with a decision regarding fees charged to colleagues, other members of the healing arts, the clergy, and relatives of the doctor. Policy varies from doctor to doctor. Fees vary from the cost of tangible items involved to a percentage of regular professional fees.

Except his immediate family, few doctors offer gratuitous or discounted services to relatives. However, if the doctor or members of his family use a relative's services or receive products at a discount, the doctor may be obliged to do likewise.

Fees presented to patients allowed professional courtesy should be by a statement for the full fee with the words "professional courtesy" indicated and the percentage or amount entered and subtracted to arrive at the net fee due. The percentage is usually taken from the total professional services fee, not including items such as supplements, supports, etc.

Inconsistency in offering professional courtesy can do more damage than the courtesy does good. Failure of the doctor to formalize an office policy in this area can cause embarrassing errors to be made by the assistant.

In regard to professional services extended to fellow doctors of chiropractic, codes of ethics of many chiropractic organizations list the following points:

1. Chiropractors and their immediate dependents are entitled to the gratuitous services of any one or more of the profession. The chiropractor is unable to care for himself when ill. The anxiety and solicitude felt when someone of his immediate family is ill may reduce his competency. In these circumstances, chiropractors are especially dependent on each other. Thus, professional

aid should be cheerfully and gratuitously afforded.

2. Should a chiropractor in affluent circumstances require the services of a distant professional brother for himself or his immediate dependents, he should pay travel expenses and such other honorarium that at least partially compensates the visiting chiropractor for his loss of time.

3. When, because of personal illness, a chiropractor refers patients to a fellow practitioner, the recipient of the references should consider it a courtesy and permit all fees incident to such services to be paid the sick colleague. If, however, a chiropractor is absent on holiday pleasures, the fees resulting from such referred practice may rightfully be retained by the colleague to whom the patients have been referred.

Each doctor must develop a personal philosophy on the proper way to handle hardship or indigent cases. Sometimes it is better to reduce a fee, sometimes to cancel it. The assistant must obtain the information needed to help the doctor arrive at a reasonable and just decision. If a patient states that he cannot pay the fee the office requires and requests a downward revision, the situation must be discussed with the doctor either by the assistant or the patient. If the patient is unable to pay any portion of the fee, patient care must be accepted on some type of charitable basis or referred to a welfare agency.

Other Professional Guidelines

At this point, it is helpful for the chiropractic assistant to be aware of other ethical codes to which many chiropractic associations adhere. Following are several points involving fees, fee policies, and fee presentations:

1. The chiropractic profession has for its objective the greatest service it can render humanity. Therefore, financial gain becomes a secondary consideration.

2. The chiropractor should attend his patient as often as is necessary to ensure con-

tinued favorable progress but should avoid unnecessary visits lest he expose himself to being accused of mercenary motives.

3. A wealthy chiropractor should not give gratuitous service to the affluent. This would injure his professional brethren. The office of a chiropractor cannot be supported as a benevolence. Hence, it defrauds the common fund when fees are refused that might rightfully be claimed.

4. It is considered unprofessional to split fees or to give or receive a commission for referring patients for a health-related service. An exception is in cases where laboratory services are required, and then the patient should be informed that there is an extra charge for such for interpretation.

5. There is no profession in which gratuitous services are more freely dispensed than by chiropractors, but justice demands some limit on the extent of such services. Poverty, professional brotherhood, the poorly remunerated occupation of some patient, and other worthy public duties should be recognized as valid justification for gratuitous services. However, services given to endowed institutions, mutual benefit societies, and for life insurance or other health certification examinations should not be provided without an appropriate fee.

Trading Services

During the depression of the 1930s, trading services was common because cash flow was small. A doctor sometimes offered health services in return for housekeeping services, repair work, yard work, or even food. There is no need for this today. Even when the practice was more justifiable, resentment arose because patients could not appreciate the high value of the doctor's time against the apparently lower value of their time. As such services must be reported as income, difficulty also arose in placing a value on the mutual services provided. Doctors have found it better for the office to pay patients for their services and for patients to pay the office for its services.

The current system is to have a fixed fee for each service and to use an acceptable fee schedule. A definite policy applied to all patients in an objective manner has proved to be a sound approach.

Hardship Cases

Patients today have a certain image in their minds of a doctor. They expect him to have made a large investment in education, to provide a modern and well-equipped office, and to maintain a standard of living proportional to his professional contributions to society. People prefer the "successful" doctor. Few have confidence in a professional whose standard of living and lifestyle are below average for the community. But this requires financial support. Equipment, instruments, furnishings, supplies, salaries, transportation, housing, insurance, and continuing education are just a few costs in practice that require constant funding.

Critics of health-care costs say doctors in past years were more charitable than today. This is not true. No doctor in good conscience will refuse care to a patient in need. It is true that doctors in past years offered more direct charity. But it must be remembered that in those days it was the common role of the professional community to offer direct help to the unfortunate. There was no Medicare, no Medicaid, few national or state or county welfare programs, and few patients had any type of health or accident insurance. In those days, the doctor's tax base was very low. Today it is very high, for much of it is used to support the charitable services and programs that were once provided directly from doctor to patient. Thus, while doctors of today may be contributing to the unfortunate in a much higher degree than their predecessors, they are frequently subjected to criticism by those who fail to relate to present realities.

Rare is the community today that does not have several social agencies, welfare organizations, and charitable institutions. These agencies are specialists in determining financial need. The doctor in private practice should not be expected to be such a specialist.

Surveys show that for some unknown reason doctors are the last to be paid. They constantly appear last on the sheet of priority to receive reimbursement. It is important here to differentiate inability to pay and inconvenience to pay. It is not unusual for an uninsured patient to ask the doctor to wait for his fee, then pay the bank payments for his new car, wife's Christmas fur, second color television set, and exotic vacation.

If a patient is under temporary financial strain and has a good credit rating, his bank or a lending agency will issue a loan. This is not the role of a health practice. If the patient has a serious problem, aid is the role of social and welfare agencies, not the role of a health practice. Another source of help is the patient's family and friends. If a patient is not willing to ask close relatives or friends for aid, he should not place this responsibility on the doctor.

There is no need today for anyone to go without proper health care whether they have the money to pay for it or not. Government aid is available.

Cash-Basis Fees

While fees are easily collected if the patient pays on each visit, purchasing on credit has become the American custom. Feasibility of a strictly cash-basis system depends on community custom, the length of anticipated care, the patient's ability to pay immediately, the doctor's practice philosophy, and how firmly the practice is established.

Even if the office is not on a strict cash basis, if patients expect to pay at each visit they should be encouraged to do so. Cash payments reduce bookkeeping chores, reduce collection expenses, and offer the greatest percentage of collection on fees charged. The alert assistant will soon realize that most patients will pay immediately *when asked*. Thus, the assistant should not hesitate to suggest it. In such anticipation, the assistant should have an "extra cash" box for making change and a receipt book immediately available. The physical presence of these items serves as a constant reminder to suggest payment by cash or check on each visit.

Patients who are paid weekly may prefer to pay a fixed amount on their account each week. When a large fee is involved, the assistant may ask the patient if this method is preferred to paying on each visit. Likewise, the patient who is paid semimonthly may prefer to pay twice a month.

While monthly statements are a common method of billing, the method creates the poorest results and the largest amount of overhead expense. This means that collection costs and losses reflect in the standard fees that all patients must assume. While this may not be fair, it is the only way a doctor's office, or any business for that matter, can remain solvent.

Patient Credit

Credit purchasing, time payments, and budget plans are a part of accepted economics that almost every office must be prepared to handle in an efficient, controlled, professional manner. If they are not, the survival of the practice may be at risk.

When a person asks for credit at any establishment, he expects to provide information that reasonably assures the lender of eventual payment. While some retail stores, hospitals, and clinics have used budget payments for many years, private practitioners are sometimes reluctantly forced by circumstances to incorporate such arrangements within their practices to fit the needs of the community. See Figure 8.1.

It is necessary here to differentiate between *qualified* and *unqualified* credit. Credit is qualified when a patient's credit rating has been verified or when payment will be made by a third party such as a Worker's Compensation Fund, an insurance company, employer, or union. Credit is unqualified when a patient's credit has not been verified, when it is not to be paid by a responsible third party, or when the doctor simply agrees to bill the patient (eg, at the end of the month). Most accountants agree that it is poor business practice to allow over 5% gross income to be on unqualified credit. This is often a goal difficult to achieve. A monthly income summary sheet is shown in Figure 8.2.

	AGE	DATE
NAME	SOC. SEC. NO.	
STREET ADDRESS	CITY, STATE, ZIP	
RESIDENCE TELEPHONE NO.	WORK TELEPHONE NO.	
EMPLOYER	EMPLOYER ADDRESS	
SPOUSE NAME	SPOUSE ADDRESS	
OWN ☐ RENT ☐	Landlord/Mortgage Holder Address	
LANDLORD/MORTGAGE HOLDER	Landlord/Mortgage Holder Telephone	
BANK REFERENCE	CREDIT REFERENCE	

NOTES: _____

_____

_____

_____

_____

Figure 8.1. Typical format for bad-debt screening form.

Offices generally have a supply of "Application for Credit" forms available for patients requesting credit arrangements. Credit is a privilege, and the patient should provide reference information freely. If a patient should ask for credit but refuse to fill out an application, it can usually be presumed that there is something wrong with the patient's credit rating or that the patient does not intend to pay the fee.

When the office extends credit, certain basic information is sought:

- Name
- Address
- Home telephone number
- Work telephone number
- Length of stay at current address
- Own, rent, lease?
- Age
- Employer's name and address
- Type of work, department
- How long employed in present position
- Previous job information
- Spouse's name, name of nearest relative
- Name of bank(s), type of account(s)
- Credit references (minimum of three).

Note that much of the above information has already been gathered on the entering patient data form. Except the name, a CA need not duplicate the information on the credit application form. A credit application form can be kept simple by requesting only the information necessary for credit that

MONTHLY INCOME SUMMARY

Month of _____ 19__

Date	Charges	Deposits	Income from Patients	Nonpractice Income		Total Income
				Amount	Description	
___	$____	$____	$____	$____	_____	$____

Month total $____ $____ $____ $____ $____

Brought forward $____ $____ $____ $____ $____

Total to date $____ $____ | $____ $____ $____

Figure 8.2. Typical format of a monthly income summary sheet.

was not asked on the entering data form. One method is to ask such questions on the back of the entering data form, rather than having a separate form. This would, however, announce to all that credit is available.

Most doctors do not find it necessary to make an extensive credit check on all those who agreeably fill out the necessary information on the application. For patients entering the practice or for whom a credit rating has not been established, a brief telephone call to the local credit bureau will usually be sufficient to judge the patient's credit rating.

When a large fee may be involved, the assistant should be aware of certain indications of a poor risk that may require more than routine checking. Here are some signals that may be cause for concern:

- Frequent change of address
- Unlisted phone, no phone, no neighbor's phone
  - Seasonal employment
  - Frequent job change
  - The emergency patient new to the practice
  - History of bankruptcy
  - The transient patient
  - Frequently missed appointments
  - Frequently changed appointments
  - Chronic complainer
  - The "demanding" patient
  - Highly neurotic personality
  - Referred by a slow paying patient
  - Patient who has been to several doctors for the same condition
  - A patient with previous credit problems
  - A recently divorced patient

A poor credit report or one or more signals of a poor risk is not an absolute indication that the doctor will refuse a patient. It means that the matter should be brought to his attention for evaluation. Signals and credit reports are but warning signs alerting the office that a firm financial policy and a clear understanding of fees be maintained at all times.

EXPLAINING FEES TO PATIENTS

The security and growth of any health practice are obviously governed by its income. Again, the principles of sound management must apply such as careful planning, establishing efficient routines, and sincere adherence to the routines. No system is any better than how it is used.

While the rationale for calculating fees is usually based on services provided, the fee presentation is often designed for patient acceptance. The fee presentation by an administrative assistant is usually conducted after entering patient data are recorded. At this time, the assistant explains the doctor's charges, what they cover, and what they do not cover. It is important that the assistant is specific, clear, and assured that the patient understands through feedback.

After this initial explanation, the patient should be asked how he wishes to pay and a method is agreed on in harmony with office policy. If health insurance is involved, this should be discussed in detail with the patient (eg, assignments accepted?). Insurance relations will be described in a future chapter.

Due to rapidly increasing health-care costs in recent years, doctor's fees have been subjected to considerable criticism. Patients complain about the size of fees, and doctors complain of the unwillingness of patients to pay them.

Studies to improve this thorny side of practice and the doctor-patient relationship underscore the need to discuss fees in advance. Yet many doctors feel embarrassed to talk about fees for their services for they look to their services as an act of humanity rather than a purchasable commodity. The assistant must be aware of the average doctor's sensitivity in this area and help him by presenting fee policy in a professional, humane, and tactful manner.

If the patient understands the doctor's charges and is satisfied with the services, the office rarely has difficulty in collections. Experience shows that failure to inform the patient thoroughly at the beginning of care of the fees involved, especially in a lengthy case, is the cause of more disagreement regarding payment for services than any other factor. Once a patient is made aware of anticipated financial obligations, he can accept them, reject them, or arrange to meet them. When fees and a method of payment have been agreed to, the major points that could lead to later misunderstanding have been eliminated.

The assistant should not wait for the patient to ask about fees. Even if they want to know, many patients are timid about discussing fees. Realizing this, many doctors post a notice in the receiving area that encourages open discussion. For example:

TO ALL MY PATIENTS

I INVITE YOU TO DISCUSS FRANKLY WITH ME ANY QUESTION REGARDING MY SERVICES OR FEES. THE BEST HEALTH SERVICE IS BASED ON A FRIENDLY, MUTUAL UNDERSTANDING BETWEEN DOCTOR AND PATIENT.

Dr. John H. Smith

Basic Economic Management

The soundness of the office's economic systems is decided largely by establishing a collection system assuring the doctor will receive the greatest percentage possible of the fees earned. A good system will exhibit these five basic features.

1. It will make certain that all patients understand all charges and appreciate that the services received fully justify the fee.

2. It will make certain that all office systems are designed to offer patients a simple and convenient method to pay at each visit.

3. It will make certain that patients with unpaid balances on their accounts are billed punctually and regularly according to a predetermined plan.

4. It will make certain that all uncollected bills be followed up punctually and regularly according to a predetermined plan.

5. It will make certain that patients comply with tactful suggestions of how problems of indebtedness may be resolved.

A health practice also must consider certain facts about human nature. People resent paying for an unwanted illness, and they resent it more when symptoms are gone. Because people who are ill are already under much stress, added financial stress must be avoided. The best way to do this is to ensure that patients understand and accept the need for the proposed services and the fee involved. The importance of reaching advanced understanding and agreement cannot be overemphasized.

Each patient is entitled to know all anticipated examination and therapy fees. The patient is a health-service consumer, and, as any consumer, he has the right to know what he is buying and how much it will cost. The itemized visit slip and the assistant's explanation of office policies are excellent ways to avoid misunderstandings.

The assistant must do more than administer a collection system. She must be in a position to understand the need for the system if she is to convey properly the office's philosophy in a humane and professional manner. Money is a symbol for services rendered. It is essentially a receipt for the health care received. The office asks nothing for which it is not entitled, and you should never feel guilty in using commonly accepted business procedures.

Once the DC provides his valuable services, he is entitled to fair payment. The assistant must understand, not only in words but in spirit, that the office's fees are just and based on the value of the services offered. Health-service costs may appear high unless compared to the cost for an emergency call to a plumber or television serviceman. What is health care worth? To answer this question one must know the value of being free from pain, to return to work and earn a living, to have peace of mind and be free of health worries. Some patients forget this. See Figure 8.3.

CAs should be aware that health care is the biggest bargain a person may have. Because patients resent being sick, they resent paying a fee to regain their health. More often than not, when they say they cannot pay, they mean they would rather not pay. They frequently resent paying a few hun-

1st visit	–I'm in terrible pain.
2nd visit	–I hope I live through this.
3rd visit	–So far, so good.
4th visit	–I think I might make it.
5th visit	–Thank heaven for that!
6th visit	–Boy, that was easy.
7th visit	–What a relief!
8th visit	–Not so bad at all.
9th visit	–I'm almost normal.
10th visit	–That doctor is a wizard!
11th visit	–Ain't life great.
12th visit	–How fortunate I was to find such a doctor.
Statement	–I guess I wasn't as sick as I thought.
Reminder	–I certainly got trimmed for that.
First notice	–Let him wait. He's got plenty.
Second notice	–I would have probably gotten well anyway.
Please remit	–Pushy, isn't he. I'll show him.
Demand for payment	–Who the devil does he think he is?
Legal action	–Swindler! Quack!
Forced collection	–I'll sue him for malpractice.

Figure 8.3. Adapted from the *Human Nature Chart* of G. S. King, MD, showing how time and debt cloud a patient's memory.

dred dollars to regain their deteriorated health and run down bodies, yet rarely resent paying thousands of dollars for orthodontics, a face lift, hair implants, or some other cosmetic but nonvital service.

Indebtedness adds to the stress of a patient's illness and tends to build a mental barrier between patient and doctor. A patient in debt to the office invariably will tend to avoid the doctor and delay attention to health needs. This is tragic, and an alert assistant with good office systems can avoid this.

Prompt payment also offers some fundamental psychologic advantages. Several studies show that patients who keep current with their accounts get better results and in less time. Dentists say that false teeth paid for fit better than those that haven't. Automobile servicemen report that a tune-up paid for is appreciated, while one that isn't is a source of chronic complaints. The reason for this is that indebtedness produces guilt resulting in projection, resentment, and rationalization. The best climate the assistant can create is to help the patient avoid indebtedness.

A General Approach

It was described earlier that payment-by-the-visit is the best procedure for most offices. It is also better for most patients because it eliminates indebtedness and its consequences. When the patient hands the charge slip to the assistant in the dismissal area, the assistant should explain office policy. She should ask, "Would you like to pay today's visit by check or cash?" Avoid the question, "Would you like me to send you the bill?" This encourages the patient to accept the offer of billing and makes immediate payment unlikely.

Once the assistant asks the question, "Would you like to pay today's visit by check or cash?" she should pause and await the patient's reply. If the patient indicates that he will pay now, the assistant then checks if the patient has any other outstanding charges at the office. If so, the patient is presented an opportunity to take care of all or part of these also.

ANSWERING QUESTIONS ABOUT FEES AND SERVICES

Questions regarding the doctor's fees require tactful handling. The assistant must remember that the chiropractor is a doctor offering a health-care service. Unlike a person engaged in a commercial enterprise, it is impossible and unwise to have a set of quotable prices. Each case is an individual matter, and the fees charged should depend on the skill, time, and technical knowledge required to treat the problem, as well as the financial circumstances of the patient. Unfortunately, some people shop around for prices and make price comparisons. Since you and the doctor are members of a professional health team, and not selling groceries or automobile parts, you cannot be expected to answer such inquiries.

Some people will inevitably ask the question, "How much does the doctor charge?" This may not be intended to be taken at its literal meaning. The question is asked merely as an opening to show a desire to arrange for professional care. An effective response to such a blunt inquiry on price would be, "How long has it been since you last consulted the doctor?" or "When did you last receive chiropractic care?" or "What seems to be the trouble?" Skirt the question by asking another question. You will be surprised how often your question leads to a discussion of the patient's problem and to an appointment without further discussion of charges. Another answer to a price question would be, "The doctor will discuss his fees with you during consultation. Would you like me to arrange a special visit with him prior to examination?"

Because we live in a price-oriented economy, you might be faced with a price question. Don't feel insulted by it or be antagonistic. One of the best solutions is your reaction. Handle it professionally: friendly, seriously, tactfully, and with understanding.

Hold one fact uppermost in your mind.

Your employer is a doctor of chiropractic, a professional. The cost of his services cannot be determined until a thorough examination reveals the individual's need for care and treatment.

Even if it were ethical to quote prices, it would be unwise to attempt to base health treatment on such an unknown factor or put it into a competitive situation. If a patient needs treatment, he should receive thorough professional care without being deluded or influenced by price.

Most practitioners have procedures for handling price inquiries. You will find that a complete rapport must exist between doctor and assistant on these matters. The establishment of a basic policy and specific course of action to follow is reached by complete and thorough discussion between doctor and assistant.

If a caller insists on knowing the doctor's "charges," respond: "There is no fee for consultation (if this is office policy). This is to determine facts about your problem and what should be done about it." If the caller persists, explain that the different examinations and therapies used in the office require different fees. There is no way of determining exact fees until the doctor has an opportunity to determine the specific type of examination and treatment necessary for a particular patient.

No ethical practitioner will ever promise a cure for anything. A patient may telephone and say, "I have severe headaches. Can Dr. Smith cure headaches?" Your response must show concern and hope but keep within an ethical framework. An example of one such response would be: "I understand what you are going through, and I'm sure that you appreciate that no ethical doctor would promise a cure. I can say that Dr. Smith has had excellent results in many cases of severe headaches in which the patients were at their wits' end. However, in your particular case, the doctor must have an opportunity to determine what the cause of your trouble might be and if the cause or causes can be corrected. Would you prefer a time reservation with the doctor at 2 o'clock pm Tuesday or 3 o'clock Wednesday for your initial consultation?"

A patient may be recommended to your

office by a mutual friend, yet the patient is apprehensive about making an appointment. The caller might ask, "How do you know when to use a doctor of chiropractic?" Respond, "Doctors of chiropractic are primary-care physicians, and so defined in federal and state regulations, who serve as portals of entry into the health-care system. Under chiropractic care, a patient is either treated or referred after a diagnosis is arrived at by using whatever procedures are necessary to determine the type care best suited for the patient's complaint. By consultation and examination, the doctor arrives at a prognosis under chiropractic care or suggests more appropriate care."

If asked whether chiropractic treatment is dangerous, the assistant should offer a reassuring response. For example: "With rare exception, the answer to your question is a strong NO. Naturally, any form of health treatment contains a degree of hazard if not conducted professionally. That is why each state requires definite educational standards prior to the doctor gaining his license to practice. Rest assured there is little danger in chiropractic care administered by a licensed practitioner. The dangers of strong drugs or major surgery, both of which are avoided in chiropractic care, represent the overwhelming concern in health science today."

"Can chiropractic do anything for cancer (or any other type of advanced degenerative condition)?" This type of question is usually posed by either the patient in a terminal state or a person seeking confirmation that chiropractors are quacks. In either case, a good response would be something like this: "While chiropractic has proved successful in a wide range of disorders, further investigation is needed concerning advanced pathology. Such cases seen are referred to appropriate physicians and surgeons who specialize in these types of conditions. However, sometimes a person suffering from cancer also has other structural/functional conditions that are contributing to pain or discomfort which are frequently aided by chiropractic care."

You may receive a call from a person who is new to your community. He has been under the care of a chiropractor who was a graduate of a certain college and used certain techniques of which the patient has grown accustomed and confident. The caller may ask in what college your doctor-employer earned his degree or what procedures he uses. Conversely, the inquiry may be motivated by the fact that he has had poor experience from a DC who was a graduate of a certain college and used certain procedures. Thus, before you can answer the question intelligently, you must first determine the patient's motivation in asking the question. It is not impertinent if you tactfully ask, "Why do you ask, Mr. Brown?" Once knowing the patient's motive, you can respond either, "Yes, Dr. Gentry is a graduate of ABC College" or "No, Dr. Gentry is a graduate of another fine college." Regarding clinical procedures, say: "Dr. Gentry is acquainted with all recognized techniques. The particular technique selected in each individual case depends on his findings, what methods have helped you in the past, and what methods he feels will help you most in the future."

Because of numerous articles in the public press, some patients may ask, "Do I have to be x-rayed?" These inquiries must be answered tactfully and honestly. For example, "Sometimes it is necessary, many times not. The doctor will only recommend a particular examination procedure if he feels it will be necessary to help in determining the cause of your trouble. While he won't take chances with your health, he won't burden you with unnecessary tests. Naturally, a decision cannot be made until after consultation and examination. Would you prefer a time reservation for next Monday morning or Wednesday afternoon?"

Probably the most common call you will receive will be that from a returning patient: "When can I see the doctor?" If you respond, "Next Friday," he may not like that day. When you do agree on a day, he'll ask, "What time?" And he may not like the time suggested. The best way to handle such calls is to give two choices. This gives the patient an opportunity to select the best alternative open. For example, "Would Wednesday morning at 11:15 or Friday afternoon at 3:30 be acceptable?" Offer the patient a chance to take part in the decision making process, yet maintain control. A closing statement should repeat the day and time to confirm the appointment and impress it on the memory of the patient.

Except this last example, which is routine, previous questions dealt with such topics as the doctor's fees, cures, education, and clinical procedures. To the assistant these questions may seem naive, but to the sincere caller they are honest and direct. Thus, it's important when callers appear nervous and apprehensive to respond frequently with, "I understand." Tactfully explain that answers to fees, examinations, or therapies used in any individual case cannot be answered by telephone. They can only be answered after the doctor has had a chance to talk with the patient and conduct at least a preliminary examination. The assistant must convey to the caller *understanding, sincerity,* and *credibility.*

Questions like those described are not always limited to telephone inquiries. An assistant may hear them from patients in the office, from a patient's friend or relative who has accompanied the patient into the office, or from friends and strangers at social gatherings.

DISMISSING THE PATIENT

After the patient has seen the doctor, receive the visit slip from the patient and total the charges for the services and supplies received. Tell the patient the total charges and open the receipt book in front of the patient. This invites payment. If the patient pays, write a receipt and present it with a friendly "Thank you!" If the patient asks to be billed, give him a copy of the visit slip and explain that it will serve as a bill. Schedule another appointment for the patient if the doctor has so recommended and set up an appointment verification according to office policy.

Dismissing the patient is the last chance for personal contact with the patient that day and the last opportunity to enhance good will. If the patient needs a taxi, call a cab. Help the elderly on with their coats and

boots if necessary, remind patients of personal packages, and offer an appropriate farewell as the patient leaves such as, "We'll be looking forward to seeing you Friday, Mr. Brown." If a patient is departing while you are on the telephone or busy at your desk, spare a moment to recognize him, smile, and say, "good-by." A courteous farewell is good manners, professional conduct, and positive human relations.

OFFICE ACCOUNTING

The business side of health care is conducted in much the same way as any business. Income and expenses must be accurately recorded in detail for tax purposes as well as to arrive at a complete picture of financial status of the practice.

Basic Requirements

Today, federal, state, and county governments and third-party payers are the doctor's silent partners. Because the Internal Revenue Service has the right to examine office records at any time and because third-party payers have the right to request clinical records, the doctor and his assistant(s) have no choice but to keep adequate records.

Taxes alone require a sound system for calculating and estimating financial data. Such a system is essential for federal income taxes, federal payroll taxes, social security deductions, worker's compensation payments, state income taxes, school taxes, personal property taxes, sales taxes, license fees, and so on. But it is not sufficient for bookkeeping just to meet taxes, for this alone would not be adequate for the doctor to evaluate practice progress. The doctor must also have a system showing the financial status and trends of the practice so professional and economic advancement can be controlled. The doctor should know at any given time how much the practice has earned, how much it has collected, what has been spent, what is still owed, and how this month, quarter, or year compares with past performance.

How a bookkeeping system is designed depends on the quantity and quality of data desired by the individual doctor. Small practices do not require the manifold records of a large or group practice.

Because doctors have individual preferences, and these preferences change with the times, the system should be designed to meet the needs of the practice. The practice should not be called on to meet the needs of a system. The important thing is that the system is adequate for tax-reporting purposes and offers the doctor the information desired to make sound economic decisions. The system used should allow flexibility to keep pace with anticipated growth and changing conditions without major redesign.

Most established doctors use the services of an accountant. It is the role of an administrative assistant to be aware of the systems established, collect fees, and make the necessary routine record entries. It's her job that financial records are accurate, up to date, and complete in terms of accounts receivable (money owed to the doctor), accounts payable (money the doctor owes), and disbursements (see Fig. 8.4). Thus, the assistant is responsible for accurately recording the fees charged, billing these fees and recording payments, recording the bills incurred by the office, implementing a system of paying bills, and properly allocating expenditures.

A doctor's basic income consists of the fees paid to him by patients in return for his services to them. It is essential that an effective cash control system be used to record services performed and the amount charged, communicate this information immediately to the patient, and collect the amount due. Ideally, all this should be accomplished by administrative personnel. The following considerations are unquestionably the basic areas involved in controlling cash flow for the typical chiropractic practice:

• Clear and efficient communications between the doctor, patient, and doctor's administrative personnel

• Accurate records reflecting the financial status of each patient and the entire practice

• Efficient administrative procedures requiring minimum attention of the doctor

• The administration of third-party payments (insurance).

The Communication Loop

Essential to successful billing and collecting is effective communication involving the doctor, patient, and administrative personnel of the practice. The most crucial communication occurs at the time of an office visit and forms the basis for administrative action.

At the time of an office visit, documentation must be initiated for each patient to be treated, and the following inputs must be generated:

• Amount owed by patient prior to current treatment
• Record of services received by patient
• Record of fees incurred for services
• Record of and receipt for any payment made
• Date and time of patient's next visit.

The most practical way to accomplish these communications and record the inputs is to initiate a separate *transaction slip* (visit slip) for each patient that is passed among the administrative assistant, the doctor, and the patient during an office visit. If an ideal transaction slip is executed completely and accurately for each patient, sufficient information is on hand for the operation of an entire billing and collecting system. The administrative assistant will have complete information on the treatment and fees involved in the visit, the patient will be aware of fees previously owed and those incurred during the visit, and the doctor will know who the next patient will be.

MONTHLY DISBURSEMENT RECORD   Month of _____ 19__

Date	Payee	Check No.	Office Supplies	Rent, Utilities, Mainte-nance	Commu-nications	Travel	Subscrip-tions, Dues
____	____	____	$____	$____	$____	$____	$____
____	____	____	____	____	____	____	____
____	____	____	____	____	____	____	____
____	____	____	____	____	____	____	____
____	____	____	____	____	____	____	____
____	____	____	____	____	____	____	____
____	____	____	____	____	____	____	____
____	____	____	____	____	____	____	____
____	____	____	____	____	____	____	____
____	____	____	____	____	____	____	____
____	____	____	____	____	____	____	____
____	____	____	____	____	____	____	____
____	____	____	____	____	____	____	____
____	____	____	____	____	____	____	____
____	____	____	____	____	____	____	____
____	____	____	____	____	____	____	____
____	____	____	____	____	____	____	____
____	____	____	____	____	____	____	____
____	____	____	____	____	____	____	____
____	____	____	____	____	____	____	____
____	____	____	____	____	____	____	____
____	____	____	____	____	____	____	____
____	____	____	____	____	____	____	____
____	____	____	____	____	____	____	____
____	____	____	____	____	____	____	____
____	____	____	____	____	____	____	____
Total			$____	$____	$____	$____	$____
Amount Budgeted			$____	$____	$____	$____	$____
Percent +/− Budget			____	____	____	____	____

Figure 8.4A. Sample format for a monthly disbursement record, left-hand page.

Taxes, License Fees	Conventions	Contributions	Insurance	Professional Services	Shipping	Advertising & PR	Payroll	
$_____	$_____	$_____	$_____	$_____	$_____	$_____	$_____	1
_____	_____	_____	_____	_____	_____	_____	_____	2
_____	_____	_____	_____	_____	_____	_____	_____	3
_____	_____	_____	_____	_____	_____	_____	_____	4
_____	_____	_____	_____	_____	_____	_____	_____	5
_____	_____	_____	_____	_____	_____	_____	_____	6
_____	_____	_____	_____	_____	_____	_____	_____	7
_____	_____	_____	_____	_____	_____	_____	_____	8
_____	_____	_____	_____	_____	_____	_____	_____	9
_____	_____	_____	_____	_____	_____	_____	_____	10
_____	_____	_____	_____	_____	_____	_____	_____	11
_____	_____	_____	_____	_____	_____	_____	_____	12
_____	_____	_____	_____	_____	_____	_____	_____	13
_____	_____	_____	_____	_____	_____	_____	_____	14
_____	_____	_____	_____	_____	_____	_____	_____	15
_____	_____	_____	_____	_____	_____	_____	_____	16
_____	_____	_____	_____	_____	_____	_____	_____	17
_____	_____	_____	_____	_____	_____	_____	_____	18
_____	_____	_____	_____	_____	_____	_____	_____	19
_____	_____	_____	_____	_____	_____	_____	_____	20
_____	_____	_____	_____	_____	_____	_____	_____	21
_____	_____	_____	_____	_____	_____	_____	_____	22
_____	_____	_____	_____	_____	_____	_____	_____	23
_____	_____	_____	_____	_____	_____	_____	_____	24
_____	_____	_____	_____	_____	_____	_____	_____	25
_____	_____	_____	_____	_____	_____	_____	_____	26
_____	_____	_____	_____	_____	_____	_____	_____	27
_____	_____	_____	_____	_____	_____	_____	_____	28
_____	_____	_____	_____	_____	_____	_____	_____	29
_____	_____	_____	_____	_____	_____	_____	_____	30
_____	_____	_____	_____	_____	_____	_____	_____	31
$_____	$_____	$_____	$_____	$_____	$_____	$_____	$_____	
$_____	$_____	$_____	$_____	$_____	$_____	$_____	$_____	
_____	_____	_____	_____	_____	_____	_____	_____	

Figure 8.4B. Sample format for the right-hand page of a monthly disbursement record.

Deferred Collections and Accounts Receivable

The inputs generated at the time of treatment must be reflected in several records that are an integral part of any billing and collecting system. These records reflect the accounts receivable of the entire practice as well as those of individual patients or family units.

The *day sheet* offers a chronologic listing of every transaction with every patient for the practice. It contains a day-by-day accounting of all services performed, all fees levied and collected, and all money still due. This record also might contain notations on each transaction useful for periodic analysis of the practice, as well as a record of deposits in the bank account of the practice. See Figure 8.5.

An individual patient financial record consists of two items: a *statement* of current indebtedness and a *permanent history* of fees and payments. A copy of the current statement (amount forward and charges for the month) is sent to the patient monthly if any fees remain unpaid. The individual patient's financial history is kept on file, usually in a *financial ledger card*. The ledger card usually shows all transactions made for a year. Thus, a patient who has been with the practice for several years may have several annual ledger cards in his file.

Thus far, the *minimum* requirements for a system of billing and collecting for the practice have been described. The system would provide the communication and documentation required to assure complete control from the start of treatment to the depositing of fees collected in the practice's bank account. It is important to the doctor, however, that operation of the system does not impose a heavy burden of time and cost on himself or his assistants.

Third-Party Payments

An increasing amount of billing and collecting for health practice involves a third party—some form of insurance, welfare, or compensation. The practice may participate partially or entirely in the claim process,

and a considerable administrative burden can result. It is not unusual for large practices to have one or more assistants exclusively handling third-party claims.

An ideal billing and collecting system includes the creation of a single record containing all the information required for filing claims for payment from insurance companies and government agencies. The subject of creating such a record during every office visit and systems for processing claims will be discussed in a subsequent chapter.

Selecting the Proper System

The doctor and accountant select the system to be used. However, the administrative assistant can be helpful by offering constructive criticisms of present systems and offering positive suggestions that she feels would benefit the practice. This will require reading business and management journals to be alert to new systems and trends.

Once the basic requirements of a practice's billing and collecting system are identified, it is important to establish guidelines for seeking improvement in a system that meet the needs of a particular practice. Basically, any system must meet the needs of controlling cash, enhancing clear communications, and providing accurate records and efficient procedures.

Pegboard Systems

One method that reduces the administrative burden involved in billing and collecting, and still offers the controls described, is a "one-write" system—often called a "pegboard" system. Using a one-write system for billing and collecting makes it possible to create most records at the time of the office visit. This system employs an accounting board designed for convenient arrangement of necessary forms and records. When (1) a *transaction slip* is filled out during the visit, the information is recorded simultaneously on (2) the patient's *monthly statement* and (3) *ledger card*, on the office's (4) *day sheet* that chronologically lists all transactions for all patients that day, or on other forms. See Figure 8.6.

DAY SHEET

Date _____   Sheet No. ____ of____

Name	Description	Office Code	A Today's Charge	B Payment Received	C Today's Balance	D Previous Balance
		Total				

Figure 8.5. Simple day-sheet format. Columns A–D offer an accounts receivable control, provide a daily cash summary, and help to proof postings.

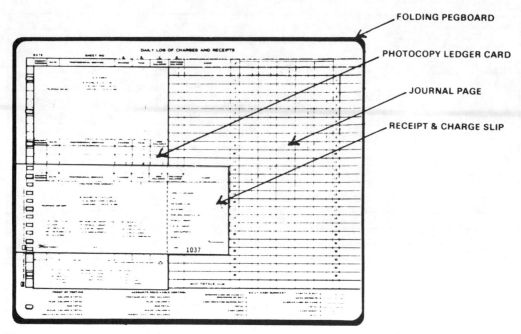

Figure 8.6. Pegboard accounts receivable system incorporating a day sheet, financial ledger card, and a visit slip/receipt (reprinted by permission of the Colwell Company).

This one-write feature saves time in establishing various records and assuring their consistency. Because entries on four records are made at a single writing, a simple daily check of day sheet entries alone provides a fool-proof check of entries on all records.

Super Bills

In recent years, the term *super bill* has appeared, and an assistant should have a clear understanding of what it is and, more importantly, what it is not. A super bill is a specific form that is commonly part of a system for health-practice billing and collecting procedures. It is usually a two- or three-part form showing current fees and services performed, treatment code, diagnostic information, and patient personal data, as well as insurance requirements. See Figure 8.7.

A super bill is, in a sense, an attending physician's statement, and usually replaces any other form designed for this use (eg, visit slip). The purpose of a super bill is to create itemized information at the time of the patient's visit. A copy of the completed

form is presented to the patient at dismissal who initiates the claim to an insurance carrier or is used by the practice to submit the claim. In either case, one copy of the super bill is attached to the insurance carrier's regular claim form. This reduces the time required when typing the claim form.

The savings of administrative time is the key to using a super bill system. The specifications of a super bill are unimportant. The arrangement of the form, the number of parts, or the process by which it is created have no significance when the results are the same. Therefore, a super bill is a method and not a form. Almost any good system can use one or more variations of a super bill.

Entry Systems

The classic double-entry bookkeeping system is often adopted in a doctor's office, and it gives the doctor the basic information usually needed. It offers built-in safeguards of checks and balances against errors in adding and subtracting and copying figures. The system also offers an excellent record of the doctor's assets and liabilities, and

RECEIPT NUMBER | DATE | PROFESSIONAL SERVICE | CHARGE | PAID | NEW BALANCE | PREVIOUS BALANCE | NAME

YOU PAID THIS AMOUNT
THIS IS A STATEMENT OF YOUR ACCOUNT TO DATE

CPT4 BC/BS OFFICE PROCEDURES FEE   Medicare: Patient's Complaint

☐ 1. 90000 09510 Office Visit-New Pat _____ ☐ Neck Pain ☐ Mid-back Pain ☐ Low-Back Pain

☐ 2. 97260 09504 Office Visit-Man. Manip _____ ☐ X-Rays Dated ___/___/___ Demonstrating a

☐ 3. 90060 09506 Interm. Ex.-Est. Pat _____ subluxation are available for review.

☐ 4. 97000 09009 Manual Manipulation _____ Treatment = _____

and adjunctive Physiological Therapeutics   DIAGNOSIS – ICD - 9 CM

A. ☐ Ultrasound B. ☐ Sinewave C. ☐ Galvanic   Cervical

D. ☐ Muscle stimulation E. ☐ Intermit Tract   ☐ A. 847.0 Sprain or Strain

F. ☐ Hydrocollator G. ☐ Cold Packs   ☐ 1 Chronic ☐ 2 Acute ☐ 3 Recurrent

H. ☐ Spinalator I. ☐ Trigger Pt. Therapy   ☐ B. 839.0 Subluxation

C 1 2 3 4 5 6 7

☐ C. 722.0 Disc Syndrome

☐ D. 723.3 Cervico Brachial Syndrome

RADIOLOGY   ☐ E. _____ Whiplash-hyperflexion-extension

☐ 5. 72040 Cervical Limited (AP & Lat) _____ Thoracic

☐ 6. 72050 Cervical AP, Lat, Open Mouth _____ ☐ F. 847.1 Sprain or Strain

☐ 7. 72052 Cervical Obliques ☐ Rt. ☐ Lt _____ ☐ 1 Chronic ☐ 2 Acute ☐ 3 Recurrent

☐ 8. 72080 Thoracic Limited (AP & Lat) _____ ☐ G. 839.21 Subluxation

☐ 9. 72100 Lumbar Limited (AP & Lat) _____ T 1 2-3-4-5-6-7-8-9-10-11-12

☐ 10. 72110 Lumbosacral-Obl. ☐ Rt ☐ Lt _____ Lumbar

☐ 11. 72020 AP Full Spine _____ ☐ H. 847.2 Sprain or Strain

☐ 12. _____ ☐ 1 Chronic ☐ 2 Acute ☐ 3 Recurrent

☐ I. 839.20 Subluxation

LABORATORY   L 1 - 2 - 3 - 4 - 5

☐ 13. 80012 12 Tests for Panel or Profile _____ ☐ J. 722.1 Disc. Syndrome

☐ 14. 800__ Over 12 Tests for Panel _____ Lumbosacral

☐ 15. 81002 Urinalysis Routine w/o Micro _____ ☐ K. 846.0 Sprain or Strain

☐ 16. 85021 CBC _____ ☐ 1 Chronic ☐ 2 Acute ☐ 3 Recurrent

☐ 17. Supportive Therapy _____ ☐ L. 839.42 Subluxation

☐ M. 724.4 Radiculitis

☐ N. 737.3 Scoliosis (acquired or postural)

☐ O. 729.2 Vertebrogenic Rediculitis

☐ 18. Supports-Orthopedic _____ ☐ P. 721.90 Spondylitis Osteoarthritica

☐ Cervical ☐ Lumbosacral ☐ Thoracic   ☐ Q. _____ Neuro Genic Syndrome

☐ Extremity ☐ _____ ☐ R. _____

☐ S. _____

RETURN M T W Th F S _____ Wks _____ Months   NEXT APPT _____

Day Month Date Time AM PM

Date of Service _____

Place of Service ☐ Clinic ☐ Dr's Home ☐ Patient's Home

Date Symptoms Appeared ☐ Accident or Accident Occurred ☐ Illness ___/___/___

Disability Related To ☐ Accident ☐ Pregnancy ☐ Industrial ☐ Other

DISABILITY

DATES From ___/___/___ To ___/___/___

OK To Return To Work ___/___/___

AUTHORIZATION TO PAY BENEFITS TO PHYSICIAN I hereby authorize and request payment to and mailing of payment directly to Physician for any Health Care Benefits due under the terms of this Insurance Policy for services rendered.

Signed Patient (Parent If Minor)   Date

INSURANCE CARRIERS – This form has been adopted to keep paperwork costs down. If any additional forms or itemized bill is required they will be completed upon the receipt of $15.00. Narrative report $50.00.

LEONARD S. TAYLOR, D.C.
2100 WEST PARK AVENUE
CHAMPAIGN, ILLINOIS 61820
Telephone 352-7658

IRS No. 123456
S.S No. 000-00-0000

1239

Figure 8.7. Super bill. The numbered super bill shown above is designed to fit a pegboard system, speeding the billing process (reprinted by permission of the Colwell Company).

profit and loss. However, a double-entry system requires many ledger books and entries and is often too time consuming for the average practice. Thus, in most offices, a single-entry system is used, and many are available that have been designed strictly for a health-care practice. They are simple, concise, easily administered, and usually combined in one volume that includes daily entries as well as monthly, quarterly, and annual summaries, and payroll records. Many styles are available, and each has its advantages and disadvantages.

The basic elements of a good bookkeeping system include (1) accounts receivable, a record of fees charged, (2) a system for billing these fees and recording payment, (3) a record of bills incurred by the office, and (4) disbursements, a system of paying bills and properly allocating expenditures. A sample monthly income and expense sheet is shown in Figure 8.8.

THE OFFICE BOOKS

The term *office books* refers to both accounts receivable and accounts payable records in particular and the established bookkeeping system and records in general.

Bookkeeping Agencies. Some doctors

MONTHLY INCOME AND EXPENSES

Month of _____ 19__

	This Month	Prior Months	Year to Date
GROSS INCOME	$_____	$_____	$_____
OPERATING EXPENSES			
Office supplies	_____	_____	_____
Rent, utilities, maintenance	_____	_____	_____
Communications	_____	_____	_____
Travel	_____	_____	_____
Subscriptions, dues	_____	_____	_____
Taxes, license fees	_____	_____	_____
Conventions	_____	_____	_____
Contributions	_____	_____	_____
Insurance	_____	_____	_____
Professional services	_____	_____	_____
Shipping	_____	_____	_____
Advertising, public relations	_____	_____	_____
Salaries	_____	_____	_____
Payroll taxes	_____	_____	_____
Miscellaneous	_____	_____	_____
TOTAL OPERATING EXPENSES	$_____	$_____	$_____
NET INCOME BEFORE DEPRECIATION	$_____	$_____	$_____
OTHER DISBURSEMENTS			
Equipment	_____	_____	_____
Improvements	_____	_____	_____
Employee taxes withheld (−)	_____	_____	_____
Employee taxes paid (+)	_____	_____	_____
Employee contributions withheld (−)	_____	_____	_____
Employee contributions paid (+)	_____	_____	_____
Personal draw (+)	_____	_____	_____
TOTAL EXPENDITURES	$_____	$_____	$_____
Total Fees for the Month	$_____	$_____	$_____
Accounts Receivable for the Month	_____	_____	_____
Starting Balance	$_____	$_____	$_____
Total Deposits (+)	_____	_____	_____
Total Expenditures (−)	_____	_____	_____
ENDING BALANCE	$_____	$_____	$_____

Figure 8.8. Sample format for a monthly income and expense statement.

use a bookkeeping service—a specialized agency serving a clientele for whom they handle the technical aspect of posting and balancing monthly books and financial statements. If your doctor-employer uses such an agency, a representative will review the office checkbook and various journals and ledgers each month and give the doctor a current financial report. The assistant, therefore, should be prepared to provide the agency with accurate records reflecting total charges for the month, total payments received, the accounts receivable control figure, and an accurate expenditure record. The agency will do the remaining accounting.

Doctor's Personal Accounts. The doctor may ask an assistant to maintain records of his personal affairs such as his property ledger where information is entered about personal property, real estate holdings, securities, professional travel, honorariums, tax-deductible expenses, and so forth. He may wish you to set up files for his insurance and/or investment programs. A sample form for recording savings account data is shown in Figure 8.9.

Vaulted Documents. The doctor also may request an assistant to see that valuable papers are properly stored in a safe or safety deposit box. Documents deserving special attention are contracts; documents concerning births, marriage, and divorce records; wills; passports; investment records; stock certificates and bonds; deeds and leases; mortgage papers; insurance papers; and property inventory lists.

Banking Accounts. Most doctors maintain two or more banking accounts, and they frequently ask an administrative assistant to maintain the records. All deposits from office fees and all withdrawals for professional expenditures are handled through office accounts. It is usually less confusing if the doctor's office account and personal account are in different banks.

Filtering Files. In all office filing systems, it is important to separate material that is outdated to avoid overcrowding office files. Keep in mind, however, that no record should be destroyed without the doctor's authorization. When destroying material that once was considered of permanent value, each item should be listed on a sheet and someone should be with you to witness and initial the destruction. This is proof of disposal in case your action is later questioned. Rather than destroying financial records, microfilming is one efficient way to save storage space should the need arise.

ACCOUNTS RECEIVABLE AND BILLING

An accounts receivable system has two parts. First, a record of money owed to the office (patient charges); and second, a record of payments made. The basic vehicles of the system are visit slips, day sheets, and patient ledgers.

Visit Slips

Many doctors prefer to use a charge slip rather than stating orally the fee for services rendered during a particular visit. The slip provides a written record. The slips are usually printed forms where the patient's name, address or file number, and date are entered by the assistant and the slip is attached to the patient's folder before the patient sees the doctor. The doctor notes services as they are given. The assistant totals the figures and quotes the total to the patient when the patient returns the slip at the dismissal desk. The slip usually shows when the doctor wishes to see the patient for the next appointment, and it may note special procedures intended so the assistant will allow adequate time in scheduling the next appointment.

When visit slips are printed, it is best that they be printed in duplicate on NCR or equivalent paper. Both original and duplicate copies are attached to the patient's folder and follow the patient through examination and therapy. When the patient is dismissed, a copy is given to the patient to serve as an invoice or receipt if payment is made at the time. The original copy is retained by the assistant as a record of the fee

BANK ACCOUNT

Account in Name of _____ Account No. _____

Name of Bank _____ Type of Account _____

Address of Bank _____

Officer Contact _____ Title _____ Phone _____

Authorized Signatures _____ _____

Custodian of Bank Book _____ Interest

                                                                    Date   %

Remarks _____   _____   __
        _____   _____   __
        _____   _____   __

Date	Deposit	Interest	Total	Withdrawal	Balance
	$	$	$	$	$

Figure 8.9. Sample format for a savings account log (courtesy of the Behavioral Research Foundation).

for services of that day. From the information on the slip, the assistant schedules the next appointment and posts entries within the day sheet and patient ledger card. It is helpful in tracking misplaced slips to have the slips prenumbered.

Content and format of visit slips vary from practice to practice. However, to save the doctor time when indicating the service and fee on the visit slip, it is desirable to have as many routine procedures and fees as possible incorporated. Then, only a checkmark is required. Refer to Figure 7.3.

Day Sheets and Summary Sheets

Charges for services and all money collected should be carefully recorded on a daily record (day sheet) for every patient conducting a transaction with the office. This daily record, which is infrequently combined with the appointment book, when totaled at the end of the day should give the amount of cash collected, the amount of money received by check, and the amount charged to patients who have not paid and must be billed. Thus, the day sheet is a running account of charges and payments made during the day from entries from visit slips, receipts, and payments received by mail.

Although the major function of the day sheet is to record financial transactions, it can be designed to give the doctor important information of his practice and practice control. For instance, the day sheet may incorporate columns for receipt numbers, visit time in minutes, office services, x-ray data, laboratory work, supplements dispensed, exercises prescribed, office library use, braces and supports sold or rented, or any other special services offered. When a sophisticated day sheet is used, a separate appointment book is used and the patient's name is entered on the day sheet only when a transaction occurs.

A typical 16-column day sheet includes:

1. *Name.* The last name and initials of all patients receiving services or with whom a transaction should be entered. If case numbers are used, they may be entered after the patients' names.

2. *Receipt Number.* Many doctors feel it is good policy to issue a numbered receipt for every transaction appearing on the day sheet whether or not the patient desires one. It offers an additional control sheet.

3. *Appointment Time in Minutes.* This column shows the time consumed by the patient in the performance of services that are to be charged to the patient. This time does not include that in the reception room. It begins in the preparation room and stops when the patient enters the dismissal area. This accounting offers the doctor data necessary in estimating average patient-visit time, preparing fee schedules, and computing time investments against income.

4. *Patient's Major Complaint.* The reason for the patient's visit is entered here. This offers the doctor knowledge about typical disorders treated, their percentage relative to common disorders treated, and trends and direction the practice may be taking toward possible specialization.

5. *Consultations.* It should be noted here if the reason for the patient's visit is for consultation. Consultations, as the term is used here, refer to potential patients who do not know whether the doctor may help them or not and seek counsel. The column provides practice development data for it shows whether public relations procedures are attracting new patients.

6. *Physical Examination.* This column offers the doctor data necessary to determine the number of patients who had a consultation and had an examination, and those who had a consultation but did not have an examination. Orthopedic and neurologic examinations may be entered here or in a separate column if the doctor desires a detailed breakdown.

7. *X Ray.* Radiographic services are entered here if they were conducted within the office or without the office by another facility unless the patient pays the outside agency directly. The number and size of films may be recorded here if desired. If the films were taken outside the office and the patient pays the outside agency directly, the doctor's film interpretation fee may be entered here.

8. *Lab.* The type of laboratory tests made and the amount charged for the tests are entered here whether they are performed within or without your office if you are responsible for paying the outside laboratory and collecting from the patient.

9. *Supplements.* Record in this column the type of supplements dispensed and the charge to the patient for vitamins, minerals, herbals, glandulars, and other prescriptions.

10. *Adjustments.* The type of spinal or extraspinal manipulation rendered is entered here. This gives the doctor knowledge of the number and type of certain manipulative procedures deemed necessary in his particular practice.

11. *Physiotherapy.* Record in this column the type of adjunctive therapy provided the patient and the amount charged for the service.

12. *Special.* Enter here any service not specifically entered in another column such as braces, supports, or home equipment sold or rented.

Note: The previous seven columns (Physical Examination, X-Ray, Lab, Supplements, Adjustments, Physiotherapy, and Special) offer the doctor a means to determine where he is deriving his income and the percentage of an individual service in relative to total income. The sum of these services represents the total services of the practice.

13. *Total Services.* The sum for all services a patient receives on any particular day is entered in this column.

14. *Cash Received.* The actual amount collected from a patient on a particular day is entered here. This figure would be the same as in Column 13 if the patient pays in full. However, the patient may make a partial payment or pay for services rendered on one or more previous visits.

15. *Transfer Check.* This column is helpful to the assistant in avoiding errors in posting entries to a patient's financial record. When information is transposed from the day sheet to the patient's ledger card, the figures should be compared for accuracy. Then a checkmark may be made and

initialed in this column, indicating that an accurate transfer has been made. This would not be necessary in a one-write system.

16. *Remarks.* In this last column, you may enter any special information or explanation of time, special charges, or patient attitude.

Some day sheets will incorporate space for additional information desired by the doctor:

1. *New Patients.* Record the name of patients entering the practice and who referred them to your office. A check box may be included to indicate that a "thank you" was sent to the individual referring the patient.

2. *Changed Appointments.* Record changed appointments and note the information within the patient's file to determine if such changes are frequent. This may indicate the need for a discussion of the necessity of regular appointments. Missed appointments may be entered here (or in a separate column) and transferred to the patient's file. Any follow-up action taken should be noted also.

3. *Periodic Checkups.* Enter here the name of patients who are returning for a periodic health examination and/or spinal analysis. Quantities here offer the doctor information about the amount of his practice devoted to maintenance care.

4. *Rechecks.* A recheck or partial examination is frequently offered to any patient who is dissatisfied with progress or not responding as the doctor anticipated. The quantity of names appearing in this column gives the doctor an overview of his diagnostic, prognostic, and therapeutic skills, as well as an indication of overall doctor-patient relations.

At the end of each day, the assistant should total each column in the day sheet and transfer the information to a monthly summary sheet. Second, she should verify the money received with the amount totaled in the "Cash Received" column and duplicate receipts and then prepare a bank deposit slip. Third, she should check to assure that all necessary information recorded in the day sheet has been properly transferred to the patient's financial records or clinical folder. A sample accounts receivable weekly summary sheet and annual comparison is shown in Figure 8.10.

Monthly and annual summary sheets may incorporate the minimal financial information necessary for tax purposes or all the information gathered in a sophisticated day sheet. Financial and practice information may be summarized on separate summary sheets. Separate sheets are usually best be-

---

ACCOUNTS RECEIVABLE SUMMARY and ANNUAL COMPARISON

Week ending _____

		This Week		Last Year, This Time	
		No. of Accounts	Amount	No. of Accounts	Amount
Direct Billings	**Days**				
Current accounts	(1-30)	_____	$_____	_____	$_____
Overdue accounts	(31-60)	_____	_____	_____	_____
Past-due accounts	(61-90)	_____	_____	_____	_____
Delinquent accounts	(91-+)	_____	_____	_____	_____
In collection		_____	_____	_____	_____
Special accounts		_____	_____	_____	_____
To be written off		_____	_____	_____	_____
Credit balances		_____	_____	_____	_____
	(Subtotal)	_____	$_____	_____	$_____
Third-Party Billings					
Private insurance assign.		_____	_____	_____	_____
Workers' Compensation		_____	_____	_____	_____
Medicaid		_____	_____	_____	_____
Medicare		_____	_____	_____	_____
Welfare		_____	_____	_____	_____
_____		_____	_____	_____	_____
_____		_____	_____	_____	_____
_____		_____	_____	_____	_____
(Subtotal)		_____	$_____	_____	$_____
Grand Total		_____	$_____	_____	$_____

Figure 8.10. Sample format for an accounts receivable weekly summary worksheet. Quarterly summary sheets would essentially be the same except that the word "week" would be replaced by "month."

cause accountants and other financial service agencies have no need for practice development information.

Financial summary sheets incorporate both income and expense information, thus arriving at net earnings information. Yearly summaries are completed in the same manner as monthly summaries. Monthly totals and balances are entered. *Depreciation schedules* are usually designed by the doctor's accountant for equipment and real estate. The purchase of these items is not considered an expense for the month in which they are purchased.

Patient Ledger Card

A ledger is any form that records a patient's charges and payments. It may be in the form of a card, sheet, or journal page. The first information recorded is identical with that recorded on the entering patient's data slip. The assistant posts charges from the day sheet to individual cards (or sheets) at the end of the day or early the next morning. Payments received by mail should be posted when they are opened, and the assistant checks off each entry in the day sheet as it is posted to the cards. The patient's balance is thus kept current as charges are added and payments are subtracted.

It should be apparent that a copy of a patient's ledger card will serve as a statement. As every visit should be recorded on the patient's record card whether it is a no-charge, cash, or money received on account, neither the doctor nor the assistant need to compute an account. The card should be maintained so that a running current balance is listed at all times. Regardless of format, the form should have a column indicating date of entry, type of transaction, fee for services, amount paid on account, and a balance column. Patient ledger cards are often called *financial cards* or *account cards*.

Posting

Ledger cards should be kept current each day with great care exercised that correct entries are made. Otherwise, a billing may

be made for an incorrect amount. If posting is current, information about a patient's account balance will be immediately available on request. Daily posting helps assure correct posting, encourages prompt payment, and speeds insurance billing. Last-minute posting to meet a billing deadline is likely to produce errors resulting in patients losing confidence in the office.

Family Cards

Some patients prefer a "family card." As the name implies, this is a single card for an entire family. The heading is directed to the head of the household, and each entry carries the name of the family member served and the type of and fee for services. The more ledger charges are itemized, the better for ease of insurance billing and patient understandig of fees charged. Office visits, adjunctive therapy, radiographs, supplements, and other services should be itemized.

Combined History and Ledger Forms

Some history forms include ledger information. Doctors who use them believe they are simpler to maintain than separate records. Most doctors, however, feel it is poor practice to keep clinical and financial information together and therefore use separate records. There is considerable objection to disclosing clinical data to an accountant or income tax agent who may have need to review financial records. In like manner, it may not be advisable to show financial information when clinical records are submitted to another doctor. Separate records also save time during the billing periods because their size makes handling much easier than the large case history forms or folders.

Recording Payments and Receipts

Every payment, whether by cash or check, made either in person or by mail, should be promptly and accurately recorded on each type of record in use (eg, visit slip, day sheet, and patient ledger card).

1. *Cash Payments Made in Person.* The assistant should: (a) Note payment on the visit slip, giving a copy showing payment to the patient as a receipt. File duplicate copy separate from visit slips that have not been paid. Those unpaid will be used for preparing itemized statements later. (b) Store cash in a special container. (c) Enter payment on the day sheet. Show both charges and payment. Note services rendered, and be certain to have the correct name. (d) Record on patient's ledger card the services, charges, payment, and new balance. (e) If duplicate visit slips are not used, make out a receipt in duplicate. Give the patient the original and retain copy in receipt book.

2. *Check Payments Made in Person.* The same procedure is used here as for cash payments made in person.

3. *Check Payments Made by Mail.* The assistant should: (a) Enter the name of the patient and the amount received on the day sheet. (b) Stamp check "For Deposit Only" and put in place provided. (c) Record in the patient's ledger the date, amount of payment, and new balance. (d) Prepare a receipt in duplicate, and either give the original to the patient on the next visit or mail with next billing or (e) make receipt and discard original, keeping the duplicate copy in the bound receipt book.

4. *Cash Payments Made by Mail.* While this practice should be discouraged, it sometimes happens. When it does, the assistant should: (a) Enter the name of the patient and the amount received on the day sheet. (b) Place cash in a special container. (c) Enter on patient ledger the date, amount of payment, and new balance. (d) Make a receipt in duplicate: one copy to be mailed to the patient or given to the patient on the next visit if scheduled soon.

5. *Recording Nonpractice Income.* Other income of a taxable nature such as dividends, interest, or honorariums received by the doctor may be deposited through the office account but separated. There also may be income of a nontaxable nature such as

insurance benefits, savings account transfers, and refunds. If there is any question on how these should be entered, check with the doctor or his accountant.

It is sound business policy to request and give receipts whenever cash payments are made or received. Although returned checks are considered receipts, it is helpful to file receipted bills. It is not always necessary to receipt bills of patients who send checks in payment of their statements. However, the assistant should pay prompt attention to patient requests for receipts. It also offers an opportunity to say "thank you."

Some doctors hold that a receipt should be given for every financial transaction occurring in the practice whether it be a charge, cash, or a received-on-account transaction. They think it is beneficial to good control that a duplicate receipt be on hand at the end of the day to verify every extension concerning finances on the day sheet. Issuing a receipt is not only sound business practice, it is required in many states to verify income and accounts receivable.

Personalized Receipts

Many offices find it helpful to have a pad of printed standard receipts in the event someone receives money in your absence. Most people dislike paying cash unless some record is being made of the transaction. Receipt forms come in a variety of styles. Most doctors use prenumbered duplicate forms that are personalized to include the doctor's name, address, and telephone number.

Accounts Receivable Insurance

Some doctors believe it is wise to carry *accounts receivable insurance* to protect against fire damage to or theft of office records. To be eligible for this insurance, records carrying a balance due must be locked each night in some type of approved cabinet or storage vault. This insurance offers protection against loss, and usually the amount of coverage is for the *average* amount of accounts receivable. This average should be checked periodically (eg, every 6 months) to verify adequate insurance is carried.

Statements

Statements should be mailed promptly on or before (preferably) the first day of the month. If the office's bills are received at the same time as others, they will be more likely paid at the same time. Many people pay their bills between the 5th and 10th of each month. If your statement arrives after this date, it may be left until the following month. Thus, prompt billing is a benefit. Many doctors believe that statements should be mailed on the 25th of each month so they will be on hand when the patient is paid on the 1st of the month. They consider it an advantage to have the office statement arrive before bills for rent, utilities, contract payments, and so forth.

Itemization. Before statements are mailed, accounts showing a balance due should be checked for accuracy. It is best to itemize bills so there will be no questions that may delay payment. Many patients may forget the details of their visits to the doctor, and a bill for a large sum that is not itemized may harm doctor-patient relations. When all major services are itemized, the patient is in a better position to see that the total balance is reasonable.

There are several methods used in chiropractic in preparing and mailing statements:

1. Standard statements are typed from patients' ledgers and mailed in either windowed or plain envelopes. These billheads are usually printed to fit the doctor's practice with his various services listed together at the bottom of the sheet with code symbols. At billing time, the amount due is shown by the service code number.

2. Self-mailer statements are frequently used. These are printed return envelopes attached to a bill. The patient separates the bill and encloses it in the envelope with the check for the balance due. The envelopes include the doctor's printed name and address and may include a mailing permit. Some doctors believe this method is an asset to collections; others feel it is too commercial.

3. Financial ledgers may be duplicated to provide ready-to-mail statements. They should be copied, typed, or carefully written. Photocopying saves time in duplicating ledger cards, avoids transfer errors, and offers the patient an exact copy of his office ledger that shows services, charges, payments received, and current balance due.

4. If a pegboard system is used, statements are prepared automatically in the one-write method.

5. Larger practices often use a centralized computerized billing service. This is a practical way to handle an extensive billing system as well as arrive at a variety of practice data. Most cities have agencies that provide these services.

Deposits

An administrative assistant responsible for deposits will need an understanding of basic banking terms, how to make office deposits and write checks correctly, and how to reconcile a bank statement. As several office and personal accounts of the doctor may be involved, she must have on file the name of each bank involved, the account number, the banks' addresses, and the type of account; viz, savings, checking, joint, or other.

Doctors managing large practices usually prefer that deposits be made daily as this allows a daily check against errors. Daily deposits will equal daily collections as listed in the day sheet.

Stamping Checks Received. Each check received should be immediately stamped "For Deposit Only" to the office account. When preparing a deposit slip, list each check—showing amount, bank's identifying number, and name of person writing the check. If the check has been written by a person other than the one who received the services (parent, guardian, third party), record this information.

Duplicate Deposit Slips. A duplicate deposit slip should be made for each deposit and kept in the office bank file. This is done so that a record will be available if a deposit is misplaced or stolen. The duplicate also serves as a reference if a patient claims to have paid on an account but your records do not show this. Thus, the duplicate can serve as a check against a recording error.

Dating Deposit Slips. Even if you do not deposit receipts daily, prepare a deposit slip for each day collections are received. For instance, if you deposit today money received yesterday, the deposit slip should bear yesterday's date. If you use today's date, future reference to the slip would be confusing.

Company Checks. When depositing a company check rather than a personal check, list the name of the company on the deposit slip and the name of the patient. For checks from insurance companies, list the name of the company as well as that of the patient involved. This is also true in situations where the signature on the check differs from the account name in which it was paid.

"Cash" Checks. Any check made out to "cash" is as negotiable as cash. Thus, it is important to get into the habit of stamping all checks as they are received and placed in your cash drawer or box. In the event of theft or misplacement, the checks are fairly well protected if they are stamped "For Deposit Only."

Traveler's Checks. Traveler's Checks are acceptable as cash. They are signed at the bank at the time of purchase and must be signed again in your presence when cashed. Again, use the doctor's stamp on the back of each as you would a regular check. When making out the deposit slip, note that the check was a Traveler's Check.

Summary of Mechanics

The tasks involved in any collecting and billing system are (1) documenting services to patients, (2) recording fees and balances, (3) collecting and recording payments, (4) proving the day sheet, (5) making bank deposits, and (6) mailing statements. If a one-write pegboard system is used, many of these tasks are combined into a single operation.

When a fresh day sheet is used, enter the appropriate date, page number if desired, and headings on the columns if they have not been printed. Store the used day sheet of the previous day in a binder after proving. The administrative assistant in charge of collecting and billing should pull the financial ledgers of patients expected and place them in sequence according to the appointment schedule. A ledger will be prepared for any new patients after the entering data have been obtained.

When a patient registers, the patient's name is posted on the day sheet and on a visit slip clipped to the clinical file folder. After the doctor sees the patient, the visit slip is returned to the dismissal desk, the doctor having indicated on the slip the services performed and the interval desired before the patient's next appointment. When the assistant receives this slip, she totals the fees and informs the patient of the services rendered, the fee for the services, and the office policy concerning payment. This simple act here of informing the patient of the services and fees involved will induce a high percentage of in-office collections. The burden is then on the patient who must either pay or ask to be billed. The assistant then records charges and collections and other necessary information on the day sheet after giving the patient a card specifying the next appointment. Later, financial information from the day sheet is recorded on the patient's financial ledger.

Payments Received in the Mail

It is advisable to set aside sufficient time to handle all mailed-in payments at once when it would not conflict with patient visits. Efficient recording of mailed-in payments on statements, financial ledgers, and day sheets can be done as follows.

1. Open all mail at once and stamp all checks with the information provided by the bank for deposit.

2. Make a tape on an adding machine totaling all checks and cash to be posted.

3. Arrange mailed-in payments in alphabetical order for convenience in selecting cards from an indexed file tray.

4. Record each payment on the day sheet and the patient's financial ledger form. You may wish to enter the letter M (for mailed-in payment) on the day sheet.

5. Prepare a bank deposit slip.

6. Compare totals posted on the day sheet and bank deposit slip with the adding machine tape. Totals must agree. Then file the patient's financial ledgers.

Balancing Accounts Receivable

Office financial transactions must be handled with exacting care. Because bookkeeping perfection is essential, it is important to account for every cent, keep accurate records, and apply receipts and expenditures to proper accounts.

If the doctor should need personal cash, he should draw a check on his personal account and cash it by replacing cash from office collections with his check. In this manner, the daily bank deposit slip will always equal the day's collections as recorded in the day sheet. If a bill must be paid by cash for some reason, use the same procedure. Write a check for cash on the office account, and place it in the receipts for the day. Some doctors, however, do not follow this accepted bookkeeping procedure; ie, they use cash on hand without replacing it with a check. For this reason, many bookkeeping systems used by doctors provide separate columns for expenditures by check or cash.

A doctor may be paid in cash during a house call or when he encounters a patient out of the office. It's easy for the doctor to forget such a transaction. When statements are prepared, the payment may not be properly recorded when the patient is billed. To avoid injury to doctor-patient relations, the doctor should be encouraged to carry a small notebook where each transaction is noted and communicated to the assistant

for proper entry in office records. The information can then be added to the day sheet and the money deposited as part of the day's receipts.

Just as one person should be in charge of the appointment book, one person should be responsible for handling office receipts. Confusion and errors multiply in proportion to the number of people involved. Because of this, the doctor will usually tell his patients to make all payments to the assigned assistant. This assistant should schedule the time necessary for balancing accounts receivable. All records should be kept in the office and never taken home to "get caught up."

The major steps involved in balancing accounts receivable are:

1. Gather patient ledgers showing a balance due, and run an adding machine tape listing each unpaid account—including those in the hands of a collection agency. Once the total balance due has been established, it is easy to maintain daily and monthly control figure. At the end of each day and month, total charges and payments are added to the previous figure to arrive at the current control figure.

2. Reduced charges such as "write-offs" or discounts are recorded by placing a red figure or a figure in parentheses on the day sheet in the "Charge" column and likewise posted in the patient's ledger. If money is received from a collection agency, the day sheet and the patient's ledger must reflect the total amount paid by the patient. The amount withheld by the collection agency as their service fee is shown as an amount "Paid Out" as an office expense.

BILLING ROUTINES

As regular billing is an essential part of a good collection system, some definite schedule for sending statements must be established within the practice. Erratically mailed statements result in erratic collections; punctual statements, prompt payments.

Professional Considerations

The common philosophy within the healing arts places on the physician the responsibility of standing above others in the practice of his art and placing the well-being of his patient above all else. Even in primitive civilizations, the witch doctor and medicine man were held in a position of awe.

Ethics. The doctor of chiropractic, as any physician, swears an oath before entering practice that places an obligation to treat all who seek his services without thought of their ability to pay. Thus, the assistant must be aware that while the financial success of the practice is determined by its economic status, the collection of fees is a delicate and sensitive area. No ethical doctor will refuse treatment to a needy patient unable to pay for services. However, a doctor must charge a fee and attempt to collect for his services if possible.

Discretion. Because of the doctor's professional oath, the assistant must use tact, sound judgment, and mature responsibility. Systems are useless unless faithfully implemented, but systems are rules and not laws. Common sense must be applied. For example, no bill is favorably received in the midst of serious illness or grief. Some patients who would like to pay if they could are temporarily unable to do so. In these circumstances, some type of time-payment plan may be considered. Special circumstances always deserve special consideration according to office policy. In situations where a large fee is involved, it would be unreasonable to ask a poor patient to meet the same payment schedule as that for a wealthy patient.

Understanding. To be an efficient assistant does not mean you must be unkind, wielding cold-blooded business tactics without consideration of human realities. Illness often strikes suddenly, finding some patients financially unprepared. Use the Golden Rule. Treat patients as you would like to be treated. An understanding assistant can set the stage for collecting amounts due in a more effective manner than a rigidly mechanical, indifferent assistant. Be human. Patients are human. Chiropractic is humane.

Attitude in Approach

An efficient assistant who develops an effective and pleasant approach in collecting fees is one of the doctor's greatest assets. The doctor is aware of this even if he does not express it directly. He is also aware that there is a type of assistant who has a high percentage of collections but is held in low esteem by patients. Such an assistant presents a cold unfeeling manner, with little regard for the problems of the patient. This attitude is resented by patients, and the resentment is projected on the doctor. When carried to the extreme, such resentment may be the motive for a patient initiating a suit for malpractice.

Keep in mind that chiropractic is a humanitarian art. The doctor is more than a health-care advisor. He is a friend to his patients, and he wants to help them meet their financial obligations. Thus, the attitude of the assistant must be to *help the patient* meet their financial obligations. In the matter of collections, the assistant must be aware of the patient's *attitude* toward the debt, the patient's *economic status*, and the patient's *social status*.

With this awareness, the assistant will come to realize that delinquent accounts represent one of three general classes of people. First, there are those patients who can pay, but they are habitually slow payers requiring several reminders. Second, there are those patients who have the willingness to pay but not the immediate ability to pay. And third, there are those patients who have neither the willingness nor the ability to pay. Unfortunately, most patients in this third class have graduated down from the first, and you usually become aware too late to handle the situation smoothly. What action is taken must be the doctor's decision. It depends on the particular circumstances involved.

The alert assistant is aware that a health-care office presents delicate human-relations situations. This is especially true with collections. Words and phrases that might irritate a patient must be guarded. See Figure 8.11. There is always a psychologic moment and a pleasant manner to approach the subject of services and fees. It is more

Avoid Using	When You Mean	Correct Example
all the farther	as far as	This is *as far as* it goes.
alright	all right	She said she was *all right*.
apt	likely	It is *likely* to hurt awhile.
badly	bad	I feel *bad*.
balance	remainder	I'll do the *remainder* later.
but what	that, but that	He didn't doubt *that* he was ill.
complected	complexioned	He was dark *complexioned*.
couldn't hardly	could hardly	She *could hardly* see the chart.
differs with	differs from	This test *differs from* that test.
differ from	differ with	I must *differ with* you on this.
different than	different from	This report is *different from* that.
don't	doesn't	He *doesn't* hear very well.
farther	further	We'll discuss it *further* tomorrow.
further	farther	We walked *farther* today.
fine	well	He walks *well* now.
good	well	She exercises *well*.
leave	let	*Let* him be.
less	fewer	There were *fewer* patients today.
liable	likely	It is *likely* to be cold tomorrow.
likely	liable	She is *liable* to injure herself.
no one never	no one ever	*No one ever* evaluated the results.
of	have	She might *have* left early.
on account of	because of	He stopped *because of* the pain.
quite	very	I felt *very* good today.
remember of	remember	I can't *remember* that experience.
since	because	*Because* it is logical.
sure	surely	We *surely* thought it would happen.
suspicioned	suspected	That diagnosis was not *suspected*.
then	than	Better this *than* nothing.
try and	try to	We will *try to* arrange that.
where	that	We read *that* he was appointed.
while	whereas	She's active, *whereas* he's passive.
without	unless	It won't work *unless*...

Figure 8.11. The faulty use of some common expressions compared with their correct usage.

important to maintain good will than prove a legal point. Ill will may lead to unfavorable publicity and even spur a lawsuit.

A positive attitude is the foundation of a good collection system. The assistant's attitude is a key ingredient. Never assume that an unequal relationship exists between the indebted patient and the office. It must be admitted, however, that it is the nature of some assistants to assume unconsciously that the office occupies a superior position

and the indebted patient an inferior one. This attitude is purely a misguided emotion that can result in strained doctor-patient relations.

The indebted patient is not a criminal. If you make him feel as one, it naturally will be resented. Financial matters must be handled in a friendly, professional manner, avoiding any possibility of enmity. Assume the patient is honest. Help him meet his obligations. Arrive at mutually agreeable solutions. If the patient is not honest, there is little chance of collecting the account despite the methods used.

There is no set policy in collecting professional services. Every doctor has the right to set his policy. But whatever it is, the assistant must be well informed.

Billing Mechanics

In preparing bills for professional services, be sure the patient's name and address are correct. Remember that overall neatness and cleanliness are important features in the physical appearance of the bill and enhance the image of the office. If a note is sent with an outstanding bill, it should be worded carefully to avoid demotivating the receiver. Gentle persuasion is better than an irritating "Please!" Use honey, not vinegar.

A sincere spirit of good will and courtesy to all patients who are indebted to the office will bring much more positive results than having an abrupt or condescending air. When in doubt about taking action, always consult the doctor about the situation.

Processing

Statements are processed in a variety of ways. Some doctors assign an assistant the task of typing statements. This can be an expensive, time-consuming process. The typewritten monthly statements of years gone by have given way in most offices to a variety of more efficient billing methods. One of these is to photocopy the patient's financial ledger. If the ledger is properly designed, the copy can be placed in a windowed envelope, thus no typing is required. Another system is the multicopy financial card, which is a series of attached replicas of the ledger. As each entry is made, carbonized paper transfers the information to all copies attached. At the end of the month, a copy is sent to the patient. Another highly efficient system is the one-write pegboard system where the statement is developed automatically. And sometimes statements are prepared and mailed by an outside service. Each system has its advantages and disadvantages and must be viewed in relation to the requirements of an individual office. Regardless of the system used, the assistant must remember that in any copying system, multicopy system, or one-write system, the system will only reproduce what has been recorded. Clear, accurate entries are essential.

Timing

When is the best time to send out statements? Some doctors prefer to send billings once a month, others twice a month as on the 1st and 15th. Some offices mail statements weekly according to an alphabetical division to spread the task over the whole month. Some prefer to bill third parties at one point in the month and personal accounts at another time. The best system is that which works best for an individual office. The important thing is to have a *system* and periodically review that system to assure it meets today's needs.

Reminder Systems

Sending a bill does not necessarily complete the collection task. Some patients must be reminded several times, some are unable to pay on request, and some are simply stubborn. The longer a balance remains on the books, the more difficult it is to collect. Thus, accounts must be constantly watched by an assistant so that continual attempts to collect are made.

Most systems start with simple reminders and increase in their emphasis as the balance ages. Typical reminders are "Please remit," "Payment on this account is now due," "Payment of this account is past due," "This is a reminder that your account is overdue and your prompt attention would be appreciated." Such notations may be typed, written, or stamped directly on the statement or on a separate slip attached to the statement. With the business side of practice placed in proper perspective to the doctor-patient relationship, these things should be done in a dignified, professional manner. Never do anything that might imply commercialism. Maintain good taste.

Tracing a "Skip"

If a credit patient has apparently "skipped town" without paying a bill, here are some steps helpful in tracing:

1. Examine the patient's original application for credit form.

2. Know (and contact) children of the family. You can call high schools or elementary schools for the child's home address (some will not give this information).

3. Send mail with return address requested. They may have a forwarding address.

4. Call the telephone number listed on card. A new number may be transferred or be available from the operator.

5. If a new number is available but unlisted, possibly secure aid of a friend of the patient or a patient who is a telephone operator.

6. Check the city directory to secure names and telephone numbers of neighbors or landlord and contact these people.

7. Check with the registry of motor vehicles. Registry must be notified of change of address.

8. Check local banks, particularly those who know the office (doctor).

9. Check place of patient's employment.

10. Check unemployment compensation agency, union, or similar organizations if special work performed by the patient is known.

11. Check with other professional people in town. They may have additional information.

12. Notify doctor's colleagues concerning the patient and family needs of health care. Do not, however, block them from receiving care.

13. If there is access, the electric company, gas company, or other utilities may have information.

14. Check city directory each year or voting lists each year.

The Problem of Discounting Fees

Discounting fees is a dilemma throughout the healing arts. Should discounts be allowed or not? Many doctors say yes, and an equal number says no. Sometimes a dissatisfied patient with a long overdue account is willing to settle if the fee is reduced. Some doctors believe it is better to receive something than nothing. Others hold that if the charges were reasonable in the first place and the patient can pay, a doctor who would reduce such an account would soon get a reputation of bargaining his services. This would be unprofessional.

Similarly, is it better to reduce a bill or cancel it in obvious patient hardship? Here again, doctors differ. Some say it is better to reduce the bill than cancel it to save the patient's pride and self-esteem. Others prefer to cancel a bill than reduce a fee—believing again that fee reduction is unprofessional as it is a form of fee bargaining. As in all aspects of collections, the decision to reduce or cancel is determined by the doctor's philosophy.

COLLECTION ADMINISTRATION

The cause of most collection problems in any office can usually be traced to the fact that the average doctor is a poor businessman because his training has emphasized science and not business. Most doctors will admit this and overcome their deficiencies by establishing generally accepted business policies and by having competent assistants and counselors. Doctors realize today that it is impossible to assure the growth or even survival of a practice without attention to the business side of clinical practice.

Collection Problems

While the assistant will readily recognize the need for accepted collection methods, few immediately grasp the importance of preventing collection problems. The less credit granted by the office, the better the doctor-patient relationship. The assistant should therefore try to detect the sources of collection problems and recommend steps to see that problem situations are quickly resolved. Here are some tips:

1. Do problems arise from a patient's lack of complete understanding of fees and terms of payment? If so, the assistant should ask the doctor how she can improve her technique of explaining services and fees to patients entering the practice, and how she can get feedback from patients to be assured they understand.

2. Do the staff and office environment reflect a businesslike, efficient, professional atmosphere? If the office appears unprofessional, careless in procedures, lax in tidiness, and too personal, the patient may gain the impression that the doctor is likewise careless, lax, and too friendly to care about payment for his services. Patients have a tendency to label a doctor by the environment he maintains.

3. Chiropractic health care is not a panacea for all ills that may befall mankind, and this is true of any healing art. Patients expecting guaranteed cures, miraculous healing, or permanent corrections of degenerated disorders will be disillusioned. Patients witnessing spectacular results in a friend or neighbor must be cautioned that such results cannot be promised. A patient receiving great improvement may be dissatisfied because the results are not 100% and feel nonpayment of the account is justified. At times, overt dissatisfaction may be a ruse to delay payment or attempt nonpayment. Patient attitude must be carefully analyzed and an attempt made to resolve the problem professionally.

A major responsibility of an administrative assistant is the explaining, billing, and collecting of fees. Naturally, no office can run without income, and the collection of amounts due is vital to the health of the practice and its ability to pay its salaries and overhead expenses. At the same time, any health practice will do a certain amount of charitable work, and there will be accounts that, for one reason or another, prove to be uncollectible.

To do her job correctly, the assistant responsible must be thoroughly aware of the procedures established for use with overdue accounts for which circumstances do not warrant special arrangements. She must know how far to go in pursuing collections, what to say in the initial request to the patient, and how to follow-up. If a sequence of collection procedures is used, it must be reviewed and changed periodically to be effective with changing times. In addition, she must know the doctor's policy of when to stop trying to collect an overdue account and at what point the account should be given to an outside collector if one is used.

Coping with Delinquent Accounts

As deficit spending has become a part of the American way of life, many offices offer some type of installment plan in cases involving a large fee or in situations where a patient's account has become grossly overdue. A conversation with a delinquent patient may sound something like this:

"Mrs. Smith, I'm sure you realize how much we are interested in you and want to help you in every way we can. I notice that your account is overdue, and I'm sure you realize that the office doesn't have provisions to carry accounts indefinitely. I feel you're as concerned about this as we are, so let's see if I can make some suggestions. First, let's arrange to pay a logical amount each month to reduce the present balance. Second, let's arrange to pay all future visits at the time of the visit so the account will not become larger. Now how much would you like to pay each month and what day of the month do you prefer?"

Most patients dislike being indebted as much as the office dislikes carrying overdue accounts. And most patients will welcome friendly, helpful suggestions to reduce their indebtedness. If they do not, their motive is questionable and may reflect unworthiness. An office filled with nonpaying patients is not a service to the community because the doctor could not afford proper equipment, supplies, maintenance, competent staff, or continuing education to provide the alert health care that the community deserves. Tax supported clinics are available for those requiring public support.

Rarely, the assistant must cope with a patient who refuses to pay a bill because of dissatisfaction. Careful evaluation of the complaint will determine if the complaint has some basis or whether it is a camouflage to avoid payment. "What he did for me was certainly not worth $200" is a common expression from such a patient. The patient will have forgotten the detailed history, consultation; the physical, neurologic, and orthopedic examinations; the x-ray and laboratory tests; the treatments, etc, and the time and facilities necessary to conduct these procedures and evaluate the findings. A quick review of each visit slip (services provided and the moderate fee charged for each) is valuable.

Avoid Unprofessional Procedures

No one on the staff should be responsible for making a derogatory remark about a patient because the patient didn't keep current with the account. Besides the fact that such a remark is antagonistic in encouraging the patient to make payment, it could lead to a lawsuit for slander, harassment, or malpractice.

Avoid harassing tactics such as telephoning a patient at odd hours at home or frequently calling the patient at work. Never threaten to inform the patient's employer about the account being overdue. Unprofessional procedures can usually be traced to becoming emotionally upset. Maintain an air of kindness, helpfulness, and calmness. When you cannot help but feel anger toward a patient because of an unpaid bill, it is usually the time the account should be turned over to a third party for collection.

Can a patient with a far overdue balance be charged for the collection fee of an outside agency? Can interest be charged against an overdue account? In most states, it is illegal for the office to add extra charges to an overdue account because of the costs involved in hiring an attorney or collection agency. Most management consultants be-

lieve that an interest charge smacks of commercialism and is not a good procedure to be used by a doctor. In some states, however, such a charge is legal, and an office is allowed to charge a monthly interest rate up to the maximum allowed by state law on delinquent accounts (eg, 20%, annually).

COLLECTION ADMINISTRATION

It cannot be overstated that a positive accounts receivable and collection program is paramount to the success of every professional and business office that offers credit. Collection efforts should start when the patient walks in the office door and engages in a financial transaction with the office and end when final payment is made. Once a positive collection routine is established, it must be maintained through discipline. Office procedures will then function smoothly and profitably.

At one time, a person's word was the only legal way to bind a credit agreement. This tenet is the basis of English Common Law. But as society grew more complex and social mores changed, another method was necessary to preserve details of a business transaction accurately. So, from simple oral common law, the practice of written agreements evolved—influenced by the fact people tend to forget when matters of indebtedness are involved.

Collection Management

A written document helps one to remember what transpired at a previous place and time. And an itemized statement of account due mailed periodically helps to keep an indebtedness fresh in the mind of a debtor to encourage discharge of his financial obligation. Systems specialists know that accurate, properly written records of daily office transactions save time, improve doctor-patient communication, and stimulate necessary cash flow.

The doctor is in practice to render a health service and earn a living. He has invested money in education, office space, operating facilities, equipment, supplies, and to keep current with professional advancements. He has payrolls to meet in order to keep competent staff. To be successful, he has to receive an adequate financial return to pay overhead expenses plus have enough left over to pay himself. Cash flow is the lifeblood of the business side of practice; therefore, it is important that accounts receivable be managed to maintain an adequate return on the investments made.

Constant control and periodic review of accounts receivable are vital to the health of the practice. Why? Even if you are confident of collecting money owed "someday," it is realistic to assess the value of these "probable" dollars. A few years ago, statistics from the U.S. Department of Commerce showed that $1 on your books today will be worth only 67¢ in 6 months. Within 1 year, this dollar shrinks to a mere 45¢. The factors involved are collection costs, inflation, plus loss and/or cost of interest if the office is operating on borrowed capital.

Supervising Effective Collections

Successful collection is a mixture of communication, timing, psychology, and persistence. Slow paying accounts must be handled with a definitive positive plan. Then you must implement the plan and follow through until accounts are paid. Each delinquent account must be made aware that you are concerned about the debt and intend to collect the balance due. At that point, you have gained the psychologic advantage and your collection task becomes easier.

The basic rules for effective collection are: (1) *Accuracy.* Maintain accurate records to keep your facts correct. (2) *Truthfulness.* Confront every indebted patient with the facts. Do not fabricate alternatives that do not exist. (3) *Persistence.* Constantly insist on immediate payment of overdue accounts. (4) *Follow-up.* Strive for a goal of 100% collections.

Tactful yet persistent collection procedures build a sound financial system. Never be too timid to ask for what is right. Inform indebted patients that the office cannot exist by offering free services. Make it known with discretion that the office is not sup-

ported by taxes as a welfare clinic and services can continue only if accounts are kept current.

Time Payments and Late Payments

An administrative assistant must be aware of the options open for handling time or late payments. More and more professional offices are faced with slow or late payments. Many indebted patients ask doctors to accept partial monthly payments instead of payment in full. When this arises, the doctor has the following alternatives in setting policy:

1. *Charge a service fee.* Regulation Z of the Truth in Lending Law stipulates that when a debtor is allowed to pay his account in four or more installments he is legally entitled to have this federal credit policy explained strictly according to the Disclosure Section of the Regulation. If the doctor wishes to set up a credit service fee, it may be helpful to suggest he consult the local credit bureau or Federal Department of Commerce for a copy of the law.

2. *Sell the "paper."* Many lending institutions and credit companies specialize in financing large professional bills. Arrangements can be made to authorize the doctor to enter the patient into a contractual agreement with a third party who assumes the collection responsibility. In essence, the doctor is selling his accounts receivable (paper) to the third party. The advantage is that the doctor receives his money immediately. The disadvantage is that the doctor's fee is discounted because of the service fee.

3. *Accept credit cards.* Accepting credit cards may be convenient, but their use can become costly because the credit card companies charge a percentage (eg, 6%) on each transaction.

Many doctors believe that selling the paper and credit card transactions between doctors and patients are not professional conduct.

4. *Accept cash only.* If after checking a person's credit, the patient proves to be a chronic slow payer, many office policies direct the assistant to explain to the patient

that the doctor will serve him on a cash basis. This must be done tactfully, but in many instances this policy can save a lot of grief for both the office and the patient.

Note: If the doctor considers the policy of adding a finance charge to accounts that extend past acceptable terms of payment, he should consult his attorney for counsel to comply with consumer credit law. Many states legally allow a reasonable charge for late payments, providing the debtor is informed in advance. The local Credit Bureau will have information concerning late fees.

While some offices have few problems with collections, others are continually short of cash due to sluggish accounts receivable turnover. The latter type office needs a positive procedure for handling accounts receivable and collections. Most positive programs are based on four basic steps: (1) preventive bad-debt screening, (2) accounts receivable aging, (3) past-due account follow-up, and (4) third-party collection help.

Preventive Bad-Debt Screening

Most potential bad-debt problems can be eliminated on the first contact with the patient. Once the patient fills out a brief credit application, you have a basis on which to determine the type of account to set up for that patient. If you have accounts receivable troubles, don't just file the form and hope for the best. Follow through. Call the patient's bank, his other references, and check his credit standing with the local Credit Bureau. If the patient proves to be a poor credit risk, tactfully explain that because of the patient's credit history all services must be on a cash basis. The doctor, of course, must be informed of the situation and agree with this method when it is used. If the patient leaves the practice, the office has lost nothing but a few minutes of productive time.

Assistants must treat all credit information confidentially. It is against the law to divulge credit information to persons other than "legally" interested parties. Use the Credit Bureau as a primary source for guidelines.

Accounts Receivable Aging

"Aging" is the classifying of accounts receivable by age from the date of the first billing. It is done with the intention of following through with an action procedure. All active accounts with an "amount due" are classified into at least five categories; eg, (1) current, (2) 30 days, (3) 60 days, (4) 90 days, and (5) over 90 days.

On the first billing day after aging the accounts, all charges for the previous month are due. These are current accounts until the next billing. On the second billing, all accounts unpaid from the first billing become 30-day accounts. On the third billing, those still unpaid from the first billing become 60-day accounts. Then they subsequently become 90-day and over 90-day accounts. This is the time to consider stern action.

Aged accounts receivable should be readily identified to facilitate billing and other follow-up action. One efficient method is to feature multicolored, self-adhesive "flags" or clips called EZ signals. Each color represents a different age category. Here are the steps recommended by Control-O-Fax Office Systems:

1. Before the billing day, review all ledger cards and attach an EZ Signal to each card with the colors corresponding to specific age groups. For instance in January, green may be used for 30-day accounts. In February, orange signals indicate charges since the green one, etc. With four colors, this cycle can be repeated three times each year.

2. Remove signal when payment is made and account shows a zero balance.

3. In 4 months, you will have a ledger tray full of flagged and blank cards. Over 90-day account ledger cards should be pulled for a special action procedure. These accounts require immediate attention because the likelihood of collecting on accounts drops sharply after 90 days.

Past-Due Account Follow-up

While every attempt should be made to receive payment as soon as possible, many doctors do not regard 90-day accounts as serious problems. Statistics, however, show that many of these accounts are already uncollectible. Most specialists in the collection field recommend in-office action on any account over 30 days past due.

From an *accounts receivable age analysis,* you will know exactly which accounts are overdue and to what extent. Then follow-up with some type of action according to office policy. Tactful positive reminders are used to focus on the time elapsed since charges were incurred. For example:

1. Enclose appropriate notices with statements.

2. Affix collection messages of good taste to statements.

3. Mail "aged" statements from 10 to 15 days after billing if a check is not received by then. Contact by telephone is often fruitful.

4. Special letters to aged accounts can be mailed.

5. Consider third-party action.

After 90 days, experience shows some type of definitive action program must be implemented. At that point, you will have exhausted most of your in-office influence on debtors.

Collection procedures are usually designed in three stages. *First,* reminders are sent to the negligent patient about his bill. *Second,* inquiries are made why payment has not been made. The reason behind the nonpayment must be known. *Third,* once the reason behind nonpayment is known, the problem can be discussed and a mutually agreeable solution worked out (eg, time payments). For this reason, the personal approach is the best way to follow-up collections. This is also a reason many doctors feel that colored stickers and other collection "gimmicks" attached to statements are inappropriate and unprofessional for a doctor's office.

Community circumstances must be considered. For instance, if the doctor is involved in a rural practice, he must frequently carry a heavy credit load until the fields are harvested. The regular billing system is maintained regardless of season, but

pressure to collect is lightened until money is available. Likewise if the doctor knows a patient has been on strike or out of work for several weeks.

Although collection stickers printed in bright colors and frequently composed in a humorous theme are often used in the business world, many doctors feel they are inappropriate in the health-care field. There is nothing amusing about being ill and financially indebted. There are, however, some innovations developed in the business world that can be applied in a chiropractic office that are considered both professional and effective. Here are some examples.

1. Whenever possible, eliminate the use of ciphers and dollar signs in totaling the account balance. When thirty dollars are written as $30.00, it appears as a much larger amount than when the dollar sign and zeroes after the decimal are eliminated, thus 30.

2. As longhand is more personal than typewritten copy, many collection specialists feel that final-stage collection attempts should have statements and collection letters addressed in longhand. This is done in the belief that the patient will treat longhand-addressed communications more seriously.

3. A stamped, self-addressed return envelope included with the statement is appreciated by many patients as convenient. It often results in a more rapid payment.

4. A small red checkmark opposite the balance due on the statement arouses the curiosity of the receiver and indicates that the amount has been specially noted by someone. Payment is often prompted. A variation of this is to underline in red the overdue balance.

While procedures are important, personal actions are more important. Attitude influences attitude. That is, the assistant who is responsible for collections must act as if she's going to collect—with tact. When she asks the patient if payment is to be made by cash or check, she should have the receipt book in front of her and pen in hand. Never allow a patient to leave with just a casual "Just bill me." Each credit account must be supported by a credit application and a complete explanation of office policies.

The assistant always tries to obtain some payment on the account, especially on the first visit. In acute transit cases, this may be all you will ever get. Rarely will a patient enter a doctor's office without at least the money for an office visit. After policy is explained and a part payment is accepted, the patient should make a commitment when the balance will be paid, and this should be recorded in front of the patient.

When speaking of office policies, use the word "customary" frequently. Few people will take exception to a policy if they feel it is *customary*. What they resent is feeling it is discriminatory.

In cases involving a large fee when a time payment plan must be arranged, the same tactful attitude must be maintained. Explain office policy, arrive at a mutually agreeable plan, establish firm dates and amounts of payment, and let the patient see you develop a written record of the agreement on the ledger sheet. This helps to solidify the commitment.

Tactful, humane, discreet discussion about the office's services and fees eliminates most potential collection problems. A lax, irregular, half-hearted approach cannot hope to succeed. An efficient assistant can handle most office collection problems in person or by the telephone, resolving many misunderstandings about services and fees, and serving as the office's good will ambassador.

There also may be times when an assistant must be strong enough in character to shoulder the embarrassment or blame of an error for which she was not responsible. The assistant can do this because the doctor is more involved in the intimate doctor-patient relationship. The doctor and patient must always "keep face" and maintain a close rapport. This is not a matter of preserving "ego." It is a matter of preserving the faith and confidence necessary for optimal healing.

Evaluating Collection Efforts

It is a simple procedure to determine if the office is doing a good or poor job at collec-

tions. It only requires a look at the practice's accounts receivable and the collection rate. When accounts receivable are more than *three* times the average monthly gross, it indicates collection procedures must be improved. A hypothetical example will explain this simple procedure:

Dr. Smith, who practices in a rural community in the Midwest, grosses $90,300 per year and has an average accounts receivable of $36,800:

$$\frac{90,300}{12} = 7,525$$

$$\frac{36,800}{7,525} = 4.89 \text{ (3.0 would be average)}$$

It is clear that Dr. Smith definitely needs to improve his collection procedures. His accounts receivable are far more than three times his average monthly gross.

Computing Office Collection Rate

About three-fourths of physicians with established practices have a collection rate of 90% or better. About one-fourth of doctors have a collection rate of 95% or better. These figures help to compare your office's performance relative to the entire field.

To compute your office's collection rate, determine the average monthly gross income, divide this figure by the average monthly charges, and multiply the result by a hundred:

$$\frac{\text{average monthly gross income}}{\text{average monthly charges}} \times 100$$
$$= \text{collection rate}$$

Dr. Jones, for example, has an average monthly gross income of $8,000, and his average monthly charges amount to $9,800. Thus,

$$\frac{8,000}{9,800} \times 100 = 82\% \text{ (92\% would be average)}$$

Dr. Jones' collection rate is 10% below average. Steps must be taken to improve the collection rate to 92% or better.

Recognize that these computations are based on averages for established practices: practices existing 3 years or more. The typical doctor should not expect to collect more than 75% of charges incurred during the first 18 months of practice. It takes a certain amount of time in establishing a practice for collections to catch up with charges made.

The Cash-Flow Factor. When collection methods are ineffective, the office is not only letting someone else use its money, it can experience cash-flow problems that affect the doctor's ability to meet payroll, rent, utility bills, supply needs, and other day-to-day expenses. If too much cash is tied to accounts receivable, the office may find itself on some company's overdue account. A doctor can never afford to have a poor credit reputation.

The Inflation Factor. If it takes many months to collect overdue accounts, the value of the overdue dollar is probably greatly depreciated when payments are finally received.

The Collection Cost Factor. Costs of contacting overdue accounts can be massive when you add all the hours, postage, and stationery necessary. In more difficult cases, legal services and collection services can take a large portion of fees earned.

The Collection Time Factor. Cash date control lets you establish definite dates when bills will be paid so you will know in advance what the cash flow will be for planning. Planning saves the doctor paying interest on short-term loans to cover current and urgent expenses. Thus, it's important to know how long it takes the office to collect its accounts receivables and to compare this figure with other practices in your area. To make this computation, start with a simple formula:

$$\frac{\text{Accounts receivable (\$)}}{\text{Net credit receipts (\$)}} \times \text{time period}$$
$$= \text{average collection period.}$$

For example, let's determine the average collection period for an office based on accounts receivable of $8,000 and net credit receipts of $40,000:

$$\frac{8,000}{40,000} \times 365 = \text{office's average}$$
$$\text{collection period.}$$

This comes to 73 days, which means it takes this office 73 days to turn over ac-

counts receivables. The average collection period for a chiropractic office in your area can usually be found by contacting several collection agencies servicing the profession in your area. These figures are useful in determining when an account actually becomes overdue and when it is necessary to make an enthusiastic collection effort.

Keep in mind that you do not have to be rude to collect. Rudeness builds resentment that can be more permanent than the debt, and it can send a worthy patient to another office while prolonging payments to your office for an indefinite period. The credit policy should be firm but fair. The more effective the credit technique, the more the office can grant favorable terms to patients when necessary.

Statement Services

Many accounting and collection agencies offer statement services, thus relieving office personnel of this responsibility. Each month a representative from the contracted service calls on your office to microfilm ledger cards and rush them to the nearest processing center. There, statements are printed from the film, inserted into personalized envelopes, and mailed directly to the doctor's patients. Billing is completed in a fraction of usual in-office time, and valuable records never leave the office.

Statement services eliminate the need for additional personnel and facilities during billing periods, and free the administrative staff for more clinical responsibilities. There is no equipment to buy, and the need for a large inventory of stamps, envelopes, statements, etc, is eliminated. The microfilm records can either be stored on the premises of the agency or returned to your office.

Collecting by Telephone

Much of this section has been taken from *How to Make Your Collection Efforts Pay Off,* an uncopyrighted publication of the Bell System. You will find it helpful in setting an effective telephone collection program in conjunction with other collection methods. If you have further questions regarding collections by telephone, contact your telephone company. They have trained collection specialists to help you.

There may be valid reasons why a patient doesn't pay on time: reasons that a dunning notice or form letter won't pick up. Besides, sending an impersonal reminder to a patient simply isn't good public relations. The personal touch through a phone call at the right time with the right attitude within a few days after the agreed on terms have expired can do much to firm a logical payment plan. The office benefits by getting its money in a given period, the patient is kept happy, and you don't have to work as hard in collections. Thus, it is important to call the patient before the account becomes long overdue. The patient may have previously agreed to a payment plan, but circumstances might have changed for the patient that require a revised plan.

A letter can be ignored. A phone call cannot. A telephone program is effective because it brings you in direct contact with the patient involved. Computerized dunning notices or form letters, while they have their place, can easily be discarded or lost. Also, courts, legislatures, and the FCC have outlawed harassment in consumer situations, and the definition of *harassment* is very vague.

A telephone approach gains personal information. Impersonal reminders will not pick up the fact that a patient has a special problem deserving consideration. By asking discreet questions on the telephone, you can determine these problems and act appropriately. Being able to treat each patient fairly and individually is a distinct advantage of a telephone collection call.

A telephone approach allows flexibility. By knowing a patient's problem, you can adapt to any situation. You can change routine procedures to meet new circumstances. But in changing, your primary concern should still be to bring an account current. The doctor's patients will appreciate the fact you are helping them to keep their accounts up to date.

A telephone approach lets you be thor-

ough. The only way you can be thoroughly familiar with every aspect of an overdue account's circumstances is through direct personal contact. A telephone call is one of the most economical ways of determining the facts. To assure a successful telephone collection call, prepare the call in advance. Determine if your office was at fault in some way (poor communications? bookkeeping error?). Ask questions that will make you aware of the patient's financial problems (past, current, long range).

A telephone approach lets you be personable. Behind every overdue account is a human being. You can show the patient how he or she can overcome almost any difficulty in bringing payments up to date. Let your voice and personality build a positive image of your office.

Using the telephone is only part of the effort. It takes training and administration to make it work, but it can be mastered in a few days. It's economical because the cost of setting your program in operation involves no special equipment except the telephone on your desk and some standard stationery material. Used with your accounts receivable records, this program can make collection efforts much more effective and efficient.

Technique

Here's how the Bell System suggests you initiate your program:

1. All necessary billing information should be readily available. You also will need the following items:

• Twenty-six 5×8-inch divider cards with tabs marked from A to Z to group accounts by name.

• Thirty-one 5×8-inch divider cards with tabs marked from 1 to 31 to group accounts by date.

• One file box to hold the index cards.

2. In addition, you'll need 5×8-inch cards called the *collection record*. Along with the telephone, these cards are the heart of the operation. You will need one card for

each patient on your accounts receivable list.

3. The *collection record card* should include space at the top to indicate the patient's name, address, and telephone number. Provide a space labeled "Contact" for the name of a parent or guardian as happens with a child patient. "Alternate" would indicate the full name of a person who also knows the reason for the overdue status and can authorize payment such as a guardian's spouse or attorney. The alternate contact should be called if the main contact is unavailable. A space labeled "Past Payment Record" records a rating system of your design to provide a history of payment performance of an account. Space for "Special Problems, Considerations" allows data to give you an awareness of any circumstances that could affect the overdue account's ability to meet payments when due such as seasonal variations in a patient's business. These suggested headings constitute the permanent record that will aid you in pre-call planning. The remainder of the card is set up as a record of the collection steps. Under "Date," indicate the date of the contact. In a space titled "Step," place a "T" for telephone call, "N" for a special dunning notice on a statement, or "L" when a letter is used. Under "Spoke to" place the initials of the primary contact or alternate. In a column titled "Results," write a brief narrative of the contact. This should include the problem encountered, the payment plan agreed on (dates and amounts), and follow-up date. You should follow-up a few days after payment is due if it has not been received. Allow for mail delays and posting of payments received. Under "Employee," enter your initials so there will be a future record of whom made the contact. See Figure 8.12.

4. The next step is to review your aging report or list of overdue accounts and fill out the headings of a collection record card for each if they have not been preprinted. You are now ready to call overdue accounts. Immediately after completing each call, record the results of the conversation, noting the patient's reason for being overdue, the agreement that was reached (dates and amounts), and the next follow-up date. The collection record card is now filed in the appropriate follow-up date card marked from 1 to 31.

5. On the next follow-up date, pull the card after determining if payment was received. If some payment was received, the card should be filed in the space of the next follow-up date. If payment was not received, call the patient to determine the reason.

6. Once all payments have been received and an account is current, the collection record card is put into the alphabetical section of your file box for reference should that account become overdue again. The collection record card is now a permanent record of collection efforts on that account.

In collecting money by telephone, the Bell System offers three steps for a successful telephone collection call:

1. *Plan Your Call.* Was your office at fault? Were previous steps taken to obtain payment? Make sure you have the name of the person who can authorize payment. Establish a scheduled payment program. Prepare an opening statement and fact-finding questions.

2. *Make the Call.* Identify yourself and your office. Give the reason for your call. Make a strategic pause—listen to what the patient has to say. Ask fact-finding questions. Suggest a payment program according to office policy. Overcome objections with logic. Obtain a firm commitment. Close your call in a friendly positive manner.

3. *Follow up Your Call.* Record your notes, update your records, and call back if payment was not received.

Although the telephone can be a valuable tool in collecting from an overdue account, the following practices must be avoided:

• Calling at odd hours of the day or night such as before 9 o'clock in the morning or after 9 o'clock in the evening.

• Repeated calling. Generally, you should not call more than once a week.

• Calls to third parties except to locate the person you are trying to reach.

COLLECTION RECORD

PATIENT _____ TELEPHONE _____

ADDRESS _____

CONTACT _____ TELEPHONE _____

ALTERNATE _____ TELEPHONE _____

PAST PAYMENT RECORD _____

SPECIAL PROBLEMS, CONSIDERATIONS _____

COLLECTION STEPS

DATE	STEP	SPOKE TO	RESULTS	EMPLOYEE

Figure 8.12. Sample format for a telephone collection record card.

• Threatening calls.

• Calls falsely asserting credit rating will be affected or that legal action will be taken.

• Calls to places of employment. Any request by an employer that further calls not be made to place of business must be honored.

After you design your telephone collection program, your degree of success can be measured in the following specific areas:

1. Have you opened new and more beneficial lines of communications with patients with overdue accounts?

2. Do you now have an increased awareness of their problems?

3. Does your average collection period compare favorably with other offices in your area?

4. Is cash flow improving?

5. Have you maintained or improved good office relationships with your overdue accounts?

When properly used, the telephone can be one of your strongest collection tools. When it is improperly used, it will fail to improve collections and create a negative public relations problem. Never make a telephone collection call if other patients can overhear the conversation.

If your doctor-employer approves a telephone collection program, be responsible. Remember that telephoning for a collection carries a greater risk for the doctor in creating ill will among patients because he does not have control how the assistant responds over the telephone. He has much greater control over what is in a letter or on a statement. Thus, honor this responsibility.

It has been stated that it is usually best not to call the patient at his place of employment unless this is the only way the patient can be reached. A good practice is to leave your number and have the patient call you back. Don't apologize for the call, but state your purpose in a friendly, forthright manner with tact. If you open with, "I'm calling about your bill," the patient is immediately placed on the defensive. A better approach is to pause after an opening remark to allow the patient to talk. Most patients will know what you are calling about and will begin an explanation why payment has not been made. Once a patient has stated his case, you can be more helpful. Be courteous, helpful, sympathetic, yet firm.

If the patient is in financial difficulty, suggest a payment schedule that is logical under the circumstances. In presenting your message, review the services provided, the charges, the dates of service, and the patient's record of nonpayment. Include the number of calls and letters sent, then pause and give the patient an opportunity to respond. Let the patient know that you do not want to add to his problems, but a regular payment would keep the account active until such time the patient could pay it in full. Remember, the purpose of your call is to get the patient to make a commitment. After a commitment is made, write the date and the amount promised on the patient's collection record card for future reference. Telephone collection calls should always be made by an assistant, never by the doctor.

Your *telephone approach* to the problem of the overdue account is the key to success. Harsh methods and irritating attitudes are seldom productive. Be friendly and tact-

ful, avoiding saying anything that might arouse the patient's anger or result in an antagonistic response. Talk directly with the patient. It is poor taste to relay credit-related messages.

After the telephone conversation, many offices send a letter to the patient outlining the agreement made on the telephone. For an example, see Figure 8.13.

Always allow the patient to save face. Let the patient know that you realize that they are very busy during your first call, and because of everyday pressures they probably overlooked the statement. Possibly remind the patient that you are aware that the mails are uncertain, and could there be a possibility that the statement became lost and never reached the patient? If a patient promises a payment and it is not received, call them on the excuse to stop payment on the check in the possibility the payment was lost in mailing. Another approach is to say that in checking the patient's records while getting ready for an office audit, you would like to know how the patient plans to handle the overdue balance so that the information can be posted in the account's record before the accountant's review.

Many local telephone companies provide free or low-cost short courses to their customers on office telephone techniques. Another training source is the American Collectors Association, 5011 Ewing Avenue South, Minneapolis, Minnesota.

Summary of Highlights

Certain telephone techniques have been established that prove to be good telephone routines. For instance, identify yourself and the office at the opening of your call. Speak to the debtor. State the problem and tactfully ask for full payment according to the original agreement. If the patient is unable to pay in full, determine the reasons and offer a solution. Suggest that the patient seek a loan from a bank, credit union, loan company, or increase an existing loan, obtain a pay advance, or consider cashing savings bonds.

Learn to differentiate between a legiti-

James C. Anderson, D.C.
167 Main Street
Anytown, Anystate 12345
(678) 912-3456

October 28, 1990

Mr. Harry D. Hopkins
78 Center Avenue
Anytown, Anystate 12345

Dear Mr. Hopkins:

We appreciate your explanation regarding your overdue account. Since circumstances prevent your paying the full balance due of $85 at this time, we shall be happy to accept the payment plan you suggested.

Your check of $35 will be expected on the 10th of next month (November), with the remainder paid in two installments of $25 each, one to be received by November 23rd and one by December 10th.

Your cooperation has been deeply appreciated.

_____
Chiropractic Assistant

Figure 8.13. Sample format for a collection follow-up letter.

mate excuse and a "put-off." Never allow a debtor to encourage you to accept partial payment. You encourage the debtor to make full payment if possible and reasonable. If full payment cannot be arranged, have the patient make a specific commitment on what date each week or month payment will reach you; the amount; whether the payment will be mailed or personally delivered; and whether payment will be by check, cash, or money order. Set a specific date for payment if the patient will not volunteer a specific date. These facts should be recorded in situations of partial payment or full payment. Once a commitment is established, ask the patient to write down the doctor's name, amount promised, and date payment will reach you.

If the patient tends to offer poor excuses, motivate payment by appealing to the patient's credit standing, honesty, reputation for fair play, and/or doing the right thing. Show the patient how he can be freed from worry by accepting a logical budget plan. If necessary, discreetly bring to the patient's attention the embarrassment of collection agency assignment of the account—but never threaten.

When a debtor breaks a promise to make full or partial payment, check previous promises and payment history. Find out why you were not informed that payment could not be made as agreed, and remind the patient that special arrangements were made as a favor to the patient. Before you suggest another arrangement, the patient should understand that this will be the last special arrangement made, that favors cannot be extended unless the patient agrees to keep promises made. On the patient's new commitment, determine how and when you will receive payment and have the patient note the dates and terms.

If payment is not received and the debtor states that payment is in the mail, ask when it was sent, from where, the amount, in what form (check, money order, cash)? If the amount is lower than that agreed to, determine why.

In cases where the patient or spouse of the debtor is not at home when you call, find out who you are speaking with and when the debtor will be home. Leave your name and telephone number, and stress the urgency of a return call.

When the debtor states that unemployment has been the cause of nonpayment, determine why the patient is unemployed, how long he has been without work, what his job prospects are, if the spouse is working, and if unemployment compensation is available. Suggest that friends and relatives may help. Ask why the patient did not let you know about his loss of employment, and emphasize that it is important that the patient keep in touch with you at specified dates.

If illness resulting in loss of income is given as the reason for nonpayment, find out who exactly has been ill (debtor, spouse, child) and why you were not informed. If it is the debtor who is or has been ill, how long has he been without normal income and when does he expect to return to work? Is sick pay or disability insurance involved? Suggest a logical solution to the situation and obtain a commitment.

In cases of separation or divorce, learn the date of legal separation, the debtor's attorney's name, and the name of his or her employer. Inform the debtor that the office must hold him responsible for the bill until legally proved otherwise. Set a specific date for him to inform you how the account will be settled.

If you learn that the debtor is deceased, determine the date and place of death, ask for payment from the spouse after a delay of several weeks, and obtain the name and address of the attorney or estate administrator

involved. If there is no estate or legally responsible survivors, determine if there is life insurance and who the beneficiaries are.

In any collection telephone call, end the conversation by verifying the debtor's employer and address, spouse's employer and address, debtor's resident address, the next payment due date, and the amount of payment.

Collecting by Office Letters

After your doctor-employer reviews the monthly accounts receivable, he will usually instruct you to telephone certain patients and discuss their overdue account or he may prefer that a letter be sent that describes the account and the method of payment. These letters are usually personalized form letters (or cards) used in a series with each successive message a little stronger in its request for payment. An activity record is shown in Figure 8.14. The process is usually administered as follows:

Account Age	Communication
30 days overdue	Notice No. 1
60 days overdue	Notice No. 2
90 days overdue	Notice No. 3
100 days overdue	Final notice

Collection communications should be as friendly and sympathetic as possible if the indebtedness is the result of an oversight. When messages are not given the courtesy of a reply, your communication should become somewhat more urgent and forceful in tone. When a response is not received from the debtor after repeated requests, the doctor may consider turning the account over to a collection agency or bring suit against the patient. Such a policy is almost never considered before an account has become 100 days overdue and no communication has been received from the patient.

The first notice is usually a short message asking whether the patient has overlooked the statement. Notices 2 and 3 often invite the patient to call or visit the office to discuss any special payment problems or questions about the bill. The messages are usu-

BILLING AND COLLECTION RECORD

Service Date		Date(s) Notices Were Sent				Remarks
From	To	#1	#2	#3	#4	

SPECIAL COLLECTION ACTIVITIES

Date	Description	Result

Figure 8.14. Sample format for a collection letter activity record, which can be printed separately or on the back of each financial ledger card. The numbers indicate the type of notice that was sent; eg, #1, regular statement; #2 statement with overdue notice; #3, first collection letter; #4, second collection letter.

ally informal, sincere, and imply confidence in the patient's honesty. Final notices usually say consideration is being given to turn the account over to a third party for collection because of the lack of response.

Some doctors believe that collection letters are the most effective method of collecting delinquent accounts. A collection letter is essentially an educational message. It can be designed to educate the patient of office policy, the state of the account, the value of services provided, and a method of payment. However, is is doubtful whether they are more effective than telephone calls.

Threatening letters or dunning letters are not only in poor taste, they have little value. A person who can pay but is unwilling to pay is accustomed to receiving such messages and pays little attention to them. Those who are not used to them may become insulted. Neither you nor the doctor can force a person to pay an overdue account. All you can do is offer motivational appeals and educate the patient to the legitimacy and age of the account. You can persuade, but not force or threaten. Properly timed soft-toned messages get better results than do harsh letters.

Sample First Notices

• Did you forget the payment that was due some days ago? We all forget things occasionally. If your payment is not already in the mail, please send it now to keep your account current. If some problem exists, please let us know. Amount due is $38.

• Perhaps you did not receive the monthly statements we mailed. I'm sure you would like to keep your account current, thus this reminder. May we hear from you before the 20th? Thanks for your attention.

• Please accept this note as a friendly reminder that your account is past due. A remittance by the 20th will be appreciated.

• Because your overdue account shows an amount of only $40, it has probably been overlooked. However, to keep your account clear, a remittance by the 20th will be appreciated. Thanks!

• As time passes quickly, you may not realize that you have not settled the enclosed bill. Please send us a check today. Many thanks.

Sample Second Notices

• We would welcome the opportunity to help you with your account. Every family occasionally has unexpected circumstances that upset well-laid plans or intentions. Thus, we are always willing to make special arrangements if needed. Please contact us immediately as we have received no word from you in response to our monthly statements. You will find our office cooperative. The balance on your account is presently $78. Thanks for your cooperation.

• In checking our records, we find your account is considerably overdue. If you cannot pay the entire amount now, please forward a part payment of $35 immediately to show good will. If you wish to handle the balance in monthly installments, contact our office for arrangements. Your account shows a present balance of $105. Thanks for your attention.

• As we have not received your check on the overdue balance of your account, we wonder if our statements or your check have gone astray because you have always paid your bills promptly in the past. If another unusual situation exists, please let us know so some special arrangement may be discussed. You'll find our office as understanding and cooperative as possible.

• We have previously called your attention to your past due account. If there is a misunderstanding about your account or if you are financially unable to make payment in full, please contact us immediately so that special arrangements can be made. Your account is now overdue $95.

• Everyone, it seems, has to meet obligations promptly these days. That is why we ask you to send your payment for the enclosed statement by the 20th. It is not our intention to make payments difficult for anyone, but we must expect cooperation from patients to whom we have extended credit courtesy. Thanks for your immediate reply.

• A review of your account shows it is past due. Our credit policy considers professional services to be due and payable monthly. Payment of the outstanding balance of $85 by the 20th will restore your account to regular handling. Thanks for your attention. We will expect your payment and appreciate your clearing this account.

• In reviewing your account, I find that it is still open and a reply to my letter of the 10th has not been received. Is this because you find it difficult to make full payment at this time? If you would prefer to pay one-third now and the balance in two monthly installments, this will be agreeable. To take advantage of this favor, please send in your check today. Thank you.

Sample Third Notices

• This is a reminder that there has been no acknowledgment of your overdue account for some time. Please let us know within the next few days how you intend to make payment. I know you will agree that Dr. Brown tries in every way to help his patients. However, indifference to obligations makes it difficult for the office to help you. Please mail your payment today or contact our office to discuss any unusual circumstances that may exist.

• To date we have neither received a check in payment of your overdue account of $78 nor an answer to our requests for payment. Because it is Dr. Smith's policy at all times to serve his patients with good conscience, we must expect similar cooperation from patients on their receipt of our statements. Thus, it is important that you forward a check for your account today.

• Our auditor reminds us that your account is considerably past due. This is our reminder that it is your responsibility to keep your account current or arrange with our office for periodic payments. It is urgent that you give your immediate attention to bringing your account up to date. Our apol-

ogies if your payment is in the mail, and our sincere thanks.

• Since this is one of several statements we have sent, we feel compelled to call this account to your urgent attention. If you have a question about your account or if full payment is impossible at this time, please contact us within the next few days. Thanks for your immediate cooperation.

• For some time we have been expecting word from you concerning your overdue account. We are at a loss in understanding why we have not heard from you concerning your unpaid balance. There must be some reason you have not responded to our requests? We cannot help you without an explanation. Because this account is now delinquent, some arrangements must be made immediately. If payment cannot be made in full, we will be happy to work out some type of budget payment if you contact us by the 20th. Please let us hear from you today.

• The auditor of our accounts has classified your account for collection processing. Dr. Jones, however, does not want your account handled in this manner. He feels you must have encountered circumstances that are unusual or your account would at least show partial payment each month. Please contact us immediately so we can understand the problem and then seek to help you make arrangements. Thanks for your immediate attention to this serious matter.

Sample Final Notices

• We have attempted in every way possible to win your cooperation regarding settlement of your account. Your failure to discuss this leaves us no alternative but to place your account in the hands of a collector. However, we still hope to hear from you within the next 10 days so this action will not be necessary. Please help us help you, as this is a final notice. Account balance is $285.

• As you didn't respond to repeated statements on your past due account, it is now time our accountant ordinarily would process your account for enforced collection.

As neither you nor we desire to have your account sent to the collector, we will hold your account for 10 days to give you an opportunity to make payment or make some type of special arrangements with the office. Account balance is $195.

• We have notified you of a balance overdue several times, yet payment has not been received. We are forced to extend one final opportunity for you to clear this long overdue account. Failure on your part to make payment or offer an explanation will force us to take action that is both costly and embarrassing. However, you leave us no option but to enforce collection. We leave the decision for such action entirely up to you. Your account balance is $425.

• Our records still indicate a balance of $245, which is long past due. As the office can no longer carry this balance, the account has been reported to a collection agency. They are to wait 10 days before commencing service. This gives you an opportunity to settle without our resorting to their methods. Your check, or arrangement for settlement, will enable us to advise them that this matter has been satisfactorily closed. A duplicate of this letter has been sent to the collection agency.

• On numerous occasions, we have notified you of your overdue balance and have asked for your cooperation. It appears, however, that you have chose to ignore our communications. As we feel we have afforded you every opportunity to settle your account on a friendly basis yet have received no response, your account is being referred to our attorney with instructions to collect the full principal plus interest if we do not receive payment by the 20th. Account balance is $175.

• We feel we have been as lenient as we could with your long overdue account— more lenient than the credit departments of the average professional practice would have been with an account as old as yours. However, we cannot continue to carry this account any longer. This is a final notice. You force us to turn the account over for collection unless definite arrangements are

made with our office by noon July 20th. Account balance is $345.

Registered Mailings

For maximum effect, many offices send their final notices by registered mail with a return receipt requested. This satisfies the office that the communication has reached the debtor. It also makes an impression on the debtor that the matter is serious. Certified mail with return requested works in the same manner at slightly less cost, but it only guarantees that the message reached the *address*.

Sample Follow-up Letters

• We appreciate your explanation regarding your overdue account. Because circumstances prevent your paying the entire bill at this time, we shall be happy to accept the monthly payment plan you suggest. Thank you for your cooperation.

• Thank you for your check of March 7th in settlement of your account. Your cooperation is appreciated.

Collection Letter Services

Collection letter services provide third-party inducement by mail and/or telephone. These are administration services and not collection agencies. The role of a collection agency will be described later in this section.

Many local, regional, and national agencies offer collection letter services for doctors. An ideal third-party service employs positive debtor psychology that elicits payments from delinquent accounts. It is designed to convert accounts receivable into cash payments while it preserves office good will with the indebted patient.

With most services, all you need do is select those overdue accounts that are not responding to your regular billing efforts. Attach a label or note that lets the debtors know you have turned the account over to a third party. Then send one final statement with this label or note attached. A percentage of people will pay at this point. For those who don't, you initiate the service.

To initiate service, fill out a form that includes the name and address of the debtor, your name and address, plus amount due. Mail it to the collection service and they will send out the first third-party letter. Payments are directed to your office, and you inform the collection service whether to stop the service after the first letter or to resume service and send out the second and subsequent letters.

Some agencies provide a third-party telephone service by which debtors may call an Adjustments Department that records debtor complaints, explanations, partial-payment offers, etc, and forwards the information to you. The Adjustments Department is trained to handle calls tactfully and record information carefully. Debtors usually respond in one of three ways: (1) they send payment to you in full; (2) they send a partial payment to you, or (3) they call the collection service and arrange for payment on a specific basis.

When payment in full is received, notify the collection service immediately so they will terminate all action and close the account. If partial payment is received, do not stop the service unless you have received a firm commitment from the debtor to arrange payment in a manner agreeable to you. If the debtor fails to live up to his promise, instruct the collection letter company to resume service.

Here are some hints and recommendations.

1. It's up to the doctor to decide who should be placed on the collection service and when. Service usually begins when payment has not been received after 90 days and your office has used all its routine techniques.

2. It is good policy to ask for a substantial first payment from the debtor. After requesting that first payment, require the debtor to make partial payments of approximately from three to six equal monthly payments depending on the size of the balance due.

3. If the debtor calls your office and is irate because you turned his account over to

a collector, you may say: (a) "The only thing I can suggest would be to pay the bill," (b) "The collection service is an independent company, but if you'll make satisfactory arrangements for payment, I can have the company suspend their proceedings," or (c) "If you mail your payment today, I can have the agency discontinue their proceedings."

Collection Agencies

An outside collection agency or attorney can be used after office resources have been exhausted. If this is done, the accounts receivable record is to be obviously marked with the date the account has been turned over to the agency. The name and address of the collecting agent should be noted in the patient's records.

A separate file for these accounts is established. One section of the file is used for credited or closed-out accounts. A notation may be made on the patient's chart to forewarn anyone using it for reference. All financial arrangements made with the collector, the assistant's part in the collection process, and just when the third party is asked to take over the account must be thoroughly discussed with the doctor in each case.

Resorting to a third party for collection may not be a sign of defeat. It is often a matter of financial survival. Every professional and business person should have a basic knowledge of available collection services and how they operate.

1. *Licensed Collection Agency.* This type of service usually requires that you assign past due accounts to them on a commission basis. The commissions run up to 50% of the amount collected, often with a minimum acceptable account amount (eg, $50). The tactics used in collecting varies from agency to agency, and you have little control over their collection methods.

2. *Local Credit Bureau.* Collection service is usually a secondary function of an established Credit Bureau. Their main function is to report credit ratings. They, too, charge up to 50% of the gross amount collected with varying account minimums.

With this service also, you surrender control of their collection methods.

3. *Flat-Rate Collection Services.* This type of service is almost identical to a collection letter service. The agency provides third-party influence over collections but you are able to retain complete control of collection methods. For a flat fee, the agency will contact overdue accounts by various methods and instruct them to make payment directly to the doctor's office. Agency fees are agreed to in advance and usually are somewhat less than the percentage required by collection agencies and credit bureaus.

Health-care fee collections call for a different approach than do collections in the business world. The agency chosen must hold high standards with a thorough understanding of the delicate nature of that doctor-patient relationship. Ideally, the agency should function as an extension of the chiropractic office, attempting to create good will while successfully collecting accounts. Turning over accounts to a third party nevertheless usually results in the loss of good will. Thus, only those accounts classed as "unworthy" by the doctor should be considered for external collection.

In selecting an agency, check with local and state chiropractic associations as they can often offer information about reliable agencies. The local Chamber of Commerce and Better Business Bureau are other sources of information. Once reputation of the agency is determined, the doctor should appraise the types of collection methods used, review communications used in contacting patients, and ask about their health-practice collection rate and specific fees for submitted accounts of various ages. Avoid signing a contract. Reputable agencies seldom require them.

The procedures and techniques used in collecting accounts must conform with the ethics and dignity of the profession in general and those of the specific doctor. For instance, legal action should not be used without permission of the doctor. The agency should also be instructed to be willing to adjust a fee in a hardship case once this has been proved.

When an account is submitted to an agency, all pertinent information should be provided by the doctor's office. Such data would include the full name of the patient and spouse or parent (or guardian), the most current address, the place of the patient's employment, a copy of the patient ledger card, and other information of interest and assistance to the agency. However, this information must be limited to nonclinical information.

When an agency assumes responsibility for the account, the doctor's office generally ceases all billings to the delinquent patient. All matters pertaining to the account are handled by the agency. Thus, if the patient calls the doctor's office about the account, the patient should be courteously referred to the agency. Payments now made to the office must be reported to the agency if agency collection efforts have begun. All payments should be made directly to the agency. The doctor's office will be copied by the agency of all transactions on a monthly basis. The patient's ledger card should then be updated according to the payments sent to the agency and the charge for its collection. The total is deducted from the patient's balance due.

Overdue bills submitted for collection by an agency are discounted. When the office uses an agency, the doctor is employing people skilled in the collection business and the doctor must expect to pay for their services. Almost all accounts turned over to an agency will be those that the doctor considers "uncollectable" by the office. Anything received is better than nothing.

One should not expect an agency to collect 100% of the accounts serviced. A 40%–50% collection rate by an agency is about average for accounts about 6 months old. If the agency is highly successful in recovering overdue accounts, it's an indication that your office should review its collection procedures. An abnormally high agency collection rate signals that the office is not doing its part in pursuing collections. Any health practice will have a number of accounts that are 30 days past due, and a lesser amount that are 60 days overdue. When many accounts run 90 days past due, you should take a hard look at your office's billing and collection policies and procedures.

The service charge made by most agencies is directed by the amount of the account. Some agencies charge a flat 50%. Others charge a third of the account if the account is less than 6 months old and 50% on older accounts or if the debtor has left the city. The average cost of collection is about 50%.

Legal Action

Your doctor-employer may prefer to use an attorney rather than an agency to collect delinquent accounts. Nonclinical records are turned over to the attorney as they would be to an agency. The usual procedure is to have the attorney proceed immediately to try to collect the amount owed. Most attorneys charge a fee of 50% of the account, as do collection agencies.

Suit can be brought, but it is usually considered unwise. Authorities advise, almost without exception, that the doctor should not go to court. One might feel that when a patient can pay but refuses to pay without sufficient reason that court action would be the most logical approach. However, lawsuits cost money and the doctor's time, and judgments are difficult to collect. In addition, some vindictive patients are likely to bring countersuit of malpractice against the doctor just for spite.

Rather than the doctor going to court, it is better that he assign the account to a third party and let the third party register the complaint and file suit. If the doctor sues and it is contested, he may have to appear in court and lose many valuable hours of clinical time, incur undesirable publicity, carry the burden of attorney's fees and the ever-present possibility of a countersuit as a reprisal by the patient.

No severe collection effort should be considered if (1) the patient is truly suffering from financial hardship, (2) there is likelihood of a countersuit, or (3) the amount is more than can be handled in a small claims court. The points that must be weighed are the clear rights of the claim, the patient's ability to pay, the exhaustion of other collection methods, and the justification of the amount by comparison with usual-and-customary fees in the area. All collection efforts must balance humanitarian principles with good business practices.

Canceled Accounts

It must be expected in health practice, as in any business, that some loss in uncollected fees will occur from "bad debts" and dishonest patients. Patients also will be encountered who find it impossible to pay the customary fee. To turn such accounts over to a collection agency would be unprofessional and only serves to harass the unfortunate. In these instances, the common procedure is to cancel the balance due and remove the debt from the books. However, when this action is taken, the act should be noted on the patient's permanent financial ledger card. Occasionally, a patient may later come on better times, remain a source of referrals, and return as a worthy patient—even to the extent of paying the long overdue bill.

The average patient who is unwilling to pay either cannot pay or may be disgruntled about the bill for some reason. More often than not, the reason is not the amount of the bill as much as it is an attitude flaw of the doctor or staff member. Thus, it's good policy to try to discuss the situation with the patient as a first step toward eliciting payment. Few patients are true "deadbeats" who don't intend to pay. However, it is these patients who cause the doctor to consider third-party action for collection.

It is important to the assistant in charge of collections that the doctor carefully explains his policy about collections. It is also important that the assistant be acquainted with the state laws involved and the Statute of Limitations in the state.

Computerized Billing Services

If a patient enters the typical office, the receptionist clips a visit slip to the patient's clinical folder, which accompanies the patient to the examining and therapy rooms.

The doctor indicates on the charge slip the services rendered so the assistant may total the fee for the visit and enter the data on the day sheet and patient's ledger card.

When outside computerized billing services are used, all charge slips along with an adding machine tape (which the assistant has run on the various charges and payments) are picked up by a representative from the computer billing office at the end of the day or week. Charges and receipts taken from the charge clips are then entered in a computer along with patient data that have previously been programmed.

Periodically, a *work sheet* is printed by the computer showing all patient visits, charges, receipts, and an aging of individual accounts. If more than one doctor works in the office, this work sheet shows which doctor has seen the patient and gives a detailed breakdown of the various procedures used in the office, the fees involved, and how much money the patient owes to each individual doctor.

At the end of the month, a master work sheet is printed by the computer. The computer also prints a monthly statement for each family with an account balance in the doctor's office. Doctors working with associates in a cost-sharing arrangement can receive a complete itemized breakdown of individual charges from the computer and an automatic computation of each doctor's share of overhead expenses for the month.

Benefits. Computerized billings allow the doctor to operate his front office with fewer personnel. It reduces the doctor's job of supervision of billing. It requires less office space and eliminates expensive bookkeeping and billing equipment outlays. It reduces duplicate billings involved in group practices and breaks down each doctor's business in multidoctor practices. It furnishes a complete and current age analysis of accounts. It reduces the chance of employee embezzlement by having all charges and receipts posted outside the office. It allows the doctor the opportunity to take advantage of the latest billing techniques and yields a greater degree of continuity in bookkeeping, billing, and collections.

Liabilities. Costs are slightly higher than in-office manual billing. Because the doctor's office does not keep ledger cards of patients' accounts, it is difficult for an assistant to answer patient inquiries concerning account status. Frequent communication between the office and agency may be required. Collection letters will be automatically mailed to patients according to aging of the account analysis—precluding the flexibility many doctors value in special circumstances. Computers do not have compassion.

Evaluation Criteria. Several factors are involved that should be considered before a decision is made to use a computerized billing service. The doctor should first carefully evaluate the efficiency, honesty, and stability of the companies offering such services in the area. He should talk with other doctors and companies using the service. Other questions that must be answered are: (1) Are qualified office personnel unavailable in the area? (2) Will patients object to impersonal billing? (3) Will prompt computerized billing improve an office's collection ratio? And (4), how convenient are the location and communications with the computerized billing service?

ACCOUNTS PAYABLE

Although a chiropractic office deals almost exclusively in services and has little dealings with wholesalers and suppliers, a systematic accounting of accounts payable or disbursements is nevertheless necessary. Because there is a limited number of suppliers and consequent bills to pay, and because almost every chiropractic office has one or more employees, it is advisable to incorporate into the accounts payable system the records required for payroll. An earnings record is shown in Figure 8.15 and an employee register in Figure 8.16.

To meet the basic requirements of most practices, an accounts payable system should (1) record total cash flow in and out of the practice and (2) require minimum attention from the doctor and his staff. The record of total cash flow includes the total income recorded from bank deposits with each deposit referenced to the billing and

EMPLOYEE EARNINGS RECORD

Name _____ No. of Exemptions _____
Address _____
Position _____ Starting date _____ Termination date _____

Year's FICA limit $_____ Rate_____
Year's Unemployment limit   _____ Rate_____

Next Review
_____
_____

Salary rate: $_____ per_____ as of_____
               _____ per_____ as of_____
               _____ per_____ as of_____

| Date | Gross Earnings | | | Taxes | | | | |
	Regular	Over-time	Total	FICA w/held	Fed. w/held	State w/held	Other	Total Deduc.
_____	$___	$___	$___	$___	$___	$___	$___	$___
Quarter Total								
Quarter Total								
Total to Date								

Figure 8.15A. Sample format of an employee's salary record, left-hand page.

Net Salary		Paid Days Off			Unpaid	
Check No.	Amount	Vacation	Sick-ness	Other	Days Off	Remarks
_____	$_____	_____	_____	_____	_____	_____
_____	_____	_____	_____	_____	_____	_____
_____	._____	_____	_____	_____	_____	_____
_____	_____	_____	_____	_____	_____	_____
_____	_____	_____	_____	_____	_____	_____
_____	_____	_____	_____	_____	_____	_____
Quarter Total	$_____	_____	_____	_____	_____	_____
_____	_____	_____	_____	_____	_____	_____
_____	_____	_____	_____	_____	_____	_____
_____	_____	_____	_____	_____	_____	_____
_____	_____	_____	_____	_____	_____	_____
_____	_____	_____	_____	_____	_____	_____
Quarter Total	_____	_____	_____	_____	_____	_____
_____	_____	_____	_____	_____	_____	_____
_____	_____	_____	_____	_____	_____	_____
_____	_____	_____	_____	_____	_____	_____
_____	_____	_____	_____	_____	_____	_____
Total to Date	_____	_____	_____	_____	_____	_____

Figure 8.15B. Sample right-hand page of an employee's salary record.

collecting system, detailed records of general accounts payable, and complete earnings and deduction records for the payroll account.

Although billing and collection systems require more attention, an accounts payable system is equally important. It should provide a complete record of total deposits (related to accounts payable) and all expenditures for the practice. In most practices, nearly all income will be from patients paying for services. Funds from other sources, however, should be recorded in the billing and collecting system so deposits to the

checking account can be accounted for by a simple reference to that system. Referencing deposit slips from the billing and collecting system into the accounts payable system provides an audit trail within the two systems.

Disbursements of checks for purposes other than employee salaries are simply those required to maintain the office and its equipment and supplies. Except regular disbursements such as for rent, utilities, telephone, and so forth, each bill should be approved for payment by the doctor before a check is drawn.

EMPLOYEE REGISTER

Name	No. of Exemptions	Hourly Rate	Hours Worked	Earnings		
				Regular	Overtime	Total

Payroll period _____

Total

Payroll period _____

Total

Payroll period _____

Total

Payroll period _____

Total

Figure 8.16A. Sample format for an employee register, left-hand page.

Taxable Earnings		Deductions				
FICA	Unemployment Ins.	FICA	Other	Total	Net Pay	Check No.
―――	―――	―――	―――	―――	―――	―――
―――	―――	―――	―――	―――	―――	―――
―――	―――	―――	―――	―――	―――	―――
―――	―――	―――	―――	―――	―――	―――
―――	―――	―――	―――	―――	―――	―――
Total	―――	―――	―――	―――	―――	―――
―――	―――	―――	―――	―――	―――	―――
―――	―――	―――	―――	―――	―――	―――
―――	―――	―――	―――	―――	―――	―――
―――	―――	―――	―――	―――	―――	―――
―――	―――	―――	―――	―――	―――	―――
Total	―――	―――	―――	―――	―――	―――
―――	―――	―――	―――	―――	―――	―――
―――	―――	―――	―――	―――	―――	―――
―――	―――	―――	―――	―――	―――	―――
―――	―――	―――	―――	―――	―――	―――
―――	―――	―――	―――	―――	―――	―――
Total	―――	―――	―――	―――	―――	―――
―――	―――	―――	―――	―――	―――	―――
―――	―――	―――	―――	―――	―――	―――
―――	―――	―――	―――	―――	―――	―――
―――	―――	―――	―――	―――	―――	―――
―――	―――	―――	―――	―――	―――	―――
Total	―――	―――	―――	―――	―――	―――

Figure 8.16B. Sample format for an employee register, right-hand page.

Because the usual transaction for accounts payable involves writing a check, a summary record of the checking account can be the basic record of any accounts payable system. A comprehensive record of deposits and withdrawals (checks) provides the doctor and his accountant with much of the financial information required to pre- pare various tax returns and useful periodic financial status reports and statements.

Checking Accounts

The typical doctor has two checking accounts. One account is used to pay bills of

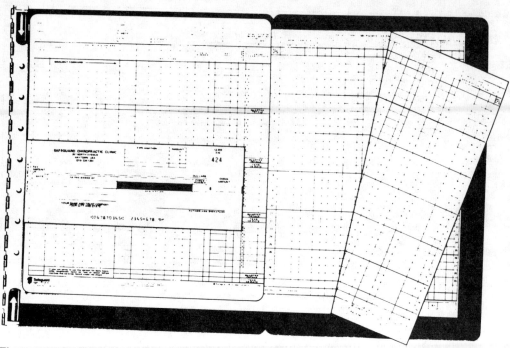

Figure 8.17. Pegboard checkwriting system (reprinted by permission of Safeguard Business Systems).

the office and the other is to pay his personal bills. These accounts are often in separate banks to avoid confusion and eliminate the possibility of mixed funds.

Daily receipts collected in the practice should be deposited in the office account. Thus, deposits shown in the office account will equal the collections posted in day sheets. Expenses concerning the operation of the practice will be issued on this account. No personal expenses or disbursements for the doctor's home or family should be paid on the office account unless an overlapping is involved such as in an office-home combination where costs are proportioned.

When bills are paid by check, the doctor has a permanent record of his expenditures as well as evidence of payment. See Figure 8.17.

It is usually the responsibility of an assistant to see that the office checkbook is current and accurate. Neatness and care are essential. Each check drawn should be clearly explained on the stub. The dates and amounts for deposits should be entered promptly and a running balance shown.

Most doctors pay themselves a salary. Once or twice a month a check is drawn and deposited to his personal checking account. Such a salary (draw) is called a *drawing account.* Office expenses are never paid from this account.

Daily Disbursement Record

Most bookkeeping systems have forms similar to the day sheets of patient services, charges, and payments on which the assistant records office disbursements. Cash or check payments are listed and placed in proper columns such as expendables (supplements, clinical supplies), maintenance (repairs, rent, utilities, laundry, office upkeep), salaries, dues, business-related taxes and licenses, communications (telephone, telegraph, telephone answering services), travel (auto, garage, parking, air travel), subscriptions (professional and business), con-

DIVIDEND RECORD							
Date	Rate	No. of Shares	Dividend Amount	Date	Rate	No. of Shares	Dividend Amount
____	____	____	$____	____	____	____	$____
____	____	____	____	____	____	____	____
____	____	____	____	____	____	____	____
____	____	____	____	____	____	____	____
____	____	____	____	____	____	____	____
____	____	____	____	____	____	____	____
____	____	____	____	____	____	____	____
____	____	____	____	____	____	____	____
____	____	____	____	____	____	____	____
____	____	____	____	____	____	____	____
____	____	____	____	____	____	____	____
____	____	____	____	____	____	____	____
____	____	____	____	____	____	____	____
____	____	____	____	____	____	____	____
____	____	____	____	____	____	____	____
____	____	____	____	____	____	____	____
____	____	____	____	____	____	____	____

Figure 8.18. Sample format to record dividends.

ventions (hotel, food, taxis), office supplies (stationery, postage, printing), x-ray (films, solutions, services), practice-related insurance and legal fees, collection fees, charitable contributions, and capital expenditures. Any expenditure in the latter column is not an operating expense. It must be depreciated and should be listed separately from tax-deductible expenses. In addition, if the doctor receives income from nonpractice-related sources (profits from sale of stocks, dividends, interest earned) this should be listed as "personal" and itemized. See Figures 8.18 and 8.19.

You may at times be uncertain whether an expense is a professional or personal one. The way in which allocations are made determines which items are deductible and which are not. This can make a difference in taxes paid, so the assistant must use great care and not guess. When in doubt, ask the doctor or his accountant.

The General Ledger

Totals from day sheets and those from daily disbursement records are usually transferred to a permanent ledger each day so that totals on all income and expenditures can be tallied at the end of each month. A monthly statement of income, expenditures, net gain and loss, and other evaluation information can be prepared from this information. As the year progresses, this forms the basis for an annual statement of the practice.

The day sheet and monthly summaries, the doctor's checkbooks and monthly bank statements, patients' financial ledger cards,

BANK ACCOUNT

Account in Name of _____ Account No. _____

Name of Bank _____ Type of Account _____

Address of Bank _____

Officer Contact _____ Title _____ Phone _____

Authorized Signatures _____   _____

Custodian of Bank Book _____   Interest

Remarks _____

Date	%
___	___
___	___
___	___

Date	Deposit	Interest	Total	Withdrawal	Balance
___	$___	$___	$___	$___	$___

Figure 8.19. Sample format for a savings account log.

daily disbursement records, and the general ledger are the key elements of a doctor's bookkeeping system. The accumulated data these records yield are used to analyze the doctor's financial status and to compute his income tax liabilities.

The responsibility of maintaining the general ledger and its categories for asset accounts, liability accounts, income accounts, and operating expenses is usually that of an accountant rather than that of a doctor's assistant.

Bills and Invoices

As bills/invoices are received, place them in a specially marked folder separated from other records. Before paying bills, check the respective statements to assure they haven't been duplicated. See if credits due are on the statement. Check the amount. If there is any question of incorrectness, do not pay it until the query is answered.

Outstanding bills are generally paid by the 10th of the month. As some bills allow a discount if paid before the due date, figure and subtract the discount before payment is made. Payment is usually made by check unless it is under a dollar, in which case it may come from petty cash if payment is made in person. Money of any amount should not be mailed. All payments for outstanding bills that are practice related should be recorded in the disbursements record.

Whenever a bill is paid, a notation should be made on the invoice or statement of the date of payment, amount paid, and office check number. An office stamp may be used that has spaces on it to record the needed information.

In preparing checks, type or write neatly. Do the stub first, then you won't forget if interrupted. Information on the stub should be inclusive such as name of person or firm paid, what was purchased, invoice number, amount of bill, discount if any, and balance remaining. If paid in full, note this on both the stub and check.

Deliveries

A "packing slip" will usually be included with each order of merchandise delivered to the office. When received, check the delivery to assure all items listed on the packing slip are included. Initial the slip and file it in the accounts payable file. When you are billed, the invoice should carry the same number as the packing slip. Be sure that you are being charged only for materials received. The invoice numbers and total amount of each invoice will be listed on the monthly statement. Check the correctness of the statement before writing the payment check. Staple the statement, invoices, and packing slips together before filing.

Credit Memos

If merchandise is returned for credit, you should receive a *credit memo* for the purchase. Note on the statement that a charge has been made on one invoice number and a credit has been issued on another invoice number for the returned items. Check the statement to see that a credit has been made in the payment column. When returning something for credit, note this in the accounts payable file so you can later check to see that credit has been given. If you are responsible for writing checks for accounts payable, assure that the doctor is not paying for items that have not been received or which have been returned.

Credit Adjustments

A credit adjustment is a revision of charges to meet special situations. Perhaps a patient convinces the doctor that a fee adjustment is warranted. There must be a method of handling such entries once the regular fee has been entered in the records. This is done by entering the amount of reduction in the charge column in red or placing parentheses around the figure to denote a minus amount when totaling the column. A credit adjustment must be placed in both the day sheet and patient's financial ledger card.

Outside Laboratory Charges

Laboratory charges can be handled in one of two ways. Your office may make the charge, collect the fee, be billed by the laboratory, and pay the laboratory. Or, the laboratory will bill the patient directly, and thus not involve your office with the charges involved. If the latter method is used for mailed-in specimens, be sure to provide the laboratory with the correct name and address of each patient for whom a specimen is sent for analysis.

PETTY CASH

While major expenses should always be paid by check, there are some small expenditures for which you usually do not write a check, or a checkbook is not available at the time. In almost every office there are occasions for very small cash expenditures such as tips to delivery men, small item purchases, newspapers, and so forth.

A small sum of money, usually from $5 to $50, should be allotted to a petty cash drawer or box and charged on the office disbursement sheet against "Petty Cash." Most offices use a simplified cash voucher system consisting of 12 special envelopes, one for each month. Receipts or sales slips are deposited in the envelope for the month each time a purchase is made. At the end of the month, the receipts and slips are totaled and balanced against the cash on hand in the envelope.

Mechanics. As the amount of petty cash is spent or runs low, it should be replenished. To bring it back to the original amount, subtract remaining cash from the base sum established. Write a check payable to "Petty Cash," which the doctor will sign and endorse. Cash it at the bank for change and small bills, and place it in the "Petty Cash" envelope.

Whenever a check is written to "Petty Cash," it should be entered under the appropriate columns in the disbursement sheet under the expense categories. This is one of the few times a check could be distributed to more than one expense column, depend-

ing on the breakdown of petty cash receipts. Care should be taken in this multidistribution to assure the total in each column equals the amount of the check.

Voucher Systems. Use a voucher system to keep track of small expenditures. When you pay a small bill from petty cash or use the money for any reason, get a receipt or make out a voucher showing the amount, date, and reason. Keep receipts and vouchers in the proper monthly envelope. A tally of these plus the remaining cash should total the original sum. All envelopes with their receipts and vouchers should be filed for tax purposes. See Figure 8.20.

Security. Keep petty cash in a safe place, preferably in a locked drawer. A small triple-column account book can be kept within the current envelope or a list can be printed on the outside of each envelope. Within the columns, indicate debts, credits, and balance on hand. No money should be removed unless the amount, reason for taking it, name of person making the withdrawal, and the date are shown.

EXTRA CASH

Extra cash is different from petty cash. It is an amount of money kept in a special envelope or drawer that allows you to have change for patients paying their bills in cash. It is usually considered poor policy to use the office's extra cash to cash patients' checks or to accommodate patients who wish to write a check for a larger amount than due and receive the balance in cash.

RECONCILING BANK STATEMENTS

When the monthly bank statement for the office account arrives, it is usually the responsibility of the assistant in charge of billings and collections to reconcile the statement with office records. The procedure is:

1. Arrange all canceled checks in numerical order, or, if not numbered, arrange by date.

```
                    RECEIVED FROM PETTY CASH

No. _____  Date _____  19__

Amount $ _____  By _____

For _____

_____

Charge to _____ _____ account.

Posted ☐ by _____ on _____
        (Initial)      (Date)
```

Figure 8.20. Sample format for a petty cash voucher.

2. Compare each check with its stub. If they match in amount, put a check mark on a corner of each.

3. List each check that has not been returned. There is usually a section on the back of the statement for this.

4. Compute an *adjusted checkbook balance* by taking the balance after the last stub was written, adding deposits that have been made but not yet entered, correcting errors made in carrying forward figures, and subtracting debit memos made by the bank (carrying charges, printing of checkbooks, etc).

5. List checks still outstanding and add them to the adjusted balance. This should be the same amount shown on the bank statement.

6. Add or subtract the difference between the adjusted balance and the amount carried in the checkbook to the running total to bring the two in balance.

FINANCIAL CONTROL

There are several ways for checking and rechecking the accuracy of bookkeeping. For example:

• Cash received from patients in the office on a given day should tally with cash received according to the day sheet.

• Income received from the practice *plus* other taxable income received *plus* tax-free income received should equal total deposits *plus* the amount on hand remaining to be deposited *plus* any cash withdrawn by the doctor before deposit.

• The total checks written should equal the total of personal expenditures when taken *plus* operating expenses *plus* capital expenditures. To reconcile payroll figures, adjust the amount withheld from gross salaries to coincide with the amount of checks written to pay net salaries.

Periodic Financial Responsibilities

Daily. Post charges and payments on the day sheet and patient financial ledger forms; bank deposit slips and deposits are prepared as required. Reconcile cash intake with receipts written. When proved at the end of the day, deposit cash in the bank.

Bimonthly. Enter information in payroll record from salary checks written.

Monthly. Reconcile bank statement to checkbook. Complete posting of day sheets, monthly summary, disbursement sheets, and permanent journal. Make office billings. Prepare monthly *profit and loss statement* if requested.

Quarterly. Analyze open accounts, putting all active accounts into the following categories: (1) less than 30 days since last date of service, (2) 30 to 60 days since last day of service, (3) 60 to 90 days, (4) 3 to 6 months, (5) 6 months to 1 year, and (6) 1 year. If an accountant does not prepare Federal Employment Forms and other quarterly forms, this may be the responsibility of an assistant.

Annually. If an accountant does not prepare the yearly reconciliation form showing withholding payments made for the quarters; W-2 forms showing total salaries paid to each employee, amount withheld, and Social Security taxes paid; then an assistant may be asked to prepare them. They must be mailed with remittance for the 4th quarter by January 31 of the following year.

Condensed Tax Form Timetable

• Near the last day of month following end of the quarter, file quarterly reports: April 30, first quarter; July 31, second quarter; October 31, third quarter; January 31, fourth quarter and year end.

• On January 31, file reconciliation of federal income tax withheld from wages during previous year (Form W-2). Attach copy A of W-2 Form for each employee. Copies B and C of the W-2 Form go to the employee, and D is retained in office files.

• January 15 is the deadline for filing final estimated tax payment and making adjustments for the year.

• Before April 15, file personal federal income tax return, and be sure that the check accompanying this return is properly prepared and signed. File first quarter estimated income-tax payment.

• June 15 is deadline for filing second quarter estimated income-tax payment.

• September 15 is deadline for filing third quarter estimated income tax payment and making adjustments.

• Check miscellaneous due dates for local or state taxes.

Payroll Records

Payroll disbursements require considerably more documentation than general disbursements and require additional records such as a statement of earnings and deductions for each employee as well as a summary of earnings and deductions for all employees. To incorporate payroll records in a single accounts payable system and by that avoid creating additional work, a more effective system for payroll than the standard three-to-a-page checkbook is desirable.

Doctors managing large or multiple establishments may have several payroll records with which to contend. Pegboard systems designed specifically for this problem combine disbursements with payroll and require just one writing to produce the payroll check and employee's statement of earnings and deductions, and to create a payroll journal and earnings record. Proving the journal automatically proves all other records, eliminating the need for separate entries and potential errors and omissions that are difficult to trace and time-consuming to adjust. This system would be similar to that shown in Figure 8.17.

Almost all payroll systems will have three parts: (1) the special payroll check, which is usually a duplicate where the duplicate is used as a voucher for a statement of earnings and deductions for the employee; (2) an employee earnings ledger form; and (3) a payroll disbursement journal sheet for the staff.

MANAGING THE DOCTOR'S PERSONAL ACCOUNTS

This chapter so far and the previous chapter have been concerned with systems designed to promote accountability and efficiency in connection with the doctor's principal business enterprise—his practice. There is another facet of a doctor's financial planning, however, that must not be overlooked; namely, the management and disposal of personal income.

Well-established doctors, lawyers, and other professionals often exercise direct control over sizable assets and engage in a diversity of outside financial interests and investments. To realize the greatest benefit from these, a systematic, uncomplicated means of keeping records is a necessity. Any enterprise, large or small, requires records that have management information available as well as adequate information for tax purposes. In the simplest case, these records can be an integral part of the doctor's personal checking account. There also are one-write systems available to meet a variety of requirements in handling a doctor's personal finances. The extent and complexity of a doctor's personal financial involvements determine which of many systems will best serve his needs.

A good system such as that recommended by Safeguard Business Systems, Inc, offers a one-write disbursement system that serves as the checkbook for the doctor's personal or joint checking account and at the same time provides an accounting of personal and investment expenses for tax purposes. It is sufficiently versatile and comprehensive to keep all necessary records and can be adapted to provide inputs for data processing if desired.

PRACTICES CAN GET SICK TOO!

As a person can become ill from either underindulgence or overindulgence, a practice can get sick from either low income or high costs. Accurate monthly reports of patient volume, collections, expenditures, and referrals offer a running record of practice growth or sickness. There are only so many hours in an office day, so many productive days in a month, and so many months in a year. Thus, periodic production analyses are important to determine practice efficiency.

High income in a practice is always proportional to high service when the practice is service oriented. When service and income are high, money is available for good salaries, equipment, and facilities necessary to conduct a quality professional service. When costs exceed income, everything suffers. If the patient volume is far below potential, there is a minus return on investment. The successful practice is that practice which does the most good for the most people at reasonable cost.

When an individual becomes ill, the doctor is able to determine certain signs and symptoms. When a practice becomes ill, a management consultant can determine its state of health by observing certain signs and symptoms. Following are a few examples noticed repeatedly in an ailing practice:

1. Office personnel who believe they are more important than the patients they serve.

2. Office personnel who fail to take the time to explain each procedure and policy carefully in terms of benefits and value to the patient.

3. Office personnel who belittle and talk down to patients when seemingly naive questions are asked.

4. Office personnel who tend to be procedure oriented rather than people oriented.

5. Office personnel who shuttle patients from here to there with little attention to the human relations involved.

6. Office personnel who believe they have something to offer that patients cannot obtain elsewhere.

7. Office personnel who are unable to look at themselves through the eyes of a typical patient.

8. Office personnel who "never have the time" to do something special, something extra, something unusually kind.

9. Office personnel who constantly talk about "serving humanity" but rarely serve the individual patient before them.

10. Office personnel who believe a good location, shiny equipment, and fancy archi-

tecture will attract patients and build referrals.

It's important to note in these ten signs and symptoms that each pertains to office personnel. One practice consultant puts it very plainly: "It's simple. The stagnant or failing practice is characterized by personnel who refuse to do those things personnel in a successful practice do. It usually is a fault in self-image. They are more interested in preserving a principle or a policy than providing a health service."

Professional aloofness, patient detachment, and self-centered behavior are often difficult to see in oneself, but the point of change can only begin at the point of recognition. Low referral rate and patient feedback are primary indicators for they measure patient motivation. The quantities of scheduled appointments and complaints are other indicators, but they may indicate *captive* patients rather than *captivated* patients.

When patients leave one practice to enter another, they rarely state why. However, public opinion surveys appear to be one medium where patients are more open and responsive to direct questions. Below is a listing taken from polls showing the seven most common complaints patients have about health-care personnel:

Indifference to personal feelings
• General attitude of superiority
• Abrupt response to questions
• Handle patients hurriedly and rudely
• Patronizing airs
• High fees without prior explanation
• Long waiting time to see the doctor for only a few moments

Note that of these seven major complaints, the first five concern personnel attitude while the last two concern poor communications. Unfortunately, those who are the most guilty are those who are most defensive.

One office that has an extremely high rate of referrals does not believe in indirect patient feedback. Periodically, patients are surveyed "in the interest of improving our health service." For instance, the office may ask, "Were all office procedures and fees explained to your satisfaction?" "Did you receive the personal and professional attention you expected?" "Did you mention the quality of service received to the person who referred you to the office?" "Would you recommend our health services to others?" "Do you have any suggestions that you feel would tend to improve the services we now offer?"

Are these questions direct? Yes. Are they blunt? Perhaps, but they are candid. And it must be said that when direct questions are asked, they are requested by people who are not afraid of the answers they may hear. Those who are afraid of honest feedback will not ask such questions.

While securing patient feedback may be new to the health professions, it is not new in the business world. Polls among consumers are an age-old practice. Good managers ask for feedback from their employees. Poor managers, afraid that their operation may not be as rosy as they fantasize, prefer Machiavellian autocracy, and the result is detrimental to their best interests. Similarly, doctors can learn much from their experienced assistants if they would just ask.

Another good source of feedback is from the entering patient who has a history of seeing several doctors for the same condition. You can tactfully learn why the patient left the previous doctors to avoid repeating the same mistakes. It should be remembered, however, that "poor results" will usually be the first reason offered. But technical competency is rarely the cause once you get to the heart of the problem. Questions concerning previous care will be accepted as normal by the patient during the recording of the case history.

Self-Appraisal. A teaching aid for both assistant and doctor is a simple tape recorder. Periodically, the doctor should record his consultations and talks with patients, and assistants should record their conversations. It is an excellent method to critique both conversational and communications skills. You can quickly learn if you are talking too slow or too fast, slurring your words, or lacking enthusiasm. You can check grammar, speech patterns, and ability to draw mental pictures. Are you too technical or too earthy? Are you convincing? Do you sound sincere? Do you get patient feedback to assure that the patient understands? These things and more can be learned in privacy.

Goal Setting and Achievement: Personal and Professional

Brainstorming and goal setting sessions among office staff are helpful functions in maintaining and progressing a successful health practice. These sessions can promote a team spirit, unify actions, define purposes, resolve problems, set objectives, and establish timetables.

One management consultant reports that 95% of people direct their courses not much better than a ship without a rudder—subject to every wind and reef. Hypnotized by the hope that they will eventually drift into a successful port, they are unaware that for every port there are thousands of miles of rocky coastline studded with shipwrecked lives. It's only 5% who have pinpointed a destination, mapped the reefs, and charted a course so that they sail straight and sure—reaching one successful port after another. Although they may not be able to view their destination in detail for fully 99% of the way, they know from the beginning of their journey what they are after, where it is, and how they will get there.

Specification. When setting a plan of action, it is important to etch vivid, detailed thoughts rather than vague generalizations. The more one can pinpoint what is wanted, the more likely it will be attained. You must formulate your personal definition of who you are and what you want.

Visualization. Learn to make desires specific and personal. They must be something you can achieve to have power—something in harmony with your nature. Analyze your basic wants, and learn to put them on paper. Be realistic. Then list the logical steps you must take to realize your desires. Whatever you can conceive, you can achieve if you are willing to pay the price. Indefinite plans produce indefinite results. Without specific visualization, we flounder.

Perception. By being specific in what we want, by vividly picturing our priority goals

and all their ramifications, we change the indefinite general into a definite specific. Specific, detailed visualization prevents anxiety and fear because the unknown is known. Without fear and anxiety, thinking becomes clear and perceptive to opportunities. Possible areas for error and obstacles can be foreseen with planning, and corrective measures can be taken far in advance. Perception enhances desire, willpower, and determination.

Develop a Plan of Action. Once you have clarified your thinking and prepared a detailed description of your goals, the next step is the construction of a detailed plan of action. Undoubtedly, certain barriers are between where you are now and where you wish to be or you would have achieved your goal long ago. Now is the time for cold analysis. Carefully list all reasons and circumstances that you can think of that have prevented success in the past. Apply fundamental problem-solving techniques. Face every obstacle squarely and recognize it for what it is. Is it a physical barrier or a mental/emotional block? Separate the real from the false, the tangible from the intangible, the facts from theories, and opinions from superstitions.

Only a few obstacles will be real such as a lack of specific knowledge. Such a limitation can easily be conquered by library research, taking a few extension or correspondence courses, or conferring with an expert in the field. It is well to find a mentor.

Set a Timetable. In addition to recognizing obstacles and preparing a course of action, specific dates and deadlines ignite the fuses of dormant energy. Besides giving a guideline to how long it will take to accomplish any task, a personal commitment is made that spurs dynamic involvement. If not, we have good reason to question our sincerity.

Here are some foundations to remember in building successful plans.

1. When you accept a plan or strategy, you automatically must accept the goal of the plan.

2. Check the effects of the goal against your personal goals to assure compatibility. Harmony is necessary for optimum involve-

ment. To assure success, personal habits (mental and physical) must be in harmony with the plan's strategy and responsibilities.

3. Maintain sufficient control. Authority can be delegated, never final responsibility. Evaluate delegated performance periodically and relate it to your plan's timetable. Control action/response in these common obstacles: (a) environment, (b) personal attitudes, (c) attitudes of personalities involved, and (d) attitudes of personalities affected by the goal.

4. Success of a plan is rarely determined by "things." Ninety-five percent of the time success is determined by people. You will usually execute the plan.

5. You must have sufficient knowledge in the field of your plan to prepare an efficient strategy that avoids barriers and hurdles common obstacles.

6. People at rest tend to remain at rest; people in motion tend to remain in motion. Thus, the first step toward doing anything is vital—the going becomes easier to overcome resistances once we get out of neutral gear.

7. If several alternative plans are available to reach the same goal, rate each plan with its pros and cons before making a final decision. Weigh personal desires and wants against all the evidence.

8. Prepare for possible repercussions. Before a decision is made, estimate what the other people's reactions will be. If the response is negative, why? Change effects by changing causes. Amend your course if necessary.

9. More is needed besides the effort of Will—and that is *leverage*. The leverage that separates the actualized from the underachiever has two basic forms, external and internal. External leverage is found in management mechanics, organization, communications, and human relations. Internal leverage is found in strategic thinking, goal setting, decision making, self-image development, and an integrated personality.

10. When properly used, a pencil and paper can be worth their weight in diamonds.

When facing a confusing choice or a complicated decision, jot down alternatives and study their pros and cons. A complicated problem can be broken into simple components easier on paper than in your head. Those "must-do" jobs won't slip by so easily. Likewise, a pocket notebook for bright ideas, appointments, and often-used telephone numbers and addresses eliminates trying to remember everything. A pocket electronic calculator is a helpful aid in computations.

It has been explained that the most successful health practices are those that put human relations as their priority. This takes planning, goal setting, constant re-evaluation, and harmonizing the goals of office personnel with the goals of the practice so everyone will be working in the same direction and mutually benefit in goal achievement. The reason for this is that organizational goals are the total of individual goals. It is almost impossible to have practice growth and improved human relations without personal self-improvement.

It is important that goals are realistic, and they become more realistic the more we can break them down into small achievable increments. For instance, to set a personal or practice goal to double present performance or income or patient volume in a few years is idealistic but often discouraging. However, these things can be doubled much more realistically by thinking in terms of a 2% increase each month for 3 years or a 1% increase each month for 6 years. Such goals are realistic and attainable by the average person.

The Art of Practice Development

Because most patients (94%) entering a practice are referred by current patients, the importance of the patient at hand is emphasized not only for present survival of the practice but also for potential growth of the practice in future years. Practices suffering a long period in getting established are those that fail to instill in each patient the value of the services provided. If this value is not instilled in current patients, it cannot be transmitted to prospective patients. A patient cannot express unless he or she has been impressed.

Doctors report that most patients who refer are those new to the practice. The reasons given are that at this time the patient is most impressed with the new services and their quality, they desire to tell others about the practice to reaffirm their decision, and symptomatic relief places them on a high level of motivation. This is a half truth. The other side of the coin is that patients associated with the practice for a long period are often taken for granted and handled hastily. Too often, the doctor and assistant radiate enthusiasm and interest in the new patient that is denied to the established patient. Thus, for a continued source of referrals and high-level patient motivation, enthusiastic interest and personalized attention must be given to each patient throughout their entire association with the practice, not just in the orientation stage.

A patient's esteem for the doctor and his assistants is the foundation for doctor-patient and assistant-patient relationships. It is the basis for patient motivation and referrals. The patient will be enthusiastic about the health care offered in almost direct proportion that the doctor and assistants are enthusiastic about the patient as an individual, a human being. When staff works hard in the best interests of the patient—physically and emotionally—the patient will reflect this attitude toward relatives, friends, and colleagues.

Patient Classifications and Codes

In the description of filing systems, several different systems for classifying patients were described. Here we shall recount a few more that are pertinent to human relations and practice development.

Human Relations Coding. Some successful doctors code different types of patients by using various colored tabs on their records to alert staff of special problems or procedures. For instance, an average patient may be coded with a certain color to indicate that routine handling is usually sufficient. Another color may indicate that the patient is temperamental, high strung, and may require special consideration and tact.

Another color may show that the patient has shown himself to be an excellent source of referrals but requires constant ego nourishment.

Social Conversation Clues. Some doctors desire a conversation guide to be included in patients' records so they may personalize their conversations. This guide could list facts about a patient's general temperament, response to compliments, patient's progress as it pertains to the patient's lifestyle, cooperativeness and its consequences, anxiety or depression, known worries and fears, hobbies and work, ability to follow instructions, or other personal guidelines.

Procurement Programs. Patient procurement programs may be classified into three distinct divisions: (1) personal, (2) regular, and (3) irregular.

• Within the *personal division* can be classified activities involving community relations, family lifestyle and activities, office location and atmosphere, personal areas of influence, personality, character, temperament, reputation, and professionalism.

• Within the *regular division* are those routine actions such as mailings, congratulatory letters, thank you notes, directory listings, periodic news releases, new-patient orientation, service club responsibilities, and all other functions that are implemented on a regular and periodic basis.

• The *irregular division* incorporates seasonal and sporadic activities defined by climate and geographic location, by urban or rural factors, and by other variables particular to the practice. These activities should be designed to augment regular activities during a predictable "slump" period.

Another type of coding involves classifying patients into the categories of (1) new patients, (2) current patients, and (3) former patients. *New patients* are those who have never been to your office before or possibly never been to a doctor of chiropractic before. *Current patients* are those now under care and the primary source of referrals if they are impressed with the services and appreciate the specialized attention. *Former patients* are discharged patients who return, often needing indoctrination to new office procedures and policies established since their last visit.

Still another type of classification system is that recommended by practice consultant Levoy which is used to let you know where and with whom to concentrate your efforts. In this system, patients are rated A, B, C, or D types:

A. Well-informed patients who understand and appreciate your services, quickly respond to your requests, pay promptly, are enthusiastic sources of referrals, and respond well to suggestions for a continuous health-maintenance program after recovery of their original complaints.

B. Enlightened but not inspired patients who are receptive to persuasion but rarely take the initiative without some urging. Patient education and motivation often develop these patients into the A category.

C. Moderate understanding and appreciation characterize these patients. Their apathy and procrastination can be overcome sometimes with persistence, patience, education, and positive human relations. Many evolve to the B category after considerable effort.

D. Cost- and time-conscious patients seeking "first aid" rather than a comprehensive therapy and preventative program. As they are not ready for it, much time can be wasted on this type of patient trying to convince them of the error of their ways. They have little loyalty to any practice, and the best that can be hoped for is to evolve them to a C category.

Each patient can be observed and assigned a rating, with your highest concentration on educating categories B and C. How long does it take to evolve a patient from one category to another? That depends on the staff's personal understanding of human nature and ability to communicate and motivate. Sometimes it will be only a matter of a visit or two; sometimes it may take much longer.

Sustaining Practice Growth

Many years of study do not guarantee a doctor a successful practice; nor does an attractive office in a nice location that incorporates modern equipment and furnishings. These factors only establish an opportunity for success. Any professional or businessman needs new people to replace dropouts and an abundance of returning people. This takes continuous positive impressions.

Funding. Seed money must be available. As a businessman must have funds available for advertising and promotion, the professional requires capital to maintain both regular and irregular practice development programs to let the public know where the office is and what services are offered. A percentage for such activities is usually incorporated into the office fee, being as high as 35% for a new practice to as low as 10% for an established practice.

Auxiliary Practice. Some young practitioners augment their income by opening an *auxiliary office* in a small community from 10 to 25 miles from their main office. Usually, an auxiliary office is minimally staffed and equipped to handle routine cases—complicated cases requiring more sophisticated equipment are referred to the main office after screening. Sometimes inexpensive accommodations can be found, and sometimes the recent graduate will serve as an associate for an established practitioner in the small community. As word-of-mouth advertising travels faster in a smaller community, a productive but limited practice can be developed in a few years.

Communication. Another procedure helpful to sustaining practice growth is to have the telephone company periodically survey the number of busy signals on office lines during several typical days. As the practice progresses, communications volume increases proportionately. As the office telephone is the major link with the outside, care must be taken not to discourage callers by making it difficult for them to contact the office.

The telephone is also an important instrument in the office's general development program. It is the medium to check on emergency cases, missed appointments, scheduled appointments, and to contact suppliers and consultants. It can be used discreetly to suggest a periodic checkup among former patients, and to remind parents of preschool examinations for their children. These are excellent methods to fill openings between current patients to maintain maximum productivity.

Patient Education. The importance of continual patient education cannot be overemphasized for two major reasons. First, repetition is usually required in the learning process. Second, continual progress within the arts and sciences requires updating and amending procedures and policies that must be communicated to each current patient as well as each patient entering the practice.

Planning. Despite what type classification system is used, each system must be tailored to meet the requirements of an individual practice and all the staff must be aware of and capable of what functions should be carried out in each division. Frequently, general classifications must be subdivided, especially if weaknesses are found. When weak areas are isolated, brainstorm, plan a strategy, set check points, and reevaluate effectiveness periodically. See Figure 8.21. Every strategy must consider the personalities and motivation involved if it is to be effective, and it must consider harmonious integration with other policies and procedures and not be considered a separate entity in itself.

In addition to evolving procedures and policies, change just for the sake of change is a motivational factor. Periodic changes in office decor, furniture arrangement, routines, professional attire, and so forth, indicate to patients the office's attempt to keep "up to date." Worthy change can turn apathy into enthusiasm, a rut into a pathway.

The Referral Practice: Key to Economic Growth

Keep in mind that patient procurement techniques are always auxiliary to and supportive of the key to practice development—referrals by current patients. Auxiliary techniques are designed to obtain attention and interest. Referrals require the development of desire and action, and these are in-office goals that require personalized attention and service.

Those of us who work in chiropractic every day realize full well the benefits of chiropractic health care. Our awareness must be communicated as a service to the sick and disabled. Because the minority health professions realize little free publicity compared to that of traditional medicine, it's the duty and responsibility of office staff to tell the "chiropractic story" to everyone, everywhere, at every logical opportunity. This takes the form of professional public relations, but these techniques should never take priority over offering the best in-office service and communications possible.

The development of a referral practice is not just the application of certain techniques although many ways and means are described in this book. The development of a referral practice is actually the result of an office's *human relations philosophy*. As such, the philosophy enters all financial, administrative, technical, and clinical functions of the practice. When it is expressed by enthusiastic personnel, the result is automatic and not the implementation of a "technique." When it is automatic, you will naturally:

• Impress patients with the results they have realized.

• Suggest to patients they mention chiropractic to their friends, relatives, neighbors, and associates when the patient is at their peak of enthusiasm.

• Use office communications such as appointment reminders, thank you notes, follow-up letters, hand-out literature, and congratulatory cards to reinforce the office's interest and concern.

• Take the initiative to suggest chiropractic health care when anyone mentions a sick or disabled friend or relative.

Enthusiasm is an indispensable ingredient of practice development and the foundation for developing yourself in your career. It is also the spice of life that makes

MONTHLY PATIENT STATUS RECORD

	A No. of Entering Patient Consultations	B No. of Established Patient Appointments	C No. of Patients Discharged	D No. of Dropouts
January				
February				
March				
April				
May				
June				
July				
August				
September				
October				
November				
December				
TOTAL				

Figure 8.21. Sample format of a monthly patient status record. Column A shows the results of a practice development program and referrals. Column B, the number of office visits made by current patient succeeding visits and returning former patients. Column C, the quantity of patients discharged; and Column D, the number of patients self-discharged. These figures provide data to evaluate the practice's public relations program (A), current patient load (A + B), attrition rate (C), and patient-satisfaction level (D/A + B).

work enjoyable. Thus, it's to your advantage to avoid factors that sap your energy and enthusiasm. Poor health, association with negative friends, indebtedness, lack of significant goals, unrealistic self-criticism or guilt, and poor personal habits are just a few of the enemies of enthusiasm.

When a patient pays a fee and receives the results anticipated, he is not obligated to refer others to the practice. He has paid for and received a health service. While he is not obligated to refer, he will if the human relationship with the practice is positive and enthusiastic. Then he wants to tell others. Again, if he is impressed, he will express.

Characteristics of a Positive Philosophy

The highly successful doctor or assistant is not necessarily an assertive personality. Nor is an abnormally high degree of technical competency a requirement, but using the competence you have to a maximum *is* essential. A sincere desire to serve plus effective human relations reinforce and maximize technical competence. Approval, praise, agreement, kindness, acceptance, understanding, interest, special attention, pleasantness—these are the easily applied power tools that turn people "on" when offered freely and honestly, or turn people "off" when denied or used as a "gimmick."

When expressing a valuable philosophy, you will automatically want to know patients better and let them know you better. In turn they will respond positively because of your sincerity. You will want to let patients know what's happening in the office—new equipment, new procedures, developments. You will want to let patients know what's happening in chiropractic education, in chiropractic research, in current public health awareness campaigns.

You will spontaneously want to deal with people as individuals on a person-to-person basis, not as "cases." As it is a contagious addiction, patients will catch your enthusiasm, spread it to others, and return to you for reinforcement. You will want to learn what people need, why they need it, when they need it, and how you can help them achieve it—because you *care*. You are sensitive and responsive, and people know it.

Whenever two personalities come in contact, an influence is made on both even if the contact is only for an instant. The longer the contact, the longer the influence—good or bad. What is said or not said, or did or not done, leaves an impression that may be positive or negative in influence. If the sway is the result of high pressure, action will be short-term and restrictive. However, if the influence is motivational, creating a "want to" response, the action will be long term and restricted very little.

People don't want to be high pressured, they don't want to be "scared" into doing even what is right for them, and they don't want to be forced into a position where they feel they have no choice in the matter. They are not deeply interested in the office's services and equipment, but they are interested in what the office's services and equipment will do *for* them. They always want to know "Why?"

Once patient motivation is established, it must be constantly fortified. Motivational reinforcement is as important as "follow through" is to a professional athlete. While it takes the most energy to get an object moving, it also takes some sustained energy to maintain momentum. This is why there should be no let up in personalized attention offered to established patients. Patients become "backsliders" as a result of poor human relations and a failure to follow through properly.

Remember that human behavior is fairly predictable. People tend to repeat their behavior and responses unless there is motivation to change. Thus, when a cooperative patient becomes uncooperative, seek a flaw in the relationship somewhere and do what you can to resolve the problem. "Thank you," deserved praise, recognition, and other simple acts may appear to be little things. Yet their lack can be the chief reason for uncooperativeness, late payments and canceled appointments, or failure to refer others to the practice as frequently as before.

Even when you have premium intentions, your sincerity and kindness may be misinterpreted by some. There is a type of individual who has suffered greatly in life. When someone is kind to them, it is almost impossible for them to accept a kindness or gift without a great deal of suspicion—feeling that there must be some "motive" behind an act appearing to be sensitive or generous. Because of past negative experiences, these people will go through life turning pleasure into pain. They learn to cope with pain, but not with pleasure; with fear, but not with faith. They would rather think the worst than leave themselves vulnerable to hope that may prove later to be a painful error. Here you have a dilemma. If you increase positive human relations, you increase their suspicions. If you decrease positive relations, you reinforce their suspicions. All you can do is what you think is right action, for it is the individual's programming and habit patterns that turn your right actions into something they are not.

When patients mention how well they are feeling, learn to embellish this. It will help the patient learn to vocalize their feelings. If they can testify before you and receive an enthusiastic response, they will be more inclined to attest before others. When patients feel better, they want to tell others yet are often timid in self-expression. Learn to be a sounding board where you can offer subtle responses that increase the patient's candid self-expression, and the patient will automatically incorporate them into his story when it is repeated.

If patients discuss a sick friend or relative, give them some appropriate literature to pass along. Rest assured that the patient will mention where they received the literature.

Satisfied patients are not those that build a practice. *Enthusiastic* patients are the centers of influence. The art of turning satisfied patients into enthusiastic patients is developed by awarding patients more than they expect. When you take time to give patients concentrated effort, they will be inclined to give extra effort for the practice—it's almost as if there is a subconscious urge to return the debt of kindness. Waitresses, bell hops, and others who offer "extra" service receive the largest tips. It's a law of human nature.

Acts resulting in recognition and appreciation are repeated. Thus, it's important that each patient who refers someone to the practice receives due recognition and appreciation if you want the act to be repeated. Even if you offer a "Thank you" in person, follow with a note for reinforcement. Never let your gratitude appear to be a standard thing, however. Be innovative, do the unexpected, yet remain within the realm of good taste. Vary your thanks with cards, notes, letters, phone calls, special acknowledgments, by compliments in front of other patients (which encourage other patients), or any other means with which you are comfortable.

Motivational Communications

Semanticists constantly remind us that what we say is not so important when we compare it with how it is said, for how it is said often determines how people interpret our meaning. This was described in the previous chapter, but it requires embellishment here. Following are four tips that help bring this point into practical application:

1. *Generalities don't motivate, specifics do.* "I see that you are feeling better, Mrs. Smith" is a pleasant remark, but little else. However, "I see a twinkle in your eye, rosy cheeks, and a lot more smiles now, Mrs. Smith, than I did five days ago" offers specifics that are reinforcers.

2. *People fear the unknown.* People can bear much suffering when they know there will be an end to it. When they don't, thoughts of suicide sometimes arise. The Communists recognized this when they instigated their "Five-Year Plans," which required much sacrifice by the common man. Dentists recognize this when they reassure a patient, "Only 5 minutes more, Mr. Anderson." Nutritionists report that people will hold to successive "10-day diets," but it takes a person with exceptional self-discipline to stay on a diet for an indefinite period. That is why people achieve when they have a plan and timetable. Because they visualize the unknown, fear lightens. This is also why after consultation and examination the doctor outlines for the patient a "treatment plan" or "health plan" with an anticipated timetable, even if it is tentative.

3. *People want to be needed.* Unless we feel we are needed by some person, some task, some cause, it is labor to justify our existence. "Mrs. Jones, I want you to. . . " is almost an order, and nobody likes to be ordered about. "Mrs. Jones, I would like you to. . ." is a request, and most people will respond. But, "Mrs. Jones, I need your help to. . ." is more than a request, it is recognition of the importance of the other person. Thus, it's good policy to use such statements as "I need your help in filling out this form" rather than, "Please fill out this form." *I need you* are beautiful words, powerful words.

4. *People become motivated when they have promise of need fulfillment.* Technical words mean little to patients unless they are translated into personal benefits and personal feelings. This is why the doctor does not explain the need for dietary supplements in biochemical and physiological terms. He will talk in patient-oriented terms such as, they'll "help give you more pep," "help you feel younger," "help reduce your

pain," "help you heal faster." Despite clinical reasons, instructions to a patient should be put in words the patient will understand from a personal viewpoint, a feeling viewpoint, whenever possible. The doctor knows that to a tennis player, "It appears you'll be back on the courts within 3 weeks" has more meaning than, "The therapy I've outlined is designed to reduce your elbow's lateral epicondylitis."

Businessmen once told their employees what to do and they did it. Teachers told their students what to study, and they did it. Doctors told patients what to do or take, and they did it. Such blind faith and obedience are not characteristic today. Today, alert businesses develop "participative management," students demand some curriculum control, and patients are rapidly developing a need to understand and participate in their health care. This implies cooperation (operating together). It means that the *whys* must be answered. It means that requests must be followed with many descriptive *becauses*.

These *becauses*, however, must be personal. For instance, the employer who says, "Do it because it's your job" spurs resistance. "Do it because I need your talent" spurs motivation and extra effort. The instructor who says, "Read it because it will be good for you" soon learns that nobody wants to be told "what's good for them." "Do it because you'll understand so much better after you do" offers a promise of reward.

Anything a doctor or assistant can do to increase patient cooperation and participation assists the healing process and helps firm the relationship with the practice. The techniques described in this chapter are not psychologic ploys to "manipulate" a patient. They are modes found beneficial in helping the patient help himself.

The doctor and his assistants are not responsible for the patient's illness or disability, thus the patient must share in the responsibility of getting well. When the patient is inspired to share this responsibility, recovery is faster, disability time is reduced, and costs are reduced—all these benefit the patient.

When a patient is impressed that he is

needed in the process and not someone to be "treated upon," he becomes actively involved. When instructions are personalized, stimulation is increased. When actions are constantly reinforced, motivation is raised higher and sustained. When *whys* are answered, the patient is inspired, cooperates, and participates because he wants to, not because he is told to.

These steps in motivational communication not only speed positive results, they evolve satisfied patients into enthusiastic patients and active centers of referral. A practice grows because it deserves to grow. If it offers exceptional service, the community will reward it accordingly.

From a psychologic learning-situation perspective, these techniques in motivational communications appear to have one common denominator—involvement of the patient's imagination. Again, when a patient can visualize the future, the unknown becomes known via imagination. When a patient can "see" personal benefits, the patient's imagination becomes motivational—a spur to action.

Besides words and gestures and acts, there are other means to stimulate a patient's imagination toward the goal of active cooperation and participation. Because we believe what we see much more than what we hear, audiovisual tools are excellent adjuncts in motivational communications. Charts, pictures, photographs, diagrams, slides, plastic models, flip charts, films and filmstrips, blackboard drawings, pencil sketches—all are excellent means to "show" the patient what you mean and how they will benefit.

Another excellent way to achieve active patient cooperation and participation is to have the patient make a personal commitment. It is imperative that the patient cooperate and participate by personal choice, as we have explained, but it is also important that the patient make a personal commitment to cooperate and participate. This personal commitment helps to establish volition deep within the personality.

How is this personal commitment achieved? Many ways. Implied consent, described in a following chapter, is a commitment. Initialing a written treatment plan is a commitment. Initialing a "budget payment" plan to resolve an overdue account is a commitment. Signing a release is a commitment. Getting a patient to do things for you is a commitment. Simply responding to the question, "Will you help me in this?" with a "Yes" is a commitment. Getting a patient to choose between alternatives is a commitment (Monday at 9:00 am or Tuesday at 3:00 pm).

Probably the most important public relations form you have in the office is the printed visit slip or super bill for several reasons. First, it openly portrays the fee schedule for office procedures—nothing is kept "secret." Second, it simplifies bookkeeping and a simple system allows you to give prompt answers to patient inquiries. Third, it advertises and publicizes most of the professional services available to every patient though a patient may now be using only a few services. Fourth, it serves as a reminder checklist for both doctor and assistant to see that all services required for the patient are accomplished, thus helping to assure that each visit will achieve its potential. Fifth, itemization of the office's full range of services implies qualification to perform a multitude of health services, thus adding to the prestige and reputation of office personnel.

Last but not least, the more you tell patients about chiropractic, the more interested and enthusiastic they become. Thus, it's valuable to carry out a constant patient education program. Many satisfied patients have little knowledge of the scope of chiropractic education and research. When they learn, they become enthusiastic patients. Many satisfied patients have no knowledge of the many postgraduate educational seminars the doctor attends to keep abreast with the latest technology. When they do, they become enthusiastic patients. Many patients who are satisfied with their personal treatment are unaware of the many types of conditions and disorders handled successfully through chiropractic care. When they become aware, they become enthusiastic patients and active referral centers.

Periodic Fee Evaluations

The establishment of fees is the doctor's prerogative. However, we will describe here the fundamentals of how and why fees are set so you will be in a better position to understand the process and need. With this knowledge, you can defend the doctor's fee with understanding and appreciation, and cope with unfair criticism in a professional and tactful manner.

When a doctor first establishes his practice, he must decide what his charges will be. He has bills to pay, equipment to purchase, and many investments to make. He enters the field at a much later age than many because of his years of education. These years without income and of self-sacrifice should be compensated. He has many financial obligations that must be met, yet he wants to be fair. He must put the clinical aspects of practice and the financial aspects of practice in proper perspective.

Setting a Fee Schedule

Before a doctor arrives at a fee schedule, he weighs the usual and customary fees of other doctors in his area, whether he is in general practice or a specialty, his personal experience as a doctor, and the costs involved in having an office. Fees set too high would burden those that he desires to serve and be incompatible with his professional oath. Fees set too low would contribute to practice instability, as well as deprive him of just compensation for many years of study and unusual skills. His fees should be standardized. As most people are covered by health insurance or government programs that pay a large share of health-care costs, financially successful patients cannot be charged high fees to offset lower fees for the poor. This practice, quite common several decades ago, is no longer applicable to today's society.

While the doctor is professionally bound to give service to anyone who needs it but cannot pay for it, such service must be limited to those unusual cases requiring special consideration. To those who can pay, he must charge a fair fee and give the best service possible for every dollar received.

Professional management consultants specializing in health-care practices say that the doctor must consider three basic factors involved in establishing fair fees. These factors are the costs involved, the doctor's salary, and a fair profit:

1. *Costs.* Expenses involved in operating the office and producing professional services represent about one-third of patient fees. These costs of overhead expenses are many and varied such as assistant salaries, outside agency fees, professional dues and subscriptions, rental or mortgage costs, loan interest, administrative and clinical supplies, maintenance and repair costs, taxes and license fees, utilities and telephone expenses, and so forth.

2. *Salary.* The doctor's personal salary (draw) represents another third of patient fees. Actually, the doctor is an employee of the practice. He must work to produce the professional services offered, and he should be compensated for this labor just as he would if he were employed by another doctor.

3. *Profit.* The doctor in private practice is also an employer and the owner of the practice, thus he is justly entitled to a profit from a successfully run operation as he would be subjected to a loss from an unsuccessful operation. This last one-third of the patient fee, profit, also must consider the investment the doctor has in equipment and facilities, the amount of money spent in obtaining his education plus the amount of what he could have earned during that time if he had been employed, the weight of responsibility of treating human health problems and accepting the risks involved, and the economic instability and insecurity of being in business for himself. Anyone who makes an investment of money and/or time deserves a fair return on that investment. Thus, profit must be considered in establishing fees. Without a profit, there is no interest on his investments and no capital for practice growth. Without a profit, the doctor would do better working for someone else. Profit is nothing more than investment yield.

Cost Analysis

If we use the formula that patient fees have three equal components of cost, salary, and profit, we can easily use gross income figures to determine if a practice is on a firm economic foundation. For example, last month's costs should be about one-third of last month's gross earnings. Likewise, last year's costs should be about one-third of last year's gross earnings. Note, however, that gross earnings represent total charges and not total money received. The difference between the two is the amount of charges or credit still on the books. When costs exceed 40% of gross earnings, the doctor should resolve (1) how to reduce costs, (2) how to increase gross earnings during productive hours, or (3) if fees should be increased.

Time Analysis

The first and last thing any doctor has to "sell" is his time. Thus, the relationship between office expenses and the number of hours the office is available to patients is a salient factor. To learn the hourly expenses of the office, one need only divide office expenses for any period by the number of productive office hours. The average hourly rate would be this figure multiplied by three (ie, costs are one-third of fees). The formula would be:

$$\frac{\text{Expenses}}{\text{Working Hours}} = \text{hourly expense}$$

$$\times\ 3 = \text{hourly rate.}$$

Thus, if it costs $3,000 a month to operate the office and the office is open 132 hours a month, the hourly rate would be $68.18 an hour:

$$\frac{\$3000}{132} = \$22.73 \times 3 = \$68.18.$$

This hypothetical office would have to earn an average of $68 every working hour to maintain a sound economic foundation. If the office averages $68 an hour and the doctor spends on the average about 15 minutes of his personal time with each patient, then the logical office visit fee would be $17 ($68/4). Income from special examinations, supplements, and other services would tend to offset losses from appointment vacancies, collection fees, and uncollectible accounts.

Let us suppose that monthly office expenses average $3,000 a month but the office visit fee is $15.00. Here, one or more solutions should be considered. First, the doctor could increase the average office visit fee to $17. Second, he could consider reducing office expenses. However, if the office is being run economically as it should be, this could be difficult. Third, he could consider various ways of decreasing his personal time with each patient so that he could see more patients per hour in an efficient manner. If through better patient flow and more efficient facilities he could see one more patient per productive hour, he would increase hourly income from $60 an hour at $15 per visit to $75 an hour ($15 × 5), thus placing the office on a sound financial basis.

It should now be obvious that appointment scheduling is an important determinant in office economics. Regardless of efficiency, only a limited number of patients can be seen in a given day. The volume of appointments should keep the doctor and staff busy all day. Allowing for emergencies and late patients, there should be at least a 15-minute break set aside each morning and afternoon to offer a buffer. This must be considered in determining visit fees. Also, the doctor's working habits should be known such as his pace with children and the elderly, emergency care, acute conditions, and so forth. The doctor must have adequate time to talk with a new patient after an examination that might take from a half hour to an hour, depending on circumstances. Routine progress care, on the other hand, may require only 10 to 15 minutes of the doctor's time. If proper appointment scheduling is made, patients will be cared for comfortably with minimum waiting.

Due to inflation and the rising cost of health-care services, doctors' incomes may be beginning to reach the maximum level of tolerance by the public. However, there are justifications for a doctor's income to be greater than that of a person in a less-demanding career. It must be remembered that education in the healing arts is more costly than that in other fields, and the doc-

tor must spend from 2 to 4 years longer in training. Also, the average doctor works about 64 hours a week compared to 40 hours for other professionals, though all the hours are not spent in patient contact (eg, in case reviews, examination analyses, reports). In addition, the doctor is subjected to pressures involved in health care not witnessed by other professionals. Finally, a doctor runs a risk of facing a malpractice suit and such a risk should be compensated.

As cost of living and overhead expenses spiral upward because of inflation, all doctors must periodically raise their fees accordingly without irritating patients and insurance companies. Many management consultants feel that when an increase is necessary, it is best to raise all fees without making exceptions for certain classes of patients and not others.

Some doctors deem it good policy to post a notice in the office announcing a change on a specific date (eg, "Due to increased costs, it will be necessary to increase our minimum office visit fee from $15 to $17, effective June 1st"). This should be posted about 30 days before the increase and removed about 60 days after the increase.

On the other hand, many doctors hold that it is not a good idea to send an announcement to patients or post an announcement in the office regarding a fee increase. The theory is that no patient is going to like a fee increase. The more it is advertised, the more it will be talked about, and the more unfavorable the publicity.

Most patients do not object to sound business principles and expect to pay a fair price for services received. Many doctors perceive that when a fee increase is necessary, it is better to start increasing charges on the visit slip and explain increased fees only when questioned by patients. Obviously, it is necessary that assistants know when a fee increase will be made and why it must be made so they can adequately answer questions.

SUMMARY OF HUMAN RELATIONS IN OFFICE ECONOMICS

The office will rarely have difficulty in collecting fees when the patient fully understands what he is paying for and is satisfied with the services. In years past, many doctors avoided discussing fees, believing that the less said the better. Today, however, uninsured patients have been accustomed to expect itemized bills each month and the opportunity for budget payments.

Misconceptions about overcharging and collection frictions are minimized when fees are frankly discussed in advance. It has been explained that a visit slip detailing the doctor's fee schedule for usual-and-customary procedures helps build positive human relations. Although a patient may not mention the subject of fees, this does not mean that the patient is not concerned.

Explaining Fees to Patients

Show interest in the patient's particular questions or problems without apologizing for the charges, which likely were set as fair as possible. There may be certain understandable or subconscious resistance to paying professional fees because patients are paying for something they *need* rather than for something they want or desire.

You may sense that the patient is questioning fees because he is afraid he cannot pay them. Your job, then, will be to elicit information concerning financial circumstances and help work out a time-payment program that will serve the double purpose of allowing the patient to retain pride and the practice to be compensated for its services.

If a patient appears angry or unreasonable, remain friendly and helpful. Mistakes sometimes happen, so first recheck the records carefully when there is a complaint of wrong billing or overcharging. If there is a mistake, correct it immediately and express regret for the error. If there is not an error, perhaps the patient merely forgot the extent of services or should be tactfully convinced of their value. Explain what the bill covers and why it is fair. Most people will understand and admit an error if allowed to save face and avoid embarrassment.

Insurance cases often put forth some difficulty. When some patients buy health-care insurance, they are convinced that their worries are over. They have the illusion that the doctor is part of their policy and all they must do is inform your office that they have a policy and all their health-care obligations will be automatically satisfied. Thus, it is the responsibility of a CA to tactfully explain to the patient that the doctor will be happy to help with the processing of the patient's claim, but the patient is held personally responsible for the doctor's bill because the contract is between the patient and the insurance company, not with the doctor.

The doctor should not be disturbed by frequent telephone calls when he is consulting, examining, or treating another patient except in an emergency. In the unusual situation where a patient will not listen to reason, insists on taking it up with the doctor, or threatens legal action, tell the patient you will refer his message to the doctor and will get in touch with him when possible. The doctor will advise you of appropriate action.

When a telephone inquiry is received about fees, explain to the caller that you can only give a general idea as your words must be based on the average patient and the usual fee schedule. Explain that every patient is a unique situation and that until the doctor has examined the patient and determined the patient's special needs, it will be impossible to state an exact amount.

If a patient calls the office and is angry because a bill was sent to him when he had insurance, listen to the patient's story. Check his file to make sure the claim has been sent, and explain that your office has completed the claim form and mailed it to the insurance company. Remind the patient that he is responsible for the bill and that the insurance company will reimburse him according to how the policy is written.

Collections of Overdue Accounts

At the completion of the initial consultation and examination, the patient should be escorted to the business desk or counter. The professional attitude here is vital to the success of the practice. An explanation of fees involved and how payment should be made is necessary. Many unpaid accounts and unhappy patients can be traced to poor initial communication about fees and payment arrangements. If the office cannot efficiently collect fees, it cannot remain open to care for the needs of the ill and disabled.

If a payment is missed, the sooner contact is made with the patient the better the chances for collection. There is no fixed time involved as each patient will have different circumstances that the doctor will want to consider. Every health-care practice has some degree of delinquent accounts and some degree of charity patients, but the degree must be controlled for the health of the practice.

In delinquent accounts, an assistant must call the patients, never the doctor. The doctor would appear "greedy," while the assistant would appear "efficient." If an assistant inadvertently angers a patient, the doctor may be able to resolve the problem. However, if the doctor angers the patient, the patient is lost to the practice.

No collection method is as effective as that of dealing with patients on a person-to-person basis. Because of the human relations involved, it is important for the assistant to make it her business to see each patient leaving the office and make an effort to collect for services whenever possible. An assistant always has an opportunity to discuss an overdue account with a patient who returns to the office at regular intervals for treatment. When the assistant shows a sincere interest in the patient as an individual and in the patient's problems, she can develop a budget arrangement for regular payments on the account.

If a patient becomes angry about fees, allow him to say everything he has to say. To interrupt serves no useful purpose. When he is finished, put things in perspective. You might respond, "You were very ill, Mr. Brown. It hardly seems possible because

you look so well now." You thus remind the patient of the serious nature of his illness and associate indirectly the doctor's role in the patient's obvious recovery. With this advantage, you can review the matter of payment by asking about health insurance and/or a budget payment plan once the patient has become more accommodating. Avoid high-handed tactics so the patient will leave the office impressed with your helpfulness. Effectively coping with angry patients is a challenge to your ability and personal charm.

Some patients live beyond their means as a matter of habit and pay their "important" bills first. Some patients simply procrastinate, and others cannot or do not wish to pay. Most patients, however, want to keep their accounts current if only so they will feel free to call the doctor when they need his skills.

It's part of a CA's job to encourage payment and to find out who needs assistance in making special arrangements, who should have special fee considerations, and who just needs tactful prodding. If effort is not made to encourage patients to make payments, statistics show that one-third will fall behind. This is obviously unacceptable and affects the ability of the practice to meet its financial obligations.

Whenever you attempt to collect an account by telephone, first ensure the privacy of your call. Do not embarrass the patient by calling where you may be overheard by others, and do not call a place of employment except to obtain basic facts. If the patient cannot be reached at home during office hours, a message may be left at his place of employment for him to return your call. The purpose of your call is to get a definite commitment to take care of the bill. You will not achieve this if the patient is angered. The patient has contracted for services received and is obligated to pay for them. Convey a sincere desire to help him in meeting this obligation.

Under no circumstances should you lose your temper. Collection follow-up requires tact, diplomacy, an understanding of human nature, and a good approach. Speak with firmness, without unpleasantness.

Sometimes patients will continue to see

the doctor though their accounts fall far behind. You may think the patient is wrong, that he is purposely dodging payment, that the doctor is being "taken"—still, do not put the patient on the defensive. Don't put the patient in the wrong. Defend the justified fee without criticizing the patient. Your attitude should be one of just concern, interest in the well-being of the practice, and helpfulness to the patient and his problems.

You can approach a patient with an overdue account with the idea that you are bringing up the matter because you want to help the patient remove any worry. You can say that the balance due has been increasing to such an extent that you would like, if possible, to help him reduce it.

After several billings or calls have been unsuccessful, you might say that you are making one last and friendly effort to find out why payment has not been received before you follow the accountant's advice that the overdue account be placed with an outside agency for collection. "Once this is done, the matter is completely out of my hands and when a third party controls collections, unpleasantness and perhaps additional expense on your part can be expected—things I would like to see avoided." This should elicit reasons (valid or invalid) for nonpayment and help you determine how to proceed.

There will always be certain cases that call for special consideration, patience, and understanding. If you sense this, gather facts such as the amount owed, funds available, future outlook, and special considerations. Then consult the doctor for further instructions. Occasionally, it will be best to write off a small delinquent charge after completing routine billing procedures. It may be that the bill is too small to warrant further effort, or the patient may be resisting payment because he thinks he has a justified complaint that the office has been unable to satisfy. Thus, pressing for payment under some circumstances may not be worthwhile. When you encounter questionable cases, discuss their handling with the doctor. He may prefer to write off a small amount, salvage human relations, and continue to treat the patient in the future on a cash basis.

When a check is returned from the bank stamped "Insufficient funds," there can be only two reasons: (1) the patient miscalculated his current balance or (2) he is trying to stall. The best policy to follow is a presumption of patient innocence. A phone call can often resolve the problem by explaining that you are holding the check returned by the bank and would appreciate his making a deposit to cover the check. State a time when you expect it is to be done; eg, a few days, a week, 10 days. At the end of that time, redeposit the check with instructions that it be forwarded for collection. If it "bounces" again, you can be reasonably sure that no "innocent" error was made. Another phone call should be made to tactfully remind the patient that it is a crime to issue a check with the knowledge that there are not sufficient funds to cover it. Diplomatically demand that payment be made immediately in cash, certified check, or money order. Under no circumstance threaten prosecution. Some courts have ruled that this constitutes extortion.

Dollars and Sense

The *Wall Street Journal* reported several years ago that bad debts left behind after a move were an increasing problem. "Skipped" accounts averaged over $100, and 59% involved doctor or hospital debts. John W. Johnson of the American Collectors Association said there has been a change in moral attitudes that makes debtors less inclined to pay their bills. "It's no longer a question whether he can pay, but whether he wants to," Johnson added. Of all the bills turned over to collection agencies, only a fourth is collected.

The Value of Itemized Statements

There is no doubt that a large part of human-relations troubles stem from a lack of clear communications in financial matters. When bills are not itemized, a patient is left to interpret and interpolate charges based on their background, experience, perspectives, and imagination. Collection agencies thrive because many offices insist on not itemizing their bills—inaccurately believing that a statement with a total "for professional services" is sufficient.

While it is true that the total is the same whether the bill is itemized or not, an itemized bill communicates "We want you to understand the charges," "Here are the details of your account," "Note the reasonable charges for each service provided." On the other hand, an unitemized statement communicates that the office is too busy to offer a clear explanation to the patient. This lack of explanation may suggest that the bill has been padded. Many complaints over total charges can be easily resolved when each service is detailed and explained to the patient. The total may be large though each service rendered was based on a reasonable rate.

Gratuitous Services. While all charged services should be itemized, it is also important to itemize services that were offered without charge. Every office provides many services without a direct charge. When these services are not communicated, patients tend to take them for granted or not appreciate their value when they receive the statement. For example, doctors spend many consuming hours without charge for consultation in the office and on the telephone. When these are noted on the statement, they help to place the doctor's bill in better perspective. When services for a second office visit the same day, special reports and memoranda, behind the scenes services, etc, are not billed, it is still good procedure to itemize them on the statement. Patients appreciate knowing what they are charged for and what they are not.

Itemizing "no charge" services has another beneficial effect. For instance, if a patient notes on his statement several "no charge" telephone consultations, their listing enhances the value of the total services and at the same time suggests the possibility that the patient may have made some unnecessary calls.

Communicating the Facts

From the patient's viewpoint, it is not important how much time is spent on his case—it is how much time the patient *realizes* is

spent on his case. Both doctor and assistant should report the facts, but in a subtle manner. For instance, the doctor might say, "Mrs. Brown, I now have your case history and findings from your physical, neurologic, orthopedic, and x-ray examinations. Your laboratory report will be in shortly. My next step will be to analyze each report, coordinate their findings in detail, and report to you my conclusions and recommendations on your next visit to the office. This is a time-consuming process, but it is necessary to be thorough."

When you *communicate* with patients, patients will talk about you. When there is a communications gap, the result is poor human relations. When patients become informed of the office's total services and facilities, they cannot help but be excellent centers of influence for referrals. Remember, before there is motivation, there must be education. Impression precedes expression. Thus, it's often good policy to show new equipment purchased to established patients so that they will be impressed with the office keeping up with advanced technology.

Some doctors and assistants exhibit misplaced modesty when it comes to their services and facilities. This is an error. While pride should not be flaunted, neither should assets be hidden from view. When offering the finest chiropractic services available, be proud of the fact and show and explain to others why you are proud. This positive attitude is contagious; not when you boast or brag, but when you show and explain and get patients caught up in your enthusiasm.

WORKING WITH AN ACCOUNTANT

Whether he is just beginning his practice or is well established, a doctor can benefit from the services of an accountant. How well the doctor and administrative assistants understand an accountant's role and how much the accountant's expertise is used will determine how much the practice benefits from these services.

A competent professional accountant can help make the doctor's practice become more efficient and therefore more profitable. An accountant can relieve many business administration duties necessary in the successful management of a practice.

An accountant can serve the doctor in two basic ways: he can set up and monitor the record-keeping system and serve an active role as a business advisor and analyst. The services a doctor receives depend on the requirements of the situation and may include assistance in the following areas:

* Design of general bookkeeping system
* Control of billing and cash receipts
* Control of cash disbursements and payroll
* Preparation of financial statements
* Analysis of financial statements
* Oversee collection of accounts receivable
* Tax planning
* Tax reporting
* Banking relationships
* Investment strategy.

Control of Billing and Cash Receipts

The most important area of concern in the record-keeping aspects of a practice is to assure that the doctor's services are properly billed and that income received from these billings is properly recorded and controlled. Invoices to patients for services should be prepared and presented to the patient as quickly as possible. This will obviously encourage prompt payment of the bill. Patients' billings should also be recorded in the books of original entry, which is commonly called in business a *cash receipts and sales journal.*

Cash received from patients should likewise be recorded on a timely basis. Individual checks should be listed in a cash receipts journal and a deposit slip prepared for bank deposit. An accountant can be helpful in selecting the proper billing and cash receipts system for the practice. He also can help with training office personnel and then monitoring the system to assure it functions properly.

Control of Cash Disbursements and Payroll

Another part of a record-keeping system required for a practice is a *cash disbursement and payroll system.* An accountant can assist in designing a system that can be used for recording the payment of vender invoices and writing payroll checks. A good system will assure the doctor that proper procedures have been established to approve invoices and prepare, sign, record and mail checks. This will limit the possibility of misappropriation of funds.

A one-write pegboard system is one of the most efficient systems for handling cash disbursements and payroll. A one-write cash disbursements journal can also be used for input to a computer center for preparation of financial statements. Refer to Figure 8.17.

General Bookkeeping System

One of the first items that must be established in any good accounting system is a *chart of accounts.* A chart of accounts is a listing of the general ledger account numbers and names that will be used for a given business unit. It is, in effect, an "index" to the general ledger. The *general ledger* is then established from the chart of accounts. It shows the dollar amount of the beginning balance, current period transactions, and the ending balance for each account. The general ledger is usually handled on a data-processing system.

At the end of each accounting period, normally monthly, transactions listed in the cash receipts and cash disbursements journals are summarized and assigned account numbers for posting to a general ledger. Each entry should be reviewed by the accountant. In addition, the accountant will normally prepare adjusting entries that assure balances in each account are proper for inclusion in financial statements.

Preparation and Analysis of Financial Statements

An important function that an accountant can perform for a practice is the timely

---

ANNUAL STATEMENT

TOTAL INCOME		$ 92,500
Fixed Expenses		
Rent	$ 2,250	
Utilities	750	
Telephone	600	
Advertising and public relations	650	
Auto and parking expense	1,000	
Bank service charges	50	
Contributions	150	
Dues and subscriptions	1,300	
Insurance	1,200	
Depreciation	2,200	
Salaries	14,950	
Taxes, general	750	
Taxes, payroll	850	
Total fixed expenses	$ 26,700	
Variable Expenses		
Supplies	$ 1,750	
Postage, freight, express	850	
Printing and stationery	1,200	
Bad debts	850	
Accounting services	900	
Legal services	650	
Repairs	1,350	
Travel and entertainment	1,700	
Total variable expenses	$ 9,250	
Total all expenses		35,950
PRACTICE EARNINGS		$ 56,550

Figure 8.22. Hypothetical annual statement, shown to portray the technique of arriving at a break-even analysis.

preparation of financial statements. These reports show the doctor what his financial position is at a specific point in time and the result of his billings and expenses for the past period. Financial statements showing an entire 1-year accounting period are then used as the basis for federal and state income tax returns. A sample format is shown in Figure 8.22.

Financial statements can answer many questions about the practice. A few are listed below:

- What areas of the practice produce the most profit?
- Is the practice treating enough patients to generate adequate revenue?
- Is the fee schedule adequate?
- What expenses are out of line as a percentage of fees?

BUDGET WORKSHEET

Revision Date					
Office supplies	$_____	$_____	$_____	$_____	$_____
Rent	_____	_____	_____	_____	_____
Utilities	_____	_____	_____	_____	_____
Maintenance	_____	_____	_____	_____	_____
Communications	_____	_____	_____	_____	_____
Travel	_____	_____	_____	_____	_____
Subscriptions	_____	_____	_____	_____	_____
Dues	_____	_____	_____	_____	_____
Taxes	_____	_____	_____	_____	_____
License fees	_____	_____	_____	_____	_____
Conventions	_____	_____	_____	_____	_____
Contributions	_____	_____	_____	_____	_____
Insurance	_____	_____	_____	_____	_____
Professional serv.	_____	_____	_____	_____	_____
Shipping	_____	_____	_____	_____	_____
Advertising	_____	_____	_____	_____	_____
Public relations	_____	_____	_____	_____	_____
Salaries	_____	_____	_____	_____	_____
Payroll taxes	_____	_____	_____	_____	_____
Miscellaneous	_____	_____	_____	_____	_____
Total	$_____	$_____	$_____	$_____	$_____

Figure 8.23. Sample format for a budget worksheet to serve as a control against accounts payable.

- If a budget (Fig. 8.23) has been prepared, are actual expenses near those expected?
- Is the level of net income equal to or above that of other practices in the community?

Collection of Accounts Receivable

The inability of a practice to collect for services is the area where the greatest financial losses incur. An accountant can establish proper office procedures that will monitor collection of accounts receivable. Some of these procedures are:

- Monthly aging of the accounts receivable balance
- Listing of large past-due accounts for follow-up
- Review of problem accounts with the doctor
- Mailing of reminder notices and statements
- Use of collection agencies or lawyers for the collection of delinquent accounts
- Comparison of the bad-debt ratio to other health-care offices
- Analysis of the reporting requirements of health plans of various insurance companies.

NET WORTH

	Year	Goal	Actual
ASSETS			
Cash on hand	$	$	$
Checking balance 1			
Checking balance 2			
Personal reserves			
Marketable securities			
Unmarketable securities			
Restricted stocks			
Partial real estate equities			
Real estate owned			
Automobiles			
Furniture			
Other personal property			
Life insurance cash value			
Other assets			
Total assets	$	$	$
LIABILITIES			
Notes payable, secured	$	$	$
Notes payable, unsecured			
Due to brokers			
Amounts payable, secured			
Amounts payable, unsecured			
Other accounts and bills due			
Revolving accounts			
Unpaid income tax			
Other unpaid taxes			
Unpaid interest			
Real estate mortgages payable			
Other debts			
Total liabilities	$	$	$
NET WORTH			
Total assets	$	$	$
Minus total liabilities			
Net worth			

Figure 8.24. Sample format for projecting net-worth growth.

Tax Reporting and Planning

There are many levels of tax reporting required on a monthly, quarterly, and/or annual basis. A few of the more important are:

• *Payroll taxes;* eg, local wage taxes, unemployment compensation, taxes withheld and accrued, and income taxes withheld

• *Personal income taxes;* eg, federal and state income taxes

• *Professional corporation taxes;* eg, federal corporate income taxes and state corporate income taxes.

These taxes must be remitted on a timely basis or the practice will likely be required to pay penalties and interest. Professional accounting can assure that the doctor is satisfying requirements of various government agencies.

The most effective way to manage the tax affairs of a health-care practice properly is through advance planning. A certified tax accountant is an expert in this area and can help the doctor avoid excessive or incorrect payment. Also, should any tax report be subject to audit, the accountant is available to represent the doctor and provide necessary financial information to the government agency (eg, Internal Revenue Service).

Banking Relationships and Investment Decisions

Accountants are constantly working with banks to help their clients in obtaining necessary funds to run their businesses. Loans may be necessary in a health practice to acquire working capital or for an installment purchase (eg, equipment or a building). A doctor will likely need advice on what financial information is required by a bank when applying for a loan. An accountant can also help the doctor develop a "Business Plan" and obtain the most favorable terms for a loan. This could include mediation of interest rates and terms of the loan. A form to compare net worth growth is shown in Figure 8.24.

Doctor's Estate Planning

Proper estate and trust planning is also an important service performed by both accountants and bankers. The doctor may want to invest profits in either income-producing or long-term growth opportunities. This could include investments in stocks, bonds, real estate, etc. Here again, it is extremely important for the doctor to discuss these financial decisions with an accountant, investment manager, and/or banker.

Selecting an Accountant

As described earlier, an accountant's role can vary greatly depending on the doctor's needs. How does the doctor select an accountant? In the same way one would select any professional assistance—with deliberation and care. It is advisable to select an accountant who is familiar with the chiropractic profession and who has been recommended by other doctors. References on qualified accountants can also be sought from lawyers and bank officers.

Chapter 9

Preparation of Professional Documents

This chapter describes the preparation of office correspondence, the use of form letters and model paragraphs, and the styling of case reports, the doctor's personal reports, narrative reports, and professional papers. The final section, "Hints and Helps," offers an abundance of suggestions in spelling conventions and word use in professional documents.

OFFICE CORRESPONDENCE

Different offices have different means to reply to or develop correspondence. Some doctors prefer to prepare a hand-written draft from which the assistant types. If the assistant takes shorthand, the doctor may prefer to dictate the letter. If dictation equipment is available, the doctor will most likely use the equipment. In other instances, especially in routine situations, the doctor may only make a few notes from which he will expect the experienced assistant to prepare a complete and more formal letter or report. As each office is judged by the appearance of its letters, preparation should be done accurately, neatly, and according to the doctor's preference of style.

Promptness

Timing and scheduling are important aspects of good mail handling. Some doctors prefer to set aside a special time of each day for reviewing incoming mail and advising the assistant on proper replies. As a chiropractic office should maintain an image of efficiency and promptness, mail requiring an answer should be responded to within a day or two of receipt if possible.

All correspondence (and their answer if necessary) should be filed promptly, with the most current letters filed at the front of the file folder. Office policy differs whether clinical correspondence should be filed with the patient's clinical records or if the correspondence should be filed in a separate file under the name of the individual, institution, or company, in alphabetical order. Filing correspondence with related clinical records is the common practice.

Signature Authorization

The signing of letters requires knowledge of office policy. Some doctors prefer to sign all letters. Other doctors wish to sign only those dictated and authorize an assistant to sign the doctor's name to certain types of correspondence that the assistant handles for them. That is, an assistant may be authorized to sign her name on certain types of office letters.

Office policy also should define how the assistant should handle correspondence when the doctor is away from the office for several days. In most instances, he will authorize an assistant to sign his name to routine correspondence, with the assistant placing her initials beside the doctor's signature. Some offices, however, do not require such initialing. Likewise, some doctors will authorize the use of a rubber stamp signature, while others will desire that all mail requiring the doctor's signature be held until his return.

Form

The proper form used in developing professional correspondence varies with what authority is used and an individual doctor's preference. Several generally approved practices are listed below:

1. *Date Lines.* The position of the date line depends on the letter style chosen and the design of the doctor's letterhead. It should be at least two to four spaces below the last printed line of the letterhead. In short letters, you may drop the date line to give better balance to the page. The date line, however, does not affect the placement of the letter on the page. If the letter is dictated, the date should indicate the date of dictation, not the date of typing or mailing. Type the date on one line; do not use *d, nd, rd, st,* or *th* following numerals; do not abbreviate or use figures for the month; and do not spell-out the day of the month or the year.

Correct Style: March 18, 1978

Incorrect Styles: March 18th, 1978
                   3/18/78

Mar. 18, 1978
March Eighteenth,
Nineteen Hundred and
Seventy-Eight

2. *Inside Address.* The inside address should be exactly as that typed on the envelope, including ZIP code (Table 9.1). In addressing an individual in a company, the address should contain both the individual's name and that of the company. In addressing a doctor within a group practice, the address should contain both the doctor's name and that of the clinic or office. Business letters may also contain the individual's business title. Correspondence to educational institutions may also contain the person's academic position (eg, clinic director). The inside address is begun not less than two spaces nor more than 12 spaces below the date line. The exact position of the first line of the address depends on the length of the letter and the letter style chosen. If the name of a company or organization is extremely long, it may be divided and carried over to a second line that has been indented on the paragraph tab. It is redundant and generally considered poor taste to precede a number with a word or sign (eg, No. or #) unless necessary for clarity. A street number is no exception.

Correct Style: 70 Main Avenue

Incorrect Styles: No. 70 Main Avenue
                   #70 Main Avenue

Spell-out the numerical names of streets and avenues if they are ten or below. Use figures for all house numbers except One. Separate the house number from a numerical name of a street with a space, a hyphen, and a space. Some correct examples are:

- 23 West Eighth Street
- 23 West 13 Street
- One Fifth Avenue
- 2 Fifth Avenue
- 563 - 49 Street

It is usually considered in poor taste to abbreviate the name of a city. States, territories, and other words may be abbreviated in computerized mailing lists. The ZIP code

Table 9.1. Postal Service State and Province Abbreviations

United States

Alabama	AL	Kentucky	KY	Oklahoma	OK
Alaska	AK	Louisiana	LA	Oregon	OR
Arizona	AZ	Maine	ME	Pennsylvania	PA
Arkansas	AR	Maryland	MD	Puerto Rico	PR
California	CA	Massachusetts	MA	Rhode Island	RI
Colorado	CO	Michigan	MI	South Carolina	SC
Connecticut	CT	Minnesota	MN	South Dakota	SD
Delaware	DE	Mississippi	MS	Tennessee	TN
District of		Missouri	MO	Texas	TX
Columbia	DC	Montana	MT	Utah	UT
Florida	FL	Nebraska	NE	Vermont	VT
Georgia	GA	Nevada	NV	Virginia	VA
Guam	GU	New Hampshire	NH	Virgin Islands	VI
Hawaii	HI	New Jersey	NJ	Washington	WA
Idaho	ID	New Mexico	NM	West Virginia	WV
Illinois	IL	New York	NY	Wisconsin	WI
Indiana	IN	North Carolina	NC	Wyoming	WY
Iowa	IA	North Dakota	ND		
Kansas	KS	Ohio	OH		

Canada

Alberta	AB	Newfoundland	NF	Prince Edward Island	PE
British Columbia	BC	Northwest Territories	NT	Quebec	PQ
Labrador	LB	Nova Scotia	NS	Saskatchewan	SK
Manitoba	MB	Ontario	ON	Yukon Territory	YT
New Brunswick	NB				

follows the state preceded by a space. If there is no street address, the city and state should appear on separate lines.

Business titles and positions (eg, President, Secretary, Clinic Director, Sales Manager) should not be abbreviated, and Dr., Mr., Mrs., Miss, and Ms. should precede an individual's name even when a position title is used. If the title is short, it may be placed on the first line; if it is long, it should be placed on the second line.

Correct Styles:
Dr. Henry Janson, President

Mr. Robert B. Smith
Technical Services Director

Miss Lillian Bergman, Librarian

Incorrect Styles:
Henry Janson, President

Robert B. Smith, Technical Services Dir.

Lillian Bergman, Librarian

It's considered correct to eliminate the position title if the address exceeds four lines. The titles of Secretary-Treasurer and Vice-president should always be hyphenated. Secretary-Treasurer is hyphenated because it represents dual positions. If Vice-president is not hyphenated, it would indicate a person who is president of vice. The one exception to this rule is not to hyphenate "vice president" when referring to the vice president of the United States. In addressing an individual in an organization, company, or group, type the individual's name on the first line and the company's name on the second line when a title position is not used. However, if a letter is addressed to a particular department in a company, place the name of the company on the first line and the name of the department on the second line.

Correct Styles:
Mr. J. P. Morgan, Vice-president
National Distributing Corporation

Ms. Janice B. Smith
Assistant to the President
Southwestern Clinical Supply Company

General Electric Company
Technical Services Department

A name should be preceded by a title (if known) unless initials indicating degrees or Esquire follow the name. The use of a business title of position or of *Sr.* or *Jr.* after a name does not replace a title. When initials, abbreviations, or acronyms indicating degrees and other honors are placed after the name of the person addressed, use only the initials of the highest degree unless the degrees are in different fields. A scholastic title is never used in combination with the abbreviation indicating that degree, but another title may be used in combination with abbreviations indicating degrees.

Correct Styles: Robert E. Smith, PhD
Dr. Ralph B. Anderson
Ralph B. Anderson, DC
Professor Henry R. Brighton
The Reverend P. D. Cole, DD, LLD

Incorrect Styles: Robert E. Smith, AB, AM, PhD
Dr. Ralph B. Anderson, DC
Professor Henry R. Brighton, PhD

Esquire or Esq. may be used in addressing prominent attorneys or other high-ranking professional men who do not have other titles. Mr. does not precede the name when Esquire or Esq. is used nor is any other title used with Esquire or Esq.

Correct Styles: Alan C. Davis, Esq.
Gerald M. Baker, Esquire
Joseph R. Smith, Jr., Esq.

Incorrect Styles: Honorable Alan C. Davis, Esq.
Mr. Gerald M. Baker, Esquire
Mr. Joseph R. Smith, Jr., Esq.

It's modern practice to eliminate the periods (and to close up letters) in abbreviated titles following a name. This is especially true in technical papers, manuscripts, formal proposals, and other lengthy documents. When you do not know the marriage status of a woman, the title Ms. is preferable to no title at all.

Modern Styles: A. C. Davis, DC
Andrew H. Martin, Jr
Henry R. Whitman, Esq
Janice H. Hartman, PhD

Contemporary Styles:
A. C. Davis, D.C.
Andrew H. Martin, Jr.
Henry R. Whitman, Esq.
Janice H. Hartman, Ph.D.

Publishers will usually state style preferences, as will government agencies. While most government agencies follow the *Government Printing Office Style Manual,* some do not. State and private agencies vary considerably in requirements.

3. ***Salutations.*** The salutation is typed two spaces below the inside address, flush with the left margin. If an attention line is used, the salutation is typed two spaces below the attention line. In typing the salutation, capitalize the first word, the title, and the name. Use a colon to close the salutation; a comma is used only in longhand social letters and notes. Titles of Dr., Mr., Mrs., and Ms. are the only ones abbreviated. The salutation should be singular if the letter is

addressed to an individual; plural if it is addressed to a company, organization, or group. Do not use any type of designation, title, or position after a salutation. If a letter is addressed to a company to the attention of an individual, the salutation is to the company and not to the individual. A title should not be used in a salutation without a surname.

Correct Styles:	Dear Miss Robertson:
	Dear Dr. Brown:
	Dear Professor Johnson:
	Dear Bobby,

Incorrect Styles:	Dear Miss Robertson, CPA:
	Dear Treasurer:
	Dear Treasurer Brown:
	Dear Professor:
	Dear Bobby:

In a letter addressed to an organization composed of men and women, the correct salutations are *Gentlemen* or *Ladies and Gentlemen.* To a married couple, the salutation is *Mr. and Mrs. Batterson.* And to one man and one woman, *Dear Sir and Madam.* A letter to a firm of men (or of men and women) may be addressed Messrs. when the names denote individuals, but do not use Messrs. when addressing business organizations bearing impersonal names. When addressing a firm of women (married or single), use *Mesdames, Ladies,* or *Mmes.* Do not use *Miss* unless it is followed by a name. It is poor taste to use either *Dear* or *My dear* with *Mesdames, Ladies, or Mmes.* If the gender of the addressee is unknown, use the masculine form.

Correct Styles:	Gentlemen:
	Ladies and Gentlemen:
	Dear Sir and Madam:
	Dear Mr. and Mrs. Peterson:
	Dear Miss Smith:
	Dear Madam:
	Ladies:
	Mesdames:
	Dear Drs. Smith and Brown:
	Dear Professors Jones and Bates:

Incorrect Styles:	Dear Miss:
	My dear Ladies:
	Dear Mesdames:

4. ***The Body of a Letter.*** The body begins two spaces below the salutation and is typed single spaced unless the message is very short. Double space between paragraphs despite the letter style chosen. For ease in making corrections, tape the left paper guide firmly so it will not move, and your sheets will always be in the same position.

5. ***Listings.*** When designing an enumerated list within the body of a letter, the number followed by a period or enclosed in parentheses should be at the paragraph tab. Begin the line at the second paragraph tab. Single space the material within each item, but double space between items. Use the same number of spaces for each tab, never less than five. From six to eight spaces are preferred in general correspondence. Indenting succeeding lines in an item is not necessary in business and professional letters, succeeding lines may be returned to the left margin in block and indented styled letters. Indention of succeeding lines is only necessary in scientific, technical, and governmental reports and proposals when specified. Numbering of items usually denotes a priority or sequence. If no priority exists or no sequence is intended, the number should be substituted with a single period. When numbers are enclosed within parentheses, the numbers are not followed by a period.

Correct Styles:	1. xxxxxxxx xxxxx xxxxxx xx
	(1) xxxxxxxx xxxxx xxxxxx x
	• xxxxxxx xxxxx xxxxxx xxxxx

Incorrect Styles:	No. 1. xxxxxxx xxxxx xxxxxx
	#1 xxxxxxxx xxxxx xxxxxx xx
	(1.) xxxxxxxx xxxxx xxxxxx
	1: xxxxxxxx xxxxx xxxxxx xx

1- xxxxxxxx xxxxx
xxxxxx xxx
-1 xxxxxxxx xxxxx
xxxxxx xxx

6. *Complimentary Close.* The close should be typed two spaces below the last line of the letter's body. It should be flush with the left margin in block form. Capitalize only the first word, and conclude the close with a comma. The form of complimentary closes differs with the general tone of the letter and the relationship between writer and addressee. The formality of a close, therefore, should be coordinated with the salutation and body of the letter. See Table 9.2.

7. *Signature.* The signature to a professional or business letter consists of the hand-written signature of the author followed by the typed name of the author and his title. The author's typed name and his title may be eliminated if it appears on the letterhead. In formal documents, the typed name of the organization, group, or company should appear above the written signature of the author. *The written signature should be the same as the typed signature of the author with one exception: the written signature should never contain titles.* When the firm's name is included in the signature, it should be typed in full capitals two spaces below the complimentary close. About four spaces should be allowed for the writer's signature. The author's name is then typed (with titles, if any), and the author's position is typed on the next line with the lines blocked.

Correct Style: Sincerely,

James E. Brown

James E. Brown, DC
Clinic Director

Incorrect Style: Sincerely,

James E. Brown, DC

James E. Brown, DC
Clinic Director

Table 9.2. Typical Letter Salutations and Complimentary Closes

Type	Salutations	Complimentary Closes
Very Formal	My dear Sir: Sir: My dear Madam: Madam:	Respectfully, Yours respectfully, Respectfully yours, Very respectfully yours,
Formal	Dear Sir: Dear Madam: Gentlemen: Mesdames:	Very truly yours, Yours very truly, Yours truly,
Less Formal	Dear Dr. Beckett: My dear Mr. Grimes: Dear Mrs. Andrews: My dear Miss Jones:	Sincerely, Sincerely yours, Yours sincerely, Very sincerely,
Personal	Dear Dr. Smith: Dear Mrs. Bickerton: Dear Professor Hanks: Dear Miss Masterson:	Yours cordially, Cordially, Cordially yours, Most sincerely,
More Personal	Dear Bob: Dear Bob and Carol:	Regards, Regards to you and yours,

When an assistant signs her employer's name to a letter with his authorization, the assistant should place her initials immediately below it. When the assistant signs a letter as an assistant to the doctor, her written signature is followed by a typed line indicating her position and relationship to the practice.

Correct Style: Sincerely,

*Henry P. Adams*ᴍᴊ

Henry P. Adams, DC

Correct Style: Sincerely,

Mary Jones

Mary Jones, CA
Assistant to Dr. Adams

8. *Attention Line.* In strictly business matters, letters addressed to a company or organization may be directed to the attention of an individual, position, or department. This marks the letter as a business matter rather than a personal letter and ensures it will be opened in the absence of the individual to whom it is directed. The attention line is typed two spaces below the address, the word *of* is not used, and the line is closed without punctuation.

Correct Styles: Attention Dr. R. M. Richardson
Attention Claims Department

Incorrect Styles: Attention of Dr. Richardson
Attention Dr. R. M. Richardson:
Attention of the Claims Department

9. *Subject Line.* A subject line serves as a convenience to both writer and reader because it eliminates the need for the writer to use the first paragraph in the body of the letter to define the letter's purpose, and it aids routine routing of the letter to the most appropriate individual. A subject line should be typed two spaces below the salutation. It should never be placed before the salutation because it is not a heading; it is an integral part of the body of the letter. Important words in a subject line are capitalized, and the line may be underscored if desired. If the subject line is preceded by *In re* or *Subject* (usually reserved for legal matters), no punctuation follows *In re*, but a colon follows *Subject*. Samples of correct styles are:

- Your Letter of June 18, 1990
- Reply to Your Inquiry of June 18, 1990
- In re Claim of Mrs. Robert T. Jones
- Subject: Claim of Mrs. Robert T. Jones

10. *Reference Line.* A reference line should be included in your reply, whether requested or not, if a file reference, case number, claim number, or another specific reference is given in incoming correspondence. Your reference should be placed beneath the incoming reference if possible. The reference line is typed on the same line as the salutation, either centered on the page or blocked on the right margin. Underscoring is optional. If your reply also has a subject line, the reference line should be typed on the same line, blocked flush to the right margin:

Dear Sir: Your File 7284   Our Case 567-C

11. *Identification Line.* In offices where more than one person may be dictating letters and more than one typing letters, an identification line is referenced. If the dictator's name appears in the signature, it's not necessary to initial the name in the identification line; only those of the typist are necessary. If the person who signs the letter has not dictated the letter, the identification line should indicate signer, dictator, and typist, in that order. Initials may be separated by either a colon or a slash. In most correspondence, the identification line is typed four spaces below the last signature line, flush left. In official documents, it may be placed two spaces below the address. Correct examples are:

AM   —When dictator is signer; typist, AM
RCS: JHD:AM —When RCS is signer; dictator, JHD; typist, AM
    or
RCS/JHD/AM

Many office policies require that an identification line should appear only on the carbon copy, never the original.

12. ***Enclosure Line.*** If a letter contains one or more enclosures, the word *Enclosure* or its abbreviation, *Enc*, should be typed flush left two spaces below the identification. If there is more than one enclosure, show the number in parentheses. If an enclosure is to be returned, it should be indicated within parentheses. A deadline for return should be stated if necessary. Correct examples (without line spaces) are:

AM
Enclosure (2)

AM
Enc Lab Report (to be returned by 4/22/91)

RCS:JHD:AM
Enc Lab Report (please return)

13. ***Special Notations.*** Special envelope notations such as "Personal" or "Confidential" should not be used as a gimmick to catch the attention of a busy person. Their use should be restricted solely to the situation where no one should have access to the information except the addressee. Special notations are typed two or three spaces above the envelope address in capitals and underscored, and in the letter two or three spaces above the address in capitals and underscored. For example:

CONFIDENTIAL

Dr. James R. Bronson
142 South Main Street
Oklahoma City, OK 73164

When a special notation is necessary on the envelope to indicate special mailing, the notation should be placed in capitals and underscored below the area where the postage would be and above the address. The same notation should be indicated in the upper right hand corner of carbon copies. If a "Personal" or "Confidential" notation is also be made, it should be typed in capitals and underscored and placed below and to the left of the address. For example:

SPECIAL DELIVERY

Dr. James R. Bronson
142 South Main Street
Oklahoma City, OK 73164

PERSONAL

14. ***Notation of Copy Distribution.*** When a copy of your letter is to be forwarded to others, note distribution flush left and two spaces below other notations. *Copy (copies) to* or the abbreviation *cc* followed by a colon may be used. If the doctor wishes one or more "blind" copies to be distributed, notation should be made in the upper-left corner of the copy or copies. This shows that the addressee of the letter does not know that another has been copied, and it alerts the person receiving the copy that the addressee is unaware that another has been copied. Examples (without line spaces) of an "open" copy notation on a letter are shown below.

AM
Enclosure (2)
Copy to Dr. R. L. Brown

RCS:JHD:AM
Enclosure (Narrative 274)
cc: Drs. Brown, Jones, Smith

15. ***Postscript.*** The use of a postscript is poor form. When it is necessary, it should be typed two spaces below the last notation and concluded with a period, space, double hyphen, and initials of the dictator (eg, xxxxxxx.—RKM). Use of the abbreviation "PS" is optional.

16. ***Alignment of Numbered Lists and Tabular Figures.*** The accepted procedure is to align numbered lists by the period and tabulated figures by the comma. If no number exceeds four digits, the comma may be eliminated.

Correct Styles: 1. xxxx
                                    10. xxxx
                                  100. xxxx

                                    1,261,423
                                       1,564.50
                                     10,000

```
            I. xxxx
           II. xxxx
          III. xxxx
           IV. xxxx
```

Incorrect Styles: 1.   xxxx
                    10.   xxxx
                  1000. xxxx

1,261,423
1,564.50
10,000

```
            I.  xxxx
           II.  xxxx
          III.  xxxx
           IV.  xxxx
```

17. *Succeeding Page Headings.* If a letter extends to a second page or more, a plain sheet (without letterhead or with a greatly reduced letterhead) is used. It should be the same size and quality paper as the letterhead. The heading should contain the name of the addressee in initial capitals set flush left, the number of the page centered and within parentheses, and the date in initial capitals set flush right. For example:

Mr. M. F. Grimes   (2)   January 16, 1990

18. *Foreign Addresses.* When addressing a foreign country, the name of the country is typed on the last line of the address. It is typed in full capitals and underscored on the envelope, and in initial capitals and not underscored in the letter. Examples are shown below:

Envelope Style: Dr. Robert F. Haynes
                   1673 South Elm Street
                   Toronto, Ontario M65
                   CANADA

Letter Style: Dr. Robert F. Haynes
                   1673 South Elm Street
                   Toronto, Ontario M65
                   Canada

19. *Addressing Government Officials.* As good citizens, many doctors of chiropractic are involved to some degree in politics and legislative matters. This requires correspondence with local, state, and national appointed and elected officials. The office should have a reference style book showing proper form in addressing these officials.

Letter Quality

Because readers judge your office by its correspondence, be careful to assure neatness, accuracy, readability, courtesy, and professionalism. Below is a listing of some errors that would make a letter unmailable in most chiropractic offices:

Misspelled words
• Transposition of letters or words
• Incorrect word division at ends of lines
• Poor margination
• Several obvious erasures or corrections
• Confusing terms
• Inappropriate expressions
• Wordiness
• Word or line omissions
• Incorrect title
• Use of uncommon abbreviations
• Incorrect punctuation
• Poor grammar, syntax, or word use
• Redundancy
• Poor paragraphing
• Incomplete sentences
• Verbs of wrong number
• Trite expressions
• Incorrect capitalization
• Lack of courtesy
• Unprofessional appearance.

Style

Because a professional office will generate letters to different audiences, at least three different styles will be used. The assistant responsible for typing correspondence should be well acquainted with the different readers. For example, the doctor will use one style of letter when communicating with a colleague, another style when communicating with businessmen, and yet another style when communicating to lay people. This is because words often have different meanings to different people with different educational levels. The "jargon" acceptable among colleagues would not be acceptable in an insurance report and would be inappropriate in writing to a lay person.

In any type of correspondence, it is preferable to avoid vague or generalized expressions when specific terms can be used:

Avoid Generalized Expressions	Use Specific Terms
in due course	by January 10th; in 2 weeks
in the near future	within 3 weeks; this month
sending	by air express; by UPS
shipping	by parcel post; by air express
under separate cover	by airmail; by first-class mail
document	contract; lease; agreement

Likewise, windy or pretentious expressions should be avoided where a simple and concise term can be used. Similarly, use terms of everyday conversational English in nontechnical correspondence rather than highly formal or archaic expressions. See Table 9.3.

Besides avoiding generalized, pretentious, and archaic expressions, doctors' letters should show good manners and professionalism. Courtesy and carefully selected words should be designed to persuade rather than criticize. It's never professional to be discourteous or is it tactful to use terms that may be unfamiliar to the reader. Frequent use of "please" and "thank you" can turn a cold demand into a warm request.

Readers are human and often egocentric. Knowing this, the alert assistant who is a courteous writer will praise the reader and show appreciation whenever possible. Examples of how an assistant can turn commonly used cold expressions into personalized phrases are shown in Table 9.4.

In a similar way, letter writers are human and will err. When an assistant must call at-

tention to an error or oversight, great tact must be used. Compare the lists in Table 9.5.

Because a health-care practice is so deeply involved in sickness, it is important that a positive atmosphere be continually generated. Healthy people also prefer positiveness to negative connotations. The alert assistant will remember this while developing correspondence. Negative expressions can be turned into positive statements as shown in Table 9.6.

Uncomplimentary words and phrases that insinuate weaknesses are not only tactless, they antagonize rather than motivate. Here are some examples that should be avoided:

- It seems *strange* to us that ...
- We do not understand *your failure* to ...
- You must certainly *know* that ...
- To correct *your error* ...
- Your *complaint* ...
- You previously *claimed* that ...
- As *only* an occasional patient at this office ...
- While we could *ethically deny* your request ...

Freshness, accuracy, appropriateness, and conformity to professional standards are the qualities that a writer should patiently attain if correspondence is to hold reader attention. Wordiness, trite expressions, inappropriate comments, and confusing terms turn readers to more interesting thoughts.

Redundancy, tautology, and circumlocution are terms indicating superfluous word use. *Redundancy* involves the repetition of meaning. *Tautology* is saying something again in different terms that do not enhance clarity such as *needless* repetition or enter *into. Circumlocution* is a roundabout way of expressing an idea.

Adjectives are redundant when they duplicate the meaning of the noun they modify. In the examples shown below, redundant adjectives are italicized:

- *final* climax
- *close* proximity
- *good* benefits
- *true* facts
- *final* outcome
- *hard* induration
- *muscle* exercise
- *first* priority

Table 9.3. Use of Conversational Terms

Avoid Pretentious, Archaic, and Inaccurate Terms	Use Simple Conversational Terms
acknowledge receipt of	thank you for
advise	explain, let know
are able to	can
are being included	are included
are in a position to	can
as per	as, according to
at all times	always
at an early date	soon, promptly
at hand	here
at the present time	now
at the present writing	now, presently
attached hereto	attached, enclosed
by personal remittance	personally
come to hand	reached us
deem	think, believe
do it on (next) Monday	do it Monday
enclosed herewith	enclosed
hand you	send, enclose
have before us	has reached us, we have received
hence	therefore, thus
hereafter	after this
heretofore	until now
his own experience	his experience
in accordance with your request	as you requested
in connection with	about, with, concerning
in re	about
in the amount of	for, of
in the manner of	among
in view of the fact that	because, although
in view of the fact that	because, as
instruct	inform
it helps in planning	it helps planning
meets with your approval	find satisfactory, you like
note	see, understand
past experience	experience
per	a, by, through
per annum	each year
subsequently	later
takes planning	requires planning
time period	period
under date of	on
under separate cover	separately
up to this writing	until now
utilize	use
whereby	by which

Table 9.4. Impersonal vs Personalized Expressions

Impersonal Expressions	Personalized Expressions
Your letter	Your helpful letter
Your reply	Your prompt reply
Your answer	Your thoughtful answer
Your explanation	Your clear explanation
Your suggestion	Your constructive suggestion
Your question	Your interesting question
Your problem	Your personal situation
Your guess	Your insight

Table 9.5. Untactful vs Tactful Expressions

Untactful Expressions	Tactful Expressions
You failed to sign the check.	The check was not signed.
You omitted the . . .	The . . . was omitted.
You forgot to enclose the . . .	The . . . was not received.
You made an error.	We need your help to correct a mistake.
You did not understand.	We did not make it clear that . . .
You are confused.	I understand your confusion.

Table 9.6. Negative vs Positive Expressions

Negative Expressions	Positive Expressions
Do not hesitate to inform us.	Please write.
Thank you for your trouble	Thank you for your help.
You won't be sorry when (if) . . .	You'll be happy when (if) . . .
To avoid further delay . . .	To speed delivery . . .
These data are insufficient.	Would you like further information?

- *important* essentials
- *invited* guest
- *necessary* requisite
- *complete* master

- *new* beginners
- *successful* achievements
- *present* incumbent
- *painful* ache

- Rio Grande *River*
- Sierra Nevada *Mountains*

Nouns can also be redundant parts of a phrase. In the examples below, redundant nouns are italicized:

Prepositions and adverbs used as part of a verb may be redundant. The redundant or tautological words and phrases are italicized in the following list:

- skin *tissue*
- undergraduate *student*
- aorta *vessel*
- radiograph *film*

- end *result*
- widow *lady*
- femur *bone*
- J. Jones, DC, *Chiropractor*

- united *together*
- attached *together*
- assembled *together*
- fused *together*
- titled *as*
- termed *as*
- fell *down*

- *still* persists
- equally *as well*
- 2 pm *in the afternoon*
- his *own* autobiography
- throughout *the whole*

- square *in shape*
- large *in size*
- lenticular *in character*
- repeated *again*
- recoiled *back*
- returned *back*
- lifted *up*
- connect *up*
- meet *up* with
- ascend *up*
- few *in number*
- blue *in color*
- amount *of quantity*
- *every* now and then
- this *same* patient
- over *with*
- all *of* the
- later *on*
- bisect *in half*
- *surrounding* circumstances

- such as *for example*
- entire *monopoly*
- are *both* alike
- *and* moreover
- *but* nevertheless
- inside *of*
- *as* yet
- anteriorly *to the front*
- audible *to the ear*
- totally *complete*
- *slightly* pregnant
- *quite* unique
- may *possibly*
- *totally* unresponsive
- so *as a result*
- the *deceased* corpse
- modern doctor *of today*
- *even* though

Circumlocution adds to wordiness though expressions may not be ungrammatical or repetitious:

- the examination in question — - this examination
- in the vicinity of — - near
- in possession of — - have
- destroyed by fire — - burned
- during the same time that — - while
- in this day and age — - today, now
- had occasion to be at — - was at
- from the professional viewpoint — - professionally
- situated along the side of — - adjacent
- an extremely large number of — - many
- It is the belief of a great many — - Many believe
- There are some places where — - At some places

Trite expressions, clichés, hackneyed quotations, overworked proverbs, and stereotyped phrases arise from a limited vocabulary. Below are some examples to avoid:

- accidents will happen
- age before beauty
- to preserve the principle
- aching void
- all in a day's work
- adds a happy note of cheer
- untiring efforts
- young comer
- watery grave
- "straights" and "mixers"
- where ignorance is bliss

- all and sundry
- abreast of the times
- acid test
- adds insult to injury
- agree to disagree
- untimely end
- weaker sex
- words fail me
- wee small hours
- no worse for wear
- vise-like grip

The use of the wrong preposition also may indicate to the reader the writer's lack of intelligence. Below are some examples of correct usage:

- abhorrence *of*
- abhorrent *to*
- abridge *from*
- abridgment *of*
- unmindful *of*
- unpopular *with*

- abstinence *from*
- abstain *from*
- unconscious *of*
- talk *with*
- variance *with*
- vulnerable *to*

Design

There are four basic letter designs and their variations. These formats are called full *block* (Fig. 9.1), *modified block* (Fig. 9.2), *indented form*, and *reverse indented form*. Any of these styles are acceptable and selected according to the doctor's preference. The block letter requires each line to begin at the left margin. The indented letter has each first line of a paragraph in the body of the letter indented to the paragraph tab. In the reverse indented letter, each first line of a paragraph in the body of the letter starts on the left margin and each succeeding line in the paragraph is indented to the paragraph tab. This style is helpful in expanding short messages.

```
                              (LETTERHEAD)



        Month nn, 19nn


        Firstname Lastname, Title
        Organization
        Department
        Street Address
        City, State, Zip

        Dear Title Lastname:

        The full block letter form requires less typing effort
        than other formats.

        In this format, the date is set from three to six lines
        above the address, depending on the length of the letter.

        The date, inside address, possible subject line, salutation,
        body, complimentary close, signature line, and additional
        information are all blocked at the left margin.

        Each line of paragraphs in the body of the letter is also
        blocked at the left margin --no paragraph tab.  Use single
        spacing within paragraphs and double spacing between
        paragraphs.

        Sincerely,

        MIDTOWN CHIROPRACTIC CLINIC

        (Signature)
        _____
        Firstname Lastname, Title


        Enclosures n
```

Figure 9.1. Full block letter format.

```
                           (LETTERHEAD)



                                               Month nn, 19nn


        Firstname Lastname, Title
        Organization
        Department
        Street Address
        City, State, Zip

        Dear Title Lastname:

        The modified block letter form presents a less rigid
        appearance than the full block letter format.

        In this modified format, the date is blocked at the right
        margin of the image area, two lines above the inside
        address.

        The inside address, salutation, and body of the letter begin
        at the left margin.  Single spacing is used within
        paragraphs, with double spacing between paragraphs.

        The complimentary close starts two lines below the last
        line of the body.  The complimentary close, office name, and
        signature line are placed between the center and right
        margin.  Additional information is blocked at the left
        margin.

                                   Sincerely,

                                   MIDTOWN CHIROPRACTIC CLINIC

                                   (Signature)
                                   _____
                                   Firstname Lastname, Title


        Enclosures n
```

Figure 9.2. Modified block letter format.

Content should be placed on the sheet artistically with equal margins. Each letter generated should have an overall appearance of neatness. Single space between paragraph lines, and double space between paragraphs despite what form is chosen.

Opening and Closing the Body of a Letter

The purpose of correspondence is to communicate, thus the need to gain immediate reader attention. By remembering seven points, even routine letters can be opened in an interesting manner: (1) keep the opening short; (2) be natural and avoid boring, pointless, dull, artificial, or stilted words and phrases; (3) go straight to the point, and reference the request or inquiry if necessary; (4) when possible, use the reader's name in the first sentence, but avoid frequent use to avoid familiarity; (5) use pleasant, appropriate statements that are not controversial to condition quick reader agreement; (6) refer to a previous contact or mutual experience; and (7) assure that your first paragraph incorporates the necessary who, what, when, where, why, and how. Authorities state that the best opening sentence is one which uses a question, makes a statement of an unusual or uncommonly known fact, presents an interesting story, offers a stimulating quotation, or makes reference to a famous name.

If your letter has been designed to capture the attention, interest, and desire of the reader to its purpose, the close of the body of the letter should be designed to motivate some type of specific action. With the following four points in mind, you will rapidly develop the habit of writing persuasive closings: (1) avoid stilted or stuffy endings; (2) suggest a major action, and be as specific as possible about what action is desired; (3) state a specific date for the action necessary—avoid generalized terms such as "as soon as possible," "when time permits," or "in a few weeks"; (4) avoid negative words and phrases or those that display a lack of confidence such as *hope, may, if,* and *trust.*

Vocabulary

Only one person in a hundred realizes that it is our ability to use our language which will decide our place in society and, to a large extent, our income. Knowledge is a power tool. The more knowledge we master, the more power we have—the more freedom we have to choose.

The favored class has always been the educated. They are immediately recognized by how they use their language. Knowledge and language are intimately related. The more words we understand and properly use, the more knowledge and power we enjoy because words are just names that label our storehouse of knowledge.

Testing of approximately a half million people from all types of backgrounds has shown that the knowledge of the exact meanings of a large number of words accompanies outstanding success in every occupational classification. Vocabulary has shown to be, time and again, the most accurate measurable characteristic of success. In one survey, a vocabulary analysis was given to executive and supervisory personnel in 39 large manufacturing plants. It was found that every man and woman tested, although all rated high in basic leadership aptitudes, showed dramatic differences in their vocabulary ratings: presidents and vice-presidents averaged 236 out of a possible 272 points; managers averaged 168; superintendents, 140; foremen, 114; and floor bosses, 96. In almost every case, vocabulary correlated with position and income.

The average person adds only about seven new words a year to his or her vocabulary. That's far inadequate for this fast-moving period in history. If we want to improve our station, we can do it with just a quarter of an hour each day. With just 15 minutes regularly applied, we could read half a book a week, two books a month, twenty a year, and about 1,000 in a lifetime. Knowledge is power.

Is the ability to communicate a real concern? A few years ago, over a thousand top and middle management executives of diverse industries were asked to list six qualities most needed in their organizations. There was little overlapping in the lists.

Some 67 different qualities were mentioned, but only one appeared on every list: "the ability to express effectively in speaking and writing."

According to Professor R. D. Scott of the University of Nebraska: "Deficiencies in vocabulary stamp one with the stigma of ignorance even more surely than do deficiencies in spelling. Of greater concern, however, to the person whose vocabulary is deficient should be the fact that a restricted or faulty vocabulary limits his or her ability to read, to acquire ideas from the printed page. Moreover, it limits the ability to express clearly and definitely one's thoughts in either oral or written discourse." In general, there is perhaps no other part of one's education that is of equal importance.

To develop your vocabulary, become word conscious and have a strong desire to add new words with their exact meaning to those already known and used. Develop the "dictionary habit," consulting the dictionary for the pronunciation and meaning of each new word you see and hear. Read good books, editorials, and articles in quality newspapers and magazines, consulting the dictionary for words for which you are not familiar. Reading aloud for half an hour or more is excellent practice that will improve your vocabulary and develop abilities in oral expression. It's helpful to read books and articles on diversified subjects to gain the broadest vocabulary. Belief enslaves the mind; knowledge frees.

While vocabulary quantity is important, it is just as essential to have vocabulary quality. Care should be taken to avoid faulty use of common words and expressions. See Table 9.7.

FORM LETTERS AND MODEL PARAGRAPHS

Every administrative assistant will find it helpful to maintain a file of form letters and model paragraphs that may be referred to in similar situations. They will save time and thought whenever a letter is not unique. They are efficient because they are usually based on much thought as opposed to a let-

ter developed "off the top of your head." However, any form letter or paragraph will need periodic review to see if it is still current with today's needs.

When you receive well developed letters that can be adapted to fulfill a routine office need, copy them and keep them in your file. If you have a typewriter that can be programmed or a computer, you will find that many letters can be made in which only one paragraph, the address and salutation, and the close and signature must be personalized.

LETTERS OVER AN ASSISTANT'S SIGNATURE

What letters an assistant will write over her signature and what letters she will prepare for the doctor's signature vary with individual office policy. If a writer would be offended when his letter is answered by an assistant, it would be poor procedure to create a negative response. However, if the writer only desires specific information regardless of source, the assistant is usually allowed to write the letter over her signature. Typical letters that an assistant writes over her signature are:

- acknowledgments in the doctor's absence
- collection letters
- follow-up letters
- letters arranging appointments
- replies to routine notices
- requests for automobile reservations
- requests for hotel reservations
- requests for plane reservations
- requests for refunds
- responses to accounts payable errors
- responses to accounts receivable errors
- responses to enclosure omissions
- responses to information requests
- responses to literature requests

Some doctors allow their assistants to write only routine letters. Others expect their assistants to handle all correspondence except those of a strictly clinical nature. Generally, the CA's responsibility will be limited only by her ability.

Table 9.7. Avoid Faulty Use of Words

Do Not Use	When You Mean	Correct Example
all the farther	as far as	This is *as far as* it goes.
alright	all right	She said she was *all right*.
apt	likely	It is *likely* to hurt awhile.
badly	bad	I feel *bad*.
balance	remainder	I'll do the *remainder* later.
but what	that, but that	He didn't doubt *that* he was ill.
complected	complexioned	He was dark *complexioned*.
couldn't hardly	could hardly	She *could hardly* see the chart.
differ with	differ from	This test *differs from* that test.
differ from	differ with	I must *differ with* you on this.
different than	different from	This report is *different from* that.
don't	doesn't	He *doesn't* see very well.
farther	further	We'll discuss it *further* tomorrow.
fine	well	He walks *well* now.
good	well	She exercises *well*.
leave	let	*Let* it be.
less	fewer	There were *fewer* patients today.
liable	likely	It is *likely* to be cold tomorrow.
likely	liable	She is *liable* to injure herself.
no one never	no one ever	*No one ever* evaluated the results.
of	have	She might *have* left early.
on account of	because of	He stopped *because of* the pain.
quite	very	I felt *very* good today.
remember of	remember	I can't *remember* that experience.
sure	surely	We *surely* thought it would happen.
suspicioned	suspected	That diagnosis was not *suspected*.
try and	try to	We will *try to* arrange that.
where	that	We read *that* he was appointed.
while	whereas	She's active, *whereas* he's passive.
without	unless	It won't work *unless* you persist.

LETTERS OVER THE DOCTOR'S SIGNATURE

The major categories of letters normally prepared for the doctor's signature are those concerning a case, contract arrangements, the legal aspects of the practice, and personal letters. See Table 9.8. Because of their content, many of these must be drafted or dictated by the doctor. On the other hand, an assistant with thorough knowledge of the doctor's desires and style may be asked to draft a letter for the doctor's review before final typing. With experience, an assistant may develop letters for the doctor's signature without specific instructions, with a few words of guidance, or from brief mar-

ginal notes on the incoming letter made by the doctor. When this occurs, keep these points in mind:

1. Familiarize yourself with the tone and style the doctor prefers in correspondence. Your aim in composing a letter for his signature is to develop it as he would.

2. When the doctor prepares a rough draft, *edit* but do not *rewrite*. In other words, correct errors in spelling, punctuation, grammar, sentence structure, and so forth. If something is not incorrect, but you would say it differently, let it be—that's the doctor's style.

3. Adapt the tone of your letter to the tone the doctor uses when he dictates. Thus,

Table 9.8. Form Letters Usually Written Over the Doctor's Signature

Acceptance of banquet invitation
Acceptance of committee appointment
Acceptance of membership invitation
Acceptance of speaking engagement
Apology for conference postponement
Apology for personal absence
Appreciation of professional expertise
Appreciation for gift received
Appreciation of patient referral
Appreciation of personal service
Appreciation of service to an organization
Appreciation of hospitality
Cancellation of accepted engagement
Confirmation of referred patient's appointment
Congratulations for business achievement
    award
Congratulations for business anniversary
Congratulations on article or paper
Congratulations on civic honor
Congratulations on marriage
Congratulations on promotion
Congratulations on retirement
Declination of invitation to banquet
Declination of invitation for speech
Declination of membership invitation
Declination of request for free literature
Declination to support charitable cause
Explanation of delayed response
Insurance claim follow-up
Introduction
Invitation to attend banquet
Invitation to dine
Invitation to give talk
Invitation to luncheon conference
Invitation to transfer records
Regret for absence
Regret for inability to visit
Reminder for periodic examination
Request for literature
Request for record transfer
Response to favorable media mention
Response to message of condolence
Response to message of congratulations
Response to message of sympathy
Sympathy for injury
Sympathy for damage or material loss
Sympathy for illness
Sympathy for loss
Year-end good wishes

if his letters come quickly to the point, compose letters in that tone. If the doctor's letters are gentle and courteous, use that tone. It is important to know whether the tone of the letter should convey friendship, a formal business relationship, or another attitude.

4. Use the same salutation and complimentary close that the doctor would use. These change with the relationship existing between the writer and the addressee, but the address does not. Thus, although your employer uses "Dear Bob" as the salutation to Senator Robbins, the address would be the same as if you were signing the letter yourself. When the doctor uses a first name or nickname in the salutation, the doctor's first name should be used in the written signature, but the typed signature should be formal. Thus, salutation and written signature should coordinate, and address and typed signature should coordinate.

Many doctors will expect an assistant to develop a letter from only a few clues such as "Thank Dr. Baines for lunch yesterday" or "Mrs. Johnson's daughter just got married. Send a note." Secretarial reference books are widely available that list several hundred types of letters designed for almost every occasion. One excellent source is *Effective Personal Letters* by William H. Butterfield, which contains over 800 letters. The reference is published by Prentice-Hall, Inc.

Timing may be important. Messages of appreciation, congratulation, and condolence should be answered immediately after the event.

A personal letter or note should be individualized for the specific reader. Be cordial and friendly but never gushy or too familiar. Use informal salutations and closes, and use the reader's name in your opening. Let the warmth of the letter convince the reader of its sincerity.

CLINICAL REPORTS

Postexamination Reports

A patient enters the doctor's office because he or she has a health problem. Most patients are under stress that is usually derived from pain or discomfort and the stress from not knowing what is wrong, what can be done, and how long it will take if the condition can be helped. Add to this basic stress the hundreds of worries and fears involved such as, "Will my career be jeopardized?" "How severe is it?" "Will I be crippled?" It is to these dire thoughts and feelings, some real and some imagined, that the doctor must direct his efforts in bringing together the facts of the case as determined by the patient's history, consultation, and examinations.

These facts must be coordinated and organized in a report to the patient in such a manner that the patient will understand what is and is not involved according to the doctor's best judgment. Essentially, the doctor will do this by discussing each finding and its significance and by responding to the patient's questions. One might term this phase of the report as a linking of cause(s) and effect(s). Even in situations of a verbal report, the doctor will likely speak from an outline so that essential points will not inadvertently be omitted.

In the second phase of a personal report, the doctor describes his working diagnosis (as few cases present a clear-cut entity on onset) and either outlines a recommended treatment plan or suggests referral to another physician. The doctor's treatment plan considers appropriate adjustive procedures, dietary considerations, nutritional supplements, adjunctive procedures, and the patient's psychological state and occupation— to name a few factors involved.

During the report, the doctor informs the patient of anticipated practices and procedures and receives the patient's consent before any necessary therapy, as he did in recommending certain examinations. The patient is informed of potential consequences so consent is given with full knowledge of inherent dangers, if any, to which the patient may be exposed. This procedure is called gaining *informed consent*.

The chiropractic physician acknowledges that the patient's condition treated is recognized and that the examinations, tests, therapeutic substances, and treatment procedures used will be based on scientific studies and principles generally accepted by the profession as needed, essential, and appropriate to properly diagnose and treat patients with that particular condition. Thus, the quality and quantity of examination and therapeutic procedures must be within the norms and/or criteria established by the profession as a whole for such a condition.

This relationship between condition and procedure is called the *medical necessity*. Third-party contracts usually call for a direct relationship between covered services and medical necessity. It also underscores why the doctor should document evidence to substantiate the need for services rendered. Besides gaining informed consent and discussing the medical necessity, the doctor should explain to the patient and differentiate between the therapeutic, rehabilitative, and maintenance care necessary in the doctor's judgment. This is especially important in third-party situations where the patient's health insurance may not cover all types of care.

Narrative Reports

Narrative reports are extremely valuable to referring doctors seeking expert counsel about insurance cases and legal claims. Because of this, it is important to note on the patient's entering data if it involves a case referred by another physician, an insurance case, or an accident (which may lead to litigation). Undoubtedly, a report of some nature will be required.

Custom directs the form in which a narrative report is developed although there is some variation in framework depending on the doctor's preference and specialty (if any). Most reports will begin with a background of the patient's condition, render details about the complaint(s), outline the patient's history, report examination findings, correlate submitted records if any, and arrive at a diagnosis or working diagnosis. The report usually concludes with a statement of the doctor's clinical judgment of the case, recommendations for therapy, and prognosis based upon the recommendations.

Before the assistant begins to type a report, she should ask the doctor how many copies will be needed. It is always best to type one extra copy than to be one short later, unless duplicating equipment is available.

Hugh G. Carruthers, DC, in *Selective Composition of Narrative Reports*, states that a typical narrative report should include most but not necessarily all headings shown in Table 9.9.

It's helpful to develop a file of narrative reports just as it is to maintain a file of sample form letters. Although each report has a unique content, reference to format and style will contribute to efficient development.

COMPLETING A PROFESSIONAL PAPER

No manual should attempt to set down a fixed edict of what you can or cannot do in preparing material for publication. It is the intent of this section to provide the necessary guidance to recognize the problems involved so efforts will be in harmony with generally accepted professional standards throughout the scientific community.

To set forth a format or style that must be followed by all for the sake of uniformity, economy, and other factors, would be sheer folly, for often the material being presented either refuses to lend itself to such arrangement or the requirements of an individual sponsor or editor forbids it. Similarly, any student of grammar will readily admit that even "authorities" disagree with many rules of punctuation, capitalization, syntax, and word use.

Overview

It is disheartening when a doctor spends several weeks in preparing a paper for submission to a professional journal and he learns that his work is rejected not because of content but because of unacceptable style, grammar, or composition. To avoid this, this section sets forth suggested styles and outlines basic systems of preparation. It

Table 9.9. Typical Topics in a Narrative Report

Introductory Statement (separate or combined
   with history of accident)
History of Accident
Past History of the Patient
Subjective Complaints
Objective Findings
Findings from General Examination of the
   Patient by Areas:
     Head
     Eyes
     Ears
     Nose
     Throat
     Mouth
     Neck
     Upper Extremities
     Chest (external appearance)
     Heart
     Lungs
     Abdomen
     Back
     Pelvis
     Lower Extremities
Orthopedic Examination
Neurologic Examination (including cranial
   nerves)
Radiographic Examination
Diagnosis or Impression
Treatment (separate or combined with
   prognosis)
Prognosis
Recommendations
Conclusion

presents a brief grammatical review aimed at achieving uniformity of interpretation of writing rules and usage of punctuation marks, prefixes, capitalizations, among others, and attempts to set guidelines that will facilitate a system for the preparation of professional material for publication.

The chiropractic assistant should adhere closely to the suggested styles and stipulations offered unless it is a requirement of a specific contract, proposal specification, or editorial preference. This is not to imply that other formats and styles are prohibited. There will be times when special formats may be desirable from the viewpoint of technical content or organizational purposes, and, on the doctor's request. These special formats and styles should be followed as directed.

The formats suggested have been derived from the study of various "Instructions to Contributors" that have been received from such organizations as the U.S. Government Printing Office, American Chiropractic Association, American Medical Association, American Osteopathic Association, National Academy of Sciences, United States Bureau of Standards, National Association of Science Writers, and the American Institute of Biological Sciences.

An assistant preparing professional material for publication should give attention to the grammatical review, which is essential in preparing a manuscript for submission. She also will find guidelines about vexations and difficult to comprehend items of style that, when properly used, greatly enhance the readability and appearance of a publication.

Deadlines are also important considerations. Before preparation begins, the assistant should ask several questions such as how long should you allow for typing drafts and proofing. Basic production questions must be answered and scheduled.

Writing Style and Format

One might say that the language used in technical publications and that used in general correspondence differ. This is a half truth. The language used in a technical publication should be chosen so it will assure clear comprehension by a person competent to understand the subject matter. The reader should not have difficulty in learning what the problem was or is, exactly what was done or what is proposed to be done, what the results were or what they are expected to be, and what the results mean. But this is also true for general correspondence: the difference being, essentially, the vocabulary used.

Writing within the chiropractic discipline is not different from that of any other type of professional writing. The elements of effective writing are the same whether one is writing a personal essay or a technical report. Science writing is not "a special way of writing." It is special only in the sense that its content differs. Following are some areas to which the assistant may help the doctor-writer pay particular attention, especially when involved in science writing:

1. The writer should know the reader's interests. He should not overestimate the reader's knowledge of the subject matter. Not all readers will be experts in the field of interest, thus the language of the writing should be free of clichés, pet phrases, and jargon common in the field of interest. When selecting a word, the writer should weigh it for both meaning and connotation.

2. The writer should try to achieve good lead sentences in paragraphs. He also should take time to break the text into small logical subtopics and paragraphs.

3. Readability and emphasis are best achieved by varying the type of sentences used. That is, simple, complex, and compound sentence structures should be incorporated into the text. Do not try to crowd a paragraph of information into one sentence by using connectives. If there can be any question of technical meaning, simplify the sentence by making several sentences from one very long sentence. In this instance, it is not always wrong to start a sentence with a conjunction. In fact, it is sometimes desirable. For example:

> It is expected that an optimum operating frequency could be determined analytically. But, in physiology, where inhomogeneous media and multiple dynamic targets are encountered, it may be more advantageous to decide operating frequency empirically.

4. Watch verb tenses, especially in a science report. Generally, the work reported *has been* done. Thus the most logical tense to use is the past tense when reporting the activity. Use present tense when a condition, a parameter, a physical law, etc, will be true, will exist, or will be in effect without regard to the information in the report. Use future tenses and other tenses as required by the conditions of the work.

5. Define unfamiliar words, abbreviations, and expressions with their first usage.

6. Assure that antecedents of pronouns are clear. Misuse of *this*, *they*, and *it* can often change or obscure technical meaning.

7. Be certain that nouns and verbs agree in number.

8. Use American spelling rather than British, and be consistent. *Webster's Dictionary*, for example, lists many words with variant spellings; i.e. usable vs useable, develop vs develope, judgment vs judgement, tying vs tieing, traveler vs traveller, etc. The first spelling shown is preferred.

A writer cannot be taught "style," but he can improve it. Like his personality, it is unique to him. However, everyone can improve style by striving to develop four qualities: emphasis, interest, meaning, and readability. In other words, the writer should say what he has to say as concise and accurately as possible. He should use words that he believes the reader knows, and explain facts and procedures in terms the reader will understand. In constructing sentences, keep them short, but do not sacrifice clarity for brevity. Do not stack modifiers unreasonably before the word they modify. Strive to save words in science writing. Flowery phrases with infinite modifiers do not add one iota to the technical content of the manuscript. Joseph Fort Newton once wrote in *The Philadelphia Inquirer* that:

In this office we do not commence, we begin. We do not peruse a book, we read it. We do not purchase, we buy. A spade is called a spade. In this town, we do not reside in residences, we live in homes. We are buried in coffins, not caskets. We have no morticians. We are not all gentlemen, but we are all men. All women are not ladies, but all women are women. All women are females, it is true, but dogs, horses, and pigs can also be females. Our priests, ministers, and rabbis are not divines. Our lawyers are not barristers. Our real-estate dealers are not all realtors. Our plumbers are not sanitary engineers! No beauticians live here. All fires, remember, are not conflagrations. All testimony is not evidence. And if any reporter writes of a body landing with a dull sickening thud, he will land on the sidewalk with a jolt, his hat in one hand and his paycheck in the other.

Goal of Research and Science Writing

The types of publications with which this section is concerned are reports, contributions to scientific publications (technical papers), and informal papers (presentations at symposia, conferences, etc).

The elements of style such as organization and typography (types of headings, paragraph indentions, spacing, margins, etc) will be considered here under the inclusive heading of "format." Experience and practice reveal that the formats suggested below are generally those which are the most adaptable and flexible in helping the doctor to efficiently present technical compositions.

An assistant is in a better position to help the doctor engaged in research if she has an overview of the two basic forms of research: applied and pure. Pure research is the type done by the scientist because he is interested in a particular activity or the results of an activity in its ultimate aspects. Applied research, on the other hand, is defined as that form of research engaged in for immediate use.

Approach

From the scientist's point of view, one does not engage in research unless he feels it will make a contribution to knowledge by discovering new principles, facts, norms, or laws. From the science writer's viewpoint, however, research consists of gathering the knowledge (state-of-the-art) that others have already uncovered. This state-of-the-art research begins by searching and interpreting the knowledge others have discovered, then giving the facts garnered from many sources to the reader in a reorganized form. An assistant knowledgeable of the many aids available in a research library can become an important asset to the DC in the preparation of professional papers, manuscripts, and reports.

The writer's research includes specialized and thorough investigation of available literature on a subject, to which he adds information acquired by experience, observations, investigations, questionnaires, or discussions with experts in the field. Usually, the greatest help is from the library: both primary and secondary sources. Primary sources are books, manuscripts, diaries, letters, journals, theses, and other published works. Secondary sources include miscellaneous periodicals and literature that report and analyze the findings of scholars, technicians, and scientists.

The developer of science writing approaches the task with high regard, if not love, for accuracy, truth, and objectivity. Scholarly care and perseverance is taken, as is care not to avoid facts and interpretations contrary to his beliefs. The true professional will not confuse facts with biased opinion— a common occurrence witnessed in writers of radical literature. The writer of science literature uses detective-like instincts and is constantly alert for inaccuracies, just as is the laboratory scientist.

Many chiropractic colleges have well-organized research departments, and the doctor and his assistants can learn to use the library skillfully. One should never attempt to develop research or a credible paper without knowing the techniques of using a research library and its potential wealth of information. Skill in library research is as important as writing ability.

As the writer or assistant gathers facts, he or she must keep in mind the purpose of the task—to inform, interpret, explain, or apply it to life. More notes are always taken than will ever be used. The writer must check to see that the basic outline holds to one specific area, that quotations are exact, and that sources used are credible to readers. Inquiring minds are needed to gather and sift the facts required, as is true for the laboratory scientist.

Talent has little to do with science writing. Skill to obtain and comprehend facts, to narrate interestingly, to describe vividly, and to write with facility are the important qualifications. "Accuracy Always," the journalist's motto, becomes "Precise Accuracy Always," in science writing. A good writer of science literature avoids generalizations. That is why pseudoscience articles are inaccurate. Their writers ignore the principles of precise accuracy.

Every good author also recognizes the need for brevity, clearness, coherence, and directness. Brevity is achieved by removing extraneous detail, eliminating unnecessary use of articles (a, an, the, that) when used as conjunctions, and avoiding long complex sentences and parenthetical expressions. The assistant involved in helping the doctor develop scientific literature will find the task stimulating and challenging.

Outlines

Because of the nature of the subject matter, the science writer should give careful thought to determining the limits of the article, the scope of the treatment, and the anticipation of what the reader may want to know. To do this requires planning. The writer's blueprint is the outline. In fact, two outlines: first a tentative outline, later a final outline before the actual writing begins. The more accurately the final outline is designed, the easier, the faster, and the more readable will be the writing.

A well-planned final outline compels the author to keep in mind the purpose of the article and aids in avoiding digressions and overlapping of information. It helps planning length and emphasis of various points, it spotlights omissions of vital information, and it greatly reduces time and energy in revision.

Contributions to Professional Journals

Many technical papers prepared by a chiropractic assistant will be those to be presented before professional societies or submitted to chiropractic journals or science publications. Contributors to such organizations or publications should follow the policies of the publisher if specified. When not specified, the suggestions offered in this chapter will be helpful.

The purpose of a paper is to convey information to others, many of whom will be far less familiar with the general subject than the author. Thus, simple terms and expressions combined with concise statements are preferred elements of style. If it is found necessary to use highly technical terms, symbols, or phraseology, they should be explained and defined at first mention. The author should attempt to write for the average reader, not the specialist. Use of the first person and references to individuals should be made in a way that avoids personal bias. Company or organizational names should be listed only in the acknowledgments.

Requirements

Many periodicals qualify that a paper should not exceed 4000 words. Therefore, long quotations should be avoided by referring to sources. Illustrations and tables are worthy if they help to clarify meaning or are necessary to show results properly. Drawings, lengthy test data and calculations, and photographs that are interesting but not necessarily important to the understanding of the subject should be omitted. Most technical journal editors are often emphatic in stressing the importance of compliance with their arbitrary requirements and usually will not hesitate to return a manuscript for revision and condensation if their requirements are not fully met.

The "Instructions for Authors" appearing in the October 1990 issue of the *Journal of Manipulative and Physiological Therapeutics* is set in very small type yet two and a half 8½ × 11-inch pages are required to list the detailed requirements for submissions. Even when these criteria are met, a paper must meet editorial approval and peer review.

It seems that some people are more interested in style than substance. Thus, an important instruction that should be carefully read and followed is the method of typing and styling. In their requirements, journals are usually quite clear whether a manuscript is desired from which they will set the type and do the layout or whether the contributor is to prepare a photo-offset makeready. For example, some simply require that:

Manuscripts should be typed double spaced on one side of letter-size sheets (nominal 8½ × 11 inches), with approximately 1-inch margins on each side. The paper should be white and of good quality and weight. Pages of the manuscript, including appendices, if any, should be numbered consecutively in the upper right corner.

Some may state that artwork should be drawn and lettered with India ink so when it is reduced to a column width of 3½ inches, the lettering will be distinct and at least ¹⁄₁₆ inch in height. The artwork should be grouped after the text with a list of "figure legends" preceding it. The same rule applies to tables unless they are small enough to be inserted into the text. The journal then sets its own type from this manuscript, photographs the artwork, and performs the necessary layout preparatory to its printout.

Camera-Ready Copy

A few science publications instruct the contributor to prepare a photo-offset makeready. That is, the copy submitted will be photographed, plated, and printed. For this purpose, they provide two-column layout sheets that have an image area of 8⅞ × 12½ inches and a column width of 4⁵⁄₁₆ inches. These sheets are reduced to 77% of the original and printed on 8½ × 11-inch paper. Figures and tables should be proportionately scaled to column width of the final printed copy. These figures and tables should also be proportionately scaled up to the makeready size so that windows will be left in the copy for their insertion. On the makeready, black or ruby-red masks are cut to the size of the layout-sheet image and pasted in the windows for any continuous tone photographs that are included as a figure. When the line (text) copy has been combined with these masks, the layout sheet becomes a "makeready." Line drawings either should be prepared the same as continuous-tone photographs (especially when they must be reduced to fit the layout sheet) or be pasted directly on the layout sheet if less than 4⁵⁄₁₆ inches in width.

General Format

If the journal or society to which your office is submitting a paper for acceptance does not spell out a preferred format, the following guidelines can be used:

1. *Title.* Place the title immediately below a 1-inch top margin and center it horizontally. It should be typed in solid caps (capitals).

2. *Author Byline.* For just one author, type the byline on two lines with the author's name on the first in initial caps. The second line should show his position or affiliation. The author byline should be double spaced from the title. For two authors, both from the same organization, place both names on the first line, and the name of the organization on the second line. If one of the authors is from another organization, a byline should be written for both authors, separated by "and" centered horizontally on the page. Thus:

John J. Jones
Mid State Chiropractic Clinic

and

Mary E. Doe
Central Laboratories, Houston, Texas

Use no titles (Doctor, Dr, Professor, etc) in the byline. Use no degrees in the byline. If it is felt that title designations or degrees are necessary, they should be described in a footnote keyed to the individual's name.

3. *Abstract.* The abstract should be started three or four lines below the last byline. It should be centered from side to side using about 2-inch left and right margins. It should be from 50 to 100 words in length and typed double spaced.

4. *Headings.* Type primary headings in full caps, centered horizontally on the page or set flush with the left margin. Secondary headings should be typed in initial capitals and centered horizontally on the page or set flush with the left margin. Tertiary headings should be typed in initial capitals, underlined, and followed by a period, two spaces, and then the text on the same line.

5. *Figures and Tables.* These may be placed either after initial mention or grouped at the end of the paper in proper sequence.

6. *Line Spacing.* The entire paper should be typed double spaced.

It is sometimes desirable for a doctor to submit a paper in final form when a society requests "preprints" of the paper for distribution at a conference or seminar. In this instance, the style of headings remains the same as described, but the spacing changes to single-spaced copy. Figures and tables must be reduced if necessary to be inserted in the text. Sometimes a sponsor will request that the entire paper be typed on oversize sheets for reduction in duplication. Manuscript papers should not be stapled together. They should remain unfastened for editorial review.

Informal Papers

On occasion, certain phases of research are reported in informal papers for the rapid exchange of information to selected groups (both professional and nonprofessional). These papers are preliminary in character, thus they cannot draw accurate conclusions. They may be of technical or nontechnical content.

GENERAL GRAMMAR AND RULES OF COMPOSITION

In the rules of English grammar set forth in this section, be aware that there are conflicts among grammarians regarding many of these rules. For example, most grammarians will state it is incorrect to split an infinitive. Yet the most famous authority on English usage in the world, H. W. Fowler, editor for many years of the *Oxford Dictionary*, stated:

We will split infinitives sooner than be ambiguous or artificial; more than that, we will freely admit that sufficient recasting will get rid of any split infinitive without involving either of those faults, and yet reserve to ourselves the right of deciding in each case whether recasting is worth while.

Rules of punctuation will vary, especially those pertaining to the use of the comma. That is, they differ in the degree of usage. Some authorities give rules and then give exceptions; others define very direct and uncompromising rules.

The grammatical rules that follow are not intended to cover all rules of English grammar. They have been compiled, based on the experience of science editors, to cover those rules most abused, misinterpreted, or with which there is disagreement.

While applying rules of grammar, one should keep in mind that they are intended to help a speaker or writer convey a message, not act as an obstruction to the transmission of thoughts and ideas. Just as civil laws are designed to maintain order, organization, and understanding in society, rules of grammar are intended to maintain order in the organization of one's thoughts so the writer might state his message clearly and concise and be understood.

Antecedents

Technical writing often involves the use of complicated sentences that have several inherent problems. The most frequently encountered is the problem of referring clearly to antecedents. Misleading constructions occur because of vague pronouns, dangling modifiers, or improperly used relative pronouns.

Vague Pronouns. The *vague pronoun* gives little or no clue about its antecedent. For example:

The cervical area was flexed severely forward while the lumbar area was extended posteriorly followed by acute muscle spasm and pain along the entire length of the spine, and *this* was considered very important.

In the above sentence, the reader lacks a way of determining what *this* represents or what was very important—the fact of the forward cervical flexion, the posterior lumbar extension, or that of the muscle spasm or pain.

When the same pronoun is used to refer to different antecedents, the meaning is particularly confusing. For example:

This assumes that the data are valid: since additional data cannot be obtained without this being done, *this* is no certainty.

Dangling Modifiers. Another common problem closely akin to the vague pronoun is the *dangling modifier.* The dangling modifier, usually a verb form, is a modifier that seems to work on the wrong word:

• Using Gundersen's method, statistics were gathered to....
• Specifying a toggle recoil, the atlas was....

The sentence structure in these examples leads the reader to conclude that the statistics used Gundersen's method and that the atlas specified a toggle recoil.

Although the dangling modifier is not as confusing as the vague pronoun, good writers will avoid it whenever possible. Sentences containing danglers can be corrected by one of four ways: (1) supplying a subject for the dangler, (2) changing the verb form to a noun so it does not need a subject, (3) changing the order of sentence elements, or (4) rewriting the sentence:

• Using Gundersen's method, *we* gathered statistics....
• *By use of* Gundersen's method, statistics were gathered....
• Statistics were gathered by using the Gundersen method.
• The team chose to use the Gundersen method in gathering statistics.

That and Which. The relative pronouns *that* and *which* are used interchangeably by some writers. However, *which* as a relative pronoun is used to introduce nonrestrictive clauses; *that* as a demonstrative pronoun serves to introduce restrictive clauses. Except *that—which* constructions, *which* will be preceded by a comma to set off an explanatory phrase. For example:

- The differential diagnostic techniques, *which* should be used with all chronic cases, will make maximum use of the doctor's ability, experience, and equipment.
- The adjusting table *that* should be used in such cases is described in Appendix A.

Note: A short discussion of the use of commas with nonrestrictive clauses is offered later in this chapter under the heading of *Punctuation.*

It, This, and These. The pronoun *it* and the relative pronouns *this* and *these* are often mistakenly used to serve for a longer phrase that would make the meaning clear. For example:

The chiropractic adjustment is designed to reduce the subluxation and release the fixation. In *this* way, *it* is a near-perfect approach.

For the above sentence, a reader is tempted to ask: which way? What is a near-perfect approach?

Verb Number

Data. Especially in science and technical writing, the word "data" is always used in the plural sense. It is the plural form of datum (the thing given) and thus signifies a collection of *facts* from which the writer is drawing conclusions. As one seldom draws conclusions from a single fact, the word is used in the plural and requires the plural verb.

Correct:	These data provide.... The data obtained were gathered....
Incorrect:	This data provides.... The data obtained was gathered....

In time, the use of "data" as a synonym of "information" or "evidence," thus a collective singular, may become conventional. Until that occurs, it should be used as a synonym for the plural word "facts."

Collective Nouns

A collective noun is a word that represents the grouping of two or more things. That is, it refers to a whole made up of parts. Some examples are *all, committee, group, majority, mass, number, pair,* and *set.* A collective noun is singular when it refers to the group as a unit. It is plural when it refers to things in a group as separate units. The verb and relative pronouns must agree with the number of the collective. "Failure to abide by the choice when made, and plunging about between it and they, has and have, is and are, its and their, and the like, can only be called insults to the reader," states Fowler.

Number. A troublesome collective noun is the word "number." A simple rule can be applied here that helps to eliminate the confusion: The article used with the word "number" shows whether it is used in the singular or plural:

- *The* number of samples is large.
- *A* number of tests were run.

Percentages and Fractions. Another rule that should be heeded pertains to collective phrases involving percentage figures or fractions: The verb agrees in number with the noun (object of preposition) or modifying prepositional phrase:

- In this regimen, 25% of the *therapy is* traction.
- About 40% of the *specimens were* rejected.
- Two-thirds of the *stock is* counted.
- In this apparatus, three-fourths of the *components are* made of steel.

Series. The collective noun "series" used to measure a "set" is used with a singular verb:

- A *series* of specimens *was* exposed to heat.
- The doctor recommended a series of exercises.

However, "series" used as a synonym of *several* is not acceptable usage and should be avoided. The problem is resolved by stating the exact number involved or avoiding the word "series."

- A *series* of five films *was* taken.
- Five *films were* taken.
- Several *films were* taken.

Compound Subjects. Compound singular subjects joined by *and* invariably require a plural verb:

- Chemistry and physics *are* closely allied disciplines.
- He and she are related.

However, a compound subject joined by *and* that is treated as one unit (a collective) takes a singular verb. For example:

Trial and error *is* a common method of testing.

Words like *each, every, everything, anybody, everybody, nobody, anything,* and *many* are called indefinite or adjectival pronouns and are singular:

- *Everybody has* finished.
- Every diplomate among the many applicants *has* been thoroughly qualified.

But words like *few, many,* and *several* require plural verbs. For example:

Many are called but *few are* chosen.

However, with certain words such as *all, more, most, some,* and *such,* either a singular or plural verb is allowed depending on the number of the noun to which it refers:

- All the *equipment was* installed.
- All the *supplies were* received.

The verb of a sentence beginning with *there is* or *there are* should agree with the substantive (noun or pronoun) following it:

- There *is* a *patient* in the reception room.
- There *are* seven *patients* in the reception room.

Words such as *neither, either,* and *none* require a singular verb:

- *Neither* of the patients *was* finished.
- *None* of the many observations *is* valid.

A compound subject connected by *or* or *nor* needs a singular verb if both substantives are singular:

- Either the administrative *assistant* or technical *assistant is* responsible.
- Neither the *doctor* nor his *assistant* was in the office at the time.

However, if the substantives connected by *or* or *nor* differ in number of person, the verb agrees with the *closer* substantive:

- Either the assistants or the *doctor was* available.
- Either the doctor or the *assistants were* available.

When two or more subjects, one positive and one negative, differ in number, the verb should agree with the *positive* element.

- It was the *editor* and not the authors who *was* at fault.
- It was the *authors* and not the editor who *were* at fault.

The number of the verb is not affected by the interposition between the subject and verb of such words as *including, with, together with, in addition to, besides, accompanied by, as well as, also, along with, with, as much as, in fact, instead of, other than, plus,* etc. Here, commas or dashes should be used to set off the intervening phrase:

- Dr. *Brownson,* assisted by Dr. Jones, *is* conducting the test.
- This *fact,* together with many other facts, *is* evidence that the prognosis is encouraging.

Verb Tense and Mode

A cardinal rule is that verb tense or mode (mood) should not be changed in the same sentence, paragraph, or passage. However, deviations from this rule are sometimes necessary when logic and meaning require a change in tense.

Splitting a compound verb also should be avoided. Splitting compound verbs with phrases or clauses, especially, often results in awkward passages. Nevertheless, logic must be applied regarding sense and ambiguity because the rule is not universally accepted and sometimes not appropriate. Both examples below are correct.

• He *would be* here now here if it were possible.
• He would, if it were possible, *be* here now.

Some authorities claim that adverbs should always be placed within a compound verb (eg, should always be, might never be); others say they should not.

The Subjunctive Mode. Another important rule that should be heeded by all assistants generating technical literature is that pertaining to the *subjunctive mode.* Today, this mode is restricted to three general uses: (1) to express a wish, volition, or motive; (2) to express doubt or uncertainty; and (3) to express a condition contrary to fact. Although Fowler states that "Subjunctives are nearly dead ... ," he obviously did not consider scientific writing. Here, its main use is with the two verbs *be* and *were.* The subjunctive *be* is properly used to express uncertainty or doubt. Note the difference in meaning of the below sentences.

• If this *be* the case, Brown's hypothesis might be proved.
• If this *is* the case, Brown's hypothesis is proved.

The subjunctive *were* is properly used to express an imaginary state (present or future) contrary fact, as in a supposition. Here, *were* should be complemented by other past forms such as *should* or *would.* For example:

If *it were* not for the fact that the ligaments ruptured, the patient *would* have undoubtedly suffered a severe fracture.

Possessives

In forming the possessive case, which signifies ownership or possession, the following seven rules apply:

1. The possessive of most singular nouns is formed by adding the apostrophe and s ('s); eg, doctor's coat, assistant's role, patient's chart. Exceptions include appearance' sake, righteousness' sake, conscience' sake.

2. The possessive of plural nouns ending in s is formed by adding the apostrophe after the s (s'); eg, doctors', assistants', patients'.

3. The possessive of plural nouns not ending in s is formed by adding the apostrophe and s ('s); eg, data's, women's, criteria's, cocci's.

4. Nouns that are both singular and plural usually add the apostrophe and s ('s) in the possessive plural; eg, deer's.

5. Nouns of one syllable ending in s or having a s sound usually form the possessive singular by adding the apostrophe and s ('s); eg, Buss's theory was. . . .

6. Modern usage also tends to omit the apostrophe in titles and names of organizations, companies, etc; eg, Southwestern Chiropractors Association, Shermans Pathology Laboratory, Wives Club.

7. Until modern times, the use of the possessive case for inanimate objects was avoided as an inanimate object cannot *possess* anything. However, modern usage attributes possession to many inanimate objects, abstractions, and measurements. For example, one day's vacation, five dollars' worth, three months' delay, a moment's notice, today's mail, at arm's length, the door's hinges, the country's flag, the adjusting table's base, life's trials.

Comparisons

Care should be taken in comparing like quantities *with* each other and quantities that are basically different *to* each other. For example, data from one test are often compared *with* the results of other tests. Blood pressure, however, might be compared *to* weight, height, age, and gender.

When comparisons are made between or among such items as properties, features, characteristics, states, etc, assure that the items are compared properly. For example:

> The blood pressure of Mr. Jones is higher than Mrs. Jones.

In the above sentence, "blood pressure" is compared to the spouse yet the writer intended to compare the blood pressures of the husband and wife. The sentence, therefore, should be corrected to read as follows:

> The blood pressure of Mr. Jones is higher than *that of* Mrs. Jones.

A comparison is made *between* two (this and that) items and *among* more than two.

• The difference in results *between* the two tests was substantial.
• The difference in results *among* the three tests was substantial.

Parallelism

Two types of parallelism are often used by science and technical writers: (1) parallelism of grammatical construction, and (2) parallelism of the development and presentation of ideas. Two examples lacking parallelism are:

• Traction was applied in various directions, pressures, and many different harnesses.
• Firstly, ... , 2nd, ... , and in the third place, ...

Parallelism is also lost by switches in verb tense and mode as discussed earlier in this section.

The second type of parallelism is more arduous to maintain because it is not as superficial and thus is more difficult to detect. Such parallelism can be obtained only by attention to a well-prepared outline.

Punctuation

The intended use of punctuation marks is to help clarify what is written. That is, punctuation identifies sentences, distinguishes questions from statements, separates words and phrases for greater clarity, and shows relationships among words, phrases, and ideas. When we speak, we pause, emphasize, and use body language. In writing, we attempt in a limited way to do these same things through punctuation.

In no other form of writing is proper punctuation more important than in science and technical writing. Improper punctuation can easily lead to misunderstanding. Punctuation marks are effective tools every good writer uses to enhance the readability of his writings. On the contrary, misuse of them disrupts the message, garbles meaning, and reduces the effectiveness of the message. The use of various punctuation marks, and their common uses and abuses is briefly described in the following sections.

The Comma

The primary function of commas is to show a pause between the context of one idea and that of another. Thus, commas are used primarily to clarify groupings of words, phrases, and clauses within a sentence.

As described earlier, there are inconsistencies in the application of the rules of grammar among various grammarians. The following rules were selected on the premise that each may be generally applied, without exception, and not be afforded the stigma of being grammatically wrong by either modern or medieval grammarians.

Because of the nature of science and technical writing, punctuation must be more accurate and more formal than that used by writers of fiction, newspapers, and other light reading. The rules presented here are not to be construed as a complete set; rather, they are intended to cover those rules most frequently violated by novice writers of science literature.

In technical writing, the comma has six principle uses. It is used (1) around parenthetic or transitional words and phrases, (2) around nonrestrictive or explanatory phrases and clauses, (3) between clauses of a compound sentence, (4) for omitted words, (5) between listed words or phrases, and (6) after inverted or introductory phrases or clauses and even after a single word if a pause is intended. Examination of each application will make the use of the comma more expli.

1. To set off parenthetical and transitional words such as *also, besides, therefore, nevertheless, however,* and *moreover,* and intervening phrases such as *in fact, as a rule, in brief, that is, in the first place,* etc:

• *However,* these results are subject to further interpretation.
• It does, *as a rule,* lend itself to interpretation, and, *therefore,* several interpretations are possible.

2. To set off nonrestrictive or explanatory phrases and clauses. Note that two commas are necessary to isolate parenthetic or explanatory words, phrases, or clauses. Note also that omission or addition of commas can change the meaning of a sentence. Care is necessary to differentiate *explanatory* phrases (which are set off by commas) from *descriptive* phrases (which are not set off by commas). For example:

Scientists, who are superstitious, will not conduct tests Friday the 13th.

Explanatory phrases, which are set off by commas, can be removed from the sentence without changing the meaning of the sentence. If the phrase "who are superstitious" is removed from the example above, the remainder is incorrect because most scientists *will* conduct tests Friday the 13th. The sentence should read as follows:

Scientists who are superstitious will not conduct tests Friday the 13th.

Some examples of nonrestrictive or explanatory phrases and clauses set off by commas are:

• Mrs. Jones' condition, *I believe,* is improving.
• It is, *without question,* a congenital deformity.
• Dr. Robert Wilson, *of Universal College,* was the keynote speaker.
• The final test, *conducted Monday,* showed further confirmation.

In the above examples, note that the explanatory phrases may be removed from the sentence without altering the meaning of the sentence. This would not be true for restrictive (descriptive) phrases and clauses, which are not set off by commas:

• He was *perhaps* busy at the time.
• The secretary *of the Board* answered the correspondence.
• In contrast, the examination *conducted Tuesday* was beneficial.

The term *for example* is an explanatory phrase by itself or may be used to introduce samples, illustrations, or cases in point. However, the term *such as (sometimes as)* introduces descriptive elements and is never preceded by a comma:

• A physical examination, *for example,* is usually conducted before laboratory tests are prescribed.
• Every other group should be given a placebo; *for example,* Group 2, Group 4, Group 6, etc.
• A comprehensive neurologic examination *such as* that for the cranial nerves is routinely conducted in cases where toxicosis is a suspicion.
• The patient manifested a high fever with notable systemic features *such as* hyperhidrosis, high systolic blood pressure, and delirium.

A comma is used after *namely (viz), that is (ie),* and *for example (eg),* whether spelled out or abbreviated, when introducing an illustration or example that is not an enumeration.

• There are three Latin genders: *namely,* masculine, feminine, and neuter.
• The patient must be positioned accurately (*ie,* centered to the beam).

• Routine examinations were conducted; *eg*, physical, spinal, postural, x-ray, and laboratory.

A nonrestrictive or explanatory phrase or clause ending a sentence is preceded by a comma, while a restrictive or descriptive phrase or clause ending the sentence is not:

• Mrs. Jones' condition is now stable, *I believe.* [Nonrestrictive]
• Examination results proved inconclusive, *however.* [Nonrestrictive]
• Tests were run in sequence *such as* Tests A, B, and C. [Restrictive]

When editing professional writing, the assistant also should be on guard to distinguish between words used parenthetically and the same word used as an adverb. While parenthetical words are set off by commas, adverbs are not:

• *However,* I shall follow the advice as given. [Parenthetical]
• *However* early he arrives at the office, his assistant.... [Adverb]
• *Thus,* the findings do not suggest.... [Parenthetical]
• *Thus* was a successful practice built from humble beginnings. [Adverb]

3. To separate *independent clauses* of a compound sentence joined by a conjunction (ie, *and, but, for, not, or, neither,* and *yet*) when it introduces a separate subject and verb conveying an additional idea:

• There is no evidence to support this claim, and it is doubtful if further investigation will prove to the contrary.
• He was schooled in strict disciplines, yet he was creative.

If an interpolation follows the conjunction, commas are usually used before and after it. Many modern grammarians, however, use a comma before the connective and omit the comma after it. Both styles are considered correct:

• The distortion was corrected, and, *as a result,* posture improved.
• The distortion was corrected, *and as a result,* posture improved.

A comma is not used, however, if the second clause is restrictive (irremovable). That is, the first is dependent on the second for its true interpretation. Usually, these clauses are adverbial and are introduced by a conjunctive adverb (eg, *after, as, before, since, until, when, where,* and *while*).

• This test must be performed *before* we can proceed.
• First aid was offered *since* the patient needed immediate attention.

However, if the adverbial clause is inverted, the comma *is* used after it:

• Before we can proceed, this test must be performed.
• Since the patient needed immediate attention, first aid was offered.

4. To indicate the omission (ellipsis) of a word or words:

• This test is easy; that, difficult. [Comma replaces *test is*]
• She was difficult, not obstinate. [Comma replaces *but*]

In a series, a comma may be used between the last and the next to last item to indicate "etc." All examples below are correct.

• ... such as the joints of the shoulder, elbow, knee, which....
• Points A, D, F, were measured.

If a series is limited for some reason, the conjunction should always be used. For example, the following sentence implies that only three points were measured:

• Points A, D, *and* F were measured.

Therefore, if a series shows only a few of many possible examples are given, terms such as "etc," "and so forth," "among other," should be used or a comma used for the missing word or phrase. All examples below convey the same meaning.

• Points A, D, F, etc, were measured.
• Points A, D, F, among others, were measured.
• Points A, D, F, were measured.

5. To separate items (three or more) of a list:

• The method used was simple, effective, and controlled.
• The three cases cited were (1) Mr. A, (2) Mrs. G, and (3) Ms. R.

Be alerted that many editors of popular literature eliminate the commas before the conjunction and. This sometimes does not make a difference in the meaning of the sentence; however, in science writing it can. For instance:

• Tests A, B, and C were run in sequence.
• Tests A, B and C were run in sequence.

In the first example above, it is obvious that the tests were run separately but in sequence. In the second example, it shows that Test A was run separately but that Tests B and C were run together. To avoid any possibility of confusion, it is strongly recommended that a comma always be placed before the conjunction unless a unity is involved.

6. To set off inverted or introductory modifying phrases or clauses from the remainder of the sentence:

• Because of the patient's pain, a complete examination was not conducted on the first visit.
• As the thrust is given, the force is directed in the plane of the articulation involved.
• In this test, all signs were negative.
• During the course of treatment, an unusual event occurred.

Another rule for which the comma is often used is to set off nouns in apposition. In science or technical writing, this frequently occurs with the definition of symbols or notations used in equations, charts, or tables. For example:

Pressure is the amount of traction, P, and leverage is the angle of pull, L, referenced to the joint.

However, be careful not to set off the callout of a specific item as a mistaken noun in apposition. For instance, if the author is speaking of circumferences of a limb at three different points, then in the sentence "The circumference C3 is twice that of circumference C1," the word circumference is no more than a modifier of the terms C3 and C1. Therefore, to set them off in commas would render the sentence meaningless.

Another pitfall that an assistant should be aware in editing copy is to avoid improper punctuation of -ing phrases. If an -ing phrase is cut, words go adrift along with their meaning. For example:

The doctor, having completed this initial examination, steps were then taken to proceed to more sophisticated measures.

The full first phrase above (an absolute phrase) is "The doctor having completed his initial examination." The sentence to be correct should have been punctuated as follows:

The doctor having completed his initial examination, steps were then taken to proceed to more sophisticated measures.

It is also important in professional writing that the word that should be kept outside commas that so often enclose an explanatory phrase or clause inserted after it. A simple test to check punctuation of the construction is to place the intervening phrase or clause at the end of the sentence. For example, if in the sentence:

It was theorized, that if the pressure were doubled, the vessel would rupture.

the intervening clause were read at the end, no sense could be derived from it. However, if punctuated correctly as:

It was theorized that, if the pressure were doubled, the vessel would rupture.

the meaning is clear. This rule holds true when it is desired that the intervening clause be read emphatically. If, however, it is meant to be read usually, the correct punctuation would be as follows:

It was theorized that if the pressure were doubled, the vessel would rupture.

The Semicolon

Although it is frequently stated that the average person may go through life without ever using a semicolon, this is not true for science writing. Here the semicolon is used for a more emphatic pause indication than the comma. It is used primarily:

1. To separate independent clauses not connected by a conjunction. For example:

No assignments will be accepted; all fees will be billed directly to the patient.

2. To separate independent clauses joined by a transitional (conjunctive) adverb such as *still, therefore, however, thus, alone, hence.* For example:

No assignments will be accepted; therefore all fees will be billed directly to the patient.

If the connecting word is to be emphasized, it is followed by a comma. For example:

No assignments will be accepted; therefore, all fees will be billed directly to the patient.

3. To separate items of a series when one or more must be punctuated by commas. For example:

The order was for printing 5000 letterheads, bond and onionskin; 5000 envelopes, No 10; and 500 copies of Form A-5 duplicate sets.

The Colon

A colon shows that more information is to be given about what has been mentioned. It is the strongest degree of break within a sentence. Its use is as follows:

1. To introduce an enumeration or explanation. For example:

• The following conclusions were drawn: first, ... ; second, ... ; third, ... ; and fourth,. ...
• He was alert and well informed: a serious student.
• Her spine at 4 years of age showed abnormal maturity: adult curvatures.
• The four principal types of examinations are as follows:

a. The physical examination
b. The spinal and postural analysis
c. The roentgenographic examination
d. The blood and urine profiles.

2. To introduce a direct quotation, especially if it is very long, begins a new paragraph, or is blocked.

3. Before an appositive phrase or clause. For example:

The doctor's advice was this: eat a well-balanced diet, exercise to tolerance, and get plenty of rest.

4. After the salutation in a business letter or an address, to separate the parts of numerical ratios or time, or between a publication's volume and number in reference citations.

• Dear Dr. Brown:
• The ratios were 4:1 and 5:2, respectively.
• The time was 10:15 pm.
• ACAJ 14:5 (1977).

Do not use a colon with the introductory phrase *such as* (either before or after) in any instance or use it with a form of the verb *to be* unless it is to introduce an enumeration or a blocked statement.

The Hyphen

In professional writing, a hyphen is a device used to connect words to achieve clarity and preciseness. Because it is applied frequently in science writing, care should be taken to use it consistently but not excessively in a given publication. The uses listed below are generally accepted and necessary for clarity:

1. With compound numbers from 21 through 99 when they are spelled out; eg, twenty-one, forty-eight, ninety-nine.

2. With a compound adjective (two or more words that express a unified idea), the adjectives that precede the noun should be hyphenated. For example:

• high-carbon steel
• up-to-date information
• state-of-the-art research.

Note: One of the better guides to proper compounding can be found within the *Style Manual* of the U.S. Government Printing Office.

3. With compound nouns that usually are transitional forms originating from separate words, often used together, that may in time be fused into one word. Words evolve from a two-word form to a hyphenated form to a closed form; eg, over all, over-all, overall. Other examples include:

- also-ran
- by-line
- burned-in
- on-site
- light-year
- go-between.

A compound adjective may be composed of adjectives, nouns, adverbs, participles, or any other parts of speech. In this context, the hyphen is *not* used if the first word is an adverb ending in *ly*, a comparative or superlative (*-er* or *-est*), if the compound is the name of a chemical compound or familiar to the general reader, or if the compound is a proper noun. For example:

- A publicly owned company
- A higher strength alloy
- A hydrogen chloride solution
- The United States flag.

4. Numerical compounds used as unit modifiers, preceding or reading back to the word modified, take a hyphen and are always singular. For example:

- 2-pound thrust
- 40-ft antenna
- 50-cc beaker
- 4-cycle, 50-horsepower engine
- Exposure: 100-amp, 300-kv, 2-sec.

5. However, a modifier consisting of a possessive noun preceded by a numeral should not be hyphenated. For example:

- 3 week's vacation
- 6 months' rest
- 1 week's pay.

6. A hyphen should be repeated in a series of separated adjectives that ordinarily would be hyphenated. For example: 3-, 6-, and 12-ounce flasks. This construction is called *suspended* hyphens. A suspended hyphen, however, is not used with *dimensions*. For example:

- Two 2 × 6-inch beams
- A 3 to 10-month program
- The 20 to 30-mile endurance test.

Dashes

The dash, in science writing, should be used sparingly. When applied, it serves to mark an abrupt suspension of the sense, a sudden change in sentence construction, or a quick change in thought. It is also used to set off expressions that demand unusual emphasis. Sometimes it is used to replace a colon. On the typewriter, the dash is typed as two hyphens without spacing between. For example:

If his diagnosis is accurate—and that means substantially better than that of the referring doctor—the patient will be in a much better position to plan his future activities.

Typesetters will use an *em dash* rather than a double hyphen. An em dash is a continuous dash equivalent in length to a double hyphen.

En dashes are also used by typesetters to separate ranges, numbers, capital letters. An en dash is a continuous dash equivalent in length to 1½ hyphens. As most typewriters do not have the capability of setting an em or en dash, a single hyphen must be used. Computer keyboards, however, do have these marks in the extended alphabet.

Thus, a combination of figures or letters should be separated by a single hyphen to indicate an en dash and not by a double hyphen. A single hyphen should also be used in the absence of the word *to* when denoting a length of time. For example:

- ACA–ICA Joint Conference
- AFL–CIO merger
- $10–$20-dollar range
- The period 1982–1988
- Model A–6
- 4–H Club
- CBS–TV Network
- May–July
- Interstate I–40

- pages 265–274
- Section 12 (h–j)
- 6–8 years
- Monday–Friday
- Public Law 85–1

Parentheses

Parentheses are used primarily to (1) enclose parenthetical remarks (ie, those not essential to understanding the sentence), and (2) enclose numerals in a listing—as in this sentence. They are also used to enclose numbers designating equations and, further, the numbers used to distinguish citations in a typed list of references.

Brackets

If your typewriter keyboard includes brackets, they are primarily used to enclose phrases or expressions, parts of which have already been parenthesized. This is most frequently encountered in mathematical texts. They are used to enclose editorial comments in text or quoted material.

Quotation Marks

Quotation marks are used to enclose direct quotations but not indirect quotations. If a quotation has several paragraphs, the marks are placed at the beginning of each new paragraph but only after the last paragraph. In many instances, quotations of great length should be additionally emphasized by blocking the entire quotation at the paragraph tab.

The marks are also used to indicate a word or phrase used in a new or unusual sense, or to introduce a new or unusual term (eg, technical jargon). In this application, the quotation marks need be used only the first time the new or unusual word or phrase is used. In this context, italic type is often used as a substitute.

Quotation marks are used to enclose titles of articles in a journal or periodical or chapter(s) of a book in references.

To set off a letter, number, or phrase for emphasis or to avoid confusion, quotation marks are often used. However, the marks are not used when the quoted matter is set in smaller type or in an indented blocked paragraph that is formally introduced with a colon. Also, quotation marks are not used to enclose familiar phrases such as *to err is human.*

The use of quotation marks with other punctuation marks is often confusing. If a question mark or an exclamation point belongs to the quoted material, it is placed within the quotation marks. If it belongs to the entire sentence, it is placed outside the quotation marks. For example:

- Did he ask, "What is your chief complaint?"
- Did he ask about your "chief complaint"?

Technically, the first example above should have two question marks for both the sentence and the quoted clause are questions: Did? What? However, quotation marks can be accompanied by only one other mark; thus, . . . complaint?"? would be incorrect.

Similarly, if a period or comma belongs to quoted material, it is placed within the quotation marks or dropped. While the same rule applies that quotation marks can be accompanied by only one other mark, commas, periods, question marks, and exclamation points are placed inside the quotation marks and semicolons and colons are placed outside quotation marks. For example:

- Our two major files are labeled "Active" and "Inactive."
- "Absolute concentration must be given," according to Boyle.

In this country but not in British or Canadian use, periods and commas have been placed inside closing quotation marks whether logically belonging to the quoted matter or to the whole sentence. This American practice was used strictly for aesthetic reasons when type was set by the "hot type" method. However, with the increasing utilization of cold type composition, the practice can no longer be justified unless it is known that hot-type composition will be used. Yet, the practice persists.

For many years, *Webster's Dictionary* tried to bring this illogical custom to the attention of publishers and journalists, but the habit has persisted and is now considered the standard in the United States. Even the current edition of *Webster's* has submitted to placing periods and commas inside closing quotation marks.

- She said, "eventually."
- He had a pain like a "knife cut."
- As the subluxation "major," it received priority consideration.

Hyphenation of Prefixes and Suffixes

One area in which grammar texts differ the most concerns the hyphenation of prefixes. For instance, The U.S. Government Printing Office (GPO) *Style Manual* states the prefix *micro* is written solid with all words except those starting with an "o"; eg, microorganism. *Webster's Dictionary*, however, writes it solid with all words including those beginning with the vowel "o"; eg, microorganism. Some technical writers choose to follow GPO style when writing for government sponsors and *Webster's* when writing for nongovernment sponsors. Regardless, care and discretion should be exercised in choosing a source to follow on the formation of word compounds. The most important thing is to be consistent in each document.

Some general rules in dealing with prefixes and suffixes are as follows:

1. Except after the short prefixes *co, de, pre, pro, non,* and *re,* which are generally printed solid, a hyphen is used to avoid doubling a vowel or tripling a consonant. For example:

- cooperation
- deemphasis
- preexisting
- nongovernmental
- posttest
- anti-inflation
- brass-smith
- thimble-eye
- shell-like
- self-confident.

An exception to this rule is invoked when such prefixes join a proper noun; eg, pre-Elizabethan, semi-Gothic.

2. The prefixes *never, self, new, vice, half,* and *quasi* are usually hyphenated. The prefix *ex* is hyphenated when meaning *former,* but closed when meaning *not* or *out of.*

Vice president when referring to the vice president of the United States is the only exception when "vice" is not hyphenated.

3. Care should be applied when using the prefix *re* as the use or lack of use of a hyphen could alter the desired meaning. For example: *re-form,* to form again; to distinguish from *reform,* to become changed for the better; or *re-cover,* to cover again as opposed to *recover* meaning to get back. The hyphenated *re* means "again."

4. Two short nouns forming a third or nouns consisting of a short verb and an adverb as the second element are usually typed solid.

- airship
- bathroom
- footnote
- bookseller
- breakdown
- makeready
- setup
- runoff.

Do not set solid short forms that would interfere with comprehension such as *cut-in, run-in, tie-in.*

5. Type solid *any, every, no,* and *some* when combined with *body, thing,* and *where;* and type personal pronouns as one word:

- anybody
- everything
- nowhere
- somewhere
- herself
- itself
- oneself
- yourselves.

6. Type as one word compass directions consisting of two points, but use a hyphen after the first point when three points are combined. For example:

- northeast
- southwest
- north-northeast
- south-southwest.

7. Unless common usage demands otherwise, use a hyphen to join a prefix or combining form to a capitalized word or when the first element is a proper name, but not in a unit modifier consisting of a foreign phrase:

- un-American
- post-Test B
- Anglo-Saxon period

- pro-ACA
- Florida-like
- Goodheart-like method

- bona fide transaction
- ex officio member.

8. Do not use a hyphen in a unit modifier containing a letter or a numeral as its second element, nor in a unit modifier enclosed in quotation marks unless it is normally hyphenated:

- article 3
- class II type
- ward D beds
- "blue sky" law

- "good neighbor" policy
- "tie-in" test.

9. A suffix is usually written solid at the end of the word it modifies. This rule generally applies to suffixes such as *like, down, fold, hand, hood, off, proof, up, wise,* and *hour.* This also is true for most Greek and Latin suffixes used in professional terminology. For example:

- wavelike
- payoff·
- galleyproof

- markup
- clockwise
- manhours.

However, as with prefixes, avoid doubling a vowel or tripling a consonant; eg, lifelike, but bell-like.

Capitalization

Determining the correct use of capitalization often results in perplexity. Although the rules set forth here were gleaned from various authorities, the sources surveyed were in close agreement. The major differences were strictly a matter of degrees of emphasis on a given rule.

The perplexity most often observed by this editor in the use of capitals arises with the use of titles before, after, and independent of a person's name; with the use of proper names used as adjectives and the words with them; with trade names; with common nouns used before a number or letter; and with catalogue names of commercial products. To help avoid these perplexities, the following rules are offered:

1. *Personal Titles.* Capitalize a title immediately preceding a personal name, but use lower-case if it appears after, removed from, or in apposition with a personal name.

- Director Donaldson. . .
- E. R. Donaldson, director,. . .
- Yesterday, President George Bush said that. . .
- George Bush, president of the United States, . . .
  - Yesterday, Chiropractor Anderson. . .
  - A. B. Anderson, chiropractor,. . .
  - It was developed by Doctor Brown. . .
  - M. G. Brown, doctor of chiropractic,. . .
  - Chiropractic Physician Smith said. . .
  - H. L. Smith, chiropractic physician, said. . .
- It was reported by Professor W. P. Michaels that. . .
- W. P. Michaels, professor of sociology, reported. . .

Dr. B. J. Palmer, son of the discoverer of chiropractic who served as president of Palmer Chiropractic College for many years, advocated capitalization of the words *chiropractor* and *chiropractic* always. However, as such use is improper according to generally accepted standards and strongly suspect of cultism within scientific and educational communities, such capitalization should be avoided.

All healing arts titles such as *chiropractor, allopath, osteopath, optometrist, podiatrist,* are never capitalized unless they begin a sentence or precede an individual's name. Such nouns as *doctor, physician, chiropractic, medicine, osteopathy,* etc, are not capitalized, nor are such adjectives as *chiropractic, medical, osteopathic.* Capitalization of these terms suggests ignorance or fanaticism.

2. *Trade Names.* Registered or proprietary names should always be capitalized and, when registered, followed by the registered trademark symbol (a small capital R within a circle) in published works. The symbol should not be placed within quotation marks.

- Chromel-Alumel® thermocouples
- Plexiglas® (but, plexiglass)

- M-19 Mylar® ribbons
- Pyrex® glass.

3. *Proper Names.* Proper names and adjectives derived from them are capitalized, but not the words used with them.

- Poisson's ratio
- Gonstead's technique
- Einstein's theory
- Rich's methodology.

4. *Catalogue Names.* Names of commercial products should always be capitalized.

- Ortho Film, Type 3
- ACA Form D-3

5. *Numbered Items.* A common noun before a number should be capitalized in science writing. It is not necessary (and is redundant) to use "No." before a number unless necessary for clarity.

- Item 10 (not Item No. 10 or Item #10)
- Series 10
- Reference 44
- Figure IX-9
- Table 20.1(B)
- Runs 6 through 11
- Tests 11, 12, and 13
- Code 102
- Volume II, Chapter 6.

6. *Directions.* Compass directions such as North, South, East, West, are capitalized when they refer to a certain section of the country or to a definite geographic location.

• the West coast	• the North Atlantic
• the Far East	• the South
• the North Pole	• back East.

As nouns or adjectives that designate natives or residents of certain geographic sections, they are capitalized.

• a Northerner	• an Eastern visitor
• a Southern gentle-man	• a Western drawl.

When used to refer to parts of the country, as simple directions or a general description, they are not capitalized.

- south of Denver
- the north of the state
- a western culture
- the southern states
- a northern winter
- off the west coast.

7. *Seasons of the Year.* Seasons are not capitalized unless personalized; eg, spring, summer, autumn, fall, or winter; but, "With Spring, her veil of green. . . ."

8. *Names of Heavenly Bodies.* Heavenly bodies are not capitalized unless used with the names of planets or stars, which are always capitalized; eg, earth, moon, stars, sun; but, ". . . travel to Mars, Venus, and the Moon from Earth."

9. *Biologic Names.* Names are capitalized for phylum, class, order, family, or genus except the name of a species, which is lower-cased even if derived from a proper name; eg, Chordata, Vertebrata, Mammalia, Carnivora, Canidal, Canis nubilus.

10. *Important Words in Titles and Subtitles.* In titles, the first word and all important words are capitalized. *Important words* are defined as nouns, pronouns, verbs, adverbs, adjectives. *Unimportant words* are prepositions, conjunctions, infinitives and articles of five letters or less (eg, of, and, or, to, the). If only one unimportant word appears in a title, it may be capitalized for the sake of conformity and at the writer's opinion. The titles below are correct.

- Nutritional Treatment of Arthritic Diseases
- Letters to the Editor
- Clinical Management of Head and Neck Dysfunction
- From Here To Eternity.

With compound words in headings or titles, the second part is capitalized as it would be if not hyphenated. For example, Cold-Worked Steel or High-Tension Test; but, State-of-the-Art.

The *GPO Style Manual* in its opening paragraph on capitalization states, "It is impossible to give rules that will cover every conceivable problem in capitalization; but by considering the purpose to be served and the underlying principles, it is possible to attain a considerable degree of uniformity." Thus, in a capitalization perplexity, the best advice is to find the correct form in a good reference if possible; if not possible, follow a similar form; if still in doubt, don't capitalize.

Numerals

The use of numbers in technical writing is extensive and for most writers a vexing problem as far as consistent and correct use. The rules described here are generally accepted as standard conventions, but again we find variation in the application of some standards. The rules listed below as preferred usage are by no means a complete treatise on the use of numbers. They treat mainly those questions found problematic in chiropractic compositions.

1. Generally, numbers representing *quantities* (not measurements) of ten and below should be written out; those above ten should be represented by numerals:

- One examination
- Nine examinations
- 13 examinations
- six doctors
- 60 doctors
- ten films
- 100 films
- five-man board
- four afternoons
- two-story building
- three-ply board
- the fourth group.

2. When two or more numbers refer to the same type of thing and occur close together in the text with only one of the numbers greater than ten, all the numbers should be written out. For example; eight, ten, and twenty; not eight, ten, and 20. However, if only one of three or more numbers is ten or less, use numerals for all; eg, 10, 16, and 19: not ten, 16, and 19.

3. One rule difficult for novice science writers and editors to remember is that numbers used with *units of measurement* (not quantities), either as a noun or unit modifier such as for dimensions, time, etc, should *always* be written as numerals whether the number is less or greater than ten.

- 20 cm
- at least 6 hours
- 3 feet
- 3-year program
- 6 hp
- 5-day test
- 300 kv
- 6-year-old female
- 1 hour
- 2-second exposure
- 57-degree angle
- 4:30 pm
- a course of 2 years
- half past 4
- 1 inch
- 3 o'clock
- 4½ percent
- multiplied by 3
- 7 meters
- about 10 yards
- 1 gallon
- 4 cents
- 2:5 ratio
- ½-inch diameter.

However, numbers expressing time, money, or measurement separated from their unit descriptions by *more than two words* are spelled out if under 11.

- two or more separate years
- 5 successive years
- either five or any number of years
- 3 or so years.

The following examples help differentiate between quantities and units of measurement.

- Each of the *six girls* earned *$6 an hour.*
- A team of *four men* ran the *1-mile* race in *3 minutes 20 seconds.*
- This requires *eight washes* in from *2 to 4 hours.*
- One engineer and *one contractor* inspected the *1-mile* road.
- The *two six-room houses* were built in *5 weeks.*

4. Numbers less than 100 preceding a compound modifier containing a numeral (quantity) are spelled out. In some instances, it is a good rule to spell-out all *quantities* up to 100 instead of ten as in Rule 1 and use numerals with all measurements and dimensions as in Rule 3.

- fifteen 3-foot boards
- three 6-passenger sedans
- thirty 5-day weeks
- 101 3-ounce samples.

5. Numbers with four or more digits should be written with a comma (eg, 2,400, 13,654, 123,997). For example:

143,562
7,943
732
20,652

To save space in tabular copy when no number is greater than four digits, the comma may be dropped from four digit numbers. For example:

673	2587.00
98	67.30
832	843.50
1256	1234.75

6. With dimensions or a series of numbers, it is not necessary to repeat the dimensions or unit of measurement. For example:

- 8, 24, and 48 hours
- a 4 × 12-inch beam
- a 12-inch × 2-foot × 1-yard container.

7. When numbers smaller than unity are used, a zero is placed to the left of the decimal point except with caliber or bore. For example:

- 0.25 inches
- 0.57 degrees
- .30 caliber rifle.

8. Rewrite the sentence or spell the number rather than begin a sentence with a numeral.

Incorrect: 20 people were surveyed in the program.

Correct: Twenty people were surveyed in the program.
In the program, 20 people were surveyed.

9. There is no need to repeat in numerals spelled numbers. This practice is a legal habit that has no place in nonlegal, science, technical, or business writing. For example: four visits, not four (4) visits. When necessary in legal documents, the correct style is five (5) dollars; not five dollars (5), five ($5) dollars, or five dollars ($5).

10. Ordinals and fractions are spelled when the fraction is part of a number of three digits or more. For example:

- first, second, third (not 1st, 2nd, 3rd)
- one-fourth, one-half, one-tenth (but, 125¾)

Numerals are used when fractions are unit modifiers. For example:

- ½-inch diameter (not one-half-inch diameter)
- ¼-mile endurance test (not quarter mile endurance test)
- ⅞-point rise (not seven-eighths-point rise)

11. With chemical formulas, full-sized figures are used before the symbol or group of symbols to which they relate and inferior figures are used after the symbol. For example:

$$6PbS \cdot (Ag,Cu)_2 S \cdot 2As_2 S_3 O_4$$

12. Indefinite expressions and round numbers are spelled.

- during the seventies (not '70s, but 1970s is allowed)
- a thousand and one reasons
- a hundred or so tests
- about a thousand doctors
- Two days, more or less
- less than a million dollars

For typographic appearance and easy grasp of large numbers, use *million* and *billion*.

- Change 12,000,000 to 12 million.
- Change 4.7 million dollars to $4.7 million.

Fractions standing alone or followed by *of a* or *of an* are generally spelled. For example:

- one-half of an inch (not ½ of an inch)
- half a dollar a piece (not $½ a piece)
- three-fourths of a dram (not ¾ths of a dram)

Calendar Dates

A calendar date is never used with a comma: 1978, not 1,978. The names of the months followed by the day and year should be abbreviated in reference footnotes, tables, bibliographies, lists of references, or when used as a citation or reference within parentheses or brackets in the text.

When the day is not given in a date, a comma should not be placed between the month and the year; eg, July 1991; not July, 1991.

It is unnecessary to use *st, nd, rd, d,* or *th* in dates unless the day is written before the month or is separated from it.

- June 29, 1991 (not June 29th, 1991)
- ... on the 1st of the month

When referring to a fiscal year, consecutive years, or a continuous period of 2 years or more, the following forms are used: *1902–3, 1945–57, 1895–1901.* For two or more separate years not representing a continuous period, a comma is used for a dash; eg, *1976, 1978.* If the word *from* precedes the year or the word *inclusive* follows it, the second year is not shortened and the word *to* is used in lieu of the dash: *from 1980 to 1988;* or *1978 to 1985, inclusive.*

In dates, AD precedes the year (AD 937); BC follows the year (254 BC).

Only in extremely narrow columns of a table, statistical composition, or informal memoranda is it permissible to use numerical abbreviations of a date slashed such as 2/10/91.

Months should be abbreviated when appropriate as follows: Jan, Feb, Mar, Apr, Jun, Jly, Aug, Sep, Oct, Nov, and Dec. There is no acceptable abbreviation for May.

Abbreviations

Although grammarians frown on the use of abbreviations (especially in correspondence), application is almost mandatory in lengthy documents that are written for a reader acquainted with the abbreviations. Their use is encouraged by such texts as the *GPO Style Manual,* which states:

> Abbreviations are used to save space and avoid distracting the mind of the reader by a needless spelling out of repetitious words or phrases.

The nature of the publication governs the extent to which abbreviations are used. In text of technical and legal publications, and in parentheses, brackets, footnotes, endnotes, tables, leaderwork, and bibliographies, many words are frequently abbreviated. Cut-in sideheads, legends, tables of contents, and indexes follow the style of the text.

Some scientific, technical, and industrial groups have adopted definite forms of abbreviations in their specialized fields. These forms, which omit internal and terminal punctuations, are acceptable for use in publications falling within the respective classes....

Standard and easily understood forms are preferable, and they should be uniform throughout a job. Abbreviations not generally known should be followed in the text by the spelled-out forms in parentheses the first time they occur; in tables and leaderwork such explanatory matter should be supplied in a footnote.

Types of Abbreviations

In its conventional sense, an abbreviation refers to any letter or short combination of letters having an alphabetical similarity to the parent word or phrase. There are three categories:

1. *Acronyms:* Pronounceable words formed by combining initial letters; eg, AUTOVON (automated voice switching network). Most acronyms, however, are formed by combining only the first letter of each word in the phrase; eg, USA, ACA, ICA, NASA, CIA.

2. *Brevity Codes:* A combination of letters designed to shorten a phrase, sentence, or group of sentences; eg, DDALV (days delay en route authorized chargeable as leave).

3. *Contractions:* An abbreviation formed by omitting certain letters or syllables and bringing together the first and last letters of elements; eg, rcpt (receipt), qtr (quarter). Contractions also link pronouns with verbs (eg, it's, we'd, I'll, you're) and make verbs negative (don't, can't). Only a few subjects like highly formal technical papers, reprimands, and funeral notices are too solemn for the occasional use of contractions.

Criteria

The source generally followed by most science writers and technical editorial units in styling abbreviations is the *American Standard Abbreviations for Scientific and Engineering Terms*. These fundamental rules apply:

1. Abbreviations should be used sparingly in text and with regard to the context and the training of the general reader. Terms denoting units of measurement should be abbreviated in the text only when preceded by the amounts indicated in numerals; eg, several inches, 12 in. In tables, specifications, maps, drawings, and texts for special purposes, the use of abbreviations should be governed by the desirability of conserving space.

2. When abbreviations are used, they should be used consistently throughout a particular manuscript. Do not use 45 cm in one place and 45 centimeters in another. One exception is to spell-out the term in the text, but abbreviate it in tabular copy; however, do not spell out in one table and abbreviate in another. Consistency is important.

In science writing, frequently used words should be abbreviated whenever placed within parentheses, brackets, footnotes, lists of references, and bibliographies. For example:

Use	Avoid
(Fig. 12)	(Figure 12)
(Ref 9)	(Reference 9)
[pp 10–12]	[pages 10–12]
(No. 32)	(Number 32)
(Vol II)	(Volume II)
(viz, . . .)	(namely, . . .)
(ie, . . .)	(that is, . . .)
(eg, . . .)	(for example, . . .)

3. Short words such as ton, day, and mile should be spelled.

4. The same abbreviation is used for both singular and plural (eg, bbl for barrel and barrels, ft for foot and feet, lb for pound and pounds).

5. Abbreviations should not be used when the meaning is unclear. If in doubt, spell out.

6. The use of conventional signs for the abbreviations of *number* (#) or *and* (&) is not recommended. Such signs may be used sparingly in tables and similar places for conserving space. The & sign should be retained if it is part of a registered corporate name (eg, Jones & Sons, Inc).

7. The period should be omitted unless the abbreviation spells a word and therefore leads to confusion. Thus, the abbreviation for inch, figure, United States, number, and collect on delivery should always be followed by a period to differentiate from the words *in, fig, us, no,* and *cod.*

8. The letters of acronyms should be printed closed without periods between. For example, USA, ACA, CCE, FCER; not, U S A, A C A, C C E, F C E R, or U.S.A., A.C.A., C.C.E., F.C.E.R., unless the acronym spells a word; eg, U.S.

9. The use in a typed text of exponents for the abbreviations of square or cube or for citing references is not recommended. Superior figures are usually not available on the keyboards of standard typewriters or some typesetting machines, thus composition is delayed.

- sq. in. (not in.^{2})
- cu ft (not ft^3)

10. Abbreviations for names of units are used only after numerical values. For example:

- 25 ft
- several feet (not several ft)

Footnotes

As a matter of good style, footnotes should be avoided as much as possible because they are a hindrance to smooth reading and add to the cost of publication. Explanatory matter is often more advantageously placed in parentheses in the text immediately after the word, phrase, or sentence to which it concerns. They also can be cited by number and included in a List of References at the end of the text or chapter. However, when necessary, footnotes should be placed at the bottom of the page on which they are cited in the text with at least a double space between the last line of text and the first notation. The first footnote should be separated from the text by a horizontal line; viz, an underscore about 1½ inches in length.

Footnotes should be keyed to the text matter to which they pertain by the standard symbols *, **, ***. It is desirable that no more than three be cited on the same page. When placing the indicator (call out) in the text, it should be placed after the text to which it pertains, not before it. For consistency, the marks should be placed after any punctuation except the dash (double hyphen in typing) or a closing parenthesis or bracket if the mark applies solely to the matter within parentheses or brackets.

The indicator should be placed immediately after the text to which it pertains without any space between it and the last word. The first word in the footnote, then, is similarly placed immediately after its indicator without any space between it and the indicator. The indicator in the footnote should be blocked on the margin with the second and subsequent lines of the note also blocked on the margin under the indicator. When several footnotes are entered on the same page, they are separated by a space and blocked or subsequent lines of each footnote may be indented a few spaces.

Remember that footnotes must be placed on the same page as their indicators and always end with a period whether they are complete sentences or a single word.

When footnoting formal tables, the same general system is used. However, when the table is inserted in the text, the notes are placed immediately below the table to which they pertain, not at the bottom of the page. If the table and its columns are "boxed-in," then the footnote divider line should extend completely across the bottom of the table.

If a document has fewer than six references cited and a separate list of references is not desired, reference citations can be arranged in numerical order at the foot of the page. The place in the text at which the footnote is cited should indicate the reference in brackets or parentheses such as [Ref 3] or (Ref 3).

A distinction is made here from the format of citations placed in a list of references or bibliography. In a List of References, the author's name is typed with forename or initials first. In a bibliography, the author's name is typed surname first followed by a comma and the forename or initials follow.

Use of the Latin terms ibidem (ibid), loco citato (loc cit), or opere citato (op cit) may be used as applicable. Abbreviations are usually preferred by most editors.

Bibliography Style

There appears to be no one acceptable method of construction of bibliographies except bibliographies and reading lists are set alphabetically by author while references are listed numerically (usually in the order of their first mention). In listing the sources used in developing the material, a bibliography entry should offer the reader information necessary to find the source in a library or bookstore if available.

Unfortunately, every editor or publisher has his or her preferred style that makes comprehension highly difficult. Some styles incorporate only commas for punctuation. Others use colons, semicolons, commas, and periods between items. Some say that the city of publication should come before the name of the publisher; others prefer it vice versa. Reasons are not given. Some have all items set in lower case except for initial letters and proper names; others have all items set in initial caps; and still others specify full caps for book titles. There is no logic behind these criteria. All one can do is follow the guidelines, if they exist. If not, select a style from a book or journal in the office that appeals to you, be consistent, and hope that it will be accepted.

Following is a common style. Include the facts when known and enter them in the order listed.

1. The name of the author(s) as it appears on the title page of the source, surname first and without usual punctuation (eg, Smith RD, Jones FW, Brown MS:)

2. The title and the subtitle, underscored. Important words are set in initial caps.

3. The edition number if other than the first edition as shown on the copyright page; preceded by a comma and followed by a period.

4. The place (city) of publication. The state should also be included if the city is not readily recognized. Cities such as New York, Chicago, Los Angeles, Philadelphia, and Boston, do not require a state reference; cities such as Springfield and Kansas City do for clarification. Small cities not widely known should also carry a state reference.

5. The name of the publisher, initial capitals, preceded and followed by a comma.

6. The volume number if more than one volume, set in Roman numerals and followed by a comma.

7. The year of publication that appears on the copyright page, followed by a comma. Do not use the date on the title page as this changes with every printing.

8. The pages cited, followed by a period.

A complete entry might appear as follows:

Smith RD, Jones FW, Brown MS: *Electrotherapy in the Treatment of Musculoskeletal Disorders*, ed 2. Boston, R.W. Smith & Sons, Vol II, 1989, pp 123–129.

The above information should be included in all book references. However, when articles are entered in a bibliography, the following style is recommended:

1. The name of the author(s) as bylined, surname first.

2. The title of the article, initial capped. Sometimes it is enclosed with quotation marks.

3. The title of the periodical in which the article appeared, underscored.

4. The volume, set in Roman numerals, and number of the periodical set, within parentheses.

5. The page numbers used in reference.

6. The month, day, and year of issue, if known.

A complete entry might appear as follows:

Smith RD, Jones FW, Brown MS: The Use of Interferential Current in the Treatment of Chronic Myalgia. *Electrotherapy*, IV(6): 123–129, May 1990.

In many publications issued by organizations, frequently an author's name does not appear. In this instance, the name of the editor should be used and identified as such. If the editor is not known, the sponsor's name or its acronym should be used.

Errata

Errata sheets (error sheets) should be issued to inform readers of errors of sufficient importance to warrant correction. Minor typographical mistakes will not usually require errata. However, they may be issued to make slight additions of information not available when the material was published. In addition to the changes, additions, or deletions involved, an errata sheet should show the basic publication number, title, and the date of publication of the original document.

Neither a cover letter nor a title page is used with an errata sheet. Use single spacing within each entry and double spacing between entries. Occasionally, the errata may require more than one page. When this occurs, the sheets should be clipped together in the top left corner of the copy. If reprints of a report having an errata sheet are required, the errata sheet should be bound in reprint copies between the front cover and the title page.

An errata sheet is constructed by first noting where the error occurs. Next, the words *for* and *read* are used as shown in the examples below:

- Page 87, line 14: *For* founder of chiropractic, *read* rediscoverer of chiropractic

- Page 92, footnote **: *For* Janze, *read* Janse
- Page 117, line 22: *For* 150 kv, *read* 180 kv

Note that punctuation is not used at the end of a correction unless it is part of the correction. It is omitted even at the end of the series.

FORMAL PROFESSIONAL PAPERS AND REPORTS

The purpose of a formal technical report is essentially to provide information on the results of a research project. To do this effectively, the writer should state the problem clearly and tell exactly what was done, how it was done, and the results of the work accomplished. Furthermore, he should use language clearly understandable to the average reader. Almost all grants and contracts require monthly progress reports and detailed quarterly and final reports to indicate how the work has met the proposed objectives.

The Basic Outline

If the writer is to present his findings effectively, he must have a thorough outline prepared that will organize the information he intends to report. This outline should divide the report into three major sections. The *Preliminary Section*, the *Body of the Report*, and the *Terminal Section*. These sections should include, as are applicable, the sequence and most of the elements shown in Figure 9.3.

Note: Some governmental agencies require special forms to be placed at the end of the terminal section, instructions for which are on the reverse side of the supplied form.

Reports should include, as a minimum, a title page; an abstract (preferably 200 words or less); an introduction; sections on approach, experimental procedures, and conclusions and/or recommendations. Documents exceeding ten text pages should be provided with a table of contents. When a report has over five illustrations, a list of illustrations is sometimes desirable. A similar standard is often applicable to tables. Other elements can be added as necessary.

Testing the Outline

Once developed, the outline will not only serve as a guide to the writer, it also will serve as a basis to construct the text. If prepared properly, the outline will show explicit transitions that are a good test for the soundness of the writer's organization. The author should write the phrase or sentence intended in leading from one idea to the next and bridging the "gaps" among successive sections. If this is not difficult, it proves a good outline and assures that each part is in the right order. If, by this test, it is discovered that the parts do not follow one another as they should, the author still has ample time to correct the trouble, whether it be major or minor.

When the outline has been satisfactorily completed, the next step is the actual writing of the report. The easiest section should be written first. For the researcher, this is usually the section(s) concerning the approach and experimental procedure.

Organization

The approach and experimental procedure sections will usually be an explanation of the theoretical basis for the experimental work and a description of the work completed. Tables and figures are often desirable and convenient to use in these sections. Their main purpose is to gather data into one convenient place and by that keep the text smoothly readable. They are preferably placed on the page following their initial mention or inserted in the text on the page where they are first mentioned. Either method may be used when the data are not extremely numerous and/or if the text is written so that the reader must refer to them frequently. However, when the data are voluminous or very complex, it may be better to relegate them to an appendix. If so, this fact should be mentioned in the text.

Preliminary Section

    Cover
    Title Page
    Foreword
    Author's Preface
    Abstract or Summary
    Acknowledgments
    Table of Contents
    List of Illustrations
    List of Tables

Body of Report

    Introduction (problem, objective, scope)
    Sections (approach, experimental procedures such as tests, results, description of equipment, future studies planned, conclusions, and/or recommendations)

Terminal Section

    List of References and/or Bibliography
    Appendices
    Distribution List

Figure 9.3. Sequence of parts of a formal professional report.

Remember that tables and illustrations are intended to aid text comprehension. To force the reader to remember the last line of a page while reading several pages of tabular and illustrative matter before the text resumes is poor design, but sometimes it is difficult to avoid.

If a report is basically a tabular and/or an illustrative presentation (ie, more pages of illustration than of text), the material should be grouped at the end of the section or chapter, or relegated to an appendix. Here they can be consulted as needed and will not interrupt the flow of the text. The writer also may extract key data and present them as tables or tabulations in the text, while putting the complete collection of data in an appendix.

In organizing the approach and experimental procedure sections, the presentation must be logical but not necessarily chronological. Also, where areas of future work are described in the experimental procedure section, they should be mentioned as they arise in the discourse.

In progress reports, the experimental procedure section should be followed with a future-work section. If the writer has mentioned, as stated above, areas of future work, it will be a simple matter to consolidate these statements into an organized general plan. The chief goal of this section should be to show that the author has a logical plan of future work that can be reasonably expected to produce results.

In final reports and certain progress reports (eg, quarterly reports), the experimental sections should be followed by the author's conclusions and recommendations. The conclusions reached should be based on the author's analysis, interpretation, and evaluation of the data obtained and an intimate knowledge of the total project. The conclusions create final impressions for the reader and, therefore, should be prepared carefully.

Recommendations should present the writer's advice for future action affecting the subject of the report. That is, if certain results were unsatisfactory or if it is felt that they could be improved, the writer should recommend modifications to the test equipment, for example, that he believes will improve the results. Or, he should suggest refinements that he or she believes will improve the results. Also, where some unusual phenomena were observed having no direct bearing on the project but considered worthy of further exploration, or where some unique test device or test method was developed that could have other important uses, recommendations for further investigation or development of the phenomena should be made.

With the easiest part of the report now written, the writer should double-back and prepare the introduction and summary or abstract of the report. The main reason for saving these sections for the last is that the writer can much more ably summarize the subject and detail its organization after he has developed the body of the text and knows what has been reported.

The Introduction

The *Introduction* should introduce the reader to the subject of the report and to the project's background. If the introduction is to the first or final report on a project, it will be somewhat longer than an introduction to a progress report. This added length usually occurs because of the inclusion of a clear statement why the sponsor has undertaken the project and how the program fits the overall program. Important here are statements showing that the writer knows and understands the sponsor's purpose in funding the research and that the author is aware of the state of the problem prior to the present research. If the report being prepared is not the first or final one for the project, the introduction can be much more specific and present only the particular aspects of conditions under which the work is being done, together with the procedure and scope of the present work.

In a series of progress reports, it is wise to sum relevant material from earlier reports and show how the work of the current report period fits the total project. Also, the report period should be indicated prominently in every report, preferably in the first paragraph of the introduction.

The Summary

The *Summary* is perhaps the key section of a complex or voluminous report. This is simply because many people will read it who do not read the entire report. Therefore, it should be thorough, concise, and conclusive. It should read independently of the report proper and be written as a concise recapitulation of information on the report as a whole.

The summary should be organized in the same order as the topics in the report proper. The most difficult part in writing a summary is keeping it brief and concise. It should not exceed three pages in length and should not be choppy. Effort should be made to keep it short, but transitions should not be eliminated. Such transitions as *finally, however, moreover, next, secondly, therefore, on the other hand, as a result*, etc, can be the useful words in the summary. To delete them would result in a seemingly confused presentation and leave a bad impression with the reader who might consequently judge the whole report to be poorly developed.

The Abstract

An *abstract*, like a summary, is a brief statement of the essential features of the report. Where the summary briefly describes *why* the work was done, *what* was discovered, *what* conclusions were reached, and *what* recommendations are made, an abstract is restricted to a concise *summation* of *objectives, results,* and *conclusions.* Its main intent is to provide the reader with an accurate impression of the contents of the report: its chief purposes are to enable the reader to decide whether he wishes to read the entire report and to provide abstracters with a statement for use in their reviews or journal announcements.

The abstract should be expressed, when possible, in terms of actual information rather than in descriptive terms, and it should not exceed 200 words (50 to 100 words preferred). All reports should contain an abstract, but the use of a summary is optional. Usually, the abstract can serve as both. However, when the subject matter is complex and voluminous, a summary should be included.

With the completion of these principal sections, all that is needed now is to add elements to complete the "whole" report. Other than those previously discussed, these elements are the *Cover, Title Page, Table of Contents, List of References* (if other publications are cited within the text but not completely referenced), and possibly lists of figures and tables.

The Cover

Copies of the finished report should be placed in an attractive binder. Cover text should be limited to a short descriptive title, the date of the report, the name of the reporting group, and a report number (optional).

The Title. An important asset to any manuscript is a well-selected title. It should be specific, describing the content of the report as explicitly as possible within the limits of reasonable brevity. Therefore, the final selection of a title for a given report should be made after the first draft is finished. By this time, the author will have acquired his broadest viewpoint regarding the contribution and be able to choose the best title for the subject matter. The most effective titles are short and informative.

Author(s). The names of authors should be shown immediately after the title, devoid of personal titles. They should be listed with the principal author first when there is more than one contributor. If there are more than three, only the top three should be shown on the cover followed by *et al* and a Foreword written to credit the others. The authors of the report are those who actually carried out the experimental work and wrote the report; authorship should never be bestowed as a courtesy. In a series of progress reports on the same project, an author's name

should be written the same way; that is; initials should not be used on one report and the name spelled out on another. Consistency on the part of an author in writing his name makes for accuracy in indexing and referencing and insures him of receiving credit for all his contributions.

Publishing Date. The date of publication shows the month, day, and year on which the report is reproduced, bound, and distributed. The month should be spelled-out (ie, February 1, 1991), and no other dates should appear on the cover.

Miscellaneous Data. Other information such as a project number, a contract number, type (progress, interim, final), identification of sponsor, and sponsor's address should not be placed on the cover but relegated to the title page along with any other helpful publishing information.

The Title Page

The *Title Page* is the first right-hand page and is unnumbered. Entries should be made on the title page in the sequence shown below:

1. Name and address of reporting group
2. Title of report
3. Name(s) of primary author(s)
4. Type of report
5. Project number and/or contract number (if any)
6. Sponsor's name and address
7. Date of issue

All succeeding pages prior to the Introduction should be numbered bottom center in lower-case Roman numerals (eg, ii, iii, iv, etc).

Table of Contents

A *Table of Contents* should be included in all reports containing ten or more printed pages. It should appear on the next right-hand page following the abstract. Entries for preliminary matter such as title page, foreword, abstract, summary, and acknowledgments need not be listed in the table of contents as these items appear *before* the Table of Contents.

List of References

A *List of References* is recommended if more than five titles are cited in the text but not completely referenced. List the sources cited in the order of initial text call-out. Each citation should be numbered with Arabic numerals. Thus, references in the text can be made by using the item number in brackets or parentheses after the subject cited; eg, (Ref 14). If five or fewer titles are cited, they may more aptly be cited in the text or listed in footnotes to the page of their initial call-out.

Optional Sections to a Report

As explained earlier, other elements such as a foreword or preface, acknowledgments, list of illustrations, list of tables, and appendices should be added to a report when applicable.

Foreword and/or Preface. A foreword or preface is used to present information about the report's subject or its preparation when the information cannot be suitably included elsewhere in the report. A foreword is usually written by a third-party reviewer; a preface, by the author. If the report is one of a series or has been prepared in several parts, a foreword may indicate this. It also may include pertinent administrative information, credit for the use of copyrighted material used by permission, names of principal researchers and scientists involved in the project covered by the report, and other related subjects not essential to the understanding of the report. Acknowledgments by the author, if he so wishes, may be made here of individuals, departments, or outside companies and organizations who materially assisted in the project if a separate "Acknowledgments" section is not included.

Lists of Tables and Illustrations. A separate List of Illustrations or a List of Tables may be given immediately following the table of contents or on the same page if possible. Such lists should be used only when there are more than five of each in the report. The wording of table captions and figure legends in the lists must agree exactly with those used on the tables and figures. Tables are titled (captioned) on top. Figures are titled (legended) below. Both are inserted in the final publication soon after their initial call-out in the text. Tables and figures are numbered in sequence, but this practice is optional in informal papers and the editor's choice in a journal contribution or book.

Appendices. Information is placed in an appendix when a report requires supplementary information not needed for understanding of the investigation or phase of it being reported. Appendices usually provide the reader with supplemental details, tables, charts, etc. Their use keeps the report from being unduly complicated in organization or excessively long because of the inclusion of details not required but helpful.

Typography of Reports

The standard page size in printing reports is $8\frac{1}{2} \times 11$ inches. The image area used in typing the report should not exceed an area of $6\frac{1}{2} \times 9$ inches, exclusive of running head and page numbers (folios). Legal size paper ($8\frac{1}{2} \times 14$ inches) *should not* be used in nonlegal literature.

Styling

Whether the report is to be double spaced or single spaced is the publisher's decision. However, it is strongly recommended that all final reports (as well as other professional manuscripts) be single spaced for the purposes of brevity, readability, and the economics accrued in processing (time and money). Whether the report is to be printed on one side of the page only (right hand) or on both sides of the sheet (back to back) is also the publisher's decision. In a single-spaced report, a double space should be allowed between paragraphs. In a double-spaced report, double spacing should be used throughout with paragraphs being shown only by indent.

When tables or illustrations are inserted in text, a triple space should be allowed before and after each insert in both single- and double-spaced reports. The caption of the table or legend to a figure should always be typed single spaced, with a double space allowed between it and the body of the table or figure to which it belongs.

In correspondence and manuscripts, it is customary to double space after a period or colon. However, this is not true for printed matter. If the document is to be photocopied from camera-ready copy, use a single space after each period or colon. This also would be true if the typesetter uses an optical character recognition (OCR) device to transfer your copy into a computer.

Primary Headings

Headings should be styled to provide continuous text style starting with the Introduction and continuing through to the appendices. An "outline format" is used, which is essentially an indentation system.

Primary heads should be enumerated with Roman numerals followed by a period and space. The title (and its number) is set in solid caps centered above the copy and from left to right with no underscore. With a full outline format, a triple space is made between the head of the first line of the text in either a single- or double-spaced report. If the report is typed using a "short outline" style, a double space is allowed.

Secondary Headings

Secondary Heads are numbered using capital letters of the Latin alphabet (A, B, C, etc), followed by a period and a tab. Headings are typed in initial caps, with the letter assigned typed flush with the left margin. The heading should be tabbed from its alphabetical designation and underscored. The first line of text begins at the same tab as the heading. Subsequent lines are typed flush with the left margin, either single or double spaced depending on the author's preference.

Tertiary Headings

Third-degree heads should be enumerated using Arabic numerals (e.g., 1, 2, 3, etc). The numerical designation is indented from the left margin to the first tab. The heading is tabbed from its numerical designation, typed in initial caps, and underscored. The

first line of text under a tertiary head starts at the second tab from the left margin, double spaced below from the heading. Subsequent lines are typed flush with the left margin using either single or double spacing as specified by the author. If additional subheadings are required, the indents (tabs) for each additional level are increased from the left margin in a full outline, typed in initial caps, and underscored. Headings below the tertiary level in a short outline format are "run-in."

The difference between a short outline format and a full outline format is a full outline does not contain run-in headings and the indentation for subheads can be far more extensive horizontally. Tertiary and subsequent headings in full outlines are set on increasing tabs and the following text begins at the same tab as the heading. See Figures 9.4 and 9.5.

Pagination of Reports

Styling and positioning of page numbers is also standardized. All prefatory pages (Title Page, Abstract, Table of Contents, etc, up to the Introduction) are numbered with lower case Roman numerals and placed about half an inch from the bottom of the page, and centered from right to left. The title page is assigned the page number of "i," but this number is not typed or printed. If the report is printed "back to back," the reverse of the title page will be numbered "ii." The remainder of the prefatory pages (front matter) will be assigned a number in sequence, even if left blank due to the requirement of starting a prefatory element on a right-hand page.

Recto and Verso Positions

The Title Page, Abstract, and Table of Contents start on a right-hand (recto) page in a back-to-back report. The foreword can be set on the back of the Title Page if it is one page or less in length. Lists of tables and illustrations are shown immediately following the Table of Contents; ie, they need not start on a right-hand page.

If both an abstract and a summary are used, the summary should be started on the

```
                    I. XXXXXXXXXXXXXXXXXXXXXXXXXXXXXXXXXXXXXXXXXXXXXXX


        A.   XXXXXXXXXXXXXXXXXXXXXXX

             XXXXXXXXXXXXXXXXXXXXXXXXXXXXXXXXXXXXXXXXXXXXXXXXXXXXXXX
        XXXXXXXXXXXXXXXXXXXXXXXXXXXXXXXXXXXXXXXXXXXXXXXXXXXXXXXXXXX
        XXXXXXXXXXXXXXXXXXXXXXXXXXXXXXXXXXXXXXXXXXXXXXXXXXXXXX

             1.   XXXXXXXXXXXXXXXXXXXX

                  XXXXXXXXXXXXXXXXXXXXXXXXXXXXXXXXXXXXXXXXXXXXXXXX
             XXXXXXXXXXXXXXXXXXXXXXXXXXXXXXXXXXXXXXXXXXXXXXXXXXXXXXXXX
             XXXXXXXXXXXXXXXXXXXXXXXXXXXXXXXXXXXXXXXXXXXXXXXXXXXX
             XXXXXXXXXXXXXXXXXXXXXXXXXXXXXXXXXXXXXXXXXXXXXXXXXXXXXXX

                  a.   XXXXXXXXXXXXXXXXXXXXX

                       XXXXXXXXXXXXXXXXXXXXXXXXXXXXXXXXXXXXXXXXXXXX
                  XXXXXXXXXXXXXXXXXXXXXXXXXXXXXXXXXXXXXXXXXXXXXXXX
                  XXXXXXXXXXXXXXXXXXXXXXXXXXXXXXXXXXXXXXXXXXXXXXXX
                  XXXXXXXXXXXXXXXXXXXXXXXXXXXXXXXXXXXXXXXXXXXXXXXXXX

                       (i)  XXXXXXXXXXXXXXXXXXXXX

                            XXXXXXXXXXXXXXXXXXXXXXXXXXXXXXXXXXXXX
                       XXXXXXXXXXXXXXXXXXXXXXXXXXXXXXXXXXXXXXXXXXXXXXX
                       XXXXXXXXXXXXXXXXXXXXXXXXXXXXXXXXXXXXXXXXXX

                       (ii) XXXXXXXXXXXXXXXXXXXX

                            XXXXXXXXXXXXXXXXXXXXXXXXXXXXXXXXXXXXX
                       XXXXXXXXXXXXXXXXXXXXXXXXXXXXXXXXXXXXXXXXXXX
                       XXXXXXXXXXXXXXXXXXXXXXXXXXXXXXXXXXXXXXXXXXXX

        B.   XXXXXXXXXXXXXXXXXXXXXX

             XXXXXXXXXXXXXXXXXXXXXXXXXXXXXXXXXXXXXXXXXXXXXXXXXXXXXX
        XXXXXXXXXXXXXXXXXXXXXXXXXXXXXXXXXXXXXXXXXXXXXXXXXXXXX
        XXXXXXXXXXXXXXXXXXXXXXXXXXXXXXXXXXXXXXXXXXXXXXXXXXXXX
```

Figure 9.4. Full outline format. In outline format, there should not be an A without at least a B, a 1 without at least a 2, etc. The limited space in this figure would not allow this to be shown.

```
        I.  XXXXXXXXXXXXXXXXXXXXXXXXXXXXXXXXXX

A.   XXXXXXXXXXXXXXXXXXXXX

     XXXXXXXXXXXXXXXXXXXXXXXXXXXXXXXXXXXXXXXXXXXXXXXXXXXXXX
XXXXXXXXXXXXXXXXXXXXXXXXXXXXXXXXXXXXXXXXXXXXXXXXXXXXXX
XXXXXXXXXXXXXXXXXXXXXXXXXXXXXXXXXXXXXXXXXXXXXXXXX
XXXXXXXXXXXXXXXXXXXXXXXXXXXXXXXXXXXXXXXXXXXXXXXXXXX

     1.   XXXXXXXXXXXXXXXXXXX

          XXXXXXXXXXXXXXXXXXXXXXXXXXXXXXXXXXXXXXXXXXXXXXXX
XXXXXXXXXXXXXXXXXXXXXXXXXXXXXXXXXXXXXXXXXXXXXXXXXXXX
XXXXXXXXXXXXXXXXXXXXXXXXXXXXXXXXXXXXXXXXXXXXXXXX
XXXXXXXXXXXXXXXXXXXXXXXXXXXXXXXXXXXXXXXXXXXXXXXXXXX

          a.   XXXXXXXXXXXXXXXXXXXX.   XXXXXXXXXXXXXXXXXX
XXXXXXXXXXXXXXXXXXXXXXXXXXXXXXXXXXXXXXXXXXXXXXXXXXXXX
XXXXXXXXXXXXXXXXXXXXXXXXXXXXXXXXXXXXXXXXXXXXXXXXXXXXXX
XXXXXXXXXXXXXXXXXXXXXXXXXXXXXXXXXXXXXXXXXXXXXXXX
XXXXXXXXXXXXXXXXXXXXXXXXXXXXXXXXXXXXXXXXXXXXXXXXX

          b.   XXXXXXXXXXXXXXXXXXXXXXXXXXX.   XXXXXXXXXXX
XXXXXXXXXXXXXXXXXXXXXXXXXXXXXXXXXXXXXXXXXXXXXXXXXXXXXX
XXXXXXXXXXXXXXXXXXXXXXXXXXXXXXXXXXXXXXXXXXXXXXXX
XXXXXXXXXXXXXXXXXXXXXXXXXXXXXXXXXXXXXXXXXXXXXXX
XXXXXXXXXXXXXXXXXXXXXXXXXXXXXXXXXXXXXXXXXXXXXXXXXXXXX

     2.   XXXXXXXXXXXXXXXXXXXXXXXX

          XXXXXXXXXXXXXXXXXXXXXXXXXXXXXXXXXXXXXXXXXXXXXXX
XXXXXXXXXXXXXXXXXXXXXXXXXXXXXXXXXXXXXXXXXXXXXXXX
XXXXXXXXXXXXXXXXXXXXXXXXXXXXXXXXXXXXXXXXXXXXXXXX

B.   XXXXXXXXXXXXXXXXXXXXX

     XXXXXXXXXXXXXXXXXXXXXXXXXXXXXXXXXXXXXXXXXXXXXXXXXX
XXXXXXXXXXXXXXXXXXXXXXXXXXXXXXXXXXXXXXXXXXXXXXX
XXXXXXXXXXXXXXXXXXXXXXXXXXXXXXXXXXXXXXXXXXXXX
XXXXXXXXXXXXXXXXXXXXXXXXXXXXXXXXXXXXXXXXXXXXXXXX
XXXXXXXXXXXXXXXXXXXXXXXXXXXXXXXXXXXXXXXXXXXXX
```

Figure 9.5. Half outline format.

reverse of the abstract. If a separate acknowledgment section is used, it should be set on either the reverse of the abstract or the reverse of the last page of the summary if it ends on a right-hand page.

Starting with the introduction, the body of the report will be page numbered with consecutive Arabic numerals, through the last page of the report, including the appendices and distribution list (when used). In a back-to-back report, all right-hand pages should be assigned odd numbers and all left-hand pages should be assigned even numbers. If the report is prepared using a "full outline" format, the introduction should start as page 1, and each subsequent primary heading should be run head to head. Each appendix, however, should start on a right-hand page. If an appendix should end on a right-hand page, the reverse of this page is assigned the next page number, but the number need not be printed. The next appendix is then started with the next odd page number, which will be a right-hand page.

If the entire report is run right-hand (one side of sheet only), all pages starting with the first page of the Introduction are assigned consecutive Arabic numerals that are placed in the upper right-hand corner about a half inch below the top of the sheet and flush with the right margin of the text.

Special Typography

Occasionally, reports are to be generated that require special typographical considerations such as special partitioning, two-column arrangements, special cover setups, and others, that can be adapted to once the sponsor's specifications are at hand.

Most contracts generated by U.S. Government agencies stipulate that certain aspects of reports generated during the course of a project, especially the final, be prepared in accord with the particular agency's report preparation handbook, guide, or specifications. Usually, the report will be published under that particular agency's cover. The formats required by these agencies are many and often vary considerably. To attempt to describe these formats here would be impractical; first because they change

frequently, and second because there are so many.

Direct Quotations

Another important element in the styling of reports is the treatment of direct quotations from another publication. Quotations are blocked on the paragraph tab and single spaced in either a single- or double-spaced report. The initial or subsequent paragraphs of the excerpt are not indented but shown with a double space. Quotation marks are placed before the initial paragraph, each subsequent paragraph, and closed only after the last paragraph in the excerpt. Many editors eliminate quotation marks in blocked quotations.

Ellipses

Line or sentence omissions within a paragraph are shown by an ellipsis, formed by typing three periods with a space between (eg, ...) within the paragraph where the omission occurs in typewritten copy. In typesetting for printing, word or phrase omissions within a sentence are shown by an ellipsis formed by typing three periods without spaces between (eg, ...). If such omission occurs after a complete sentence, do not consider the preceding period as part of the three ellipsis marks. A double space in typewritten copy should be used before the ellipsis as between sentences when this occurs (eg, xxxxx....). Similarly, if the omission occurs at the end of a sentence, do not consider the succeeding period as part of the three ellipsis marks (eg, xxxx....).

Listings (Enumerations)

An important element entering the styling of almost every report is the treatment of listings. This is not to be confused with headings or the "heading style" previously described with full and half outline formats. Enumeration numbering and spacing have little to do with the numbering or spacing of headings. Confusion arises because both the outline format and lists may contain numbers.

When items of a list are referred to in the text or when they follow a definite order or sequence, each item should be numbered in parentheses with the description of each item blocked after the number. Format is shown in Figure 9.6.

The opening parenthesis of the first item's number is typed on the paragraph tab. The text of each item is blocked on the next paragraph tab for both single- and double-digit numbers and is single spaced within each item in either single- or double-spaced reports, with a double space inserted between items. However, blocking of enumerations is a style reserved fairly exclusively to technical and scientific reports. In informal papers, books, and contributions to professional journals, succeeding lines of an enumeration are not blocked, they are brought to the left margin. This is for appearance of the printed page and to conserve space.

If a listing occurs within an item of the main list, the subitems should first be enumerated with lower case letters in parentheses, with a subsequent division in lower case Roman numerals in parentheses. The opening parenthesis of the subitem's letter is typed on the item's tab, and its text begins on the next tab. Refer to Figure 9.6. Parentheses are not generally used in book style.

Punctuation of enumerations requires careful consideration. A period is placed after an item only if the item forms a complete sentence. If the items are not complete sentences, a period should be placed following the last item in the list as the whole list is then a complete sentence. Each item in a list should start with the first letter of its initial word capitalized whether the item is a complete sentence. If none of the items in the list is a complete sentence, no punctuation is used. However, if one or more of the items is a complete sentence but the remainder of the list is not, either a semicolon or a period should be placed after each item in the list with a period after the last item. Here, it is the author's choice whether to capitalize or lower case the first letter of the initial word in each item. Book style uses different conventions than typewritten copy.

Where items in a list are not referenced later in the text or no sequence preference is intended, they can simply be shown by a dot (period), called a bullet in printing, as follows:

- The period is typed on the paragraph tab, centered on the line, and the text is blocked on the next paragraph tab.
- The same rules apply here as with numbered lists.

Where items are included as part of the text, remember that (1) numbers in parentheses are used to indicate each item, (2) commas separate each item, and (3) this structure should be used only if the sentences can be kept relatively short. Where individual items contain commas, semicolons are used to separate numbered items.

For run-in enumerations within a single sentence, one should observe the relative values of comma, semicolon, and colon. If one of the items listed is a simple sentence, semicolons should be used between each item listed. However, if each item listed is of simple character, not a sentence, with little or no punctuation within the elements, comma separation is sufficient. Within each item, as between them successively, punctuation should be based on the desire for emphasis and clearness. In sentence style, the first word of each item is capitalized only if the list has been formally introduced and every item listed is a complete sentence.

In a typewritten document containing many enumerations, it is often desirable to maintain uniformity of style throughout the manuscript. That is, if several lists contain complete sentences and, therefore, are punctuated after each item, then it is permissible to punctuate at the end of every item in every list contained in the manuscript for the sake of consistency.

Where items within an enumeration are all single line entries, it is permissible to single space the entire list. However, if one or more items listed is multiline, then the text of each item should be single spaced, with double spacing between each listing. Here again, for the sake of consistency in a given publication, the enumerations may be single or double spaced whether they are

```
        xxxxxxxxxxxxxxxxxxxxxxxxxxxxxxxxxxxxxxxxxxxxxxxxxxxxx
xxxxxxxxxxxxxxxxxxxxxxxxxxxxx (TEXT) xxxxxxxxxxxxxxxxxxxxxxxxxxx
xxxxxxxxxxxxxxxxxxxxxxxxxxxxxxxxxxxxxxxxxxxxxxxxxxxxxxxxxxx.

    (1)  xxxxxxxxxxxxxxxxxxxxxxxxxxxxxxxxxxxxxxxxxxxxxxxxxxx
         xxxxxxxxxxxxxxxxxxxxxxxxxxxxxxxxxxxxxxxxxxxxxxxxxxx
         xxxxxxxxxxxxxxxxxxxxxxxxxxxxxxxxxxxxxxxxxxxxxxxxx.

         (a)  xxxxxxxxxxxxxxxxxxxxxxxxxxxxxxxxxxxxxxxxxxxxxxx
              xxxxxxxxxxxxxxxxxxxxxxxxxxxxxxxxxxxxxxxxxxxxxx
              xxxxxxxxxxxxxxxxxxxxxxxxxxxxxxxxxxxxxxxxxxx.

         (b)  xxxxxxxxxxxxxxxxxxxxxxxxxxxxxxxxxxxxxxxxxxxxxxx
              xxxxxxxxxxxxxxxxxxxxxxxxxxxxxxxxxxxxxxxxxxxxxx
              xxxxxxxxxxxxxxxxxxxxxxxxxxxxxxxxxxxxxxxxxxx.

              (i)  xxxxxxxxxxxxxxxxxxxxxxxxxxxxxxxxxxxxxxxxx
                   xxxxxxxxxxxxxxxxxxxxxxxxxxxxxxxxxxxxxxxx
                   xxxxxxxxxxxxxxxxxxxxxxxxxxxxxxxxxxxxxx.

              (ii) xxxxxxxxxxxxxxxxxxxxxxxxxxxxxxxxxxxxxxxxx
                   xxxxxxxxxxxxxxxxxxxxxxxxxxxxxxxxxxxxxxxx
                   xxxxxxxxxxxxxxxxxxxxxxxxxxxxxxxxxxxxxx.

         (c)  xxxxxxxxxxxxxxxxxxxxxxxxxxxxxxxxxxxxxxxxxxxxxxx
              xxxxxxxxxxxxxxxxxxxxxxxxxxxxxxxxxxxxxxxxxxxxxx
              xxxxxxxxxxxxxxxxxxxxxxxxxxxxxxxxxxxxxxxxxxx.

    (2)  xxxxxxxxxxxxxxxxxxxxxxxxxxxxxxxxxxxxxxxxxxxxxxxxxxxxx
         xxxxxxxxxxxxxxxxxxxxxxxxxxxxxxxxxxxxxxxxxxxxxxxxxxxxx
         xxxxxxxxxxxxxxxxxxxxxxxxxxxxxxxxxxxxxxxxxxxxxxxxxx.

         (a)  xxxxxxxxxxxxxxxxxxxxxxxxxxxxxxxxxxxxxxxxxxxxxxx
              xxxxxxxxxxxxxxxxxxxxxxxxxxxxxxxxxxxxxxxxxxxxxx
              xxxxxxxxxxxxxxxxxxxxxxxxxxxxxxxxxxxxxxxxxxx.

         (b)  xxxxxxxxxxxxxxxxxxxxxxxxxxxxxxxxxxxxxxxxxxxxxxx
              xxxxxxxxxxxxxxxxxxxxxxxxxxxxxxxxxxxxxxxxxxxxxx
              xxxxxxxxxxxxxxxxxxxxxxxxxxxxxxxxxxxxxxxxxxx.

    (3)  xxxxxxxxxxxxxxxxxxxxxxxxxxxxxxxxxxxxxxxxxxxxxxxxxxxxx
         xxxxxxxxxxxxxxxxxxxxxxxxxxxxxxxxxxxxxxxxxxxxxxxxxxxxx
         xxxxxxxxxxxxxxxxxxxxxxxxxxxxxxxxxxxxxxxxxxxxxxxxxx.
```

Figure 9.6. Format for typewritten listings in professional reports.

single or multiline. If all are to be single spaced, however, those items that are multiline should have the subsequent lines of each item indented a few spaces to show separation of the listings.

TYPING HINTS AND HELPS

Preparing a Typewritten Table

Tabular material is common in professional manuscripts, proposals, reports, and papers. Good organization of the material requires concern for measurement, arrangement, vertical and horizontal spacing, headings, and margination.

Measurements

• An 8½ × 11-inch sheet contains 66 vertical lines. If a 6½ × 9-inch image area is used, there will be 54 vertical lines in the 9-inch area; ie, six lines in each vertical inch.

• An 8½ × 11-inch sheet can contain 85 pica characters and 102 elite characters. A 6½ × 9-inch image area can hold 65 pica characters and 78 elite characters; ie, ten pica characters per horizontal inch and 12 elite characters per horizontal inch.

An easy way to plan a table is to think of each table having three major parts: (1) a title, (2) column headings, and (3) the columns themselves. The left descriptive column (stub) may or may not be titled, but all other columns must be. Headings may be centered over their column or blocked left. Figures are usually blocked right, with decimals aligned, but infrequently it is more appropriate to center them.

Vertical Spacing

In arranging vertical spacing, allow three spaces between the title and the column headings. If a subtitle is necessary, allow three spaces between the title and subtitle, and two spaces between the subtitle and the column headings. Two spaces should be inserted between column headings and the first entry in the column. Double space all

column entries in short tables, single space in long tables.

Margination

Most tables require a rough draft to determine the number of vertical lines necessary, the character width of each column, and how many spaces you wish between columns.

If you wish to center a table on the sheet, count the number of line spaces in the table including lines between title, subtitle, headings, and entries. Subtract this total from the total number of vertical lines in the image area and divide this number in half. This gives the number of lines for the top and bottom margin. For example, if you are using a 9-inch vertical image area (54 lines) and the table requires 30 lines, the calculation would be $54 - 30 = 24/2 = 12$. Thus the table would be centered vertically in the image area, with even margins top and bottom of 12 lines each.

To center a table on the sheet horizontally, count the number of characters and spaces in the longest line of each column; then total. If you are using a 6½-inch-wide image area, the total area will fit 66 characters in elite type, for example. If the total for the number of characters and spaces in the longest line of each column is 42 characters and spaces, the calculation would be $66 - 42 = 24$ spaces remaining. You must now decide how you would like to divide these 24 spaces between the right and left margins and the spaces between each column (gutters). If the table has three columns, you may wish to allow four spaces between each column and eight spaces for each margin. In a three column table, you would have a left margin, the first column, a gutter between the first and second column, the second column, a gutter between the second and third column, the third column, and a right margin.

Setting Tabs

Before typing, space over from the left margin of the image area the number of spaces you allot for the left margin in your table and set the tab. This will be where the first column begins. Then, space over the number of spaces required for the first column and its gutter, and set the tab. This will be where the second column begins. Repeat this process for each column, but keep in mind that the last column will not have a gutter.

Standard Rules for Spacing

One space is used after a comma, after a semicolon, after a period following an abbreviation or acronym that spells a word, after an initial, after an exclamation point used in the body of a sentence, and before and after the multiplication sign " × ," meaning "by" (eg, 3″ × 5″ card).

Two spaces are inserted after a colon, after every typed sentence, and after a period following a figure or letter at the beginning of a line in a list of items (unless tabs are used).

A space is not used before or after a hyphen, an apostrophe, quotation marks, words enclosed between parentheses, or impersonal initials and acronyms.

Never separate punctuation from the word it follows. For example, do not set a dash at the beginning of a typed line.

Labeling Drafts

When preliminary work is being developed, write "Draft," "First Draft," or "Final Draft" in capitals or initial caps in parentheses and centered at the top of the first sheet.

When a rough draft is retyped, examine the corrected page to note portions marked for omission, where new material is to be inserted, and necessary corrections. Assure that additions and corrections are grammatically correct.

Tabulator-Key Uses

The "tab" key on a typewriter can be used for more purposes than setting-up tables. Some other primary uses are (1) placement of dateline, complimentary close, and signature lines in correspondence; (2) paragraph

indentations; and (3) setting an outline format in reports.

Centering Headings and Titles

First count all letters, spaces, and punctuation marks in the heading or title. Then divide this number in half and space over this amount from the center of your image area. For example, if your image area extends from 30 to 106, the center will be at 68 on the scale. If a heading contains 30 characters, the starting point will be at 53 $(68 - 30/2)$.

Word and Line Divisions

Word division avoids great unevenness at the right margin. The break should come between syllables, but one- or two-letter divisions such as e-vil, en-velope, entire-ly, consecrat-ed, are rarely acceptable. As a general rule, compound words should be divided according to their major parts; eg, uneven rather than une-ven, volley-ball rather than vol-leyball. Never divide a word between pages in typewritten copy.

A person's given name and surname, initials and surname should not be divided in typewritten copy. Letters of a radio station or government agency, dates, parts of an equation, combinations of monetary expressions, and hours of a day should not be divided. Following are some examples:

WKBW	525 BC
$1,378.50	6x + 4y = 27
March 2	4:00 am

Orphans (single lines) at the top of pages should be avoided if possible, and paragraphs should not start on the last line of a page.

Proofreading

No matter how often a doctor and an assistant check a manuscript for errors, at least one always seems to escape detection. One reason is that it is difficult to see errors in

MARK	EXPLANATION	EXAMPLE
ℂℏ	Start new paragraph	ℂℏ fine papers ‸Mead grades are
no ℂℏ	No paragraph. Run in	no ℂℏ fine papers.⤸ Mead grades are
⊐	Move to right	⊐ Mead grades are
⊏	Move to left	⊏ Mead grades are
⊔	Lower letter or word	⊔ Mead|grades|are
⊓	Raise letter or word	⊓ Mead |grades| are
tr.	Transpose	tr. Mead are|grades|
wf.	Wrong font	wf. Mead grades are
lc.	Lower case letter	lc. Fourscore and $even years ago
Cap.	Capital letter	Cap. The united States
C+SC.	Caps and small caps	C+SC. The united states
C&lc.	Caps and lower case	C&lc. The United States
rom.	Put in roman type	rom. The United States
ital.	Put in italic type	ital. The United States
bf.	Put in boldface type	bf. The United States
stet	Let it stand. Disregard previous correction	stet Fourscore and seven years ago
e	Delete (take out)	e Fourscore and and seven years ago
sp	Spell out	sp the U.S.
X	Broken or imperfect type	X The letter "t" is broken
?	Turn a reversed letter	? Fourscore and seven
#	Insert space	# Our fathersbrought
Eq#	Equalize space	Eq# Our fathers were brought
‿	Less space	‿ Our fathers were brought
=/	Insert hyphen	=/ It happened in midweek
(/)	Insert parentheses	(/) Prepositions at, in, of are
▢	Indent one em	▢ Romeyn rode away
⌄⌄	Insert quotation marks	⌄⌄ Sing Yankee Doodle Dandy
sp?	Spelling questioned	sp? The city of Springfield

Figure 9.7. Proofreader's marks.

one's own work—the mind seems to make a correction and perceive what should be rather than what is. Thus, objective parties make the best proofreaders. Most errors will be found in spelling, poor word divisions, inaccurate verb numbers, and the use of superfluous words or phrases. Common proofreading symbols used in editing drafts and galley proofs are shown in Figure 9.7.

Spelling

There should be no need for guidance in the area of spelling because the dictionary should serve as the authority. Unfortunately, dictionaries differ, and different sponsors and publications use different dictionaries. The majority, however, use *Webster's Ninth New Collegiate Dictionary.*

Many spelling errors come from the improper use or nonuse of hyphens in compound words, inconsistencies observed in plurals and possessives, and the use of British rather than American spelling. These subjects have been described earlier and deserve periodic review.

As explained in the chapter concerning chiropractic terminology, an understanding of Latin and Greek prefixes and suffixes, along with Old English and Latin and Greek roots and derivatives, is helpful in forming correct spelling habits.

Verb Endings

The suffixes *ed* and *ing* are usually added to the basic verb without changing its spelling. But when a verb ends in a stressed syllable in which the final consonant is preceded by a single vowel, the consonant is doubled (eg, fitted, referring). When c is the final consonant, k is added instead (eg, frolicked, picnicking). When a verb ends in *e*, the e is dropped as in changing. Some exceptions to this are dyeing, singeing, agreeing, eyeing, stymieing, trueing, canoeing, hoeing.

Contractions

An apostrophe is used in such verb contractions as they're, isn't; and in such coined verb contractions as OK'd and KO'd. An apostrophe is also used to denote the omission of letters as in rock 'n' roll, fin 'n' claw; and it is used in contraction of years as in Class of '65. Contractions such as from telephone to phone have been used so long that an apostrophe is not used.

Foreign Words

When foreign words or phrases are used or quoted, they must be spelled according to the rules of their own languages. Should an occasion demand the quotation of Greek, Russian, or another language that does not use the Roman alphabet, the quotation must be transliterated.

Chapter 10

Brief Introduction to Computer Science

Having use of a small computer can improve an assistant's working life by doing many routine duties much faster, minimizing peak work-load periods, and automating many laborious tasks. It saves the office money by reducing task manhours, increasing individual productivity, and reducing the required number of administrative assistants. It increases office income by automating an efficient accounts receivable system. It improves management control by controlling costs, having detailed information instantly available, developing a variety of reports from numerous files automatically, monitoring patient data and the doctor's investments, and providing customized planning and budgeting signals.

Of course, there are some horror stories associated with the use of a computer. One reason is poor understanding of what a computer is and what is does. If input is erroneous, output will be false: "garbage in, garbage out." Another reason is that a computer cannot do anything that cannot be done manually—however, it does it in a fraction of the time. If the original manual system was inefficient, the computerized model will be rapid implementation of a flawed system. The purpose of this chapter is to provide the reader with the understanding necessary for common errors to be avoided.

THE BEGINNING

Computing by machine started (as near as we now know) in the Mideast with the use of counting stones in channels. This was the precursor of a counting instrument invented by the Babylonians but usually associated with the Chinese. It is called an *abacus*. The abacus reigned supreme for centuries because its use did not require knowledge about the theory of numbers. The uneducated could be trained to use it easily.

Early Contributors

Mathematics with Arabic numbers entered Europe in the 8th and 9th centuries. It did not become popular because the user had to understand theory. To help, various mechanical devices were invented. In the early 1600s, Napier (the inventor of logarithms) developed a series of rods that could be used for multiplication. Partial products appeared on the rods so all the user had to do was add them to get the final product. This led to ever more complicated mechanical devices based on gears and rods, with Blaise Pascal's mechanical Pascaline being the most famous.

These inventions led to the work of Charles Babbage and the Countess of Lovelace in 1791. Babbage was an English mathematician and inventor, and the Countess of Lovelace was Ada Byron, daughter of Lord Byron, the famous poet. Babbage is often thought of as the Father of Computers because of his inventions. Ada is usually considered the first computer programmer because of her analyses and explanations of Babbage's work.

Babbage achieved fame by developing the ideas for two "engines" (mechanical calculators). The *difference engine* solved polynomial equations by the method of differences. The *analytical engine* was designed to be a general purpose computing device. Neither machine was produced because tooling of the day was not advanced enough. Babbage nevertheless left detailed designs that contained within them the heart of modern computers. The analytical engine, in particular, was designed with five parts common to today's computers:

1. An *input device:* borrowing an idea from textile mills, a form of punched cards was the input.

2. A *processor (calculator):* a mill containing hundreds of vertical axles and thousands of gears, 10 feet tall.

3. A *systems control unit:* a barrel-like device with slats and studs, operating like a complex player piano.

4. A *data storage unit:* the store, containing more axles and gears. This device could hold 100 40-digit numbers.

5. An *output device:* plates designed to fit in a printing press.

A Need Is Met for the 1890 Census

The 1880 census of the United States took some 7 or more years to complete because all processing was done by hand from journal sheets. Because the population was growing rapidly, hand tabulation in 1890 would likely take longer than the 10-year period to the next census. A competition was held for a better method, and Herman Hollerith, a Census Department employee, proposed a "better mousetrap."

Hollerith's method incorporated the punched card—the "do not fold, spindle, or mutilate" card many of us remember. It entered the world of numbers with the 1890 census, which announced within 6 weeks the nation's population (62,622,250). By using the cards, the Census Department could produce many different statistics for the nation—so many that despite the speed and use of the information, the cost almost doubled that of the 1880 census. This was a vision of times to come when instant information demands processing, whether the data are useful or not.

Hollerith went on to found the Tabulating Machine Company, which later became International Business Machines (IBM).

Enhancements During World War II

As usual, the war effort was a spur to the development of technology. Computers were no exception—in fact, it was this era where the first true electronic digital computers were introduced. The most foremost were:

• The Mark I: An electromechanical device using relays, built for the Navy by IBM. Last of its breed. Overtaken by electronics.

• The Colossus: A special purpose code breaker built for the British to decode German radio codes.

• The ABC: For Atanasoff-Berry Computer, built at Iowa State. Now considered the first electronic digital computer.

• The ENIAC: Most famous of the early computers, containing 18,000 vacuum tubes. Built for the U.S. Army for ballistics.

• The Manchester Mark I: Built by Manchester University; the first "stored program" computer. Before this time, all computers had to be told what to do by rewiring. This was a breakthrough.

The Postwar Periods

The period from World War II to the present can be divided into roughly four generations for computers:

1. From roughly 1951 through 1958, generation one computers featured the use of vacuum tubes. The standout of the era was the UNIVAC (UNIVersal Automatic Computer), which was the first true general purpose computer in America designed for both alphabetic and numeric uses. This made the UNIVAC a standard for business, not just equipment for science and the military. Punched cards formed the input to the machines, and all programming was through machine language (ie, numbers interpreted by the machine as commands).

2. The transistor dominated computers from 1959 to 1964. Computers became smaller. There were no outstanding computers during this period, but it is noted for the development of higher order languages. Computers could now be programmed with English-like commands instead of strings of numbers. Programming efficiency improved greatly. FORTRAN for scientists and COBOL for business became the two major system languages of the era.

3. The years from 1965 to 1970 saw the introduction of the integrated circuit. Instead of large boards, circuits (electronic roadways) were developed on single chips of silicon. Two devices stand out during this period: IBM introduced its 360 series mainframe computers, and the smaller minicomputer made its debut. The latter was similar to a large computer but with smaller memory and slower processing speed. The introduction of the minicomputer made computers available to the small businesses.

4. Microprocessors derived from integrated circuits put computers on the office desk. Beginning in 1971 and running to the present, generation four is characterized by the development of the microprocessor and its derivative, the personal computer (PC). Computers of the fourth generation are roughly 100 times smaller than those of generation one, yet more powerful.

Microcomputers

The history of computing can be compared to a large tree. Early computing is fairly easy to trace with few branches to worry about. As one moves up the tree, the branches become more numerous and more difficult to follow. The history of microcomputers, being fairly high on the tree, is arduous to follow with many related or competing things happening near the same time. Here are the highlights:

• In the 1950s, several semiconductor companies were founded to produce transistors. At least one attempt to design a small computer using these vacuum-tube replacements was made, but it failed. The Intel Corporation received a commission to produce integrated circuits for Japanese calculators in 1969. This led to their decision to build the first microprocessor: the 4004. John Kemeny and Thomas Kurtz developed the first version of BASIC programming language at Dartmouth College in 1964. The computer industry was now primed for greatness.

• The 1970s were years of rapid advancement. The 8008 was developed by Intel in 1971. The *People's Computer* Company published practical information about computers for the public in 1972. The Community Memory project was started by Lee Felsenstein and others to allow people access to a public network and see the power of computers. The 8080 microprocessor was developed by Intel in 1974. The July 1974 issue of *Radio Electronics* published an article showing how to build the Mark 8, a computer based on the Intel 8008. They called it "*your personal minicomputer.*" In 1975, Microsoft Corporation developed the first

BASIC system language for the Altair computer. This was a giant step forward. IBM, Apple, Commodore, Tandy/Radio Shack, and others who manufactured "clones," firmed their roles in the PC market.

We are now at the point where microcomputers became available to the public—not just to "hackers" who were willing to put up with the unfriendly user interface presented by the first "micros."

Steven Jobs visited the Xerox PARC laboratories in 1979 and got ideas for the Macintosh desktop PC. The TRS-80 Model II was announced by Tandy, and WordStar, the first practical word processing program, was introduced by MicroPro.

VisiCalc is largely credited for the microcomputer revolution. This popular spreadsheet made desktop analyses easy and allowed anyone to write what amounted to programs without having to learn a complex systems language. The program was truly a "visible calculator" that took its name from a shortening of those words.

Microcomputer development and sales continued to escalate during the 1980s. IBM introduced their first PC in 1981 and quickly took over the corporate marketplace. Apple attempted to make inroads into corporations with the Lisa in 1982, but the closed architecture (little ability to add features from other vendors) and other factors caused Apple to drop the Lisa eventually in favor of their Macintosh line, first introduced in 1984. The popular IBM-architecture machines use a character interface; the Macintosh uses a graphical interface. Each type of interface has its proponents and opponents. When the 1980s closed, versions of past computers based on ever more powerful microprocessors were quickly giving the user the power of older minicomputers (and some mainframes) at their desk.

A Look Ahead

It's difficult to predict the future, but there are some projections that can be made based on extensions of current technology. In the early 1980s, Japan announced a 10-year program to leap-frog technology a generation. The outcome is not certain, but one thing we can look forward to are advances in artificial intelligence. The computers of today do not "think"; they obediently respond to logical commands. Whether a machine will ever have true "intelligence" is a matter for philosophers to debate. There is no doubt, however, that as computers get faster and contain more storage, their responses will become more complete and take on the demeanor of "intelligence." Every week, we read of the development of smaller, lighter, faster, and more powerful PCs. The revolution continues. The Computer Age is here.

The author purchased his first desktop computer in 1979 at a cost of $15,500. A smaller, lighter, yet more powerful computer can be purchased today for less than $800.

WHAT COMPUTERS DO

Besides common business applications, the computers can take the image of a CAT (Computerized Axial Tomography) scanner and provide a three-dimensional image of any joint. They can compose music and sculpture sound, test locomotor reactions (eg, in automobile driver's training or air-traffic control), simulate flying an airplane under normal and abnormal conditions, explore "what if" scenarios in business and engineering models, gather data from a multitude of "sensors," draw architectural designs, guide robots in building automobiles and other machinery, and transcend a multitude of limitations and boundaries of the past.

A common misconception is that computers can do almost anything. Actually, they are quite limited. Most computers are held to four mathematical operations and three comparison operations. The four basic mathematical operations are addition $(+)$, subtraction $(-)$, multiplication $(\times)$, and division $(/)$. The three comparisons are equal to $(=)$, less than $(<)$, and greater than $(>)$. Everything the computer does is done with one or more combinations of these functions. Programming ingenuity makes the computer just seem "intelligent."

Many things can be done with a computer; some, however, are more efficiently done by hand or with four-function calculators. Table 10.1 shows just some areas in which PCs are highly efficient.

Hardware Software

When people talk about computers, one quickly hears the terms *hardware* and *software*. The difference is important to understand. Hardware is everything that you can put your hands on. It is just what the name implies, all physical parts of a computer.

Software includes all instructions and data necessary to make a computer function. Software is divided into two subcategories: operating systems and applications programs. An *operating system* is a set of housekeeping instructions. It keeps track of instructions and data in use. An *applications program* is a specific set of computer instructions to perform a given task (eg, word processing, accounting, searching).

Computing power greater than that found in the 5-ton computers of the 1950s with their vacuum tubes and punched paper tapes can now fit on a silicon sliver the size of a fingernail. Forecasts are made that this

Table 10.1. Common Uses of Desktop Computers

Repetitive typing	Nutritional analyses
Correspondence	Planning
Outlining	Budgeting
Manuscript preparation and editing	Cost estimating
Report development	Quotations
Instant dictionary, thesaurus, famous quotations	Project tracking
Spelling, grammar, style critiques	Loan amortization tables
Literature scanning	Legal guidelines
List sorting (eg, alphabetically, numerically, by date, etc)	Preparation of wills
Form designs	Automatic banking
Sheet printing	Automatic bill paying
Envelope addressing	Control factory operations
File management	Monitoring energy use
Accounting and money management	Airline/rapid transit control
Bookkeeping ledgers (spreadsheets)	Crop and weather information
Invoice and billing	Corporate stock and bond data
Payroll records	Stock and bond purchases and sales
Checkbook management	Drafting
Check writing	Training and grading
Mathematical calculations	Business diagnosis
Scientific equations	Data analysis
Inventory control	Experiment modeling
Cataloging	Helping disabled study
Mailing list management	Preparation of engineering designs
Tickler files	Development of slides and animation
Instant calendar revisions	Instant news service
Tax records	Statistical data processing
Development of graphics, artwork	Data searches
Development of charts and graphs	Personality analyses
Automatic telephone dialing	Tutors on a large variety of subjects
Communication with other computers internationally	Music composition
Indexing and bibliographing	Decoding
	Entertainment (eg, games)

power will shortly be increased many thousands of times in the same space. The secret lies not only in hardware that stores data for easy access but also in improvement in software that abolishes ambiguity, calls for mathematical rigor, and matches computer language to the job.

The 1980s saw a software explosion, with many thousands of programs developed by companies and independents to solve almost any imaginable problem in text manipulation and checking, calculation, graphic presentations (drawings and paintings) with text, animating, information organization, communications and networking, and management of input and output.

Computer Hardware

Computer systems vary in how the hardware is configured, but what that hardware does is similar in all systems. The most basic differences among computer systems are size and use. Below are four different sizes and their descriptions:

• *Mainframes:* Computers built to minimize distance between points for very fast operation. Used for extremely large complicated computations.

• *Microcomputers:* Large computers with fast processing speeds and access to billions of characters of data.

• *Supercomputers:* Moderately-sized computers. Used when a desktop computer is not powerful enough to do the job.

• *Minicomputers:* Smallest computers (desktop PCs). They are inexpensive and largely owned by individuals.

Basic Hardware Elements

As explained previously, all computers regardless of size perform similar tasks. The basic hardware elements that perform these tasks are:

• *Input:* Some method of getting software information into the computer. For a microcomputer, this is usually a keyboard, storage unit (disk), modem, or scanner.

• *Output:* Equipment to get data out of the computer. Usually a video display (monitor) or printer.

• *Memory:* A temporary storage location within a computer for software and data. This memory (RAM) is cleared when the computer is turned off.

• *Secondary Storage:* Permanent storage for both data and software. This can be recorded on computer chips (ROM), tape, magnetic disk, or other media.

Hardware elements often pass data/instructions to and get instructions from the CPU. Sometimes this is not necessary, and those tasks can be given to "coprocessors."

The major electrocomponents of a PC are:

• A *power supply*, which serves as the interface between a building's electric service and a computer's components. It converts alternating current to direct current.

• A *clock* that pumps electronic impulses through the control bus, synchronizing all computer activity.

• *Buses* (internal pathways for information) where control signals travel on the control bus. Data travel on the data bus to a destination whose address is carried on the address bus.

• *Ports* to mediate the flow of data into and from the computer. They may be either input, output, or dual-purpose input/output ports operating either in serial or parallel.

• The *CPU* (Central Processing Unit chip) that serves as the brain or heart of the entire computer system, performing the machine's arithmetic and logical operations. The CPU processes data in response to software instructions. Small amounts of memory in the CPU, by RAM circuits optimized for speed, are called *registers*. They hold the location in main memory of the next program instruction. An instruction register holds the instruction being executed.

• *ROM* (Read Only Memory). Permanent memory bank that remains intact even when the computer is turned off. Access time is between 50 and 200 billionths of a second. Use is typically to hold start-up information to prepare the machine for use.

• *RAM* (Random Access Memory). A temporary memory bank that serves as a repository of data and programs which can be altered by the CPU at the will of an operator.

• An *address decoder*, located between the CPU and ROM, and DIP switches set to record important addresses help direct the electrical pulses to their destination.

• *Disk drives* that store programs and files.

The Factor of Time

Shortly, we'll describe the CPU and other hardware elements in greater detail. Before we start, there are some basic terms that require understanding. The first set of these deals with time.

In the human world, the smallest time element usually dealt with is the second. Rarely do we need to think smaller. In the computer world, however, time increments are much smaller and events occur much faster: (1) millisecond, one thousandth of a second, associated with smaller computers and early PCs; (2) microsecond, one millionth of a second, associated with microcomputers, some mainframes, and most PCs; (3) nanosecond, one billionth of a second, usually seen only in supercomputers and modern mainframes; (4) picosecond, one trillionth of a second, a barrier to be broken.

A Byte Is Not a Bite

One might bite when eating, but with computers, bytes and nibbles are terms having special meaning in defining how characters are handled by the computer. Because computers are made of digital electronics, they respond to only two types of electrical states: "on" or "off." These may actually be high or low voltage, positive or negative voltage, or some other combination. The key is that there are only *two* conditions.

They are represented by two numbers: 0 and 1, and the arithmetic that deals with these two states is called *binary* arithmetic.

A computer "chip" is an electronic powerhouse consisting of hundreds of thousands of microscopic electric circuits etched on a tiny sliver of silicon, and tolerances cannot exceed $\frac{4}{100,000}$ of an inch. A microprocessor chip works by responding to electric impulses that open and close its circuits thousands or millions of times per second. Each opening or closing represents a unit of information (eg, a typed character, number, or symbol) encoded with the digits 0 or 1 (binary number system). Thus, each chip is a "digital" device that can only interpret information presented as individual bits, or binary digits, rather than perceiving it as a smooth "analog" wave form.

Each 0 or 1 in the binary system is called a *bit* (short for binary digit). Like the dots and dashes of Morse Code, opened and closed circuits of a microprocessor can combine to provide instructions for almost any electronic machine. This commonly occurs unknowingly when we make a telephone call, use an electronic thermometer or digital blood-pressure instrument, start a modern car, use a modern camera, pass through a supermarket check-out counter, install unobtrusive sentries for a home, or glance at the time on a digital watch.

A 19th Century British mathematician, George Boole, theorized that a proposition is either true or false, just as a switch is either open or closed or a binary digit is either 1 or 0. Circuits on computer chips are usually designed according to Boolean principles.

Strings of bits are used to represent numbers larger than 1 (much like combinations of digits are used to represent numbers larger than 9 in our decimal numbering system). A string of eight bits is called a *byte*, and one byte usually represents a single character of information in the computer (eg, a numeral or letter of the alphabet). It's a rarely used term, but you might be interested in knowing that a nibble is half a byte (usually, 4 bits).

Think of binary numbers in terms of switches. With two switches, you can represent up to four different numbers:

0	0	= Decimal 0
OFF	OFF	
0	1	= Decimal 1
OFF	ON	
1	0	= Decimal 2
ON	OFF	
1	1	= Decimal 3
ON	ON	

In the above, note the decimal number versus the number of numbers. Two binary numbers give up to decimal 3, but there are four actual numbers. In our decimal system, we rarely think of the zero; with computers, however, zero is always thought of as a number. Thus, a single bit represents 2 numbers, two bits give 4 numbers, three bits show 8 numbers, four bits represent 16 numbers, and so forth up to a byte, or eight bits, which represent 256 potential numbers. Each additional bit doubles the total numbers.

Table 10.2 shows the correspondence between several binary and decimal numbers. Binary numbers are formed just like decimals, except there are only two numbers to work with. Exhaust those two numbers, and you must start over with the next position

Table 10.2. Correspondence Between Binary and Decimal Numbers

Decimal	Binary
0	0
1	1
2	10
3	11
4	100
5	101
6	110
7	111
8	1000
9	1001
10	1010
11	1011
12	1100
13	1101
14	1110
15	1111

to the left filled with a "1." Once you arrive at 111, simply start the entire marked series again with a 1 in front of it. Thus, every time a binary digit is added to the string, the total decimal digits available for use is doubled.

Examine Table 10.2. One bit counts to two numbers, two bits count to four numbers, three bits to eight numbers, four bits to 16 numbers, five to 32, six to 64, seven to 128 and finally, one byte (8 bits) counts to 256 numbers.

It's easy to be confused over the point of zero being a digit. A byte with all digits ON represents the decimal number 255, and it may be difficult to visualize this as the 256th digit in a series, but that's exactly what a computer does. Computer language starts counting from zero, not one.

The first situation where this concept is used is in explaining computer memory. Most manufacturers state memory capacity in terms of kilobytes. In the decimal system, the prefix *kilo* means 1000. In the binary system, however, kilo means 1024, the closest number of digits to 1000 that can be represented by a number of bits that are all set to one. That number is 10. Thus, ten ones in a row represent the decimal number 1,023 and the 1024th digit. With this terminology, a computer has 256K (256 kilobytes) of memory: when it really has $256 \times 1,024$ or 262,144 bytes. Similarly, computers are described as having megabytes and gigabytes of memory, though there is somewhat more than a million or billion actual bytes available.

Addressing

To understand addressing, each memory location can be thought of as a post office box containing one character (letter, digit, or special character). Each box has an "address" that makes it unique. An 8-bit binary number has 256 boxes. A 16-bit binary number can specify 65,536 boxes. If we think of memory as a series of 256 pages, each number contains 256 bytes of information. This is what a 16-bit number can address: $256 \times 256 = 65,536$—or 64K.

Of course, the maximum amount of memory any computer can have depends on how many bits the CPU has in its address bus (the wires the CPU uses to send out addresses). Most computers had a 16-bit bus or 64K memory a decade ago; current computers have a larger bus.

The CPU

The Central Processing Unit (CPU) is the control center for the computer. It carries out all instructions sent to it by the operating system or applications software. But what makes it do its job? The CPU has two circuit elements that perform tasks and contain memory locations where data and instructions are held temporarily while actions are performed. They are:

• The *control unit,* which directs and coordinates all elements of the computer. The control unit does *not do,* it *only directs.*

• The *arithmetic/logic unit,* where the basic mathematical and logical operations explained previously take place.

Registers

Registers are temporary storage areas within the CPU that are used when data must be manipulated or instructions carried out. There are at least four registers, often more. The most common are:

• *Accumulator,* an area used to "accumulate" the results of calculations.

• *Storage,* a holding area for information taken from or to be sent to memory.

• *Address,* an area holding the *location* of information or instructions the computer needs for processing.

• *General purpose,* an area that can be used for multiple functions to include arithmetic or addressing.

Registers vary in length (number of bits) depending on the computer. Personal computers have 8- or 16-bit registers; larger PCs, 32-bit; and mainframes, up to 64-bit registers. This length is commonly known as a word; and the longer it is, the more powerful

the computer. Sometimes registers have different lengths, depending on their use.

THE KEYBOARD

The PC keyboard has three sections that are briefly described below:

1. *Function keys:* The group of 10 keys on the left side of the keyboard.

2. *Alphanumeric keys:* The large center section that works and looks much like a standard typewriter's key arrangement.

3. *Numeric keypad:* The right group of keys that switches function from numbers to cursor control. It resembles the keys on a simple hand calculator.

Each of these sections contains keys with special meaning to the PC. Only these special keys will be described in this chapter. The standard typewriter keys will not. See Figure 10.1. We assume that the reader knows how to type or at least "hunt and peck."

Before keyboard function is described, an operator should understand the concept of a buffer—something the keyboard and other parts of the computer use.

Buffers

A *buffer* is a temporary storage area in the computer's memory. It is necessary because activities requiring input or output are generally much slower than those that only interact with memory. Text input from the keyboard is therefore placed in a buffer until the operator signals the computer that he or she is done. The computer then acts on what was entered. The signal is usually made by pressing the Carriage Return (Enter key). Buffers vary in length. The disk operating system command line buffer, for example, can contain up to 127 characters.

When text enters the keyboard buffer, it usually stays there until replaced, even if brought into the computer as a command and acted on. The DOS allows limited editing of the buffer using "function keys."

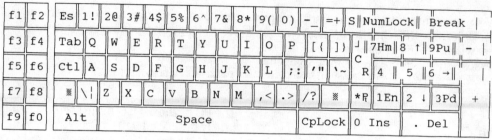

Figure 10.1. Layout of a standard PC keyboard.

Function Keys

The 10 function keys on the left side or top of a PC keyboard assume different roles for different programs. F1 through F5 have special meaning within DOS. They help in re-issuing/editing the last DOS command typed.

Some keys redisplay characters previously typed and help in editing the line currently in the buffer:

1. *F1* redisplays (automatically types) the buffer one character of the last command at a time each time the F1 key is pressed.

2. *F2* redisplays the buffer up to the character typed after pressing F2.

3. *F3* redisplays the entire contents of the buffer.

4. *F4* deletes all characters in the buffer up to the character typed after F4 was pressed. The buffer is not displayed. To see the buffer on screen F3 must be pressed.

5. *F5* stores the current line for further editing. This key is used with the other four keys to fix errors in long command strings. When F5 is pressed, the typing line is marked and the cursor (location pointer on the screen) is moved to the next line without showing a new prompt. A *prompt* is a displayed data, instruction, or a question by the computer.

Keys *F6–F10* can be programmed to initiate a series of commands by a single key stroke. This programming is called creating an *alias, synonym,* or *macro.*

Numeric Keypad

The keys on the right side of the keyboard assume a dual role. The *NumLock (Number Lock) key* is the toggle between numbers and cursor control; ie, key functions change each time NumLock is pressed. The default on starting (booting) the computer is cursor control mode in XT computers; off in AT computers. The *ScrLock (Scroll Lock) key* by itself has no function.

Cursor Control Mode

The *cursor* (usually a *blinking underscore* character) indicates where the next action will be displayed on the video screen. It moves in response to keys pressed on the keyboard, keeping just ahead of the last character typed. In cursor control mode, many programs assign the following meanings: The *Arrow keys* move the cursor one character at a time in the direction the arrow points; ie, upward (8), to the right (6), downward (2), and to the left (4). Keys 9, 3, 1, and 7 point diagonally in direction mode.

The *Home key* moves the cursor to the upper left corner of the screen. The *End key* moves the cursor to the end of a line or to the bottom of the screen depending on the program used. The *Break key*, if available, stops computer action.

The *Ins (Insert) key* sets an insert mode so text enters at the cursor position and pushes existing text to the right. This is helpful if a word is typed with a letter missing. The *Del (delete) key* deletes the character at the cursor position. This is helpful in editing a word typed with an extra character.

The *PgUp (Page Up) key* scrolls the

screen display about 18 lines "up" so the cursor appears to move toward the start of the file. The *PgDn (Page Down) key* reverses this action so the cursor moves toward the end of the file. Assume an operator has a file of text with the screen placed midway in the file. Pressing the PgUp or PgDn keys will usually have the described up or down effect on the display.

Two keys modify the effect of others. For an operator to use them, either must be held down and then the key whose function is wanted is tapped. These keys are the *Ctrl (control)* key and the *Alt (alternate) key.* The Control key is often used to produce codes many programs recognize as valid commands. The Alternate key is also used by many programs to issue commands or make typing easier through macros (strings of frequently used keystrokes assigned to a single keystroke).

Three keystroke combinations can help in times of trouble: (1) Pressing Ctrl + NumLock simultaneously causes data scrolling past to *pause* until another key is pressed. (2) Pressing Ctrl + Break simultaneously causes a program to stop execution completely. (3) Pressing Ctrl + Alt + Del simultaneously causes the computer to reboot (start again *as if* the power were switched off and then on again).

The *CapsLock (capitals lock) key* is a toggle that causes all letters (only) to be upper case. If CapsLock is on, a shift key can be used to change any single letter back to lower case.

The *Esc (Escape) key* is used for various purposes. In DOS, Escape deletes the current line. In programs, it might be used to stop activity or signal the program to be alert for special commands to follow. The *Enter← (carriage return) key* tells the computer the operator is done typing the entry.

The *Tab key* on a PC often performs like the tab on a standard typewriter. Tabs are normally set each eight spaces, but any number is acceptable. Pressing Control + Tab simultaneously moves the cursor to the next word on a line, and Control + Shift + Tab (Reverse Tab) finds the previous word. These functions, however, are not standard with all PCs.

The *←Backspace key* moves the cursor one space left, deleting the character to the left while dragging the rest of the line left to fill the space.

The *PrtSc (Print Screen) key* when pressed simultaneously with the Shift key causes text on the screen to be dumped (sent) to the printer. If Control + PrtSc is pressed, everything appearing on the screen will be echoed to the printer until that key combination is pressed again. However, if the screen contains some special characters or graphics, the operator may not be able to print that screen.

The keys not described function like those of the standard typewriter. They have lower and upper case characters as indicated on each keycap.

Do not confuse the Virgule (slash) and Backslash (reverse slash), the apostrophe and Grave Accent, or the capital "Oh" (O) and Zero (0). In most computer applications, a zero is displayed with a slash through it to aid differentiation.

Enhanced Keyboard

With the introduction of the Personal System/2, IBM made their "enhanced" keyboard the standard for their microcomputer line. This keyboard design relocates many control and function keys and introduces status lights in the upper-right corner for CapsLock, NumLock, and ScrLock keys. The function keys (12) are located on the top row of the keyboard rather than placed on the left.

STORAGE AND INPUT/OUTPUT DEVICES

Storage is a term describing how a computer retains data in a form that can be used later. For a personal computer, storage is generally in the form of either a hard or "floppy" disk. These disks work similar to a common tape recorder where music is recorded by taped magnetic impressions. Computer data appear as magnetic bits (1s or 0s) placed on a flat magnetic surface.

Floppy disks are portable, but hard disks can store many more bytes.

Floppy Disks

Music is recorded on up to four tracks on a cassette tape recorder (left and right channels, both sides). Data are written similarly on computer disks except there are many more *tracks* and they are arranged as concentric circles on a flat surface.

Tracks are written to and read from by one or more read/write heads that move across the surface of the disk in steps. Most disks today have 40 tracks (steps), which are numbered from 0 through 39. The lower numbers are on the outer surface of the disk. Tracks are placed on the disks electronically by a *formatting* program provided with the disk operating system (DOS).

Tracks are divided into smaller units called *sectors*. The number of sectors per track differs with the exact operating system used. With PC-DOS version 2.0 and higher, there are 9 sectors per track. The old Version 1.1 used 8 sectors per track. While new versions of the DOS can read 8-sector disks one should not generally use an early DOS version to write to a disk formatted by a newer DOS. Version 3.3 is in common use, but version 4.1 has been released. Version 5.0 is scheduled for release in 1991.

Because each track is divided into the same number of sectors, one may think of them as pie-shaped sections on the disk. Each sector is labeled by the operating system's format utility. These electronic labels enable the DOS to find information on the disk.

Floppy disks have two major grades: single- and double-sided. This means a single-sided disk is certified by the manufacturer to be good on one side only. It does not mean that there isn't a magnetic surface on the other side of a single-sided disk, just that the manufacturer does not *guarantee* that the surface will reproduce magnetic pulses at their true intensity, resulting in possible data errors. A double-sided disk is certified to store information on both sides.

One should never use a single-sided disk in a double-sided drive. It may work for awhile, but the risk of eventually losing data is great. There is also a temptation to turn a single-sided disk over to use the second side. Avoid this because the disk will spin in the opposite direction and this could result in scratching the reverse side or other problems that will cause loss of data.

The final factor in the equation to find the amount of data on a disk is the *density* or number of bits per inch. Single density records at 2768 bits per inch (bpi) and double density is 5876 bpi; some special disks, over a million bpi.

While the number of bits per inch is the technical definition of density, usually a more practical way to solve the question is to look at the number of bytes stored in each sector. Early computers used 128 bytes per sector, some new use 256, and the IBM-PC uses 512. By using this information, it is possible to calculate the capacity of IBM disks.

	512	bytes per sector
$\times$	9	sectors per track
$\times$	40	tracks per side
$\times$	2	sides per disk
	368,640	bytes stored per disk

The example above assumes a DOS version 2.0 or later. High-density 3.5-inch disks differ.

Disk Safeguards

At the top of a floppy disk is a small notch. If this notch is covered with a piece of tape, the drive mechanism *will not* write to the disk, thus protecting it (making it *read only*). If an operator wants to write information on the disk, she must make sure that the notch is *uncovered;* ie, open.

Remember that bits are recorded rather closely. When the disk is spinning, the read/write head(s) travels a few thousandths of an inch from the disk. Any obstruction will cause the head to jump parts of the data, or if an obstruction is caught by the head, it might scratch the disk. What's large enough to do this? Fingerprints, smoke, a small piece of hair. It doesn't take much! Other things to keep away from magnetic materials are TVs, magnets, x-rays, paper clips, cats and dogs, and liquids.

Other Formats

The 360K 5.25-inch floppy disk has long been the standard for removable storage on IBM-architecture equipment. The AT-class (80286 and 80386) computers introduced a new high-density format: 15 sectors per track, yielding 1.2 megabytes (M) on a 3.5-inch disk. The magnetic properties and often the design of these 1.2M disks make them unusable in 360K drives, but for a little more money they provide four times the storage capacity.

Since its introduction, the Apple Macintosh computer has used the smaller 3.5-inch disks with hard plastic shells. Since the introduction of the IBM PS/2 computer line, 3.5-inch disks are becoming the standard for IBM-architecture as well. Many of today's computers offer at least one 3.5-inch drive. The basic 3.5-inch drive yields 720K per disk, with a high-density version packing 1.44 megabytes on a 3.5-inch disk.

There are new floppy disk formats under development that include optical media or a combination of magnetics and optics to pack 20 megabytes or much more on 3.5-inch or smaller disks. Within a few years, expect cost per megabyte to drop dramatically.

Hard Disks

Hard disks work much like floppy disks. They just store more files and operate faster. Instead of thin mylar-coated materials, a hard disk uses an aluminum (or other rigid material) platter covered with a magnetic coating. Also, there is more than one disk in any drive. They are stacked like music records with the number determining the capacity of the disk.

Because a hard disk spins faster and has increased density compared to a floppy disk, environmental controls must be stricter to prevent dust, smoke, or other damaging agents from contacting the disks. A hard disk is in a sealed unit and the technology associated with sealed units is termed *Winchester* technology. Hard-disk capacity ranges from a usual minimum of 10 megabytes up to several hundred megabytes or more. Less than 40 megabytes is impractical.

If a hard disk is used, be prepared to spend some time backing-up files frequently. Even with a sealed unit, problems develop that may destroy all data on the disk or make it inaccessible. This is called a hard-disk "crash." Actually, frequent backup should be exercised with any work disk, hard or floppy.

Monitors

Operators interact with a computer largely through its monitor (video display). A monitor resembles a television screen. Because of its construction, the monitor is often known as a cathode ray tube (CRT). There are inexpensive monochrome monitors limited to displaying black and white and monitors that display in 4 colors (CGA), 16 colors (EGA), or 256 tints and shades (VGA). Quality of display is determined by resolution (pixels per inch) not color.

Input Devices

Two input devices are the primary interfaces with a PC: the *keyboard* and a *mouse*. The keyboard has been previously described. Keyboard input is by typing commands and pressing the Enter key for execution. This is called a *character recognition* system. Of the two interface systems, typed commands are executed faster by the experienced operator but a graphic interface is much easier to learn and use. A graphic interface requires a "mouse."

A *mouse* is an electromechanical device. Underneath the body of this device is a ball, which when rolled along a desktop or other flat object transmits position information to the computer. In this manner, a mouse replaces the cursor with a pointer on the screen that moves along a "menu" of commands. When the desired command label is found, a button on the mouse is "clicked" for execution. This process is called a *graphics interface*. Position is achieved in some versions by using a special pad with grid marks so optical sensors can derive position information from the grid. Note that the plural of a computer mouse is not mice; it is mouses.

There are other special input devices that are usually reserved for specific tasks. A *scanner* is one. A scanner "reads" information from sheets of paper, artwork, or photographs and transfers the information into the computer. This can save laborious retyping or redrawing time. There are also *digitizers*, where external illustrations can be traced or drawn with a pencil-like stylus and stored in a computer.

Output Devices

There are many output devices for a computer. Most have specialized uses and will not be discussed here. A few deserving mention are plotters, printers, modems, and internal fax machines.

Plotters. A plotter is a device that uses some mechanism to drive pens in defined horizontal/vertical motions to produce combined text and graphic figures. Most are driven by software that controls pen motion and ink color, with different colors available depending on the model purchased. Most plotters used with personal computers come with a flat bed. Other models are available with a pen that moves back and forth and wheels that drive the paper back and forth for the second dimension of motion. Some plotters move the pen back and forth and roll a drum with paper attached to obtain the other dimension.

Printers. By far, paper is likely the single largest output an operator will have from a computer. Despite claims for "paperless" offices, it is rare not to see printers frequently outputting reams of paper.

Modern printers come in a variety of types, with many capabilities. One class is called *nonimpact* printers because the printing element never touches the paper. In the other class, the print element does touch

the paper, sometimes quite hard. It is called an *impact* printer.

Types of impact printers include (1) *dot matrix* (characters made of dots), (2) *daisy wheel* (single-character impacts), and (3) *line printers* (print an entire line by a single stroke). Types of nonimpact printers include (1) *ink-jet* (dots of ink make-up characters), (2) *thermal* (wires burn special paper), and (3) *laser* (full-page print).

Nonimpact Printers

An *ink-jet* printer "shoots" individual dots of ink to the paper, calculating the location of each dot to form individual characters or dot graphics. A *laser printer* is noted for producing an entire page of text at a time. With this printer, a laser scans a photoactive plate to build an image of the printed page. Like in a photocopy machine, the plate is then dusted with toner that sticks to exposed areas. Paper is then placed in contact with the plate, transferring the image to the paper. Final heat-bonding seals the toner to the paper. All this takes just a few seconds.

Thermal printers used to be popular, but their need for special paper was subject to extraneous marking (not to mention a high cost). The use of thermal printers has dropped significantly since 1980. Daisy wheel and dot matrix impact printers were highly popular in the period 1977–1987. Today, ink jet and laser printers are the standard in professional offices.

Impact Printers

There are two types of impact printers you may see with a personal computer: dot matrix and daisy wheel.

The difference between dot matrix and daisy wheel (thimble) printers is the quality of output from the impacting device. Dot matrix printers form characters from individual dots whereas a daisy wheel printer imprints fully formed characters, much like those of a typewriter. A dot matrix printer is the more versatile of the two but its quality is less likely to be acceptable for professional correspondence. Both printers impact the paper through a ribbon to transfer ink to the paper by the hitting element. Dot matrix printers use from 9 to 24 individual wires. The more wires the higher the quality.

Modems. A modem connects a computer with another computer via telephone lines. In this manner, two-way communication can be established with any other computer in the world having a modem and telephone service. In this manner, a PC can "tap into" a very large computer and the operator will then have available any of the data contained within the mainframe's databases. Modems may be installed within or without of a PC; ie, internal and external types.

Internal Fax Machines. Rather than having a stand-alone fax machine, a less expensive internal fax can be installed in a PC by using a fax board. A stand-alone fax machine sends messages by scanning a document and sending pixel (dot) signals via telephone lines. In contrast, an internal fax board sends computer files via telephone lines. Several types of data conversion are involved: binary in the sending PC, analog over telephone lines, binary in the receiving computer; and vice versa in two-way communications.

Interfaces

Whatever printer is used, it must be connected to the computer. The connecting cable is an *external interface* and interacts with the computer by a communications "Port." There are two types of ports: one is called *serial;* the other, *parallel.* These names describe their function. Recall that there are eight bits to a byte (character) of data. In a serial interface, each bit is sent to the printer individually. A parallel interface sends all eight bits at once. Each interface has its quirks; the key is assuring sure to have the correct one. They will not intermix. A printer or scanner will likely use a parallel (LPT) interface; a mouse or modem, a serial (COM) interface.

By no means has this been a complete education in computer storage and input/output terminology, but it should be enough to understand your friendly(?) computer salesperson.

OPERATING SYSTEMS AND COMMANDS

Remember that the disk operating system (DOS) on any computer is the general manager for that computer. It directs files and data throughout the system and serves as the interface between the operator, the program being run, and the remainder of computer operations. Most anything done with a computer will be done through its operating system.

As described earlier, there are two general types of operating systems: character recognition and graphics. DOS is the standard character recognition system for IBM PCs and clones. Apple computers use a graphic interface. Microsoft's popular "Windows" program is a graphic interface that works as a subsidiary of DOS.

DOS

Personal computers usually have a certain generic operating system that is a version of the same operating system built for different sets of hardware to allow a programmer to have a standard set of commands to do similar things on different machines. PC-DOS, the disk operating system for the IBM-PC computer is similar to the more general MS-DOS, developed for other microcomputers. DOS is used by more than 90% of PCs. Remember, the acronym "DOS" means *Disk Operating System.*

Parts of DOS

The DOS has an input/output system, a command processor, and several utilities. *Utilities* are specific program files found on a DOS disk. While part of DOS, these files are not needed often enough to make it necessary or practical to keep them in the computer's ROM (permanent memory). FORMAT.COM, the program that formats (prepares) blank disks, is an example of a DOS utility. Utilities are called external commands, which are temporarily held in RAM computer memory, as opposed to internal commands that are always in ROM whether the computer is "on" or not.

Once read into a computer's RAM memory, the command processor (typically a file called COMMAND.COM) usually resides there. But some programs provide their own command processor, and there are times when the DOS command processor will be overwritten by a program and must be reloaded when the program stops executing. This unloading and reloading is done automatically by the program.

The input/output system has two files and a ROM chip. While the two files are on "boot" (starting) disks and loaded into memory when the computer starts, they are normally hidden from view and not available to editing except by the highly experienced. These two "hidden" files are labeled IBMBIO.COM and IBMDOS.COM. These two files plus COMMAND.COM must be on a formatted disk for it to be a boot disk.

Input/Output System

This most primitive of DOS systems has two parts:

1. *BIOS (Basic Input/Output System):* fundamental routines controlling the keyboard, video display (monitor), and other peripherals (eg, printer, scanner, modem). The BIOS has a ROM chip on the computer's main circuit board and the file IBMBIO.COM, one of the two hidden files on a boot disk.

2. *Operating System:* the main file-handling system for the computer. Actually, two systems exist: one for disk-based files and one for nondisk peripheral devices. They are in hidden file IBMDOS.COM. IBMBIO and IBMDOS are IBM names; MS-DOS uses IO.SYS and MSDOS.SYS. The two systems are necessary because nondisk peripherals demand their data as strings of

characters, while disks move information in large groups, known as blocks.

Command Processor

The command processor (file COMMAND.COM on the start-up disk) performs four major tasks:

1. It handles critical interrupts; ie, COMMAND.COM manages all demands for attention by parts of the computer. A user processing Control + Scroll Lock keys simultaneously is an example of initiating an interrupt.

2. It handles critical errors; ie, COMMAND.COM takes care of problems. For example, if the disk drive door is left open during a disk operation, COMMAND.COM is responsible for the error message displayed: "Not ready error reading Drive X."

3. It performs end-of-program housekeeping; ie. COMMAND.COM manages the computer's memory available for other programs and reloading parts of itself if the program wrote over them.

4. COMMAND.COM places the "Drive:\>" prompt on the screen and interprets any command typed. In short, the command processor tells the remainder of the DOS what to do.

Starting the Computer

The process of starting a computer is given the special name *booting*. When a PC is started, it must literally pick itself up by its bootstraps when switched "On." Once current flows, the computer first checks its memory and some other components. After this, individual disks in the computer will sequentially begin to spin and the boot process will begin:

1. ROM BIOS loads Track 0, Sector 0 of the disk. This sector contains a short program that can read the rest of the input/output system.

2. The boot loader read in step 1 loads the input/output system (files IBMBIO.COM

and IBMDOS.COM, or IO.SYS and MSDOS.SYS).

3. IBMBIO.COM *initials* the hardware of the computer, runs the file CONFIG.SYS (if found on the disk), and then moves IBMDOS.COM into its proper location in RAM (temporary computer memory).

4. IBMDOS.COM loads COMMAND.COM and turns over control to it. COMMAND.COM runs the file AUTOEXEC.BAT (if found). When all necessary housekeeping chores are done, command control is relinquished to the operator.

Default Drive

Typing always occurs are the cursor, which is initially displayed after the symbol ">." The prompt shown on the monitor consists of the cursor preceded by the > symbol and drive letter (eg, A>, B>, or C>). Other information such as the date or time may be incorporated.

The *default drive* is the disk drive on which PC-DOS will look for a program if no drive specification is given with the filename. It is the drive that appears at the prompt on start-up. For example:

- A> shows that drive A (a floppy disk drive) is the default drive.
- C> shows that drive C (a hard disk drive) is the default drive.

DOS supports many more than drives A through C. In fact, if a computer has them, the operator can specify up to 63 drive names. But rarely will more than half a dozen be necessary (A–F). Drives are easily changed by typing the desired drive letter(s) followed by a colon at the prompt. To change from Drive B to Drive E, for example, just type E: and press the Return key. B> will be instantly replaced by E>.

Device Names

Character-oriented devices can be addressed by DOS through their names, and each device has a unique name. For example:

- CON:—The name for the video display (terminal) and keyboard (console). See Figure 10.2.
- PRN or LPT1:—The first parallel printer port. PRN comes from PRiNter and the LPT is an old designator derived from Line PrinTer. A colon on PRN and all device names is optional in later DOS versions. The second parallel port is LPT2:; the third, LPT3, etc.
- AUX: or COM1:—The first asynchronous communications port, which usually has a modem or other serial device connected to it. The second communications port is COM2; the third, COM3, etc.
- NUL:—This is a test device. Anything sent to device NUL goes into the "bit bucket" (ie, it is thrown away).

Rules for Filenames

Disk files also must be identified so that the DOS can address them. Some specific rules for naming files are:

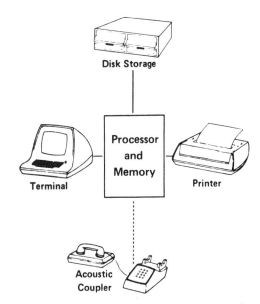

Figure 10.2. A typical small business computer system includes a processor and memory manager (the computer), a disk storage device (floppy and possibly hard disks), a printer, a modem or acoustic coupler, and a video terminal.

1. Each filename must have a *root* name. The root can be from 1 to 8 characters in length. The file name or abbreviation may consist of any combination of letters and numbers and most symbols: viz, A–Z, a–z, 0–9, $#&@_!()-', but *device* names (eg, CON, PRN, AUX, NUL) and names of the *DOS commands* (eg, FORMAT, COPY, ERASE, etc) are illegal. The symbols <> + = ?/[]",^* and a few others (eg, space) also are illegal.

2. For subdivision, a filename may include an optional *extension*. An extension must not exceed three characters in length and a period must be used to separate the root from the extension.

DOS Commands

DOS commands are issued at the prompt; eg, C>. Whatever is typed after the prompt (at the cursor) that is not in the COMMAND.COM standard library is assumed to be the name of a file on the default disk, and the DOS will search for it under one of three names in the order listed.

If only FILENAME is typed at the prompt, DOS will look for FILENAME.COM, FILENAME.EXE, or FILENAME.BAT. The first example is a command file (note the COM extension). The second is an execution file (EXE extension). And the third is a batch file (to be explained later). The first file found will be read into the computer's memory and the command processor will start the program. Both .COM and .EXE files execute programs. The difference between the two relates to how memory is allocated and how certain parameters in the computer are set.

Command Syntax

Each DOS command has a mandatory part, and some have optional portions. In our examples, the mandatory parts will be shown in CAPITAL LETTERS and the optional parts in lower case. In actual practice, however, either capitals or lower case may be used.

Note the following typed command:

DIR d: /p/w

This is a command for a list of files on a disk directory. Note that only DIR is necessary if a list of files on the default drive is desired. The instruction "d:" is necessary only if not currently at Drive D; "/p" instructs the computer to scroll the list in 23 line segments; and "/w" instructs the computer to display the list in five short columns rather than one long column.

With some commands, wildcards may be used. A wildcard, like the joker in a deck of cards, can stand for any character or group of characters.

- ? represents any single character; eg, FILE? = FILE1, FILE2, etc.
- * represents any group of characters; eg, *.* = all files despite name or extension.

Listing a Disk Directory

Thus, to see a complete list of what is on the default disk, issue the DIRectory command: DIR. To see a listing of what is on a different drive (Drive E, for example), type "DIR E:" To see all files on the current drive beginning with the letter a, type "DIR a*.*" without the quotation marks. To list all files on the current drive having a ".com" extension, type, "DIR*.com" without the quotation marks. By "issuing a command," we mean to type the command and then press the Return key (Enter) to execute it.

The command DIR lists the filenames requested plus the size of the file, the date it was created, and the time it was created. However, it will not execute any of these files. Several lines in a directory list might be:

BACKUP	BAT	41	7-17-90	3:00p
BROWSE	EXE	958	10-02-86	12:45p
CPANEL	COM	19858	9-28-87	10:15a
FAX	BAT	37	7-27-90	2:50p
FIND	COM	18734	2-05-89	11:30a
MOUSE	COM	14668	8-01-88	1:37p
PRINT	COM	9011	3-22-88	3:54p

At the end of the list, the DIR also tells how many files are in the total list and what free space remains. Note that the period separating an extension from its root is not shown in a directory display. The sample list above is set in filename alphabetical order; however, by using a SORT command, the directory may be displayed by extension, size, date, or time in ascending or descending order.

Internal DOS commands are not displayed in a directory list; they must be memorized (thus one advantage of a graphics interface) because they are not a file that has been created on or copied to the disk by an operator.

Date and Time

These two commands show and/or set the system date and time. When the computer boots, the operator is expected to set these (or have software and a clock that sets them automatically). If they are not set, the default values will be 1-1-80 for the date and 00:00:00.00 for the time. However, on some computers, new commands will change default settings.

The date is entered as month/day/year with hyphens or slashes; ie, 03/01/91 or 03-01-91 are acceptable dates. The day of the week is not entered though it shows on the screen. The computer calculates it for the operator. A two-digit year assumes dates between 1980 and 1999. After 2000, an operator must put in all four digits.

The time setting requires a 24-hour clock; ie, any time after noon has to have 12 added to it. For example, 3:00 pm is entered as 15:00.

When typing the command DATE or TIME, the following will be displayed on the monitor:

DATE
Current date is Tue 01-07-1991
Enter new date (mm-dd-yy):

TIME
Current time is 13:08:55.28
Enter new time (00:00:00.00):

Formatting Disks

Disks removed from their package usually need to be formatted; ie, tracks and sectors must be defined so the DOS can find programs and data on the disks. If the operator is working from Disk C: where FORMAT.COM resides and wishes to format a disk in Drive A, he or she would type "FORMAT A:" without the quotation marks. The DOS will examine the new disk for type and format it correctly.

The FORMAT.COM can be written so that other information is added during formatting. For example, if the disk is to be used as a boot disk and the disk is to be named, systems files and a label must be copied. The command would then be FORMAT A: /s/v, where "/s" puts the DOS hidden files and COMMAND.COM on the disk and "/v" puts on an identification label.

If a disk in Drive A has been formatted without a label and the operator later wishes to add a name, she types LABEL A: The computer will display the line, "Volume in drive A has no label." Then the name is typed and the Return key is pressed. To check that it has been recorded, "VOL A:" is typed and entered, and the computer will display "Volume in drive A is (name assigned)."

When formatting is complete, DOS will display what has occurred, such as

Formatting complete
System transferred

362496 bytes total disk space
40960 bytes used by system
321536 bytes available on disk

Format another (Y/N)? N

Extreme caution must be taken to ensure that a disk to be formatted does not contain information that should be retained. Formatting *erases all information on the disk* to provide the operator with a "clean" formatted disk. A hard disk may contain data that has taken years to develop. Typing "FORMAT C:" in error would erase all this information. This is one reason disks should be backed-up (duplicated) frequently. Rest assured that an extra copy will likely not be needed unless there is none.

Erasing Files

Files no longer needed can be easily erased from the disk to make room for more current files. The ERASE (or DELete) command is used for this purpose. For example:

ERASE FILENAME.ext
or
DEL FILENAME.ext

Be careful, typographic errors in this command can cause disaster!

An operator is allowed to erase all files on a disk with the wildcard * (eg, ERASE A: *.*), but the DOS will question the user and ask for confirmation. This is a safety factor.

Programs are commercially available that allow recovery of deleted files if nothing else has been written to the disk after the erasure. UNDEL.COM is one example.

Renaming Files

An operator may need to change the name of a file on a disk. This usually occurs when she wants to change a backup file to another name in order to return it to active status. The command is:

REName OLDNAME.ext   NEWNAME.ext

The original filename is called the *source* file; the new filename, the *target* file. The REName command will produce an error message if NEWNAME exists. Wildcards are allowed, but they can cause trouble if the operator is not careful.

Copying Files

The COPY command is a powerful command in DOS. With it, an operator can create duplicates of any file, join several files into one, or even use the computer like a standard typewriter by "copying" from the device named CON: to the device named PRN. The latter is inefficient, but permis-

sible for short notes that do not require editing.

When copying a file to one that has a different name, copy from filename1 to filename2:

COPY FILENAME1.ext FILENAME2.ext

To copy a file named ACT-1.TXT and rename it ACT91.TXT on the same drive, type

COPY ACT-1.TXT ACT91.TXT /v

The "/v" option in a copy command means to verify (confirm check) the copy as it is written on the disk. This adds confidence at the cost of slightly slower operation. Wildcards are allowed. There are many other options beyond the scope of this chapter, but a few examples are:

- C>COPY ABC.LST B: —Copies the single file ABC.LST from Drive C to B
- D>COPY *.*   B:/v —Copies all files on Drive D to the disk in Drive B and verifies
- C>COPY A:*.*   —Copies all files from Drive C to Drive A: but does not verify.

If COPY ADDRS.LST is typed, an error message will appear: "You can't copy a file to itself."

The COPY command can also be used to concatenate (join) two or more files by combining file names with the "+" symbol. For example

COPY FILENAME1.ext + FILENAME2.ext
FILENAME3.ext /v

1st FILENAME + 2nd FILENAME =
NEWFILENAME

Note that a space does not precede or follow the "+" symbol in the command.

All specified filenames (1st, 2nd, etc, source files) will be copied and combined into the new filename (target file). If a new filename is not specified, the first source file named will be used automatically. Options are the same as with the standard copy command. Wildcards are dangerous with this command. If an operator has complete subdirectories to copy, the XCOPY command should be considered instead of COPY. It works much like COPY but has a richer assortment of command options.

The COPY command can be used to create text files by copying from the screen (device CON) to a file. The procedure, which must be issued before the text is typed, is:

COPY CON (FILENAME)

Anything typed will go into the text file being created. As each line is typed to the screen, it will be saved in a buffer for later transfer to the file. Each line may be corrected as it is typed, but it cannot be changed after a carriage return. Also, if the operator happens to type beyond column 80 on the screen, she cannot correct anything on the line above. Each line must be ended by a carriage return (pressing the Return key). She signals when finished by typing a Control + Z or ^Z to indicate the end of the file, followed by pressing the Return key. This flushes the buffer and copies the file to the disk. The computer will then display "1 File(s) copied."

Typing a File

Any text file saved in character format can be easily seen on the video display. Use the type command:

TYPE FILENAME.ext

All characters in the file will then be displayed on the screen, including any control characters. Any Control + I characters found will be interpreted as a tab, and spaces will be added to get the cursor over to the next 8-character boundary so some output may appear as tables. Entering Control + Z will cause output to stop. Attempting to TYPE a .COM or .EXE file will result in garbage on the screen and should be avoided.

Backing-up a Disk

Floppy disks wear out after several hundred spin hours. Well before that time, she should have made a copy of the disk to preserve the integrity of its contents. The operator can, of course, FORMAT a new disk and then copy files on the old disk in Drive A to the new disk in Drive B or C, for example. If she does not give drive specifications, the utility will ask for them. If a file exists on the target disk, the file on the source disk will be added to the directory of the target disk.

A standard DOS comes with a back-up program, but there are several commercial programs available that are superior.

Checking a Disk

Now and again it is useful to check the integrity of the disk directory and File Allocation Table (FAT). The FAT is so important to the DOS that there are two copies of it on each disk. The FAT can be checked, for example, by entering the command:

CHKDSK C: /f/v

CHKDSK will then examine the drive for continuity (ie, files stored on contiguous sectors on the disk for efficient access). The signal "/f" tells the DOS to repair the FAT and other problems automatically, and "/v" orders a verbose mode that shows progress as disk checking takes place. When evaluation is completed, DOS displays the results in a description similar to:

Volume	MYDISK created Feb 3, 1991 7:58 p
362496	bytes total disk space
22528	bytes in 3 hidden files
316416	bytes in 42 user files
512	bytes in bad sectors
23040	bytes available on disk
131072	bytes total memory
106064	bytes free

Only the version of CHKDSK that came with your version of the DOS should be used. Other versions can damage a disk severely.

Concluding Remarks

Every operator should understand what the DOS contains, what constitutes a file, and how to run several useful DOS commands. By no means have we described all DOS commands. Some commands are rarely needed and may be looked up in the DOS manual as required. A list of DOS commands is shown in Table 10.3.

Some PCs have 1.2 megabyte 5.25-inch disk drives. There is the temptation to use 360-kilobyte disks in those drives—don't do it. The track width is smaller and if an operator puts 360K disks in a 360K drive, they may not work properly. Likewise, she cannot use high-density floppy disks in 360K drives. The magnetic properties are such that 360K drives will not format them.

With the introduction of 3.5-inch drives, higher versions of a DOS are required to support the new formats correctly. The 3.5-inch drives come in two sizes: 720K and 1.4M. Unlike 1.2M/360K disks, it is possible to format to 720K in a 1.4M 3.5-inch drive. All an operator must do is tell the FORMAT command the track/sector combination needed. For example: FORMAT A: /N:9/T:80. This tells the DOS to set 9 sectors per track and 80 tracks for a total of 720 kilobytes.

THE ROLE OF SUBDIRECTORIES

Many commands previously described contained filenames as either part of the command or an option to the command. To find the necessary filename, all the operator must do is call up a DIRectory. With the large storage capacity on a hard disk, however, a directory listing could take considerable time to review if an operator must go through every filename of possibly hundreds on the disk. The solution incorporated in DOS 2.0 or later is the addition of subdirectories and *pathnames*.

A pathname is similar to an interstate expressway number that shows DOS the route to a particular file. This lets the operator divide files into groups and place each related group into its own directory. This means that an operator needn't search an entire disk to find one file.

Remember that each file on a disk is represented as an entry in the directory, put there so both the operator and the DOS can find the file on disk. If, instead of data, a file was created that pointed to other files on the disk, the operator will have built what amounts to a subdirectory. All she must do to make the subdirectory display like those in the root DOS is to tell the DOS not to display the files in the subdirectory unless the operator specifically directs it. The DOS does this through directory commands that use a *pathname*.

Tree Structure

The DOS directory structure can be thought of as a tree, with the master disk directory the *root* and subdirectories thought of as branches. Actually, the name *trunk* would be a better describer than *root* for the master directory. Nevertheless, the root is the disk's main directory, and each subdirectory may contain subdirectories (branches from branches). The root directory may contain up to 512 subdirectories and files. Subdirectories may contain any number of entries (until the disk is full).

In the brief example shown in Figure 10.3, there are five files in the main root directory (Files 1–5) and two subdirectories (SubDirA and SubDirB). SubDirA has six files (Files A1–A6) and one subdirectory (SubDir AA) that contains 3 files (Files AA1–AA3). SubDir B has four files (Files B1–B4) in it but no subdirectories. If all these files were in the root, the list would comprise 18 files in one directory. Eighteen files would not be a problem but 180 would in locating a specific file. This structure can be extended until the disk is completely full, subject only to the constraint of 63 characters for the pathname that an operator must use to find a particular file.

The rules for a subdirectory name are just like those for filenames (eight characters, possibly followed by a period and a maximum three-character extension). They show up in a directory listing with the designator ⟨DIR⟩.

Each subdirectory in the path is sepa-

Table 10.3. DOS Commands

APPEND	Instructs DOS to seek files in a specified drive and directory.
ASSIGN	Refers requests for one disk drive to another disk drive.
ATTRIB	The attribute command allows an operator to protect files by making them read-only (unable to be altered or deleted), or to set or erase a file's archive flag for use with an XCOPY or BACKUP command.
BACKUP	Makes duplicate copies from one disk to another.
CD	The change director command displays the name of or changes the current director.
CHKDSK	The check disk command evaluates the allocation of storage on a disk and displays a summary report of (1) the space used by directories and files and (2) the number of bytes available, and alerts the operator if noncontiguous files exist.
CLS	The clear screen command erases the screen and places the prompt at *Home* (upper left corner of image area).
COMMAND	Lets the operator invoke a copy of the parent command processor or editing. The command processor is that part of DOS that interprets commands and batch files, issues prompts, and loads and executes application programs.
COMP	The compare command compares two files or sets of files to see if they are identical.
COPY	Allows the operator to (1) combine files, (2) copy from a device, (3) copy a file to a device, and (4) copy a file to a file.
CTTY	The change I/O device command specifies the character device to be used as the standard input/output device (eg, COM1, COM2).
DATE	Shows or sets the current date according to the computer clock.
DEL	The delete command erases a file or group of files. Functions the same as ERASE.
DIR	The directory command lists files in a directory and their size and date of creation.
DISKCOMP	The disk compare command compares two floppy disks in different drives.
DISKCOPY	Duplicates a floppy disk from one drive to another.
ERASE	Erases one or more files.
EXE2BIN	The executable to binary conversion command changes an executable file (viz, one with an .exe extension) to a binary-image file (viz, one with a .bin extension). If the source file meets certain specifications, the .bin file can then be converted to a command file (viz, one with a .com extension). Command files run faster than executable files.
EXIT	Ends a secondary copy of the command processor invoked so that control returns to the parent program or the command processor from which it was initiated.
FC	The file compare command compares two text files of similar type (ASCII or binary) and displays differences on the monitor.
FIND	Searches a specified file for a particular word or string of characters.
FDISK	The fixed disk command is used to partition a hard disk into two or more letter-designated drives after low-level formatting.

Table 10.3. *continued*

FORMAT	Prepares a disk so DOS can store files on it while simultaneously erasing all existing data on the disk.
GRAFTABL	The graphics table command allows DOS to display special graphics characters (extended ASCII 128–255) when a color graphics adapter is in the graphics mode.
GRAPHICS	Allows DOS to print graphic images on a printer.
JOIN	Enables an entire directory, and substructure if any, on a drive to be spliced into an empty subdirectory of a disk in another drive.
KEYBxx	The keyboard command changes the keyboard to match a specific language. For example: KEYBgr for German, KEYBfr for French, KEYBsp for Spanish, KEYBit for Italian, KEYBuk for British (United Kingdom).
LABEL	Changes, assigns, or erases the volume name of a disk.
MKDIR	The make directory command creates a new subdirectory.
MODE	According to options, aligns display (color/graphics adapter), configures a printer, configures a serial port, redirects to a printer, and selects the active display and controls characters per line.
MORE	Scrolls 23 lines of input to standard output (eg, monitor), and waits for any key to be pressed before scrolling the next 23 lines.
PATH	Instructs DOS to seek a command file in a specified drive and directory.
PRINT	Prints a file or several files in queue while the system is executing other commands or programs.
PROMPT	By itself, returns to default prompt. When the command is followed by specifications data can be added such as date and/or time of day, and/or DOS version number.
RECOVER	Attempts to reconstruct a file having bad sectors or a damaged directory structure.
RMDIR	The remove directory command deletes a specified empty directory.
REN	The rename command changes the name of a file.
REPLACE	Selectively replaces or adds files so a target disk can be updated with a more recent version from the source disk.
RESTORE	Restores files backed-up with the DOS BACKUP command.
SELECT	Formats and configures a country- and language-specific system floppy disk that includes a CONFIG.SYS file.
SET	The set environment variable command defines an environment variable's name and value.
SHARE	Loads a module into system memory that supports file sharing and locking in a network environment.
SORT	Sorts lines typed at the keyboard so they will be displayed on the monitor or used with redirection characters as a filter to sort the contents of a file or the output of another program.
SUBST	The substitute command accesses a directory by a drive letter and then automatically replaces any reference to drive1: with drive2:path.

Table 10.3. *continued*

SYS	The system command transfers DOS system files from the default drive to a disk in a specified drive; eg, from C⟩ to A⟩.
TIME	Shows the current time according to the computer clock or sets a new time.
TREE	Displays the path and optionally scrolls the contents of each directory and subdirectory on a disk. Works best with the MORE command.
TYPE	Scrolls the contents of a file. Works best with the MORE command.
VER	The version command shows the DOS version number; eg, DOS 3.2. Type VER and then press Return key (carriage return). The answer would be something like "MS-DOS Version 3.30."
VERIFY	Toggles an internal command on and off that controls disk write verification.
VOL d:	Where d is the drive number, displays the disk's name (volume label) if one exists. This name was issued during formatting and is used optionally for identification purposes (eg, in cataloging disks). Type VOL and drive number (eg, VOL C:) and then press Return key. The answer would be "Volume in Drive C is (Name)."
XCOPY	The extended copy command copies files and subdirectories, if they exist, to another specified disk.

rated by a backslash. The single backslash at the beginning of the pathname indicates the root. All pathnames must originate in either the current directory or root.

When the root directory is displayed, subdirectory names are shown but not the files within them. When an operator is in a subdirectory and issues the DIR command, he or she will see something like:

```
        <DIR>    3-15-85   11:48-a
..      <DIR>    3-15-85   11:48-a
FILE1  COM  16256  3-08-83   12:00-p
FILE2  TXT    458  9-10-84   11:20-a
```

The dots to the left in the first two columns above indicate that the operator is working from a subdirectory. The single dot represents the current directory and the double dots, the parent to the current directory.

All directory paths and their relationships are called a tree. If the operator doesn't remember the various subdirectories (and optionally the files in them), DOS provides a way to see them with the TREE command:

TREE X: /f

where X represents any drive and the "/f" option requests seeing all files in each subdirectory. This command lists all paths from the root on the disk. But unlike DIR, only filenames are shown, not their size or creation date/time. For a permanent record, pressing the Control+PrtScr keys before and after issuing the TREE command will order printing of all text scrolling on the screen.

Directories are not free. Each consumes disk space. A disk can become so burdened with directories that there won't be room for anything else. Operators should use subdirectories as needed, but overuse should be avoided. It is easy to get lost in a complex directory structure if one is created with many levels of subdirectories. Third- or deeper-level directories should be rare because they require an extremely long pathname. This fault, however, can be corrected with a batch file: the subject of the next section of this chapter.

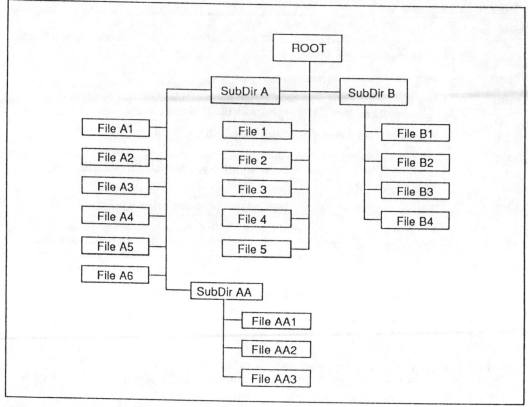

Figure 10.3. Simple subdirectory tree.

BATCH AND CONFIGURATION COMMANDS

Batch File Commands

A batch file is a collection of DOS commands that execute multiple commands in sequence via a simple command. When DOS executes a batch file, each line in the file is treated as a DOS command and executed as if the operator had typed the command at the system prompt. The primary use for a batch file is to automate multiple DOS command sequences that are repeated often. If not for this capability, operating a PC would often be drudgery.

Besides standard DOS commands, batch files have their own subset of commands that allow an operator to write a batch file as a small program. Branching and iteration are allowed in these programs. Batch commands may also have external parameters passed to them at the time a file is executed.

A batch file label must have the ".BAT" extension. Commands are executed in it as any other DOS command: by typing the file's root name without the extension at the system prompt. All executing files (.BAT, .COM, and .EXE) require only that their root name be typed and entered.

Autoexec.bat File

The file *Autoexec.bat* is a special batch file name that, if found in the root directory when a disk is booted, will automatically run before control of the computer is turned over to the operator. This is a great "time saver." An operator might wish to always load several files into memory on start-up, and the commands to do this would be in AUTOEXEC.BAT. An example might be:

```
C:
date
time
prompt $P$G
verify = off
print /b:4608 /d:1pt1
mode 1pt1:,,p
cls
```

In the example above, this autoexec.bat file would first set the date and time, install the information desired in the prompt, turn off read/write verify, set criteria and mode for a printer, and clear the screen. Thus, seven instructions are issued automatically when the computer is turned on. The date and time commands are needed because if autoexec.bat is found then the DOS request for date and time is not issued. However, most PCs have a program that sets time and date automatically via an internal battery operated clock.

If an operator wishes to terminate the execution of an autoexec.bat file (or any other batch file) before it is complete, the break command (Control-Break or ^C) is executed. Changes in an autoexec.bat file can easily be made with any text editor that does not implant hidden codes (ie, an ASCII-file editor).

Parameters

Command parameters are extra pieces of information than can be typed after many DOS commands. For example, DIR B:/W contains the parameters B: and /W. These modify the basic operation of the command but are not required by the command. The "B:" order specifies the B drive, and the "/W" tells the DOS that the operator wishes the directory displayed in *wide* (multicolumn) format.

Parameters can be passed to a batch file in the same manner—by typing the information after the batch command but before tapping the Return (Enter) key. Parameters may be used in a batch file anywhere a parameter would normally be used as part of the DOS command to be run. *Markers* are used within the batch file to signify what parameter goes where. A marker is a percent sign (%) and a single digit between 0 and 9

(that's a potential of ten markers in use at any one time). Remember, zero is a number.

Batch Subcommands

In addition to normal DOS commands, batch files have their own subcommand structure. Table 10.4 shows the subcommands that can be used in a batch file.

Figure 10.4 shows a sample batch file one might use to backup and clear a word processing data disk periodically. It assumes that all word processing backup files are named with the extension ".BAK," the operator does not want them, and that they are on the disk in Drive B. This sample batch file is called BAK.BAT and is also on the word processing data disk in Drive B. The operator starts it by typing a batch file labeled B.BAK. Clever use of DOS by using numerous batch files will save time, effort, and money by not having to purchase scores of programs. The limits in using batch files are found only in an operator's imagination.

A batch file can call another, but the original file will lose control of the computer. Thus, an operator should not expect the first batch file to do anything of use after a second is activated. However, DOS reference books show tricks to get around this limitation and others.

The DOS "remembers" the disk that contains the batch file and the drive it is in. If the operator removes the original disk, the DOS will ask her to replace it before going on. Also, if a batch file contains a syntax error in any of its commands, the file will stop execution at that point and the operator will be returned to the DOS prompt.

Configuration System Commands

DOS commands and batch files tell the system *what* to do; configuration commands tell DOS applications *how* to do it. Configuration commands are not entered at the keyboard. They are sought, loaded, and executed automatically on start-up by a file called CONFIG.SYS just before AUTOEXEC.BAT is executed. Both CONFIG.SYS and AUTOEXEC.BAT must be located in the

Table 10.4. Batch Commands

ECHO   Controls whether batch-file commands are shown on the monitor as they are executed. Also allows an operator to display messages or notes.

FOR   Enables the operator to carry out a DOS command on one or more files within the batch file.

GOTO   Instructs DOS to seek a specific line in the command file, rather than go to the next command in the sequence established, and resume execution with the line following the label. A label is a string of characters identifying the line in a batch file where DOS should go next.

IF   Checks whether an established criterion is met.

PAUSE   Makes a DOS execution stop and displays the instruction "Strike a key when ready," allowing the operator time to read a message or perform some task as turning on the printer.

REM   The remark command displays a message (string of characters) if ECHO is on or allows the operator to insert explanatory notes in a batch file if ECHO is off.

SHIFT   Discards the contents of the %0 replaceable parameter and shifts the contents of each subsequent parameter to a lower number. For example: %1 and %0, %2 become %1, %3 becomes %2, etc.

```
ECHO OFF                                        <— Screen echo off
CLS                                             <— Clear the screen
ECHO ***Word processing cleanup***             <— Display a label
ECHO                                            <— Skip a line
ECHO Put backup disk in drive A:               <— Display instructions
PAUSE                                           <— Wait for key press
ERASE B:*.BAK                                   <— Erase all .BAK files
COPY B:*.* A:                                   <— Copy files to backup disk
DEL A:BAK.BAT                                   <— Erase batch file from A:
ECHO The backup is complete. Label your disk.  <— Terminate with message
```

Figure 10.4. Sample batch file used to periodically erase word processing files with a .BAK extension in Drive B, copy all other files in Drive B to Drive A, and delete a file in Drive A called BAK.BAT. Your situation might be different and you may not want to delete .BAK files first, but this should give an idea of what can be done.

root directory. In fact, these two files and the hidden DOS files (eg, IBMBIO.COM and IBMDOS.COM) are the only files that *must* be in the root directory.

Configuration commands are shown in Table 10.5. If an operator wishes to make a change in the CONFIG.SYS or AUTOEXEC.BAT files, the file must be edited, stored on the disk, and the system re-booted for the new file run. Following is a sample CONFIG.SYS file:

device = himem.sys
device = hardrive.sys
device = ansi.sys
device = tvgabio.sys
buffers = 20
files = 20

Table 10.5. Configuration Commands

BREAK	Break = On instructs DOS to check to see if Control-C or Control-Break has been pressed every time a disk is written to or read. Break = Off disables.
BUFFERS	Buffers = number defines the quantity of work areas in memory (from 1–99) that DOS can use to store data when writing to or reading from a disk. Twenty is average. If a "cache" is used, five is sufficient.
COUNTRY	Country = code directs DOS to follow local conventions for a specified country in matters such as format, currency symbols, and decimal separators. For example: Country = 033 for French, Country = 034 for Spanish, Country = 039 for Italian, Country = 044 for British, Country = 049 for German, Country = 972 for Israel. United States (001) is the default and need not be set unless the default has been changed.
DEVICE	Device = [drive:]pathname specifies a file with the extension .sys that tells DOS how to use a particular device such as a mouse, scanner, video system, cache, or ram board.
FILES	Files = number tells DOS the quantity of files (from 8–255) it can have open at the same time. Twenty is average. Some accounting programs require 40.
LASTDRIVE	Lastdrive = letter specifies the last drive letter DOS will recognize as valid. Drives A–Z are valid; Drive E is the default. Specifying the least letter necessary saves memory.
SHELL	Shell = [drive]pathname defines the name and location of the command processor (the interface to the operating system). Command.com is the default. "Shell" is necessary only when command.com is not located in the root directory.

Note that all configuration commands are followed by the equal symbol and a specification.

stacks = 0,0
lastdrive = E
break on

PROGRAMMING

Programming can be simply defined as the method used to "talk" to a computer abstractly. Operators rarely get involved in programming except possibly the simple programs that can be incorporated in a batch file. Programming takes much training to become efficient. It's easier to purchase an application that has been programmed by others. Thus, this section will not describe *how* to program. Rather, it will briefly explain *what* programming is so an operator can have a fundamental understanding of its need and scope.

What Is Programming?

A computer is a tool that requires both hardware and software to do anything useful. Without software, the computer is functionally useless—like an automobile without a steering wheel, brakes, or an accelerator. Software is a series of electronic instructions that the hardware must carry out. A specific set of instructions to implement a given task is called a *program*. Although programs can be written in a variety of "languages," all are reduced to a series of ones and zeros (binary instructions) when the computer executes the program.

The methods used to program the first computers of the world were as cumbersome and primitive as the 5-ton hardware they served. Programming instructions were fed from spools of punched paper tape that were hand fed by technicians—a far cry from the magnetic floppy disks used today.

A programmer's job is to convert user needs into a set of instructions for execution by a computer. Converting a problem to computer code is a five-step process:

1. *Define the problem.* Before starting, it's important that the programmer completely understands the nature of the problem to be solved and its related assumptions. Precise statements are made.

2. *Plan the solution.* Separate the problem's solution into the smallest steps possible and decide how they are logically linked. A logical outline is created.

3. *Code the program.* Translate the logical solution to a programming language that the computer will understand.

4. *Test the program.* Check the program logic on paper and then by machine using various scenarios.

An important process in each of the above points is to document everything; ie, develop a "sequential how-to" manual. Recall will frequently fail when a person is involved in complex configurations.

Translators

Computer hardware does not understand anything except binary electronic pulses; ie, Ons and Offs, 1s and 0s. To get from programming language to binary representations that the computer understands requires some form of translator. Translators come in two general types: compilers and interpreters.

The first step with either system is the development of a source program that embodies the computation and logic required to solve a problem. It must conform precisely to the rules followed by the interpreter or compiler that does the translation. With both interpreters and compilers, a program passes through (1) a type of *scanner* that converts a segment of source code into symbols, (2) a *parser* that arranges the symbols into a hierarchy reflecting program logic, (3) a *type checker* that analyzes the rearranged

symbols to locate program errors, and (4) a *code generator* that sends a set of binary machine-code instructions to the CPU.

Interpreters translate *one program line* at a time while executing. Interpretation translates in one step, and interpreters must be in the computer while a program is running. CPU execution is immediate.

Compilers translate an *entire program* once and then execute it. Compiled programs execute rapidly, are usually a multistep process, and do not require space in memory when programs run. CPU execution is not immediate; the computer stores instructions from the code generator in memory. A part of the compiler (an optimizer) refines the translation to make it as efficient as possible before execution. Compiler output (target code) may be either a set of low-level binary machine-code instructions (object code) or assembly language instructions. If of the latter, it must be further translated by an assembler before execution.

Programming Language

There are a variety of programming languages that fall into several classes. These classes range from actual machine code through languages with very English-like structure. Trade-offs include ease of use and efficiency. A language provides a list of instructions and other words that, when translated into binary machine code, trigger certain sequences of computer operations to execute a particular task. Every language has a set of rules called its *syntax.*

Once the programmer has selected how he will set up a program, a language must be chosen. Common languages are:

• *FORTRAN:* FORmula TRANslator, introduced in the late 1950s primarily for scientific use; eg, when long equations are involved. Essentially, FORTRAN is an automatic coding system for precision applications. Once a breakthrough in programming by IBM researchers, but now considered a relic number problem solver by many. Yet, it is still being taught for nuclear physics and engineering applications.

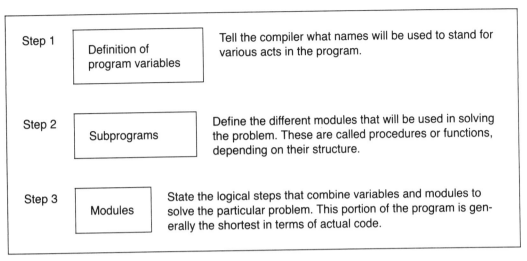

Figure 10.5. Program structure.

- *COBOL:* COmmon Business-Oriented Language, introduced in 1959 as an easy-to-read English instruction machine-independent business-oriented program. It is a verbose and cumbersome "number cruncher" like FORTRAN, yet used widely internationally for adding, subtracting, dividing, multiplying, and manipulating percentages and ratios. It is versatile in dealing with enormous quantities of simple data (eg, sales, inventory, and payroll records).

- *FACT:* Fully Automatic Compiling Technique, introduced by Honeywell researchers in 1960 as a better (but disputed) alternative for COBOL.

- *ALGOL:* Algorithmic Language. Like FORTRAN, this is a numerical problem solver, especially popular in Europe during the 1960s. Sometimes called "the first elegant but not necessarily practical program" by Americans.

- *BASIC:* Beginners' All-purpose Symbolic Instruction Code. This is an easy to learn language introduced at Dartmouth College in the 1970s; an evolving standard in most microcomputers (BASIC or GWBASIC) that allows programming by nonscientists.

- *Assembly:* A step away from the binary minutiae by using symbols more easily understood and remembered.

- *Pascal:* Named after Blaise Pascal, the French mathematician. It is a highly structured, relatively simple high-level language.

- *C:* Released by AT&T in 1972 as a rapid low-level assembly language.

- *Ada:* Named after Lady Augusta Ada Lovelace (who worked with Babbage). A large complex "do-everything" language becoming a popular Department of Defense and NATO standard for big projects.

- *LISP:* LISt Processor. Often used for artificial intelligence applications.

- *Logo:* A derivative language from LISP, designed in the late 1960s, that's so easy to use that 3-year-old children have learned to create programs with it to draw simple geometric figures.

Program Structure

Most structured programs are organized in a manner similar to that shown in Figure 10.5. LISP and other newer languages have somewhat different structures.

Chapter 11

Insurance Considerations

This chapter portrays insurance considerations from two viewpoints. First, coverage for the office; second, the administrative aspects of handling some type of patient health-care insurance involving a third-party payer.

INTRODUCTION

Physician Coverage

The category of physician insurance includes protection of personal and office risk. This is necessary to safeguard against potential financial loss. The common types of personal coverage frequently considered are residential public liability, fire and theft, automobile liability and collision, accident and health, extended disability, major medical, and life insurance.

Practice coverage might encompass office public liability, office fire and theft, office overhead, practice liability (malpractice), automobile liability and collision if a business-owned vehicle is involved, and employee fidelity bonds. Employee benefits may include major medical insurance and likely worker's compensation and unemployment benefits.

Patient Insurance

Many patients carry third-party payment plans that cover all or part of the costs for health-care services and the replacement of income lost as the result of disability. These accounts have a distinct relationship with a practice's billing procedures, financial account aging management, record maintenance, and data confidentiality. To be handled profitably, efficient claims processing procedures must be established. Concern should be given to office policies, data storage and retrieval systems, insurance coding and nomenclature, forms, communications, reporting, and billing procedures.

AN OFFICE'S INSURANCE INVENTORY

The types of policies to have and the amount of coverage to finance are not easy decisions for the doctor. The answer depends on individual circumstances, capabilities, and the degree of risk involved. Total coverage is financially impractical. To become "insurance poor" is as imprudent as underprotection. Potential risks must be assessed and reduced to approximate a fail-safe level.

The level of protection is not static. Due to inflation and practice growth, insurance needs must be assessed annually. They cannot be fixed and forgotten. Some areas might need a substantial increase periodically, and other areas might require pruning.

An Overview

Events occur in any practice or business that are beyond the control of management. Risks such as resulting from an accident, a fire, or a natural disaster (eg, a severe storm) can result in a great hardship on a property owner. The loss might be in health, money, property, or valuable documents. With a practice, other factors become involved such as a loss of a key employee or associate. A practice interruption for any reason can shackle productive time and fetter good will. The same is true for criminal risks such as embezzlement, theft, burglary, fraud, and vandalism. Such losses can have a great impact on a practice; thus, insurance coverage is a good investment if kept in balance with the risks involved. See Figure 11.1

To enhance protection against criminal acts, well-lighted premises, deadbolt door locks, jimmy-proof windows or window bars, alarm systems, and hidden vaults discourage or minimize burglary losses. Valuables should be locked and secured and only accessible to certain key people.

Despite the scope of insurance policies, good coverage is no excuse for poor precautions and safeguards. An insurance policy does not assure a riskless environment. Constant vigil should be maintained against hazardous conditions by being "safety" conscious. Slippery steps and floors, stairways without hand railings, overloaded electric circuits, incautious use of inflammables, careless techniques, etc, should not be allowed to occur. They invite accidents and suits for negligence. Still, some risks to a

INSURANCE CONSIDERATIONS

Patient Risks

    Malpractice
    Premises liability

Practice Risks

    Fire and theft
    Renter's protection
    Criminal, vandalism
    Fidelity bonds
    Key-person

Personal and Family Risks

    *Social Security contribution
    Automobile liability
    Automobile collision
    Homeowner's insurance
    Accident and health
    Major medical
    Disability
    Business interruption and
       office overhead
    Life
    Mortgage
    Retirement plan
    Special property

Employee Risks

    *Social Security contribution
    **Worker's compensation
    **Unemployment
    Accident and health
    Major medical
    Life

*Involuntary.
**Usually involuntary.

Figure 11.1. A listing of insurance coverage considerations. These are listed in the general order of their priority, but this may change with individual needs.

practice are beyond control such as a long strike in a one-industry town or the street in front of the office closed for extended repairs. Such events require a strong financial foundation and innovative thinking.

Maintaining Coverage

Insurance premiums are usually paid quarterly or annually, and a policy should never be allowed to lapse unknowingly. Assure that you inform the doctor immediately when premiums become due and that all policies are filed in a safe place (eg, a bank vault, with copies held in the office). Liability policies (personal, practice, public) should be kept indefinitely or at least up to the statute of limitations as claims may be presented many years after an accident was supposed to have occurred.

The typical doctor will carry a number of different insurance policies that become due at different dates. A *personal insurance log* helps ensure that premiums are paid on time so protection does not lapse (Fig. 11.2). Important data should be recorded. If space does not permit all information to be included on the log sheet, some facts may have to be recorded elsewhere. Following is a listing of the vital facts:

- Policy holder (if more than one DC is involved in the practice)
- Title and number of the policy
- Name of the insurance carrier
- Carrier's address and telephone number
- Due dates and amounts of premium partial payments
- Effective date of the policy
- Expiration date of the policy
- Type of coverage and limits
- Dollar value of the policy
- Renewal date of the policy
- Amount of annual premium
- Name of the insurance agent
- Agent's address and telephone number
- Names of the beneficiaries.

Malpractice Insurance

Malpractice (professional liability) is the risk resulting from the actual practice of chiropractic. Alleged claims are one of the greatest hazards in practice today. Malpractice is a serious problem, reflected in increased claims and increased premium costs. No health-care practitioner is immune. The dangers are real, and the consequences are severe for those who fail to take reasonable precautions. Although the vast majority of cases are unsuccessful, they still are costly to the doctor financially and emotionally. To be subjected to suit for professional negligence, whether merited or not, is an experience to be avoided. If a suit is decided in favor of the patient, the insurance company pays damages up to the amount insured but the doctor is liable for any additional damages if awarded.

Negligence vs Judgment Errors

Because a patient was not cured or a patient's condition became worse under treatment is not cause for malpractice if usual and customary procedures were followed. If a doctor prescribes or administers a wrong treatment, this is not necessarily malpractice. It may be considered an "error in judgment" and not negligent unless it can be proved that the doctor or an assistant did not use reasonable care in examining or treating the patient. If an assistant were responsible for the negligence, both the assistant and the doctor may be found at fault.

If a patient is injured during health care because of an accident or negligence by the doctor, an associate, or an assistant, the patient can sue the doctor for damages. Most accidents result when some form of therapy or diagnostic procedure is used incorrectly or an unsterile or unsafe instrument results in harm to a patient. To prove malpractice, the patient must prove negligence.

Prevention

Even frivolous suits cost a defendant money, time, reputation, and peace of mind. The money involved far exceeds that for insurance. Regardless of a jury's decision, it can affect the doctor's entire future. Thus, prevention rather than defense is the priority. The office environment should be made as safe as possible to guard against accident claims as the result of negligence and accidents. Special care must be used in handling sharp and pointed instruments, following directions of use, avoiding the unlabeled containers, and lifting or moving disabled patients. Equipment should be maintained in good working order and applied only by au-

Insurance Summary

Company	Dur. of Policy	Type	Guide-lines	Non Canc.	Guar-Renew	Indemnity Period and Amounts		Elim. Prd.		Death or Disab.	Annu. Prem.	Due Dates
						Accid.	Sickness	Acci.	Sick			

Figure 11.2. A sample form to log a doctor's various insurance policies. Premium due dates are then at hand for quick reference.

thorized personnel following operational instructions. Clinical instruments used in body contact (eg, speculae, needles) should be sterilized prior to use.

Protection Against Liability

If a doctor does not carry malpractice insurance, he might be obliged to pay damages, court costs, attorney fees, and other costs involved in a suit if it is decided in favor of the patient. In most situations, the effect would be bankruptcy. Even if a suit is decided in the doctor's favor, defense costs could be staggering.

Public Liability Insurance

Several hazards to public safety are involved in health care besides those of professional liability. Liability insurance covers actions by the doctor or his employees that cause harm or financial loss to others. Although the incidence of fires, accidents, claims of negligence, etc, is quite low, just one $100,000–$500,000 suit can easily bankrupt a physician not adequately protected. Juries are not too sympathetic to doctors and assistants when they are at fault.

Public liability may arise by owning or leasing real property such as an office building, a lot, residential property, or vacation property. As any owner or lessor of property may be held responsible for an accident occurring on the premises in which neglect can be proved, liability protection should include accidents both within and without the office such as on the office grounds and parking areas. A suit or broken rapport may arise from an injured employee, patient, friend, solicitor, or salesman visiting the office.

Physical Hazards and Office Equipment

Patients preoccupied by worry and pain or disabled in some manner require special safety considerations. A cane or a crutch may catch something that a shoe would not. Electric cords should never be placed where they might cause someone to trip,

and stairways should be well lighted, dry, and free of unnecessary objects. Throw rugs should be avoided. Children should not be left in a room alone. Their imaginations can become overactive. Dangerous substances should be locked in cabinets and properly labeled. Precautionary vigilance is imperative if accidents are to be prevented.

Roentgenographic Considerations

Diagnostic x-ray procedures offer inestimable benefits to clinical knowledge of a case, yet there are risks and possible detriments that must be weighed against the benefits. Optimal measures for patient protection must be used. Personnel training should include safe procedure factors, continuing exposure monitoring, protection during patient exposures, and protection of the skin from chemical exposure during film processing.

Infection and Contagious Diseases

The rules of good hygiene should be maintained at all times. Precautions should be made in the sterilization of instruments that enter a body cavity, venipuncture needles, and acupuncture needles, and in the care of open wounds. Although infection cannot always be prevented, the physician and assistants involved are liable if usual and customary precautions are not taken such as the proper sterilization of instruments and the use of sterile bandages.

Medical Expense Insurance

The benefits of health insurance are available in two general types: medical expense insurance and disability income insurance. Many variations are found within these two general types.

Coverage. Basic policies usually cover hospital care, diagnostic services, surgical services, operating room services and supplies, in-hospital physician services, and certain forms of outpatient service. Benefits are typically based on usual and customary fees or an amount set by a fee schedule.

Hospital expense insurance provides

specific benefits for daily hospital room and board and usual hospital services and supplies during hospital confinement. *Surgical expense insurance* provides benefits for the cost of surgical procedures (and often the related anesthesia) performed because of an accident or sickness. *Physician's expense insurance* (once called "Regular Medical Expense Insurance") provides benefits to help pay doctor fees for nonsurgical care in a hospital, home, or doctor's office.

Major medical expenses policies often provide broad benefits for practically all types of health care whether performed in a hospital, in a doctor's office, in an institution (eg, nursing home), or in a patient's home. The benefits are broad, but a deductible is usually required.

There are two major forms of major medical expense insurance: (1) *Supplemental:* This form of coverage is supplemental to a basic hospitalization insurance policy (hospital/surgical/physician's expenses), and it comprises about 80% of major medical coverage in the United States. (2) *Comprehensive Major Medical:* This form of coverage is used when a basic health insurance policy is not in effect, offering comprehensive protection where both basic coverage and extended health-care benefits are integrated. The exact coverage, however, varies extensively with how the policy is written.

Exclusions. Some common exclusions of most health insurance policies are costs of routine physical examinations, hearing aids, eyeglasses, cosmetic surgery unless related to an accident, charges for attention to a pre-existing condition, charges covered under government-sponsored programs (eg, Worker's Compensation, Medicare), or injuries suffered from an act of war. Routine dental and optometric services and prescription drug costs are usually covered under separate policies or special provisions.

Disability Income Insurance

Disability income insurance provides periodic payments when an insured is unable to work because of injury or sickness. Within the insurance industry, the term *disability*

generally refers to the inability to engage in one's occupation for 1–2 years and after that the inability to engage in any gainful occupation for which the individual is reasonably fitted by experience, training, or education.

Disability policies provide protection designed to replace a substantial portion of an individual's income status to finance a near-normal life-style during illness or disability from an accident. Policies are inevitably previous income-related, and benefits range between 50% to 80% of normal income. In general, benefits apply in situations where legislated workers' compensation programs would not apply, such as for self-employed individuals.

The subject of patient disability coverage will be described later in this chapter. However, it is appropriate to mention here that there are disability health-care programs under the Social Security system, the Railroad Retirement Act, worker's compensation state statutes, and the Veterans Administration, to name a few. For needy individuals who cannot qualify for Social Security disability benefits, the Social Security system also administers another public assistance program called Assistance to the Permanently and Totally Disabled (APTD). These programs, of course, are besides group and individual insurance coverage.

Other Types of Coverage

An assistant may be asked to supervise a variety of the office's and doctor's personal insurance policies.

Employee Protection

All states have worker's compensation laws that explain an employer's responsibilities if an employee is injured as the result of an occupational accident. Besides employee protection established by law, many doctors voluntarily make available to their employees various types of life insurance, disability insurance, and hospitalization and medical benefits, as part of their Employee Benefit Plan via a group comprehensive plan.

Fidelity Bonds

Doctors are very trusting of their employees, yet most practice consultants suggest that a doctor carry employee fidelity insurance in the event some employee proves to be dishonest. The purpose is to protect the practice against internal theft. Employee bonding should not be considered an insult to any assistant. It is just good business practice and does not reflect adversely on any individual's integrity.

Fire and Criminal Insurance

Fire and theft insurance should include the complete inventory list of all buildings, furnishings, clinical equipment, instruments, supplies, business office equipment, and all records and files. It is good procedure to keep duplicate inventory lists: one in the office and one at another location (eg, a bank vault).

Many fire insurance policies automatically cover losses from both fire and lightning, and some also include coverage against explosion, smoke, wind, hail, and riot damage. If not, additional coverage can be purchased if the doctor deems it necessary. Patient charts, tax records, and accounts receivable files are especially valuable records that should be protected against loss. Most damages in a typical office or residential fire are not caused by flame; they are the result of smoke and water. Several companies offer fire, burglary, theft, and malicious mischief coverage under a single comprehensive policy where extended coverage can be added to include smoke, explosion, wind, hail, vehicle, and riot damage.

Burglary, robbery, and theft insurance should include damage to property and equipment as well as the potential financial loss involved. In recent years, doctors' offices have had a rise in burglary incidence. Although chiropractic offices do not contain narcotics, they do contain expensive clinical and business office equipment (eg, diathermy, ultrasound, computers).

Vehicle Liability Insurance

Besides normal automobile personal and property liability, medical payments, and collision coverage, any assistant who uses an office automobile in performing a service for her employer should be co-insured in the doctor's policy as she may be sued as well as the doctor if an accident should occur while she is driving the doctor's automobile. The doctor should also consider coverage while driving a borrowed or rented automobile. Liability may also result from the use of a corporate-owned vehicle by either an officer or employee of a corporation. Besides automobile liability, a motorcycle, a recreational vehicle, a boat, an airplane, and other types of vehicles present a potential source of liability.

Business Interruption and Office Overhead Insurance

More is involved than property if the office should suffer severe damage from fire or a natural disaster. Considerable income can be lost when repairs are being made, equipment is being replaced, or a new location must be found. This financial loss may be far greater than the property loss. Business interruption insurance reduces the risk of a prolonged downtime in which fixed expenses must go on but no income is received. Typical coverage includes both the loss of profits as well as the practice's fixed expenses.

Office overhead expenses continue though the doctor's income may cease. These expenses are not usually covered under the typical disability policy. Because of this, many doctors obtain protection through a form of insurance that is based on verifiable office overhead expenses such as salaries, rent, utilities, and other fixed expenses. Several companies offer business interruption and office overhead insurance under a comprehensive policy.

Accounts Receivable Insurance

Accounts receivable insurance is not expensive compared to other types of coverage, but it is not commonly carried by most doctors. Specific criteria in extending credit that have been established by the insurance company must be followed, and most insurers require a copy of the office's monthly aging list. When a claim is made, it is usually paid in 90 days. The insurance company uses this time to see if the debtor will respond voluntarily.

Key-Person Insurance

The unexpected moving, retirement, pirating, disability, or death of a key assistant or associate can sometimes impose a severe hardship on a practice. Personnel depth and a contingency-oriented training program can safeguard against such an event in a group practice, but such depth is rarely possible for the small practice and the only logical safeguard is key-person insurance.

Life Insurance

The primary purpose of life insurance is to protect a family in the event of the insured's death. Many doctors carry some type of term, ordinary life, endowment, or annuity life insurance policy to protect their families and creditors (eg, debts, security, mortgages) when death occurs. It is also beneficial protection in partnerships and corporate practices involving two or more associates.

THIRD-PARTY RELATIONSHIPS

Third-party payment for chiropractic care is increasing in volume each year. In 1960, only a few major private insurance companies incorporated chiropractic health care in their policies as standard procedure. By 1970, well over 600 private companies included chiropractic in their policies. By 1980, it was estimated that approximately three-fourths of patients receiving chiropractic care were covered by some type of health-care benefit program.

Chiropractic inclusion within programs operated through state and federal agencies for special groups are also expected to increase. Some of these programs are designed to help veterans, servicemen, and their dependents, and some are for the aged and the indigent. For many years, the American Chiropractic Association has tried to assure that all citizens will have the right to avail themselves of chiropractic care.

Administrative Control

In years past, the relationship between doctor and patient was a simple one-to-one agreement. Today, because third-party payers are involved extensively in health care, this relationship has become more complex. It need not, however, jeopardize the one-to-one relationship between doctor and patient.

Fee-for-Service Arrangements

A good method to maintain control of the doctor-patient business relationship is the *fee-for-service* practice; and this concept is followed by most private practitioners in the United States, regardless of discipline. That is, the intimate one-to-one doctor-patient relationship need not be diluted just because the patient has health-care insurance. The business and professional relationship between the doctor and patient is a matter for determination by those two parties; provided, of course, that the terms do not violate established laws.

In the fee-for-service practice, many doctors consider the contract between doctor and patient complete when services have been provided, the related fees have been paid by the patient, and the patient has been dismissed. They will usually provide the patient with a completed form that indicates the diagnosis, treatment rendered, itemized charges for each service provided, and the amount paid. This information is attached to the insurance form that a patient sends to his insurance company for reimbursement. In this simplest of arrangements, the patient receives the service, the doctor receives the professional fees involved, and the patient is reimbursed by the insurance company. Complicated collection efforts are not involved.

Simplifying Claims Processing

If the doctor chooses to defer collection of fees from the patient until third-party benefits due the patient are collected, efficient claims processing is a necessity. The key is to keep the system simple and standardized. This way, you can explain office policies the same way to every patient entering the practice.

An efficient claims processing system begins with complete and accurate data gathering, uncomplicated forms administration routines, accurate in-office forms filing, and the maintenance of a current patient insurance log.

Data Gathering

Each patient should be asked about health insurance or company coverage during the initial visit. The name of the company, type and extent of coverage, dependents covered, policy numbers, and recent claims are important facts to be recorded. This information should be rechecked and updated if it has been 6 months or longer since the patient's last visit. A running record may be kept on the patient's entering data form or history form, or on a separate sheet.

If a patient cannot supply all necessary information on the first visit, they can be asked to check their contracts or bring them with them on the next visit. It is usually best, however, to get all pertinent information on record before services are provided to a nonemergency patient.

Form Processing

Proper claim forms, usually in multicopy sets, are commonly obtained from the patient; if not, from the insurance company or the patient's employer. Some commonly used forms can be stocked in the office.

Neat, accurate, complete records are the first step in proper handling of claims. Forms should be completed and filed without delay. Sometimes a "rough copy" is prepared as an initial draft prior to final typing. All blanks on the form must be filled. When not pertinent, "N/A" (not applicable) should be entered so it will not appear as if the entry has been overlooked.

The typical procedure is for the doctor to review or dictate the professional section. An assistant fills in the general information from the patient's permanent record files and processes claim forms. The assistant can obtain the patient's name, address, age, place of employment, dates of treatment, and other basic data from the patient's chart. Diagnosis, therapy, prognosis, and other necessary clinical data can be obtained from the patient's clinical records or the doctor's dictated notes. However, the doctor should review the finished form before signing it, for it is the physician who is responsible for the accuracy of all information entered on the form. The doctor's name should be typed below his signature to assure legibility.

Proper processing of claim forms will be one of an administrative assistant's more time-consuming tasks. In group practice, it is not unusual that one or two assistants do little else but process claims.

Data Release Authorization. All patients should sign a records release form early during initial care (Fig. 11.3). This legal requirement will be necessary to provide progress reports and the final claim form to the insurance company after case dismissal.

Ledger Coding. When an insurance statement is given to a patient or mailed directly to an insurance company, it should be noted in the patient's financial ledger and initialed by the CA who mails the statement. A simple code is often used to indicate the type of insurer (eg, MC for Medicare, MA for Medicaid, WC for Workers' Compensation, BS for Blue Shield, and PI for private insurance). Related date, charges, and balance should be entered in the regular columns of the patient's financial ledger.

Maintainence of Current Information. Many carriers periodically mail newsletters explaining changes in policy and procedures. These should be carefully reviewed and kept on file for future reference.

In-office Forms Filing

Proper filing is vital to efficient management. For reference, at least one duplicate copy should be filed of all forms completed.

AUTHORIZATION FOR RELEASE OF RECORDS

To..
Doctor or Hospital

....
Address

I hereby authorize and request you to release

To..
Doctor or Hospital

....
Address

any and all health records in your possession, including x-rays, concerning the undersigned.

Date...   Signed...
(Patient or Nearest Relative)

....   Relationship...
Witness

ACA Form 16

Figure 11.3. Sample authorization for release of records form (ACA Form 16).

tained for all blank claim forms and related literature. Duplicate copies or an original used for photocopying can be stored here.

Insurance records may be filed separately or with the patient's clinical or financial records. The former method is the simplest, but patient folders sometimes become quite bulky and difficult to handle. If a separate insurance file is maintained, it should be divided into three parts:

1. *A holding or pending file*, for current forms received but not completed. All forms received in the mail or delivered by a patient should be dated when they are received. This date will direct the general priority for completion.

2. *An active-completed accounts file*, for duplicate copies of forms submitted to insurance companies and/or attorneys that may be needed for reference. Depending on the volume of cases attended, many offices subdivide this file into categories. For example, (a) private insurance and group plans, (b) worker's compensation claims,

(c) Medicare claims, (d) Medicaid claims, (e) Medicare/Medicaid claims, and (f) other claims. The Medicare and Medicaid categories are best set-up with monthly dividers.

3. *An inactive-completed accounts file*, for those records unlikely to require follow-up reference. Essentially, this file holds inactive records until the statute of limitations or office policy is met, whichever is longer.

Patient Insurance Log

Some offices keep a source book in which a patient's name and address, employer's name and address, type of insurance coverage, type of claim (service or indemnity), name of insurer, contract number, date claim was received, date claim was submitted, recording assistant's initials, and other helpful information concerning insurance claims are listed. A sample is shown in Figure 11.4. Years later, the doctor may have reason to review old records if the patient suffers another accident or illness.

PATIENT INSURANCE LOG

Date Claim Filed	Follow-up Date	Patient's Name Guarantor's Name	Insurance Co. Address	Assignment		Amt. of Claim	Amt. Paid	Balance
				Yes	No			

Figure 11.4. Sample patient insurance log sheet.

Processing Fees

Years ago, it was considered unethical for a doctor to levy a charge for completing necessary insurance forms, but that was when an "insurance case" was somewhat a rarity. Today, however, the proliferation of insurance claims and the introduction of sundry complicated government programs has made this chore a major concern in health-care practice. Some offices charge either the patient or the insurance company a small fee for processing routine claims, and some offices do not. However, because of the time involved, at most offices charge for the time involved in preparing a narrative or medicolegal report. Such charges should be itemized on some type of transaction slip (Fig. 11.5).

Blue Shield prohibits a charge for filling out a routine insurance form, and at least one state has a statute preventing physicians from charging patients to complete insurance forms.

Coding Systems in Insurance Claims Processing

In recent years due to the massive increase in computerized data processing, coding of diagnosis, treatments, and procedures has become increasingly important. Coding of procedures and the diagnosis or the nature of an illness is provided for in most claim forms. The two most commonly used systems are CPT and ICD 9-CM codes.

CPT Procedural Codes

To speed the reporting of professional services, a coding system was developed called *Current Procedural Terminology* (CPT). It lists standardized terms, eponyms, acronyms, and descriptors. Samples are shown in Figure 11.6. A common reference, published by the American Medical Association, is the *Physicians' Current Procedural Terminology*. Every office should have a current copy and see that it is kept current.

Any standard 5-digit CPT number can be modified by using a 2-digit code number preceded by a hyphen. The number 22 means

"more than," and the number 52 means "less than." For example, 72052 is the code for the standard radiographic Davis series of seven views of the cervical spine. The number 72052-22 indicates that eight views were taken, while the number 72052-52 shows that six views were taken. This would justify a higher or lower charge, according to the number of films.

Using CPT code numbers does not automatically ensure prompt payment of claims, but it does save time and space. If code references are not appropriate, written descriptions can be added to explain the procedures administered. However, this disrupts the computerized process, which usually requires further explanation and delays payment. When the necessary services are charged at reasonable rates, the doctor will probably be paid if a procedural code number is used.

ICD Diagnostic Codes

Diagnostic codes are also popular. The most universally accepted diagnosis coding system is the *International Classification of Diseases (ICD), Clinical Modification*. This is a modification of the World Health Organization's *International Classification of Diseases*. Some samples are shown in Figure 11.7, but due to revisions their accuracy may be in question at this reading. Current ICD volumes are available from the Superintendent of Documents, U.S. Government Printing Office, Washington, DC 20402.

Since the Health Care Financing Administration (HCFA) of DHHS gave its approval for mandatory use of the CPT-4 procedural codes and the supplementary alphanumeric HCFA Common Procedure Coding System for government financial health-care programs, many authorities predict other procedure codes will become increasingly less popular.

CLAIMS CONTROL

All patient health-insurance policies are direct agreements between the individual

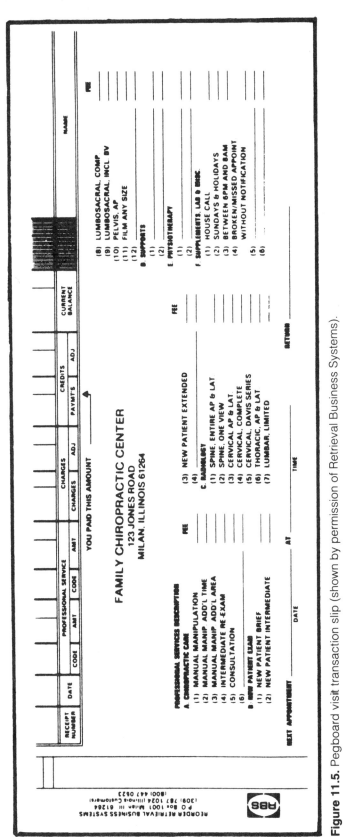

Figure 11.5. Pegboard visit transaction slip (shown by permission of Retrieval Business Systems).

SAMPLE CPT NUMBERS

Code	Clinical Procedure
97260	Manipulation, performed by physician, one area
97261	Manipulation, performed by physician, additional area
90000	Visit, new patient, brief history and examination
90010	Visit, new patient, additional examination time
90015	Visit, new patient, intermediate examination
90017	Visit, new patient, extended examination
90040	Visit, established patient, new condition, brief service
90060	Visit, established patient, intermediate service
90070	Visit, established patient, extended service
97799	Unlisted service or procedure

Code	Radiologic Procedures
72010	Entire spine survey, AP and lateral
72020	Spine, one view
72040	Cervical, AP and lateral
72050	Cervical, comprehensive, 4 views minimum
72052	Cervical, complete, including oblique and flexion and/or extension studies
72070	Thoracic, AP and lateral
72100	Lumbosacral, AP and lateral
72110	Lumbosacral, complete, with oblique views
72114	Lumbosacral, complete, including bending views
72170	Pelvis, one view only
73020	Shoulder, one view
73030	Shoulder, complete, two views minimum
73560	Knee, AP and lateral

Code	Laboratory and Miscellaneous
80012	Automated multichannel test, 12 clinical chemistry tests
81000	Urinalysis, routine, with microscopy
85022	Hemogram, automated, and differentiated wbc count (cbc)
85014	Hematocrit
85018	Hemoglobin, colorimetric
85007	Differential blood count
93000	Electrocardiogram with interpretation and report
90030	Blood pressure and/or weight check and diet
90100	House call
99054	Sundays and holidays
90052	Between 6 pm and 8 am
99049	Broken/missed appointment, without prior notification
99070	Braces, nutritional supplements, diet evaluation

Figure 11.6. Some typical CPT code numbers applicable in chiropractic practice.

SAMPLE DIAGNOSTIC CODES

Code	Diagnosis/Symptom
789.5	Abdominal pain, colic
724.9	Ankylosis of the spine*
493.4	Asthma
723.4	Brachial neuritis or radiculitis*
784.0	Cephalalgia or headache*
722.0	Cervical disc disorders
756.2	Cervical rib anomaly
847.0	Cervical sprain or strain
839.0	Vertebral subluxation or dislocation
723.2	Cervicobrachial syndrome
755.30	Congenital short leg
564.0	Constipation
923.0	Contusion of shoulder, upper arm
719.7	Difficulty in walking
781.3	Disturbed coordination
626.2	Excessive menstruation
213.0	Exostosis of unspecified site
351.0	Facial paralysis
E883	Fall into hole or other opening
E881	Fall on or from ladder, scaffolding
E880	Fall on or from stairs, steps
535.0	Gastritis, acute
477.9	Hay fever or allergic rhinitis, cause unspecific
455	Hemorrhoids
V65.2	Malingering
E826	Pedal cycle accident
722.1	Lumbar or thoracic disc disorder
847.2	Lumbar sprain or strain
839.20	Lumbar vertebra subluxation or dislocation
846.0	Lumbosacral sprain or strain
839.42	Lumbosacral subluxation or dislocation
E929.0	Motor vehicle accident, late effect
783.0	Osteoporosis
724.4	Radiculitis, neurogenic, lumbar
724.5	Radiculitis, vertebrogenic, back*
737.30	Scoliosis (acquired, idiopathic)
721.90	Spondylitis osteoarthritis*
E916	Struck by falling object
847.1	Thoracic sprain or strain
839.21	Thoracic vertebra subluxation or dislocation
454	Varicosities, lower extremity

*NOS - Not otherwise specified (or unspecified)

Figure 11.7. Many insurance companies prefer a diagnosis listed by its International Classification of Disease (ICD) number. A few examples are shown above.

insurance company and the individual patient, not between the doctor and the patient or the doctor and the insurance company.

Policy Coverage

There are many types of health-care insurance. Most pay for chiropractic services; a few do not. A knowledge of coverage and the differences in methods of payment is an important aspect of health practice today.

Financial Responsibility. If some services are covered but others are not, it is the patient's responsibility to pay the doctor what the insurance company does not. It is the insurance company's responsibility to pay only those claims or losses according to the specific type of policy for which the patient is paying. Sometimes a patient buys a limited policy to avoid paying a higher premium that does not include chiropractic coverage. This is poor economy.

Private Insurance Companies. Almost every major insurance company in the United States includes chiropractic services in its policies. However, this does not mean that every policy written by the company includes chiropractic services. As the result of insurance equality legislation, the majority of states requires the inclusion of chiropractic services under *all* commercial health and accident policies written in those states.

Self-Insurers. Major industrial employers have included chiropractic in the health plan for all their employees. Many major international, national, and local unions also include chiropractic in their health and welfare plans (eg, railroad workers, rubber workers).

Federal and State Programs. The federal government has authorized the provision of limited chiropractic services under federal law for all eligible Americans in Medicare, Medicaid, and the Vocational Rehabilitation programs. The National Conference of Insurance Legislators adopted a model bill for state health insurance programs that defines "physician" to include the doctor of chiropractic.

Federal-Employee Programs. Chiropractic care is authorized in Federal Employees Health Benefit (FEHB) programs, in federal employee worker's compensation, and in leave approvals for federal employee excuse of illness. Out of 17 FEHB employee organization plans, 13 include chiropractic benefits.

The U.S. Internal Revenue Code has long recognized chiropractic care as a medical deduction, and the U.S. Public Health Service classifies doctors of chiropractic among "medical specialists and practitioners" and includes DCs in its *Health Manpower Source Book.* However, some governmental programs such as those of the Veterans Administration and the Civilian Health And Medical Program Uniformed Services (CHAMPUS) do not as of this writing offer chiropractic care or such care must be upon the prescription of an allopathic physician. National chiropractic associations are actively encouraging legislation to help remedy this situation. A trial study is now in progress.

Helping Patients Process Claims

Most large businesses have a personnel department or have assigned someone to be in charge of health-care insurance benefits. This person has the job of helping an employee fill out his claim form when he has incurred eligible expenses. For smaller employers and individual plans, the patient is usually given a form that the patient and doctor complete to send to the insurance company. Regardless, the patient must file a claim with his insurance company before any action is taken on this claim.

Most misunderstandings about coverage can be avoided if the patient fully understands what his policy provides. If there is doubt, the patient should contact his agent or carrier and request an opinion in writing.

Inappropriate Advice. It is inadvisable to attempt to interpret a patient's policy. Only the carrier or the patient's agent should attempt to do that. A CA's good intentions might easily backfire. It is also inadvisable to recommend a specific company to a patient seeking health-care coverage. If the patient follows your suggestion and later becomes dissatisfied, the doctor might lose the patient and potential referrals.

Office Guidelines. Many frequently asked questions about claims processing can be answered by having printed guidelines available for patients entering the practice. These guidelines should give patients step-by-step instructions so that their claims can be processed efficiently.

The Processing Procedure

After a patient's health claim has been submitted, it is evaluated by claims analysts and screened for eligible expenses. Usually, this means subtracting the deductible and assessing 80% of the remaining eligible charges. The patient's bills are screened to see if all items are covered; and sometimes the doctor may be asked to submit additional information to substantiate the necessity for the diagnostic and therapeutic procedures provided.

Most health-insurance companies make their determination on the experience of their claim analysts, but many request reviews by their medical and chiropractic consultants. They review claims based on the limits of the policies. This sometimes results in less payment for a claim than the amount submitted. A policy that is highly controversial.

If a patient disagrees with what has been paid, he may request the carrier to reevaluate the payments made. Ultimately, of course, if the patient strongly disagrees, he may contact the office of his state insurance commissioner for resolution of the problem.

Routine In-Office Checkpoints

It should be the responsibility of an administrative assistant to periodically remind the doctor of all insurance cases pending. All completed or even partially completed forms should be proofread carefully. Following are some common checkpoints that

help to avoid delayed payments and follow-up reports:

• Monitor discharge dates closely so forms can be sent in promptly.

• Verify that all treatment dates and charges agree and are itemized. This will be automatic if a superbill is used (Fig. 11.8).

• Verify the accuracy of the date and time of the original injury.

• Verify the spelling of the patient's name and address.

• Verify the patient's policy identification and group numbers.

• Verify that fees correlate with usual, customary, and reasonable rates.

• Verify that all codes used correspond to the procedures or diagnosis described.

• Verify that all necessary related documents are attached to the form.

• Assure that each form is fully completed, accurate, and signed before it is mailed. Do not use ditto marks for identical entries on different dates. Another person may sign the doctor's name only if that person is *legally authorized* to do so.

• Check to see that the doctor's identification numbers are properly entered (eg, license number, Social Security number, federal ID reporting number, or a number assigned to him by the carrier).

• Submit the claim form immediately on case dismissal or monthly if this is permissible with the carrier.

Refunds

It sometimes occurs that an insurance company will send the doctor a check to cover services for a patient's account that has already been paid by the patient. This need not cause an accounting problem: (1) issue an office check payable to the patient for the overpayment; (2) enclose this check in a letter of explanation to the patient; and (3) credit the amount of the company's check and debit the office's check in the patient's financial ledger and in your usual in-

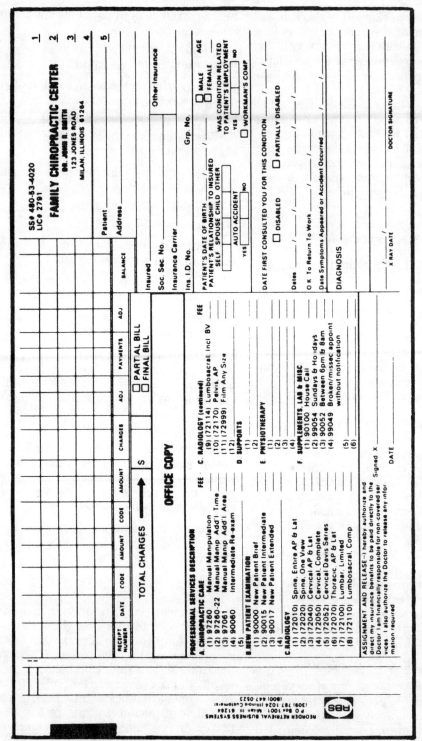

Figure 11.8. Office copy of a superbill serving as both a transaction slip and statement. The bottom left portion of the slip contains an authorization for assignments of benefits if that is desired. The right portion provides spaces for basic insurance, auto accident, worker's compensation, disability, and diagnostic data. The slips are usually made in three-part sets: a copy for the patient, a copy for office files, and a copy to attach to an insurance report (shown with permission from Retrieval Business Systems).

come and disbursements records. This will save the patient the trouble of requesting another check payable in the patient's name and protect you from an accusation of receiving double payment.

Telephone Contacts

Specific contract provisions vary considerably, and it will be unlikely that the doctor or assistants will be familiar with them all. Insurance is a highly complex subject, and policy phrasing is not always clear. Frequently, telephone contact must be made by an assistant with a carrier to clarify some facts. Here are some tips:

• Whenever you are completing a form for an insurance program that you have not processed before, call the carrier to find out what they may prefer. Have your questions organized in a list, but ask one question at a time. Allow space on the sheet to complete the answers.

• Respect the other person's time and expertise. Offer to call back if a different time would be more appropriate.

• Get the name and title of the person you are speaking with, and record it. Use the person's name frequently during the conversation. Also record the telephone number and extension number for future reference. Record all the facts of the conversation. Don't try to rely on memory alone.

• Try to learn the procedures used for applying benefits and processing claims whenever it can be done diplomatically. Once they are learned, record them for future reference.

Insurance Terms

Several common terms used in the insurance and/or legal community have quite limited interpretations. Following are some examples of which you should become familiar.

Medical Necessity. Insurance contracts usually call for a direct relationship between covered services and medical necessity. This means that the patient's condition

treated must be a recognized one and that the examinations, tests, therapeutic substances, and treatment procedures used must be based on scientific studies and principles generally accepted by the profession as needed, essential, and appropriate to properly diagnose and treat patients with the condition involved. The attending physician must document in all records and reports facts to substantiate the need for the services provided. The quality and quantity of examination and therapeutic procedures used must be within the norms and/or criteria established by the profession as a whole for such a condition.

Fee Terminology. A health-care provider can charge any fee for service and select any manner of billing felt to be appropriate and within legal bounds. However, an insurance company is only obliged to pay what *they* decide are usual, customary, and reasonable (UCR). The terms "usual," "customary," and "reasonable" have rather limited interpretations within the insurance industry. According to the Health Insurance Association of America, the following definitions are believed to be accurate and reflect the insurance industry's definition:

• A "usual" fee is that fee usually charged for a given service by a physician to patients; ie, the doctor's usual fee.

• A fee is "customary" when it is within the range of usual fees charged by physicians of similar training and experience for the same service within the same geographic or socioeconomic area of the country. Sometimes the word "prevailing" is used rather than the word "customary."

• A fee is "reasonable" when it meets the above two criteria or, in the opinion of the responsible local, district, or state professional society review committee, it is justifiable, considering the special circumstances of the particular case in question.

Some insurance policies use only the two terms "usual and customary" or "reasonable and customary" when professional fees are mentioned. Others may use a disclaimer that "benefits are not payable for charges that are not medically necessary or are unreasonable."

Major Medical Accounts

The most common form of health insurance Americans have today is "major medical" insurance. About 85% of Americans today have a major medical policy protecting their health costs. Most employers provide a major medical coverage for their employees and their families. This type of health insurance covers a significant portion of hospital and physician's expenses. Chiropractic benefits are usually covered in the physician expense benefits of major medical contracts. This coverage, like other physician services, is made near 80% after a specified deductible amount has been met by the patient.

It may be important to remind some patients that *major* medical insurance was not created to cover *all* health-care costs, merely *major* costs. In most contracts, there is also a provision for paying only *reasonable* fees for *necessary* services.

Personal Injury Accounts

Personal injury is related to almost all non-job-related injuries, but it is most commonly associated with automobile injuries, falls on public transportation, falls in stores, etc. These cases require an extremely detailed case history that deeply explores the circumstances surrounding the accident. These cases invariably involve some type of litigation, but many cases are resolved outside court.

Doctor's Lien. Because the patient's attorney lacks responsibility to pay the doctor and many patients become unappreciative months after professional services were provided, professional supply houses have available a "Doctor's Lien." This document is signed by the patient at the beginning of care and directs the patient's attorney to pay the doctor's fee from any settlement *before* the patient receives the balance. Two copies of the signed agreement are sent to the patient's attorney. The attorney signs the copies and returns one to the attending physician. See Figure 11.9.

Blue Cross and Blue Shield

The Blue Cross and Blue Shield Association is the coordinating body for the nation's Blue Cross and Blue Shield plans. Blue Cross and Blue Shield are allopathic-oriented autonomous nonprofit corporations, directly or indirectly sponsored by various state medical associations and designed to help in payment of health-care expenses. These plans are the largest health-care program in the nation, and they have contracts with both member subscribers and member providers.

Blue Cross is the hospital portion of the system. Its plans provide benefits on essentially a "service type" basis under which the organization, through a separate contract with member hospitals, reimburses the hospital for covered services rendered to an insured patient. *Blue Shield* is the medical and surgical portion, whose plans provide benefits performed by a physician. Well over a hundred different plans are available.

Blue Shield does not always pay the total doctor's fee involved, but it usually covers most expenses. In some areas, Blue Shield does not cover chiropractic services; in several other regions, it may cover all or a part of chiropractic services. Inclusion of chiropractic services has increased rapidly during the last 15 years.

A participating physician must sign an agreement with Blue Shield to provide subscribers with services and abide by Blue Shield regulations. Regardless of the type of Blue Shield policy the subscriber might have, the doctor cannot make a charge for completing and processing the forms involved.

A large variety of contract arrangements are available to its subscribers, but basically there are two general types of policies sold: balance billing and UCR contracts.

The Balance-Billing Contract. This is the most popular Blue Shield policy. It provides partial payment of fees according to the Blue Shield predetermined fee schedule. The allowance usually runs from 25% to 50% less than usual fees. In this type of policy, the doctor can bill the patient for any balance remaining after Blue Shield has paid the benefit due. If a patient has this type of

TO: Attorney..

....

....

RE: Health Reports and Doctor's Lien

Doctor:

I hereby authorize the above doctor to furnish you. my attorney, with a full report of his examination, diagnosis, treatment, prognosis, etc., of myself in regard to the accident in which I was involved.

I hereby authorize and direct you, my attorney, to pay directly to said doctor such sums as may be due and owing him for professional services rendered me both by reason of this accident and by reason of any other bills that are due his office and to withhold such sums from any settlement, judgment or verdict as may be necessary adequately to protect said doctor. I hereby further give a lien on my case to said doctor against any and all proceeds of any settlement, judgment or verdict which may be paid to you, my attorney, or myself as the result of the injuries for which I have been treated or injuries in connection therewith.

I fully understand that I am directly and fully responsible to said doctor for all professional bills submitted by him for service rendered me and that this agreement is made solely for said doctor's additional protection and in consideration of his awaiting payment. And I further understand that such payment is not contingent on any settlement, judgment or verdict by which I may eventually recover said fee.

Dated:.. Patient's Signature:...

The undersigned being attorney of record for the above patient does hereby agree to observe all the terms of the above and agrees to withhold such sums from any settlement, judgment or verdict as may be necessary adequately to protect the said doctor named above.

Dated:.. Attorney's Signature:...

Attorney: Please date, sign and return one copy to doctor's office at once.

Reply envelope attached.

Keep one copy for your records.

Doctor's Lien
ACA Form 19

Figure 11.9. Health report release and doctor's lein (ACA Form 19).

contract, the physician is prohibited from sending the patient a bill until the patient has been paid his Blue Shield benefits. This is true though the patient is responsible for paying the doctor's full fee.

The UCR Contract. This second type of policy provides payment according to usual, customary, and reasonable rates of the area. The doctor must accept whatever Blue Shield allows as the full fee. The patient cannot be billed for any remaining balance. However, the doctor may request a review.

Workers' Compensation Accounts

Most employed people have protection by law for injuries sustained at their jobs. "On the job" injuries involving industrial accidents are covered by worker's compensation laws in all states, and chiropractic services are covered in these laws. In addition, the federal government has recognized chiropractic in on-the-job injuries for all federal employees. Laws have also been established by the federal government to cover railroad employees, longshoremen, and harbor workers.

Structure

Workers' compensation programs vary in structure, rules, and regulations from state to state. In some states, private insurance companies do the underwriting; in other states, there is a compensation fund established and administered by the state. Guam, Puerto Rico, and about 10 states require employers to insure in a noncompetitive state fund. About a dozen states permit employers to purchase insurance from a competitive state fund or a private insurance company. In addition, many states allow large organizations and businesses to be self-insured. Premium rates for worker's compensation insurance are based on accident experience and are collected by an agency recognized by all states and insurance companies: the National Council on Compensation Insurance.

Extent of Coverage

Most industrial occupations are covered, even those usually conducted by minors. In the private sector, about 30 states require coverage for all jobs while others exempt those employers with fewer than a specific number of employees. Most jurisdictions exclude certain farm labor jobs, domestic servants, and casual employees. Public employees are automatically required to be covered in all jurisdictions except in a few states where compensation is voluntary on the part of the employer.

Employee Protection

Workers' compensation laws have generally imposed an absolute, but limited, liability on employers. The benefits paid to injured employees are an attempt to cover most of a worker's economic losses. These losses include both loss of earnings and extra expenses incurred because of the injury. Specific benefits are: (1) *cash benefits*, which include payment for physical impairment and impairment with loss of wages; (2) *medical benefits*, which are usually provided without limit (a few states have fixed-dollar limits); and (3) *rehabilitation benefits*, where severe disabilities can include both medical and vocational rehabilitation benefits. Thus:

• Medical and chiropractic expenses incurred by the patient are paid by the insurance company or state fund involved. No deductible is involved, and there should be no cost to the patient for the health expenses covered by the worker's compensation insurance. Many state laws prohibit billing the patient.

• If the patient's injury is substantial and he is unable to work, the insurance company or state fund pays a sum of money in weekly disability benefits. The amount varies from state to state. Health-care expenses are paid on a *reasonable* basis for medically *necessary* services, as previously defined, as the result of on-the-job injury.

An important point for each involved patient to remember is that his medical benefits, which cover 100% of his health-care expenses, are only for injuries sustained on the job and conditions related to those injuries. Thus, benefits are usually paid only for a short period; ie, until the patient recovers and can return to work. For example, if a patient has a long-standing disorder for which he is being treated (eg, diabetes), the expense involved for treatment of that chronic condition would not be covered.

Administration

When an employee suffers an industrial accident, the first step is to notify the employer. In many states, the employer must authorize treatment. The employer is paying the insurance policy's premium and usually has quite a lot to say in these matters. The doctor's office should verify this authorization before the case can be considered a worker's compensation case. This can usually be accomplished by a telephone call. If authorized, the employer will mail the necessary report forms if you do not stock them. This can be requested when you verify authorization for treatment.

The CA involved should understand that promptness and accuracy are important requisites in handling compensation cases. If she prepares a letter that acts as a supplement to the standard report, its content is important and should be verified by the doctor. Each form and supplement must be accurately filed for quick retrieval.

Because programs covering workers have lost considerable money in recent years, patients and their doctors may encounter a delay in payment when carriers closely scrutinize the claims. Also, the patient may be subjected to an examination by an insurance company doctor at times, although such services do not usually apply to treatment. The injured employee is usually allowed the freedom to select the doctor of his choice.

In-Office Filing. Most offices store in-process compensation forms with the most current form at the front of the patient's file folder. Past forms may show a relationship between the patient's present condition with past claims. As many questions on report forms are fairly routine, the doctor may

be able to obtain information on one form that will be helpful in other forms.

Data Release. An exception to previous instructions should be noted. A signed authorization is *not* required for reporting a worker's compensation case to a carrier. This exception refers only to the carrier, however. You should not release information to anyone else without a written authorization. In fact, authorization is often needed from both the patient *and* the carrier if another party desires information of a compensation case.

Claims Processing. Both the doctor and an assistant should check each report carefully before it is mailed. Note that all pertinent questions are answered such as those concerning the patient's injury, the doctor's prognosis of the patient's disability, and the date that the form was completed. Care must be taken in reporting the patient's condition, symptoms, and examination findings to show some relationship between the job-related accident or illness to the patient's complaint(s).

Problem Areas

Inclusion of chiropractors in the compensation system resulted from dogged persistence of many chiropractic patients and injured workers bringing pressure to bear on legislatures through labor groups and through the courts. Some problems existing earlier in the care provided injured workers still exist today. For example: (1) discrimination against DCs by company physicians; (2) use of panel physicians rather than complete freedom of choice by the injured party; and (3) the insurance company covering workers' compensation claims paying far less than usual and customary fees or limiting services for which it pays.

If the employer refuses to authorize chiropractic services and your doctor-employer is a registered provider, most states have an elaborate complex of state Workers' compensation claim offices that will help in processing a claim. Personnel in these offices can often be helpful and may make it unnecessary for a patient to seek a legal resolution.

Automobile Accident Cases

Almost every American family has automobile accident (liability) insurance. In some states, it is called No-Fault Auto Insurance. In several states, liability coverage is mandatory.

Automobile insurance is often written as a comprehensive policy that includes coverage for liability, collision, and medical expenses. Chiropractic services are usually included under the medical expenses provisions. In "No-Fault" states, medical expenses are sometimes called "personal injury protection. (PIP)"

As the patient has enough problems after an automobile accident, protection is offered to receive proper health care as soon as possible. Hospital and physician services are usually covered for a year (if necessary) following an automobile accident.

Personal injury cases, regardless of type, can be an important aspect of practice income. Some doctors specialize in these type cases alone. However, any type of personal injury case that is involved in litigation has two major drawbacks: (1) it may be a year or longer before the case is settled in court; (2) narrative reports will undoubtedly be necessary; and (3) there may be some court time necessary for the doctor.

Claims Processing

All reasonable chiropractic expenses are usually covered for necessary services related to the patient's injuries. There is no deductible involved in the medical benefits; thus, 100% of the actual expenses are insured. For this reason, most DCs will accept an assignment from the patient and bill the insurance company.

Typically, the insurance company requests certain information from the patient shortly after the accident is reported. The patient may then give them the name and address of the attending doctor. The insurance company will then send the physician a form to complete and submit with a copy of his bill. When the insurance company fails to send a form, the patient should ask his insurance agent to forward the proper form. Once this has been done, the paperwork involving health-care expenses is usually between the doctor and the insurance company.

Cost Control

Most insurance companies (particularly No-Fault carriers) make fairly rapid payment of health-care benefits. However, you should be aware of a growing concern that may delay payment. Automobile insurance companies have lost considerable sums of money in the past decade or so. They are concerned about this, and many have added extra claims analysts, examiners, and professional consultants to their staff. It also appears that some patients and doctors have taken advantage of the system by submitting excessively high claims. This has resulted in significant losses by some companies, and they have begun to scrutinize claims more closely than in the past. Eventually, this procedure should save us all premium dollars.

Health Maintenance Organizations

A Health Maintenance Organization (HMO) is a geographically based group that provides health care for enrolled patients on a prepaid or capitation basis. In some HMOs, members pay membership costs directly; in others, sponsors pay costs (eg, cooperatives, employers, labor unions, employer groups, state Medicaid Departments); and in still others, members and sponsors share the expenses involved.

Comprehensive medical care, including hospitalization, dental care, maternity care, and mental health care are usually provided when determined necessary by a plan physician. Although most services are provided without additional payment, some plans now require a small co-payment with some services. Health education, preventive care, and routine physicals may be provided because it is more economical to keep enrollees healthy than to treat them for illness. Relatively few HMOs offer service by a chiropractic physician. If an enrollee desires a health service not offered by the HMO, service expenses must be borne by the enrollee.

GOVERNMENT-SPONSORED PUBLIC PLANS

Several types of federal and state government-sponsored programs have been developed to cover some or all costs of health care for eligible individuals. Approved beneficiaries can be recognized by their identification cards.

Medicare

Medicare is a federally created and sponsored program financed through payroll deductions and premiums paid by enrollees. It is administered by the Social Security Administration, a branch of the Department of Health and Human Services (formerly HEW). Unlike some other plans, there is no requirement for the doctor to wait to bill the balance of his fee until a patient has received a check from the Medicare agency. In nonassignment cases, patients are billed immediately and are reimbursed by Medicare for a substantial portion of the physician's fee.

Medicare was established in 1966 to cover citizens over the age of 65 and amended in 1973 to include younger citizens eligible under the Social Security Disability Insurance Program and citizens undergoing kidney dialysis or transplants. The program was never intended to provide reimbursement for all medical expenses of eligible beneficiaries. Participants must pay a deductible and 100% of disallowed expenses.

The program is composed of two parts: Part A, hospital insurance; Part B, medical insurance. Chiropractic services are covered as physician services under Part B for manipulation of the spine to correct a subluxation shown by roentgenography to exist. Thus, it is necessary at this writing for a chiropractor to have a recent x-ray film of the patient's spine that discloses the presence of a subluxation when filing claims for Medicare benefits. To prevent the patient from being exposed to unnecessary radiation, current legislation is pending to make the x-ray requirement not mandatory.

The Blue Cross Association is presently the major administrator intermediary for Part A (hospital co-payment coverage) nationally. Blue Shield plans and other insurance companies have been appointed to administer Part B (surgical/medical co-payment coverage) in the various states. The Social Security Administration is the primary source for information about Medicare. A telephone call to your local Social Security office will direct you to specific sources of assistance helpful in resolving particular problems.

Identification. Each Medicare patient should have an identification card indicating whether the patient is covered under Part A (Hospital Insurance), Part B (Medical Insurance), or both Parts A and B of the Medicare program. The assigned claim number is usually the person's Social Security number. Many patients carry "supplemental" insurance, and these data should also be recorded.

Printed Guidelines. Each Medicare patient receives a booklet titled *Explanation of Medicare Benefits*, yet many of them either fail to read it or understand it. You should be acquainted with this booklet as well as the *Physicians' Guide*. Take care to explain to patients that while payment for certain services may be *disallowed*, this does not mean that the services were not necessary or appropriate.

Fee Determination. Medicare uses two combined processes for determining professional compensation. First, an individual fee profile is developed for every doctor who treats patients covered under Medicare. This is established by analyzing the claim forms submitted. Second, a community fee profile is developed for every doctor in your area of the country who treats patients covered under Medicare. The fee profiles of all physicians in your area in the same type of practice or who render similar services are averaged. The result is a UCR profile for the area. Medicare then pays 80% of whichever is lower, the doctor's individual fee profile or the UCR profile.

Claims Processing. Submitted claims

are screened by Medicare for eligibility. Guidelines are established for the number of office visits and treatments for all physicians. If a patient's claim exceeds these guidelines, payment of the claim will be delayed for several weeks, and additional information will likely be requested from the attending physician whether the abnormal number of treatments provided were necessary. While this is a nuisance for all involved, it is a mechanism to assure that federal funds are spent only for necessary services. At times, Medicare will initially disallow a portion of a claim after review. This could occur for a number of technical reasons. There are two types of appeals: informal and formal.

Medicaid

Medicaid is a state-sponsored federally supported welfare program set up to cover part of health-care costs for the needy. It became effective in 1966; and by 1977, all states and the District of Columbia were included in the program. Each state administers its own program within general guidelines established by the federal government. Each state has a great deal to say about whom is eligible and what types of health care will be covered. The extent of coverage varies widely from state to state.

The program is designed to help those in dire need—people with almost no income. The fee schedule is substantially lower than UCR rates, and it must be accepted as the full fee. Patient billing or balance billing is not allowed. Most states issue eligible recipients of benefits an identification card or coupon showing the bearer's current eligibility status. Besides this, some states require a telephone verification of *each* visit before care is provided to obtain authorized multidigit transactions numbers.

Medicaid patients should verify eligibility on a visit basis because they sometimes "bounce" in and out of the program at various times. This requires careful, usually separate, filing and refiling between Medicaid files and current accounts receivable files at involved doctors' offices.

Medicaid 65 is a special type of Medicare/ Medicaid assignment. It establishes the total fee and pays 80% of it direct to the doctor, as is typical in any assignment. However, the remaining 20% is paid by Medicaid rather than the patient.

FEHB

The Federal Employees Health Benefits Program (FEHB) offers health-care protection for active and retired federal civilian employees, their dependents, and the employee's surviving spouses and dependent children. This voluntary program is administered by the U.S. Office of Personnel Management but underwritten by various private insurers. Two general options are provided: one that offers a few benefits at a low cost and one that offers broad benefits at a higher premium.

CHAMPUS and CHAMPVA

The Civilian Health and Medical Program of the Uniformed Services (CHAMPUS) finances the cost of civilian-provided health care for dependents of active duty and retired personnel of the armed services. The program is administered by the U.S. Department of Defense. Participating physicians must meet specific requirements outlined in the official regulations and be authorized to care for patients under this program.

The Veterans Administration offers medical care and disability compensation to armed service veterans. This program is called the Civilian Health and Medical Program of the Veterans Administration (CHAMPVA). Presently, primary chiropractic services not the result of a referral from an MD or DO are not covered under CHAMPUS or CHAMPVA, but legislation is pending to correct this. Until inclusion becomes effective, there is no need to describe the complicated rules and administrative procedures involved.

Welfare

There are scores of welfare programs operating in the United States but rarely does the word "welfare" appear in their titles. They are usually state programs, often federally supported, that are administered on the county level. These programs are primarily of a financial or social nature, but they often extend health-care benefits to needy people who do not qualify for Medicaid.

The health needs of these people are usually conducted in authorized facilities such as a county hospital. Rarely is ambulatory private practice care authorized. However, it is important for your office to have knowledge of what programs are available in your area so that you can refer possible beneficiaries to the proper agency. Few practices today can afford to duplicate the tax-supported welfare services already established in the community.

STANDARDIZED CLAIM FORMS

A patient who files a claim for health-care benefits is obligated to give the insurance agency whatever information it may require. Likewise, a doctor is obliged to give a patient whatever medical information is necessary to file a claim for benefits. This information is usually communicated by a fill-in type of claim form. However, unless there is a contract between the doctor and the company, the courts have held that the doctor is not obliged to use a particular insurance form unless the doctor practices in a state that has passed a uniform claim law.

The paperwork involved in processing an insurance-related account represents a vehicle to a major potential source of a physician's income. This mandates that prompt and accurate completion and processing be made to assure minimal follow-up procedures. Routines should be established for handling related forms, records, releases, and reports. Many office procedural manuals have a separate section just for this purpose.

One problem in insurance relations has been that on the many hundred insurance companies in the United States each company has its own claim form. This has been confusing for both doctors and assistants. Fortunately, a standard health insurance form has been adopted that satisfies the needs of almost all health insurance organizations and agencies.

The approved claim form (as of this writing) is shown in Figure 11.10. It can usually be substituted for a nonstandard form a patient may submit. Thanks to standardization, this form generally satisfies health-provider requirements and is easier to complete than many nonstandard forms. It has been designed so it may be typed-in with either pica and elite type sizes or used as a computer print-out. Although typing is preferred, it may be completed by hand.

A standard form reduces total costs of claims processing and simplifies office reporting and third-party communications in an efficient and controlled manner. Note that certain sections are only applicable if the patient is entitled to disability benefits, if the patient is hospitalized, or if the patient is entitled to Medicare or Medicaid benefits. A separate form must be used for each patient though the doctor may be treating several members of a family whose policy was written for a combined family deductible. Thus, services are always itemized for each patient on separate forms.

A doctor should not be required to do any more than review and sign routine insurance forms. A trained assistant should be able to gather all necessary data from the patient's entering, financial, and clinical records.

Statements to Private Insurance Companies

Form HCFA-1500, refer to Figure 11.10, will be used in this section to explain the typical information needed.

The Patient Information Section. It is good policy to have this section completed by or with the help of the patient. All blanks (1–13) should be filled. Point 13 should *not* be signed by the patient unless the doctor desires assignment of the patient's benefits. Verify the accuracy of spelling and recording of numbers.

Physician Information Section. Those areas of this section that have caused the most confusion are mentioned below:

HEALTH INSURANCE CLAIM FORM

READ INSTRUCTIONS BEFORE COMPLETING OR SIGNING THIS FORM

☐ MEDICAID   ☐ MEDICARE   ☐ CHAMPUS   ☐ OTHER

FORM APPROVED
OMB NO. 88-R0012

PATIENT & INSURED (SUBSCRIBER) INFORMATION

1 PATIENT'S NAME (First name, middle initial, last name)

2 PATIENT'S DATE OF BIRTH

3 INSURED'S NAME (First name, middle initial, last name)

4 PATIENT'S ADDRESS (Street, city, state, ZIP code)

5 PATIENT'S SEX   MALE ☐   FEMALE ☐

6 INSURED'S I.D. MEDICARE AND/OR MEDICAID NO. (Include any letters)

7 PATIENT'S RELATIONSHIP TO INSURED   SELF   SPOUSE   CHILD   OTHER

8 INSURED'S GROUP NO. (Or Group Name)

TELEPHONE NO

9 OTHER HEALTH INSURANCE COVERAGE Enter Name of Policyholder and Plan Name and Address and Policy or Medical Assistance Number

10 WAS CONDITION RELATED TO

   A PATIENT'S EMPLOYMENT   YES ☐   NO ☐

   B ACCIDENT   AUTO ☐   OTHER ☐

11 INSURED'S ADDRESS (Street, city, state ZIP code)

12 PATIENT'S OR AUTHORIZED PERSON'S SIGNATURE (Read back before signing) I Authorize the Release of any Medical Information Necessary to Process this Claim and request Payment of MEDICARE Benefits Either to Myself or to the Party Who Accepts Assignment Below.

SIGNED   DATE

13 I AUTHORIZE PAYMENT OF MEDICAL BENEFITS TO UNDERSIGNED PHYSICIAN OR SUPPLIER FOR SERVICE DESCRIBED BELOW

SIGNED (Insured or Authorized Person)

PHYSICIAN OR SUPPLIER INFORMATION

14 DATE OF ILLNESS (FIRST SYMPTOM) OR INJURY (ACCIDENT) OR PREGNANCY (LMP)

15 DATE FIRST CONSULTED YOU FOR THIS CONDITION

16 HAS PATIENT EVER HAD SAME OR SIMILAR SYMPTOMS?   YES ☐   NO ☐

16a IF AN EMERGENCY CHECK HERE ☐

17 DATE PATIENT ABLE TO RETURN TO WORK

18 DATES OF TOTAL DISABILITY   FROM   THROUGH

DATES OF PARTIAL DISABILITY   FROM   THROUGH

19 NAME OF REFERRING PHYSICIAN OR OTHER SOURCE (e.g. public health agency)

20 FOR SERVICES RELATED TO HOSPITALIZATION GIVE HOSPITALIZATION DATES   ADMITTED   DISCHARGED

21 NAME & ADDRESS OF FACILITY WHERE SERVICES RENDERED (If other than home or office)

22 WAS LABORATORY WORK PERFORMED OUTSIDE YOUR OFFICE?   YES ☐   NO   CHARGES

23 DIAGNOSIS OR NATURE OF ILLNESS OR INJURY RELATE DIAGNOSIS TO PROCEDURE IN COLUMN D BY REFERENCE NUMBERS 1, 2, 3, ETC OR DX CODE

A

1

2

3

4

B EPSDT   YES ☐   NO ☐
FAMILY PLANNING   YES ☐   NO ☐

PRIOR AUTHORIZATION NO. _____

24 A DATE OF SERVICE	B* PLACE OF SERVICE	C FULLY DESCRIBE PROCEDURES, MEDICAL SERVICES OR SUPPLIES FURNISHED FOR EACH DATE GIVEN — PROCEDURE CODE (IDENTIFY)	(EXPLAIN UNUSUAL SERVICES OR CIRCUMSTANCES)	D DIAGNOSIS CODE	E CHARGES	F DAYS OR UNITS	G* TOS	H LEAVE BLANK

25 SIGNATURE OF PHYSICIAN OR SUPPLIER (I certify that the statements on the reverse apply to this bill and are made a part hereof.)

SIGNED   DATE

32 YOUR PATIENT'S ACCOUNT NO.

26 ACCEPT ASSIGNMENT (GOVERNMENT CLAIMS ONLY) (SEE BACK)   YES ☐   NO ☐

30 YOUR SOCIAL SECURITY NO.

33 YOUR EMPLOYER I.D. NO.

27 TOTAL CHARGE

28 AMOUNT PAID

29 BALANCE DUE

31 PHYSICIAN'S OR SUPPLIER'S NAME, ADDRESS, ZIP CODE & TELEPHONE NO.

I.D. NO.

*PLACE OF SERVICE AND TYPE OF SERVICE (TOS) CODES ON THE BACK

REMARKS

APPROVED BY AMA COUNCIL ON MEDICAL SERVICE 8-90
APPROVED BY THE HEALTH CARE FINANCING ADMINISTRATION & CHAMPUS
Form AMA-OP-088
Form HCFA-1500 (4-90)
Form CHAMPUS-501

PRINTED IN U.S.A.

Form 1223   BRIGGS, Des Moines, Iowa 50306

Figure 11.10. Health insurance claim form HCFA-1500 (ACA Form 1223).

1. *Diagnosis.* In point 23, it is better to enter only one diagnosis per claim in major medical claims because they do not usually allow the listing of more than one diagnosis on a single claim. However, concomitant conditions can be entered on the same dates. The diagnosis must be complete and phrased in standard nomenclature. Do not confuse findings (eg, subluxation) with a diagnosis, and such phrases as "for diagnostic support" or "diagnosis not established" are unacceptable. If a diagnosis has not been confirmed, it is preferable to record the patient's chief complaint. When extended care is provided and a previous claim for the same diagnosis has been filed, a notation should be made in parentheses after the diagnosis: eg, (Continued treatment. See previous report, dated February 5, 1991).

2. *Procedures.* Procedures itemized in 24.C should be numbered to correspond to the numbers used in 23 (diagnosis). Only one procedure per line should be used. CPT codes are usually used in column 24.C, and ICD codes are used in column 24.D, if this is agreeable with the carrier. Unusual circumstances should be listed such as extraordinary time used by a severely injured patient, multiple visits on the same date, or treatment provided late at night or on a holiday.

3. *Fees.* In column 24.E, itemize usual charges. In column 24.F, explain unusual fees if a modifier has been used. If the doctor is a member of the Preferred Provider Organization (PPO) or has a contract involving a specific fee schedule, the related schedule fee is the fee for those patients involved. One should not bill the patient for one fee and the insurance company for another, although you do not anticipate full payment from the insurance company. To do so would alter the office's "usual" fee schedule.

4. *Pertinent Reports.* Attach a copy of any consultation or laboratory report that might help the insurance company's examiner in processing complicated claims.

Whenever the format of a printed form is altered (eg, changing words or blocking out printed words), the doctor should initial the changes.

Blue Shield

A Blue Shield claim form may require certain 5-digit procedural codes, which are essentially refined CPT codes. Each member physician is given a loose-leaf *Manual for Physicians* showing the codes currently in use and offering samples of the various contracts and agreements in use that Blue Shield has with physicians, individuals, and groups.

Medicare Statements

The standard Medicare Claim Form is used for chiropractic as well as other physician services. As an alternative, Form HCFA-1500, refer to Figure 11.10, can sometimes be used. The patient is responsible for filling in the upper part of the claim form, but this information is usually typed in by a CA. The DC supplies the information necessary in the lower portion.

Licensed practitioners are assigned special provider numbers. In some states, it will be the doctor's state license number prefixed by the letters DC. This number should be entered in the form and with any correspondence directed to the intermediary.

It was explained previously that chiropractic coverage under Medicare presently is limited to treatment by manual manipulation of the spine to correct a subluxation proved by roentgenography to exist. No other service rendered by or furnished on the order of a DC is currently covered. That is, only an office visit with manipulation is paid for. Adjunctive care and diagnostic procedures are not covered.

X-Ray Films. A specific certification must be included stating when the x-ray films were taken and that copies are available for review on request. These films, which must be of acceptable quality, must have been taken within 3 months in acute conditions and 12 months in chronic conditions of the date care was initiated to be applicable. Unless this certification is provided, the patient's claim for reimbursement will probably not be accepted.

Although the law currently requires x-ray

films to prove the presence of a subluxation, Medicare benefits do not cover their cost, nor will the patient's payment for the mandatory x-ray films apply against his deductible. Duplicate, not original, films should be submitted with the claim.

Professional Services. Specific treatment procedures must be spelled out, as well as the complete diagnosis and fees involved. The diagnosis must be identifiable as related to one or more subluxations, and the precise level of the subluxation(s) must be specified. The necessity of chiropractic care provided must be closely related to the patient's symptoms and the level of the subluxation. This currently implies a musculoskeletal relationship, and most diseases and other pathologic disorders would not provide grounds for chiropractic treatment according to the current guidelines issued by the HCFA.

Medicare restrictions to chiropractic care have long been considered an injustice by the chiropractic profession. National organizations have continually sought revision. Hopefully, this will occur soon.

For patient convenience, it is good policy to have a stock of Medicare forms on hand in the office. However, completing a form does not make a person eligible for Medicare benefits. This is a complicated process, and eligible individuals should be referred to the nearest Social Security Administration office if they do not have proper identification cards.

Medicare Receipts

For patients covered by Medicare, a special receipt is often necessary. This requirement can be noted on the visit slip, in a color-coded folder, or a label can be used as a signal. The special receipt is intended strictly to cover one-visit claims. A superbill will often suffice. It is important that the following data appear on each receipt: (1) the patient's name and address; (2) the type of visit (eg, office, house call); (3) the diagnosis; (4) the itemized clinical and diagnostic services rendered; (5) the doctor's total fee, the amount paid, and the balance due; (6) the doctor's name, address, and tele-

phone number; (7) the doctor's identification numbers; and (8) any other information routinely required by the processing carrier.

Medicaid Statements

Medicaid statement forms, and even procedure codes, vary from state to state. However, the forms described in this chapter can be used as a guide. Almost all health insurance agencies seek the same information. As a standardized alternative, Form HCFA-1500 can sometimes be used. Refer to Figure 11.10.

Two important elements of a Medicaid statement that differ from most other forms are that the recipient's Medicaid identification number must be included and documentation showing evidence of patient eligibility for health-care service must be provided monthly. This last point varies somewhat from state to state.

For *Medicaid 65* beneficiaries, the standard *Medicare* "Request for Payment" form is used as if it were an assignment. The *Medicaid* form is not used. The word "Medicaid" is typed in the box titled "Other Health Insurance Coverage" (9).

Workers' Compensation Reports

Standardized worker's compensation claim forms are supplied by various insurance companies, the State Industrial Commission/Workers' Compensation Department, or they may be duplicated. While forms vary from state to state, they are always standard within each state. The official fee schedule, if the Department has one, should always be referred to when fees are listed. Form HCFA-1500 may or may not be applicable in situations of workers' compensation injuries.

Some states require two separate forms: (1) a preliminary report, and (2) a final report to be filed by both the injured employee and the attending physician (Figs. 11.11 and 11.12). Other states combine the two reports into a single form with the top portion being the preliminary report and the bottom portion for the final report. The *Physician's*

FORM NO 3

WORKERS' COMPENSATION COURT
JIM THORPE BUILDING
OKLAHOMA CITY, OK 73105

Send copies to:
3 to W.C. Court

In re claim of:

____
Name of Claimant (Injured Employee)

____
Name of Employer

____
Name of Insurance Carrier (To Be Added By Court)

EMPLOYEE'S FIRST NOTICE OF ACCIDENTAL INJURY AND CLAIM FOR COMPENSATION

Court Claim Number ______________ (To Be Added By Court)

(Please type or print in ink legibly all information.)

EMPLOYEE

Name ____________ (Last) ____________ (First) ____________ (Middle) Social Security # ____________ (Must Be Filled Out)

Address ____________ (Number & Street) ____________ (City) ____________ (State) ____________ (Zip Code)

Telephone ____________ Age ______ Sex ______

Average weekly wage $ ____________ Was your employment agreement made in Oklahoma? ______

INJURY

Date of accident ____________ Time ____________ (To Nearest Hour (am-pm))

Place: City ____________ County ____________ State ____________

Last day worked after injury ____________ Were you paid full wages that day? ______

Have you returned to work? ______ If so, on what date? ____________

Treating physician ____________ (Name) ____________ (Address)

Nature of injury ____________ (Example Burn, Cut, Sprain or Amputation)

List parts of body injured ____________ (Example Eye, Finger, Arm or Back)

How did the accident occur? ____________ (Describe Fully The Events Which Resulted In The Injury. Tell What Happened and How it occurred)

____

Name object or substance which directly injured you ____________ (Be Specific. Example Hammer, Saw, Box, Floor or Desk)

____

EMPLOYER

Name ____________ Telephone ____________

Address ____________ (Number & Street) ____________ (City) ____________ (State) ____________ (Zip Code)

Were you at the time of this last injury a physically impaired person on account of a pre-existing disability as a result of accident, disease, birth, military or other cause? If the answer is "Yes", then you may be entitled to additional benefits from the Special Indemnity Fund. ______ If so, please describe the impairment and give the dates of the injuries and of any court orders.

____

You are required to elect where you want any future hearing to be held regarding this claim. Hearings must be in Oklahoma in ONE of the counties you choose UNLESS the parties mutually agree upon a different location or the Court orders otherwise. You should make your selection by writing in the name of the county you prefer on one of the blank spaces below:

______ a) county of your residence AT THE TIME OF THE ACCIDENT,
______ b) county in which the accident occurred,
______ c) county in which employer's principal place of business is located,
______ d) county in which the contract of employment was entered. (This last county is available ONLY to non-resident claimants who were injured outside Okla.)

I declare under penalty of perjury that I have examined this notice and claim, and all statements contained herein, and to the best of my knowledge and belief, they are true, correct and complete.

Signed this ______ day of ____________ 19 ______

____
Signature of Claimant

COMPLETE THIS FORM IN TRIPLICATE AND MAIL DIRECTLY TO THE COURT. THE COURT WILL THEN SEND A COPY EITHER TO YOUR EMPLOYER OR TO ITS INSURANCE CARRIER.

Name of claimant's attorney if represented:

Name ____________
Address ____________
____________ (City) ____________ (State) ____________ (Zip Code)
Telephone ____________

NOTICE: IF YOU HAVE NOT ALREADY NOTIFIED YOUR EMPLOYER OF THIS ACCIDENTAL INJURY, DO SO AT ONCE. NOTIFICATION WITHIN 30 DAYS IS REQUIRED BY LAW, AND FAILURE TO GIVE SUCH NOTICE MAY RESULT IN BARRING YOUR CLAIM FOR ANY BENEFITS UNDER THE WORKERS' COMPENSATION ACT.

Do you want the court to send you information regarding rehabilitative services? ____________

WCC 7-18-81

Figure 11.11. Sample preliminary report of a worker's compensation case filed by an employee.

O   O

FORM NO 9

WORKERS' COMPENSATION COURT
Jim Thorpe Building
OKLAHOMA CITY, OK 73105

In re claim of:

_____
Full name of claimant (injured employee)

_____
Name of Employer or Respondent

_____
Name of Employer's Insurance Carrier

MOTION OF CLAIMANT TO SET FOR HEARING

Court Claim Number _____

Claimant's Social
Security No. _____
                                    (Must be filled out)

Claimant respectfully requests that the captioned cause be set for hearing at the earliest available docket. Claimant states:

1. Issues to be tried: (Circle all applicable issues below.)
    a.   Temporary disability from _____ to _____
    and Medical treatment from _____ to _____
    b.   Permanent disability
    c.   Motion to commute.
    d.   Motion to reopen on change of condition.
    e.   Form 19 proceeding.
    f.   Liability of Special Indemnity Fund.
    g.   Other (Specify): _____

2. Indicate any material amendments that will be offered to the previously filed Form 3: _____

_____

3. List the names of all witnesses who may be called by claimant at trial. The names of any additional witnesses must be submitted to the court and respondent no less than five (5) days prior to trial.

_____   _____

_____   _____

_____   _____

4. Claimant hereby certifies that a copy of the medical report written by Dr. _____

and dated _____ was attached to a copy of this Motion and mailed to respondent on

_____ . (Identify on a separate attached sheet any other written medical report or medical evidence which claimant may offer at trial and likewise certify when same was mailed to respondent.)

                                                                    Yes   No

5. Will claimant consider the case submitted at the conclusion of the hearing?   _____   _____

6. Will this case take an unusual amount of time to try?   _____   _____

7. The parties hereto have mutually agreed that the hearings may be held in _____ .
                                                                                      City

Signed this _____ day of _____ , 19 _____ .

_____
Signature of claimant or claimant's attorney

_____
Typed name of attorney

Telephone number of attorney _____

Figure 11.12. Sample final report of a worker's compensation case filed by an employee.

Preliminary Report, usually required to be filed within a few days, provides the insurance company or compensation fund with the facts concerning the job-related accident or illness, the working diagnosis, and the initial treatment (Fig. 11.13). It is sometimes called the *Doctor's First Report of Work Injury.* The *Physician's Final (or Monthly) Report* is filed when the case is dismissed or when extended services are necessary. This report includes the attending doctor's final or monthly bill for the services provided (Fig. 11.14).

Frequently, supplementary forms and reports are required. These self-explanatory documents are mailed to the attending doctor by the carrier when necessary.

Requests and Follow-up Activities

While a doctor does not have an obligation to follow-up on a claim that does not involve an assignment of benefits, it is obviously conducive to good doctor-patient relations. Helping a patient to obtain reimbursement is a SOP (standard operating procedure) in most health-care offices.

If a patient reports that he has not received reimbursement and the time is nearing the end of the usual processing time, you should file an inquiry with the insurance company or state fund. This procedure is sometimes necessary to decide if the patient has been reimbursed. The same might be true if a check was received that was far below that anticipated, whether the benefits were assigned or not. Besides lack of response and a reduced payment, a follow-up inquiry is in order when procedural codes have been changed or certain services were disallowed that were not anticipated. Some form of clarification is needed.

One of the best sources of information for avoiding insurance disputes is to ask the advice of CAs in other offices, many of whom process a large volume of insurance claims. Weigh this advice carefully, however, and always seek the opinion of several respected colleagues so that you will obtain a wide viewpoint. District societies frequently have meetings on this subject to keep their members informed of new policies, procedures, and regulations.

ASSIGNMENTS

When a patient enters a doctor's office or clinic, it should immediately be established for billing purposes whether the patient has health insurance protection and explained whether the doctor is to be paid by the insurance company or the patient for the services provided. Refer to Figure 11.8.

There is sometimes a choice whether payment will be made to the patient or assigned directly to the attending physician. Even when assignment is not accepted, all offices should help a patient prepare necessary reports and itemizations on request. Extensive help is considered proper in cases concerning the elderly and severely disabled.

Some doctors never accept assignment on any case, some accept assignment on some types of claims but not on others, and some accept assignment at every opportunity. Each doctor has a long list of reasons to support his individual policy, and each policy is the prerogative of that doctor.

Cases Accepted on a Nonassignment Basis

When an assignment is not accepted, all treatments, x-ray examinations, laboratory services, and other fees are charged directly to the patient, and the patient is responsible for payment. In this situation, the office does not render any service on the assumption that charges will be paid by any insurance company or agency. If the doctor complies with a patient's request to "wait until the insurance company settles up," that is his choice, but he has lost control of the doctor-patient business relationship. He may subject himself to delayed income, aging accounts receivable, endless forms and reports, and frustrating review procedures.

When a patient is billed directly for all services provided, payment is usually received faster. Of course, the typical causes of late payment must be faced. Just because an insurance company issues a check to a

Figure 11.13. Sample preliminary report of a worker's compensation case filed by the attending physician.

FORM NO 18

WORKERS' COMPENSATION COURT
Jim Thorpe Building
OKLAHOMA CITY, OK 73105

(FILE IN TRIPLICATE)

In re claim of:

_____
Full name of claimant (injured employee)

_____
Name of Employer or Respondent

_____
Name of Employer's Insurance Carrier

REQUEST FOR REVIEW OF CHARGES
FOR MEDICAL OR REHABILITATIVE SERVICES

Court Claim Number _____

Claimant's Social
Security Number _____
(Must be filled out)

1. Full name of employee _____
2. Address of employee _____
3. Name of employer _____
4. Address of employer _____
5. Date of injury _____
6. Was employee's first treatment rendered by you? _____ If not, state the names
   and addresses of other physicians _____
   _____
7. Describe treatment or services rendered _____
   _____
8. Were prescriptions ordered? _____ If so, indicate what they were _____
   _____
9. Has the employee refused recommended treatment? _____ If so, when? _____
10. When were treatments terminated? _____
11. Has employee been released as able to return to work? _____ If so, when? _____
12. Is the employee capable of doing the same work as before the injury? _____
13. If not, why? _____
14. Does the employee have any permanent disability? _____
15. If so, describe same _____

PLEASE FILL OUT THE INFORMATION BELOW REGARDING CHARGES:

Use following characters for filling out record below O for office visit, V for house visit, H for hospital visit, N for night visit, X for X ray, S for operation

MONTH	1	2	3	4	5	6	7	8	9	10	11	12	13	14	15	16	17	18	19	20	21	22	23	24	25	26	27	28	29	30	31

$

_____ Office Visits   @ $ _____ each _____
_____ House Visits   @ $ _____ each _____
_____ Hospital Visits   @ $ _____ each _____
_____ Night Visits   @ $ _____ each _____
_____ X-Rays   @ $ _____ each _____
_____ Operations   @ $ _____ each _____

Other charges must be itemized and explained fully.

Total Expense for Medical Aid $

I declare under penalty of perjury that I have examined this request, including all statements contained herein, and to the
best of my knowledge and belief, it is true, correct and complete

Signed this _____ day of _____ ,19 _____

Type or print name of
physician or other person
or company who has rendered
medical or rehabilitative service

Signature of authorized
person making request   _____

Address   _____

If the party making this request is not a physician, questions 6 through 15 may be disregarded.

Figure 11.14. Sample final report of a worker's compensation case filed by the attending physician.

patient does not automatically mean that the patient will pay the doctor's bill.

Cases Accepted on an Assignment Basis

When a doctor chooses to relinquish the fee-for-service concept in favor of accepting an assignment of benefits, the validity and scope of the protection should be verified by a telephone call to the insurance company or employer. Although a patient may authorize the insurance company to make payment of benefits due the patient directly to the attending physician, this does not alter the basic contractual relationship between the patient and the insurance company. Nor does it necessarily alter the obligation of the patient to pay the attending physician for services not paid by the insurance company.

If it is office policy to accept cases on assignment, the patient must approve the assignment of benefits. When a policy ordinarily pays the patient, an assignment of benefits form is used to assign payment directly to the doctor. Such a form is usually called an "Authorization to Pay Physician." It is not good policy to accept a case on assignment that is not first supported by such an authorization (Fig. 11.15), because it is unlikely that you will be paid by the insurance company and the result is misunderstandings with the patient.

There is some financial safety in accepting cases on assignment because the credit rating of insurance companies is typically better than that of individuals. An authorization to receive payment directly from the insurance company prevents the patient from being paid, going on a spending spree, and failing to pay the doctor's bill. However, claims processing takes time, and it is not unusual to wait 90 days or longer for a claim to be paid by the company or agency. This means that the doctor must wait for fees earned and relinquish the interest on that amount until he is paid.

It is good policy to flag financial ledgers of all cases accepted on an assignment basis. Some offices also use color-coded folders and signals on related records.

Private Insurance Company Assignments

Assignments for private health-care benefits in most practices are taken only in cases of firmly established need or when required by a contractual arrangement. However, assignments from private insurance companies are considered good policy when the patient is in obvious financial need.

Blue Shield Assignments

If a participating physician has been assigned benefits under any type of Blue Shield contract, the doctor may not be allowed to bill the patient. The physician must accept whatever amount Blue Shield pays as his full fee. When a UCR contract is involved, this makes little difference because it usually covers the doctor's full fee anyway. However, if a no-balance-billing contract is involved, the doctor's UCR fee will be reimbursed only partially.

Medicare Assignments

An assignment of a Medicare account means that the doctor will accept the determination of the fee made by the Medicare intermediary. This does not mean, however, that the patient will not be responsible for (1) the deductible, (2) the percentage not covered by Medicare, and (3) any disallowed procedures that were necessary. However, amounts for other than these cannot be billed; ie, the difference between the doctor's actual charge for a service and what Medicare determines the UCR fee to be.

Posting Procedures in Assignment Accounts

When a check arrives in payment for an account accepted on assignment, the amount should be recorded in the day sheet and patient's financial ledger. Frequently, the payment received is for less than the amount of the charges for the services rendered. The patient's account is posted for the amount

```
┌────────────────────────────────────────────────────────────────────┐
│                                                                      │
│              AUTHORIZATION TO PAY PHYSICIAN                          │
│                                                                      │
│   I hereby authorize the.................................................Insurance Company │
│   to pay by check made out and mailed directly to:                  │
│                                                                      │
│                                                                      │
│                                                                      │
│   the medical and surgical expense benefits allowable, and otherwise payable to me under my current │
│   insurance policy, as payment toward the total charges for Professional Services Rendered. This │
│   payment will not exceed my indebtedness to above mentioned assignee and I have agreed to pay, │
│   in a current manner, any balance of said Professional Service charges over and above this insurance │
│   payment.                                                           │
│                                                                      │
│   Date......... ...................... 19.........    Name................................................ │
│                                                                      │
│                                              Address....   ...................................... │
│                                                                      │
│                                              ..................................................... │
│                                                                      │
│                                                          ACA Form 17 │
└────────────────────────────────────────────────────────────────────┘
```

Figure 11.15. Sample authorization to pay physician form (ACA Form 17).

received, and the balance due is the responsibility of the patient.

When a patient signs an assignment statement, it should be carefully explained what this actually means. Some patients have the misconception that when they assign benefits to a doctor, this relieves them of all health-service costs provided and they feel they should not be billed for any remaining balance. It may only mean that the doctor will receive the insurance company's check rather than the patient, and any charges beyond that amount is the patient's responsibility. Thus, the patient should understand that he will be billed for the *full* amount of services provided until the insurance company's check is credited.

Write-offs

Many elderly patients on Medicare or people on other public assistance programs have meager income and/or savings resources. Some must survive strictly on Social Security benefits, unemployment benefits, etc. In this event, some doctors adjust the account to zero by placing the balance in the "charge column" in parentheses to show a negative charge. In essence, this "writes off" whatever balance would otherwise appear on the account.

This charitable act, however, may suggest to some investigator that the reduced fee is the doctor's customary fee. To avoid this accusation, many doctors carry the balance due on their books without billing the patient, and then forgive the debt at the end of the year with an explanatory cover letter. This procedure, when warranted, avoids a hardship on the patient, allows a consistent fee schedule, and maintains positive public relations between the doctor and the patient. The same procedure can be used for cash accounts of indigent patients.

Medicolegal Considerations

There are a few unscrupulous people who promote the use of unprofessional, unethical, and sometimes quasi-illegal schemes to cheat an insurance company or deceive a patient. Often, these practices involve interference in the contract between the patient and the insurance company.

A doctor should not be seduced by promises of more money for the same services by clever use of CPT code numbers. The misuse of code numbers will eventually cause problems for those involved. In fact, such schemes can easily jeopardize many hard-fought gains achieved by the individual physician and the profession at large.

Another device questioned by many is that of advertising "free examinations." One may question how often recipients of these examinations are ever told that they do not need treatment. A more recent scheme being promoted is to accept assigned insurance benefits as payment in full for services where the deductible or co-payment is waived by the doctor. This practice might be considered a conspiracy in which the doctor and patient have entered to mislead an insurance company inasmuch as the patient is not complying with the agreed-on contract.

Never falsely alter a claim to satisfy a patient's request. For example, a patient may say his insurance coverage will not take effect until next week and he asks you to alter dates when services were provided. This would likely constitute fraud and conspiracy.

Rarely, you may be asked by a patient to include the costs of your services for his wife or a relative in his claim so that the insurance company will pay more. If you agree, it would constitute a fraudulent claim and subject you and the doctor to prosecution. Never compromise ethical conduct.

Whenever in doubt of the legality of any action or you are considering pleasing a patient by entering an unusual business arrangement, it is always good policy to consult with the doctor. It may save you considerable stress, embarrassment, and harm to your reputation and that of the office.

COST AND UTILIZATION CONTROL

The government, the public, and insurance companies are becoming increasingly concerned with the rising costs of health care.

Several approaches have been taken to hold costs at reasonable levels. The two major approaches involving ambulatory care are Health Maintenance Organizations (HMOs) and Preferred Provider Organizations (PPOs). More are developing, especially "closed panel" health provider groups that may or may not include DCs.

Professional Standards Review Organizations

The review of professional activities by peers within the health professions is not a new concept. It has been an integral part of professionalism for many years. It has been a major consideration within the legal, educational, and military professions since their sophistication within civilized societies.

PSROs involving hospital health care developed because of Social Security Act Amendments of 1972 concerning Medicare and Medicaid. The original purpose was to develop methods of determining, reviewing, and evaluating the medical necessity for institutional health care in an attempt to reduce unnecessary diagnostic and therapeutic procedures by developing standards and protocol. Under the provisions of a law passed in 1982, PSROs were supplanted by Professional Review Organizations (PROs) under contract to the secretary of HHS.

Peer Review Objectives

Peer review is essentially a process of evaluation by other practicing physicians in the same discipline of the quantity, quality, and efficiency of services ordered or performed by a licensed physician. It is more than claims review because it includes not only utilization but also the necessity and appropriateness of care. The peer review function is not intended to be disciplinary but to be valuative, analytical, consultative, and educational. It is generally agreed that peer review reveals deficiencies responsive to remedial education. Most peer review guidelines state that the objectives are: (1) to assure high quality health services; (2) to ensure high standards of professional conduct and ethics; and (3) to provide assistance to the doctor in improving his services.

Independent Consultants

Some third-party payers seek the advice of independent chiropractic consultants on questionable chiropractic claims, just as they seek the advice of allopathic physicians on questionable medical claims. Third-party payers using this type arrangement usually do so to reduce the processing time span for questionable claims.

Preferred Provider Organizations

PPOs gained national attention in the early 1980s. The concept is essentially a system of providing health-care insurance in which an employer either purchases insurance or self-insures with a "stop loss" provision. The incentive to hold down costs is that beneficiaries who use specific *panel physicians* (who have agreed to a discounted fee schedule) suffer no additional cost. However, those beneficiaries who choose other providers must co-pay a flat sum or a portion of the charges. There may or may not be a pool funded by the discounts that could be shared by the employer, the insurer (if any), and the health-care providers if the plan operates with a profit.

Obviously, such plans are attractive to insurers outraged by increasing health-care costs. From the chiropractic viewpoint, however, there is always danger that there may be a temptation to adopt some strategies not conducive to professional parity, thus circumventing state insurance equality laws, medical service corporation acts, HMO enabling acts, etc. From the viewpoint of the patient, the quality of health care is restricted to the quality of services offered by the closed-panel physicians. From the viewpoint of the panel physicians, participants are subjected to discounted services. Also, they may be subjecting themselves to various antitrust violations, charges of unfair competition, and other legal implications, according to some authorities.

Chapter 12

Medicolegal Considerations

This is likely one of the more important chapters in this book. While it is not designed to improve the technical aspects of an assistant's career, it will offer guidelines that can save her from committing an error leading to great grief.

There have been many points in previous chapters that were repeated several times, and the reader may have questioned the need for this repetition. Although these points were described in topics of records management, human relations, and communications, the student of this chapter will understand the importance for their emphasis: the underlying legal implications in professional and paraprofessional actions.

INTRODUCTION

An old saying containing much truth is "Ignorance of the law is no excuse." Thus, anyone engaged in a business or profession has a responsibility to acquire a reasonable knowledge of general law and a thorough knowledge of those laws that relate directly to one's career.

Jurisprudence is the science of law. We are concerned here with that portion applied to the practice of chiropractic. Within this context, the first part of this chapter describes the advantages of fail-safe record management from a medicolegal viewpoint, patients' rights, the doctor-patient contract, and the sometimes misunderstood subject of patient consent. The second part of the chapter explains malpractice and safeguards against it, some precarious situations to avoid, the consequences of criminal behavior, and court actions. This chapter also offers general guidance in common medicolegal topics, but the reader should be aware that sometimes there are wide variances in state statutes, area assiduity, and court opinions. When in doubt, immediately seek your doctor-employer's advice and direction.

The Legal System

We all desire protection of our person, health, welfare, reputation, property, and our agreements with other people. The purpose of law is to determine the rationality of our desires and those desires that are to be recognized in the interest of social progress.

Law also judicates conflicting interests of people and assists in giving effect to such interests.

While justice and law are different, they are intimately intertwined and interdependent. Justice is that relationship existing between individuals and between the individual and society. Law, on the other hand, is that collection of statutes and principles used to ensure the administration of justice and by that further the ends of the social order. Laws are designed to protect the rights of the state and society, yet they may appear unjust in terms of the individual. Thus, justice is "blind" and its symbols are often depicted blindfolded.

Common liabilities in health care can result from an accident occurring on the office premises, a malpractice suit, a female patient's misinterpretation of a routine examination as an unwarranted personal advance, or the errors involved in privileged communications and patient authorizations. Other common legal situations involve probate claims, depositions, medicolegal reports, etc.

RECORD MANAGEMENT

The integrity of professional health care is determined largely by the quality of the doctor's data gathering and retrieval systems. Quality health care is the result of accurate observation, analysis and synthesis of information, and appropriate action. This implies that good decisions are the result of accurate and complete facts being recorded from which a logical course of action can be taken.

To be aware of patients' problems is the doctor's first step in logical health care. The second step is to have capable assistance to systematically develop records of patients' problems and the care administered to monitor progress.

If a doctor is faced with an unwarranted charge of malpractice, it is almost impossible to offer an adequate defense if case records are incomplete or illegible. Thus, more is needed besides a memory of patients' problems for judges and juries will find it extremely doubtful that all patients' histories, complaints, symptoms, signs, and laboratory data could be remembered without a record. Most likely, a jury would consider total recall from visit to visit of existing problems and their ramifications over a period of weeks or months to be incredible.

Confidential Communications

What transpires between a doctor and patient is considered by law to be extremely privileged information, and each state has laws protecting its confidentiality. This even includes information obtained in casual conversations, notes, and data that do not concern a patient's clinical or financial records.

The concept of privileged communications between doctor and patient is not a modern idea. The Hippocratic Oath states: "Whatsoever I shall see or hear in the course of my profession in my intercourse with men, if it be what should not be noised abroad, I will never divulge, holding such things to be holy secrets."

This atmosphere of secrecy must be highly respected by DCs and CAs so that a patient will feel confident in disclosing personal information. Revealing confidential information without the patient's authority may be grounds for suit (breach of confidentiality). Both state and federal statutes prevent a doctor or paraprofessional from disclosing or testifying about the health care provided to a patient unless that patient has given specific permission or if the patient has behaved in such a manner that the law no longer protects the information.

Requests for Privileged Information

Just about all clinical data are considered privileged information. For example, case history data, examination reports, test results, diagnosis, prognosis, progress notes, descriptions of treatment procedures, narrative reports, consultation reports, or other clinical data in office records are considered privileged information. A patient's telephone reports, direct communications, memory of events, or discussions of therapy applied should not be divulged without proper authorization by the patient. Nor are DCs and CAs at liberty to mention whether the patient *is* a patient of the practice.

The law states that such secrecy even includes disclosing information to the immediate family of the patient. Exceptions to this would be in instances of informing a parent or guardian of the condition of a minor or incompetent adult or informing unknowledgeable family members that may contact a contagious infection.

Telephone Requests. Each CA must be on guard against disclosing confidential information on the telephone, despite how the person identifies himself, in the belief that it is being disclosed to an authorized person. People desiring information they are not legally entitled to can often be quite clever and subtle in getting the information they want. A CA's good intentions are not a defense in the eyes of the law. To protect the patient's and the practice's best interests, telephone inquiries should be responded to with the suggestion that (1) the information requested can be mailed to the patient and

can be obtained from the patient, or (2) the request can be put in writing and accompanied by the patient's signed authorization (Fig. 12.1).

Third-Party Requests. Common third-party requests are received from attorneys, insurance companies, and health agencies. They should never be processed without a release from the patient—unless allowed by law. When clinical records are requested by a third party and authorization is not given by the patient, the documents must be subpoenaed. Unauthorized requests for patient information by a third party should be tactfully discouraged by referring them to the patient.

Exceptions

The major exceptions to strict data confidentiality are in criminal cases, personal accident cases, and situations involving public health or welfare.

Criminal Cases. The rule of privilege regarding clinical data in criminal cases does not apply in most states. This is another reaffirmation for the need for constant

AUTHORIZATION FOR RELEASE OF RECORDS

To..
          Doctor or Hospital

....
          Address

I hereby authorize and request you to release

To..
          Doctor or Hospital

....
          Address

any and all health records in your possession, including x-rays, concerning the undersigned.

Date..   Signed..
                                                     (Patient or Nearest Relative)

                                                 Relationship..

....
          Witness

                                                                    ACA Form 16

Figure 12.1. A sample slip authorizing the release of patient records to a third party (ACA Form 16).

accuracy, neatness, legibility, completeness, dating, and initialing of record entries.

Personal Injury Cases. Patients waive their privilege of confidentiality when they place their physical or mental condition "at issue" in a personal injury case. Also, the rule does not apply to accident cases when a patient is examined by a physician representing the defendant.

Public Health and Welfare. Depending on laws of a specific state, there are events in which a doctor is legally obliged to report to certain authorities: usually the health department such as with births, deaths, certain communicable diseases, child beating, drug addiction, and so forth. In many but not all states, the fact that a patient is afflicted with a highly contagious disease must also be reported to members of the immediate family. The purpose of this communication is to help avoid acts that might spread the infection throughout a community.

Office Procedures

Office procedures should be planned to be efficient and well organized to support the best interests of each patient and designed and administered to aid the practice's services and types of cases seen. Thus, the best interests of the practice will be served, from both a clinical and a jurisprudence standpoint. All financial arrangements should be resolved prior to examination and therapy. See Figure 12.2. Record quality can mean the difference between winning or losing a legal action.

Keep in mind that office systems and procedures are never an end in themselves. Office policies, procedures, records, forms, systems, supplies, equipment, furnishings, etc, are but vehicles to reach the goal of efficient, safe health care.

Office Forms

Records and forms help to provide quality patient care through gathering and preserving information. They also protect the doctor by documenting what was or was not said or done during care. A plaintiff's attorney will exploit whatever weakness may appear in the records and experience no compunction in winning their cases for the wrong reasons.

The most crucial rule on the keeping of records relating to actual treatment is that the doctor faithfully, accurately, and thoroughly record what was done, the reasons it was done, and the patient's response. Entries in patient progress notes should include the date and time and be as concurrent as possible. "DNKA" (did not keep appointment) should appear in the patient's chart whenever the patient didn't keep an appointment.

Many doctors use patient progress slips that are filled in, dated, and signed by the patient at each visit as they sign-in. Excellent evidence of a patient's subjective appraisal of progress is then provided by the patient's signed list of symptoms and complaints and degree of improvement noted. Regularity and orderliness enhance credibility when the patient can find no support for his allegations later in either the subjective or the objective portion of case notes.

Most physicians believe that nonclinical data do not belong on the same form or even in the same file with treatment-related information. Doctors who routinely gather accident, insurance, and referral information should do so on a separate form. The same would be true for financial data.

When fill-in forms are used, each condition that a patient marks on a form should be addressed in some way. Every potential entry on a form should be completed—showing no spaces, blanks, or omissions that may imply some error or oversight. When an entry is not appropriate, enter "N/A" (not applicable).

Two words that should not be used in reports and records except for some compelling reason are "routine" and "inadvertent." Routine has little meaning except to suggest impersonalized care. "Inadvertent" infers a careless, unconcerned, reckless, hasty, inattentive, lax, lackadaisical, or negligent act.

Record Changes

No matter how thorough and accurate, office records will be of no benefit to the doctor involved in malpractice litigation if they

Medicolegal Considerations

CONFIDENTIAL PATIENT INTRODUCTION

Date _____

Patient's Name _____ Phone No. _____

Mailing Address _____

Age _____ Date of Birth _____ Soc. Sec. No. _____

Occupation _____

Employer _____

Name of Wife or Husband _____ Phone No. _____

    Occupation _____

    Employer _____

Patient's Nearest Relative _____
                    (not at patient's address)

    Address _____

Have you had previous chiropractic care? _____ When? _____

ARE YOU INSURED? _____   (PLEASE CHECK BELOW)

____ Blue Cross/Blue Shield   ____ HMO

____ Group Health and Accident Insurance   ____ Disability Insurance

____ Union Health Benefit Plan   ____ Owner's Landlords & Tenants Insurance

____ Accident & Health (Individual)   ____ State Workers' Compensation

____ Medical & Surgical Service Plan   ____ Federal Workers' Compensation

____ Medicare/Medicaid   ____ Federal Employee Health Benefit Plan/
                                CHAMPUS/Veteran's Administration

____ Interscholastic Insurance   ____ Other

PAYMENT IS EXPECTED AT TIME OF VISIT

    Name of person responsible for payment _____

HEALTH AND ACCIDENT INSURANCE POLICIES ARE IN ARRANGEMENT BETWEEN THE CARRIER AND THE PATIENT WHICH ARE USUALLY DESIGNED TO OFFSET A LARGE PORTION OF THE TOTAL COST. THIS OFFICE WILL PREPARE ANY NECESSARY REPORTS AND FORMS TO ASSIST IN MAKING COLLECTIONS FROM THE INSURANCE COMPANY TO THE PATIENT. ANY AMOUNT AUTHORIZED TO BE PAID DIRECTLY TO THIS OFFICE WILL BE CREDITED TO THE PATIENT'S ACCOUNT. IT SHOULD BE UNDERSTOOD THAT ALL SERVICES FURNISHED ARE CHARGED DIRECTLY TO THE PATIENT WHO IS PERSONALLY RESPONSIBLE FOR PAYMENT, INCLUDING THE SMALL CHARGE FOR COMPLETING THE FORMS.

    Patient's Signature _____

                                                                ACA Form 18

Figure 12.2. Confidential patient introduction form. This is an entering data form offering third-party information and stating office policy regarding financial relationships (ACA Form 18).

are not perceived by judge and jury to be a faithful and honest account. Whether an erasure is done because an error is recognized or made later for the sake of accuracy in a crucial part of the record, it has a high potential to damage a doctor's credibility. When entries are squeezed-in, scribbled in margins, inserted with arrows and wedges, written between existing lines, etc, it may be impossible to tell what was original and coincident with time and at what time various changes were made. Any inaccurate or obsolete statement recorded should be lined through, corrected, initialed, and dated. The error should not be erased, painted with liquid paper, or hidden beneath an adhesive label.

Medicolegal Reports

Most medicolegal reports are prepared by doctors at the request of an attorney representing a patient of the doctor who has been involved in some type of accident. The objective of the report is usually to aid non-physicians in settling a medical claim out of court by offering a comprehensive report of a patient's injuries, physical condition, mental status, and prognosis.

The report is necessary to the patient's attorney so that he will be aware of the nature and extent of the patient's injuries and have the basis for planning legal arguments. A lucid report holds great weight in settlement negotiations and seeing that a fair settlement is reached. If an out-of-court settlement is reached, the doctor will have saved himself valuable time from a court room appearance. If the doctor is required to appear in court, a review of the report will help to refresh his memory before he takes the witness stand. The report should make clear those details of the accident that are not factual to the doctor but were related by the patient or an observer.

Medicolegal reports of an accident are similar to a narrative report. The major items covered are:

• Patient's name, address, age, occupation, and marital status
• Date and place of injury

• What first-aid was provided at the scene of the accident and who rendered it
• History of the patient
• Nature of injuries and a description of any complications
• Findings of the doctor's physical, neurologic, and orthopedic examinations
• Findings of auxiliary studies such as roentgenography and clinical laboratory
• Consultations (if any)
• Diagnosis
• Treatment
• Follow-up visits
• Prognosis and evaluation of permanent impairment
• Concluding remarks
• Review of the doctor's fees for services provided to date and estimated fees for future services deemed necessary.

To protect privileged communications, an attorney's request for a report must be accompanied by a release signed by the patient for the information deemed necessary. Refer to Figure 11.9. Whenever possible, medicolegal reports should be submitted within a few days of the request.

The attorney is responsible for reimbursing the doctor for his time in preparing the report. Charges, agreed on by the attorney and the doctor, vary with the time necessary to prepare the report and its comprehensiveness. The report is usually submitted in duplicate, along with the doctor's statement for preparing the report. However, an increasing number of doctors request payment before the final report is released.

Subpoenaed Records

On occasion, your office may receive a telephone call from a legal service stating that they have a subpoena to photocopy one of your patient's charts. You normally will have several days to comply with the subpoena. This will allow time to collect the information requested and give the service a specific appointment when the records may be photocopied. Take care not to provide information not specified in the subpoena.

Record Ownership, Disposal, and Transfer

Ownership of Records

Case records, test results, x-ray films, etc, concerning a doctor's patients are the property of the doctor. Patients pay for professional services that usually include examination, diagnosis, treatment, and counsel, but the patients involved do not own the records that emit from or from which these services are based. To firmly establish this right of ownership, many doctors ask patients to sign a form that clarifies the doctor's ownership of all clinical records, laboratory reports, x-ray films, ECGs, EMGs, etc.

Patients are legally entitled to, on request, copies or summaries of records forwarded to a subsequent physician or institution. However, patients, other physicians, and institutions are not entitled to the original documents.

Disposal of Records

Most patient records should be preserved for four major reasons: (1) to provide continuity of care; (2) to fulfill statutory or regulatory requirements; (3) to serve as legal evidence; and (4) to fulfill research, educational, and teaching needs.

Physicians have the legal right to destroy records at any time or to keep them as long as they desire, unless specific state regulations or Chiropractic Board rulings apply. Most doctors keep all records as long as they feel they will be of value to a patient's health care. It is good procedure to retain records at least until the state's statute of limitation applicable to the course of treatment has expired.

It is sometimes difficult to be assured that some record might not be needed in the future. They may be helpful to somebody in the future for reasons that may not be apparent earlier. Thus, records should not be destroyed until the necessity for retaining them is no longer pertinent.

To maintain confidentiality, records to be destroyed should be shredded or burned with a witness present. A record of the act should be kept on file.

Transfer of Records

When doctors retire or relocate their practices to another area, they may wish to provide a doctor selected by the patient with certain reports. The record owner may choose to transfer complete records or only summaries of specific and pertinent data. These record transmittals, as all patient records, should only be released by the signed authorization of the patient.

The same is true when a practice is purchased by another doctor. Each patient should be given the opportunity to have his records forwarded to another doctor. *When one doctor buys another doctor's practice, the physician purchasing the practice is only entitled to receive the records of those patients whom have chosen to transfer their records to the new doctor.* The remaining records should be preserved by the doctor selling the practice until an authorization for release has been provided.

On the death of a physician, the rights to the doctor's records are extended to the surviving spouse, if there is one. Many doctors, however, arrange for disposition of patients' records in the event of their death to a colleague to spare their spouse the responsibility involved.

THE PATIENT'S RIGHT TO PRIVACY

The law recognizes that health service is an intimate and private service. Sick people deserve uninterrupted care and privacy from unnecessary observers.

A patient under a doctor's care has the same right of privacy as any individual has under different circumstances. The patient should not be subjected to unwarranted and unwanted personal contact or publicity that may effect possible invasion of privacy, shame, mortification, or humiliation. In most states, this privilege survives the patient's death and may be claimed by the executor of the estate.

Typical Information Releases

As mentioned previously, patients have the right to have any facts pertaining to their state of health kept confidential and not made available to others without proper authorization. A patient may desire that some information but not all information is released to certain individuals.

Referral Data. If a case is referred to another doctor or institution for consultation, diagnosis, or treatment with the patient's permission, the release of records must be preceded by a consent form signed by the patient. It is important that this disclosure be limited to only those individuals or institutions specified on the release form.

Employer Data. A question sometimes arises if an employer has the right to a report after he has sent an employee to the doctor for examination, the employee consents to the examination, and the employer pays for the examination. Even in this situation, the employer should receive no information unless the employee gives consent. Payment by the employer does not negate the patient's legal right of privacy.

Collection Agency Data. A collection agency or attorney may be provided data concerning an indebted patient's financial records. However, it does not relieve doctors from safeguarding patients' clinical data rights. It is not pertinent that service charges were not paid.

Naive Disclosures. Some examples of unintentionally violating a patient's right of privacy might include discussing a specific patient's interesting or amusing physical or mental condition with another person without prior authorization or offering patient data to an attorney or private detective, who "represents" himself as acting for the patient, without signed authorization.

Medicolegal Reports. Even for the benefit of a patient's attorney or insurance company, a signed consent form should precede the release of any information. An oral request is not sufficient to give the doctor ade-

quate protection. If the request initiates from a third party, a signed request (not a telephone request) should accompany a release signed by the patient for the necessary information.

Unessential Observers

Patients have the right of not being viewed or examined by people who are not necessary to the carrying out of a procedure. When patients disrobe for a procedure or treatment, they do so solely for the professional benefit of the doctor. Thus, the presence of an unessential person (eg, in view of another patient) without the specific consent of a patient can be a violation of the patient's right of privacy.

Aid is often necessary to help a doctor with various examinations and treatments. A member of the office staff (eg, an assistant, associate, consultant) would be considered an essential person. However, the presence of unessential persons could be considered a violation of a patient's right to privacy. A chiropractic extern, for example, who is in the doctor's office for educational purposes is there for the student's benefit, not the patient's benefit. Whenever the presence of an unessential observer is desired, it is good policy to have the patient's authorization via a signed consent form (Fig. 12.3).

Photographs

Some doctors frequently use photography to have a permanent record of a patient's posture during the various stages of structural correction. At other times, before-and-after photographs of a patient are sometimes helpful for progress reports or to portray damages in an accident case. Photographs are sometimes helpful in the development of a scientific paper or book. Nevertheless, the unauthorized taking of photographs for clinical or professional purposes, even if they are not published, can be grounds for suit. Legally, publicity of a patient's condition can only be given if specifically agreed to by the patient (Fig. 12.4).

AUTHORIZATION TO ADMIT OBSERVERS

I, ____(Name of Patient)__ , authorize Dr. ____(Name of Doctor)___ to permit the presence of such observers as he may deem fit to admit in addition to associate doctors and assistants while I am undergoing examination and treatment.

Date: _____   Signed: _____

Witness: _____   Relationship: _____

Figure 12.3. Sample consent form authorizing the admittance of nonessential observers in the presence of a patient.

AUTHORIZATION TO TAKE AND PUBLISH PHOTOGRAPHS

I, ____(Name of Patient)__ , authorize Dr. ____(Name of Doctor)__ , or another person authorized by him to take and publish photographs of me for clinical records. Such photographs may be published and re-published for the purpose of scientific and/or clinical research, chiropractic education, and health science when in the above-named doctor's judgment such publication will benefit these goals.

It is understood that the photograph(s) may be presented in part or in total at the discretion of the above-named doctor and may be modified or retouched if he so desires. It is also understood if such a photograph(s) is published in any publication or use I shall not be identified by name without additional authorization.

Date: _____   Signed: _____

Witness: _____   Relationship: _____

Figure 12.4. Sample consent form to take photographs of a patient to be used in a professional paper or book.

THE DOCTOR-PATIENT CONTRACT

Professional Responsibilities

In the view of law, health care is a contractual arrangement. It is not the type of contract usually based on a formal document; rather, it is often an implied contract of an oral transaction to purchase health services. A health practice involves many such transactions between the doctor, or an assistant acting in his behalf, and the health-care consumer.

There are four major requirements that must be met to fulfill the implied terms of any contract: (1) there must be two or more competent parties involved; (2) an offer must be made; (3) an acceptance by both parties to the conditions is essential; and (4) some form of consideration by each party is mandatory. When these requirements have been met, a contract has been established.

The doctor-patient relationship does not depend on the charging of a fee. The requirement of "some form of consideration" does not always mean that money must be exchanged. For example, "Good Samaritan" acts or services rendered without charge do not necessarily insulate a doctor from the liability if malpractice is involved. The doctor is obliged to use the required standards of skill, care, and diligence necessary, and the patient is obliged to faithfully cooperate with and follow the instructions of the physician.

The Professional Contract

A doctor may accept or refuse to accept a patient who seeks treatment. This is true even if there is no other doctor available. The actual doctor-patient relationship begins when the doctor starts to provide services to the patient in response to the patient's (or guardian's) request.

At times, a doctor may wish to limit his services to one or more particular treatments or procedures or to a particular time or place. All that is necessary in such instances is a qualified agreement with the patient. This is not to say, however, that doctors can escape liability from their negligence or that of employees simply by forming a contract with patients. Doctors are held accountable for the skill and knowledge that they represent themselves as having, despite a contractual disclaimer.

Once the doctor-patient relationship is established, a contract is established. As mentioned, this is true whether a fee is charged or not. In consenting to treat a patient, a physician automatically implies that: (1) a reasonable degree of knowledge, skill, and training such as that ordinarily retained by typical colleagues in practice is held; and (2) reasonable care and diligence will be used in the exercise of skill and the application of training to accomplish the purposes of the contract. These obligations affect examination, diagnosis, and treatment, and in giving proper instructions to the patient regarding daily activities that may affect the patient's condition.

PATIENT CONSENT AND ITS LEGAL IMPLICATIONS

A doctor who administers services without a patient's consent, expressed or implied, is liable for damages. An exception would be during an emergency; otherwise, the law states that the doctor can be charged with assault and battery. The fact that services were performed with professional skill and care is not a legal defense because negligence is not the point. The point is that services were provided without the patient's consent.

There are two types of consent: simple consent and informed consent. Sometimes the concepts of simple consent and informed consent are erroneously combined. This occurs because both concepts involve a degree of rational consideration by the patient. The *simple consent* to a procedure is usually a physical thing (eg, a signed form). The *informed consent* to a procedure, on the other hand, is more difficult to secure. It involves a thorough understanding by the patient of the ramifications of the procedure. Because of this, we shall consider them separately.

Simple Consent

The term *simple consent* refers to the consent of the patient to the fact of the procedure. For example, if a patient has a general understanding of what the doctor intends to do and agrees to the procedure, then the patient's simple consent has been obtained by the doctor.

Spoken words are not necessary if obvious actions show simple consent. Implied consent of this nature is the customary consent given in health care. For example, the courts have held that an adult of sound mind has implied simple consent when he has been made aware of what is to be done and/or cooperates by acquiescence. In controversial situations, however, it is difficult to provide implied consent. Just because a patient followed directions does not prove he was aware of the possible consequences.

Informed Consent

Simple consent can probably be secured and proved by the patient signing a form, reading some literature, viewing a videotape, etc, but such media cannot be used as a substitute for obtaining informed consent. These means of education are no substitute for a face-to-face discussion with a patient and for office personnel to make themselves available after such discussions to answer any questions that the patients may have.

In situations involving accusations of malpractice, evidence that simple consent was obtained is rarely sufficient. Proof of *informed consent* is a much better defense. To meet the legal requirements of informed consent, the patient should be made aware in nontechnical terms:

• Of the risks inherent in the recommended treatment and the probability of those risks occurring (eg, statistical percentage) so that the patient's consent is given with full knowledge of any inherent dangers involved. Risks that are not inherent (foreseeable or frequently associated) to the recommended procedures need not be discussed.

• Of alternative courses of action available, when appropriate, and the potential risks associated with them.

• Of the risks and dangers attendant to remaining untreated.

It must be the *patient*, not the doctor, who makes the decision whether to proceed or not in view of the possible consequences and alternatives. This disclosure procedure is called "gaining informed consent." It is not the patient's responsibility to ask for information.

There is always the possibility of unusual circumstances that excuse a doctor of advising a patient of possible dangers if the doctor felt such disclosure would result in detrimental patient anxiety or apprehension. Such "good intentions," however, may be difficult to prove in court later. It is the patient's *right to know*, and the physician must provide this knowledge and its ramifications whether it is requested by the patient or not.

Related Factors

The importance of gaining a patient's simple and informed consent to a procedure cannot be overemphasized. Both types of consent are important. Without them, a doctor can be held either criminally or civilly liable if he treats a patient without proper consent and the patient can prove resulting damages. When damages cannot be proved, failure to obtain consent may be cause of a suit for assault and battery. Here, malpractice would not be involved.

Qualified Consent

Anyone of legal age and sound mind has the right to say what should happen to his or her body. Physicians cannot substitute their judgment against that of their patients. Likewise, although a patient has given prior consent, he may withdraw consent at any time. While doctors may feel justified to do so, they have no duty to withdraw from a case if some patient refuses to consent to particular procedures deemed necessary by his doctor. In such situations, however, a signed release is essential.

In most situations, the courts have held that it is the natural right of individuals to choose whether to risk the chances with a suggested procedure or risk living without it. This applies except in cases of death-threatening conditions of a minor or compulsory procedures (eg, state-mandated vaccination) where the State steps in as a sovereign power to dictate that which is thought best for society.

Written Consent

There is no law requiring a signed consent to perform a health-care procedure. However, such records offer the physician a degree of protection against later charges. To be valid, a signed consent should clearly state the exact nature and extent of a procedure and be signed by a legally qualified individual (Fig. 12.5).

Various types of general or "blanket" consent forms are available and in use that appear to give the doctor almost unlimited au-

---

CONSENT TO CHIROPRACTIC SERVICES

1. I, _____ (Patient's Name) _____ , authorize the performance upon myself of the following procedure(s):

_____
(State nature and extent of diagnostic/therapeutic services)

_____

to be performed by or under the direction of Dr. (Doctor's Name).

2. I also consent to the performance of other diagnostic and therapeutic procedures in addition to or different from those stated above, whether or not arising from presently unforeseen conditions, that the above-named doctor, associates or assistants, may consider necessary or advisable in the course of my health care.

3. The nature and purpose of the procedures, possible alternatives, the risks involved, the possible consequences, and the possibility of complications have been explained to me by the above-named doctor and/or his associates and assistants.

4. I acknowledge that no guarantee or assurance of the results that may be obtained from the procedure has been given by the above-named doctor, his associates or assistants.

Date: _____   Signed: _____

Witness: _____   Relationship: _____

Figure 12.5. Sample consent form authorizing chiropractic services. Be aware that no form, including that shown above, is a satisfactory substitute for a personal discussion with the patient in securing informed consent.

thority and discretion. However, courts have held that such general authorizations are so ambiguous to be almost worthless because they fail to specify the exact nature of the procedure authorized.

Invalid Consent

Even if consent is given, it can be held invalid for a number of reasons. For example:

• Consent is invalid if it was given by a person not considered legally authorized to give consent.

• Consent is invalid if it was obtained by fraud or misrepresentation. To persuade a patient to give consent for a procedure that cannot be clinically justified is to perpetuate a fraud on the patient that violates the patient's consent.

• Consent is invalid if in gaining consent the physician's explanation was made in technical terms that would not be understandable to the average lay person.

• Consent is invalid if the service performed is illegal. Informed consent and signed authorization are necessary whenever any procedure is considered "experimental."

Whether a procedure is standard or normally contains an inconsequential risk is not the major consideration but whether the procedure might have an adverse effect on the patient because of the patient's particular condition.

Quality of Care

Once consent is given, physicians are obliged to use diligent judgment and exercise the requisite degree of skill. That is, doctors and/or assistants can be held liable for injury to patients that result from substandard knowledge or skill or for failing to exercise reasonable judgment. This means that doctors are held to the standards of care "commonly held and generally possessed and exercised" by their colleagues, as long as the doctor-patient contract exists. While a professional relationship does not guarantee a good result, it is implied that physicians will use the knowledge and skill held by at least typical colleagues in the area and to exercise reasonable care and their best judgment to bring about a favorable result.

Medical Necessity

Medical necessity was explained briefly in the previous chapter, but it is well to review a few points here. A CA must realize that when a patient is accepted by a physician for health care, the doctor automatically acknowledges that the patient's conditions to be treated will be recognized ones and that the examinations, tests, and treatments used will be based on scientific studies and principles generally accepted by the profession at large as necessary and appropriate. This relationship between condition and procedure is termed the "medical necessity," and third-party contracts usually call for a direct relationship between covered services and medical necessity. It also underscores why accurate office documents are necessary to substantiate the services rendered in cases involving litigation.

Objectives of Care

Besides gaining informed consent and explaining the medical necessity, the doctor should explain to the patient and differentiate between therapeutic, rehabilitative, and maintenance care necessary in the doctor's judgment and what is covered in the patient's insurance policy. If a patient later receives a bill for services not covered by insurance that was believed to be covered, the unforeseen financial burden could possibly serve as motivation to bring legal actions against the doctor.

Treating Minors and Incompetents

Consent should be obtained from a parent or guardian when professional services involve a minor. In situations involving simple procedures, however, many courts have stated that a mature child may offer consent in his behalf.

A typical exception to the necessity for parental consent would be an emergency where delay in seeking parental approval might involve serious risk to a patient. In such situations, some courts have held that a minor's consent is sufficient if the minor is mature enough to understand the full significance of the suggested procedure.

Age cannot be used as a sole criterion of maturity or intelligence. If a child is immature for his age or of maturity but of unsound mind and thus incompetent to understand the nature, purpose, and risks involved in a proposed procedure, consent must come from a parent or guardian. Any patient obviously under the influence of a drug would not likely be considered competent. Authorization must come from a spouse, parent, or legally appointed guardian when an incompetent patient has attained legal age.

Clinical Releases

In recent years, the use of diagnostic and therapeutic consent forms has increased greatly in an attempt to reduce the increasing number of suits against doctors. While no state requires signed consent forms by law, their use is highly recommended. This is especially true if a diagnostic or therapeutic procedure is not usual and customary.

All consent forms need not be printed. When a rarely used form is necessary, it may be typed or photocopied as needed. A carbon copy, however, should never be used as an original.

Even the best designed consent form is not the total answer. That is, the mere signing of a consent form by a patient does not prove that a patient had all the pertinent knowledge on which to give consent intelligently. Juries are well aware that a patient under stress of pain or illness might sign almost anything. The procedures described in the form and their implications must be *explained*. To verify this, it is good policy to document in the patient's records a note to the effect that the consent form was explained in detail and the patient agreed to proceed prior to signing the form. This is not foolproof if the patient later denies it, but it is better than the signed form itself.

In recent years, informative literature, films, videotapes, slide/tape programs, etc, have been used in patient orientation. They are helpful in explaining basic concepts, but their use is far from as good as a face-to-face discussion in gaining informed consent. They should only be considered as complementary procedures.

PROTECTION AGAINST MALPRACTICE CLAIMS

It should be well-established at this point that professional negligence producing a wrong against a patient is grounds for a claim of civil malpractice. In simple terms, *negligence* results from failure to have done something that ordinarily ought to have been done or to have done something that ordinarily ought not to have been done.

Although positive human relations can help assure but not guarantee lawsuits will never occur, poor patient relations are sure to create them. Litigation might be avoided simply by acknowledging a patient's grievance and taking steps to resolve the problem.

The detrimental effects from being involved in a malpractice suit are much more than money. The psychologic implications, the affect on social and peer relations, and the encouragement of harmful behavioral effects can be overwhelming. But with alertness and skill, potential problem patients can be immediately referred or possibly some potential problems can be defused early during the informed-consent process.

Background

Professional malpractice is defined in the various states in different ways. Thus, practitioners and their assistants should know the local definition and its implications in the area of practice. In general, the law requires that physicians exert a reasonable degree of knowledge, skill, and care in their professional endeavors, as are ordinarily possessed and exercised by other members of the profession under similar circumstances.

Basis for Legal Action

Physicians have a legal duty to their patients to act in a reasonably prudent manner in their professional conduct. If this duty is breached by a doctor, the injured party has cause for legal action against the negligent doctor. However, factors as those described below must be established and certain evidence of malpractice must be at hand before suit is justified.

1. The doctor-patient relationship must be firmly established prior to suit. That is, a true doctor-patient relationship must be proved to exist at the time of injury.

2. The patient must prove negligence to prove malpractice. It must be established that health-care personnel failed to perform a duty with reasonable skill and care or did something that was not authorized. Because a patient was not cured or a patient's condition became worse under treatment is not in itself cause for a malpractice suit. It may, however, be cause for another type of legal action, depending on the circumstances involved.

3. It must be established that the act of negligence must be the direct or indirect cause of the damages suffered by the patient. Thus, malpractice can be established from either negligent diagnosis or therapy when damages to the patient are related to a negligent omission or action.

If there is more than one accepted method of conducting a procedure, physicians cannot be found negligent if they select a method that retrospectively turns out to be in error or unsatisfactory. This is not considered malpractice; it is simply an error in judgment. Negligence is not involved unless it can be proved that the doctor or an assistant did not exercise or direct reasonable care in examining and treating the patient.

Establishing Proof

The burden of proof is invariably on the plaintiff during litigation. Malpractice may be proved by (1) testimony of the defendant, (2) testimony of expert witnesses, or (3) self-evident knowledge that the injury could not have resulted unless negligence was involved.

The defense must present its side of the case during litigation, and a doctor's own statements may be used against him. For example, a doctor or assistant may have openly admitted to a patient or another employee that an error in judgment had been made. It is not unusual for a patient bringing suit to use statements, opinions, or promises made by the doctor or one of his assistants. A doctor's assistant may be called to testify to this. Malpractice can also be established by expert witnesses if one or more testify that the defendant failed to use ordinary skill and care and/or failed to apply usual-and-customary procedures.

Although it is usually the testimony of expert witnesses that establishes the extent of injury, the effects of some injuries may be judged self-evident (eg, burns). For example when expert witnesses are not used, the doctrine of *Res ipsa loquitur* can be used. This means that "The thing speaks for itself" and implies that a jury may be expected to appreciate that a certain injury could not have resulted unless lack of skill or care was involved. If an assistant administers physiotherapy to a patient, for example, and the patient is obviously injured, many states hold that the burden of proof is on the doctor and assistant to prove that negligence was not involved.

The plaintiff's attorney in some states must establish that there was no contributory negligence on part of the patient. When the defense claims there is contributing negligence by the patient, usually the defense must prove (show evidence of) contributory negligence.

Statute of Limitations

Each state has a statute of limitations on malpractice claims and other legal actions pertinent to health-care practice. The time limit for filing malpractice cases is usually from 1 to 3 years, but it may be as long as 6 years in a few states. If the injured party is a minor, a statute of limitations does not start until the minor becomes of legal age (usually 18 years old). The Statute of Limitations is a dangerous defense against charges of malpractice because it can be readily waived by subtle signs of concealment or fraud.

Professional Standards

Every health-related profession has its standards of care. Some criteria are determined by law, others by the profession itself.

Acceptable Procedures

The standards of chiropractic care are judged relative to their consistency with scientific knowledge and to what is generally accepted within the "area" by the profession at large. These standards are never established by insurance companies, professional associations, or a single chiropractic college.

Professional standards are usually established by expert testimony during malpractice litigation, and this testimony is commonly based on what is currently taught in accredited colleges. That is, the standard of chiropractic compels that diagnostic and therapeutic procedures used should be those based on the academic and clinical training received in and through accredited chiropractic colleges. These standards depend on what is in general use and what is taught today in credible institutions, not what was in general use or taught several years ago. A procedure taught throughout the nation in "weekend seminars" that is not taught in or approved by an accredited college would not likely be considered a "standard," despite its popularity among some practitioners.

Some courts have restricted the definition of "area" to mean the doctor's local community; while other courts, in increasing numbers, have defined it as the entire state or nation. Thus, a rural practitioner may be held to the same standards as a practitioner close to highly sophisticated diagnostic facilities. A recent graduate may be held to the same standards as a physician in practice for many years, or vice versa. Diplomate status or advertising that one "specializes in ..." will hold that DC to a higher standard than that for a general practitioner.

Unusual Procedures

Even the most conscientious doctor can make an error in judgment. A difficulty arises in trying to prove that the error was one of judgment and not one of procedure. For example, doctors are constantly seeking means to facilitate patient care, and it's always an ego boost to be the most "modern" doctor in an area. However, there is a potential danger in applying innovative procedures not widely accepted. Thus, diligent care must be used in using a procedure that has not been adequately tested and generally accepted. If an injury results from a procedure that is not used by a respectable minority of the profession, the law is especially stern against errors. Novel therapeutic approaches are dangerous practices if a doctor and/or an assistant is to avoid a claim of malpractice.

Whenever procedures are suggested that would not be considered usual and customary, physicians are legally obliged to inform their patients that the proposed service is novel and unorthodox. The patient must be made aware of the possible risks involved while gaining informed consent, and it is always good policy to have on record a signed release.

Common Causes of Suit

The precipitating motive for a suit is often rooted in several real or imagined discourtesies, ego-deflating acts, and irritations leading to ill will that could have easily been avoided. The development of trust and an air of accessibility between health-care providers and patients encourage patients to speak openly and voice concerns.

We communicate in many vocal and nonverbal ways, as well as through gestures and facial expressions. The chiropractor has a special advantage by being able to communicate by touch.

In most malpractice suits, defendants feel they had carried out competent care and that the legal action is unjust. It is not unusual that the involved doctor is "astonished" when named a defendant in a legal action. The reasons some patients sue without cause and others do not with cause is a complex subject yet to be resolved. However, certain generalities will be described below.

Professional Negligence

Our system of justice holds that patients are entitled to usual and customary skill and care from any doctor, and patients injured through negligence are justified in bringing suit for compensation. These injuries may be physical, emotional, or both. A general release of liability for negligence from patients will not protect a doctor from malpractice.

Some malpractice situations are surely the result of avoidable negligence as with an adverse effect of some form of treatment or procedure that is applied incorrectly, faulty equipment, careless handling of equipment, improper work habits, or an invasion of the patient's rights. Proper steps taken to avoid the common pitfalls inherent in the doctor-patient relationship would most likely prevent a majority of such malpractice cases.

Personalities Under Stress

Typical patients entering a doctor's office do so because they have health problems. Most of these patients are under exceptional stress usually derived from pain or discomfort and not knowing what is wrong, what can be done, how long it will take to get better, how much will it cost, etc. Added to these are the basic stresses of everyday living. These accumulating worries and fears must be reduced to the satisfaction of the patient if good doctor-patient relations are to be furthered.

It is a common experience that people under severe stress do not always act rationally. Thus, it is not difficult to appreciate that the precipitating motivation for a suit is frequently not the reason given on the formal complaint. As described, the precipitating motive often involves numerous real or imagined discourtesies and irritations leading to ill will that could have been easily avoided. This is one reason the importance of building positive human relations has been stressed in previous chapters of this book.

The National Chiropractic Mutual Insurance Company (NCMIC) reports that many suits are filed after patients have had their accounts placed with a collection agency. Collection actions appear to precipitate retaliation by some patients when they are placed under severe pressure.

Misguided Intentions

A "Good Samaritan" attitude is often a common pitfall. This liability should not be confused with the "Good Samaritan" statutes of various states that involve emergency care for a stranger in distress. We are referring here to the physician who is tempted to save a patient the cost of a necessary x-ray film or the inconvenience of a helpful laboratory test. Such a "considerate" doctor may later find that same patient confronting him in court in a malpractice litigation. Thus, the direction and scope of recommended procedures should be determined by the nature and extent of the disorder presented. They should never be sacrificed for the sake of time or economy. Another factor is that the rising number of malpractice litigations has forced many doctors to practice "defensively."

Therapeutic Contraindications

It is well recognized that any therapeutic procedure or agent having a potential for effectiveness has a potential for danger. Every therapy has its clinical indications, contraindications, and precautions that must be observed if the procedure is to be applied safely and effectively. This requires knowledge of the biomechanical, biochemical, and physiologic factors involved and their pros and cons in achieving a specific therapeutic purpose. Before any therapy is applied, the physician is expected to inform the patient of what to expect from the therapy and what safety measures should be observed by the patient during treatment.

When a patient is advised to exercise, he should be given adequate instruction and *personal demonstration* of the correct way to do each exercise, and a review of the patient carrying out each prescribed regimen should be made. Any prescribed therapeutic or rehabilitation apparatus to be used in the patient's home must be fully explained and demonstrated, its use by the patient observed and monitored, and its application periodically reviewed.

Public criteria for professional performance are established by usual and customary practices, but this fact does not mean that there is not more than one acceptable method to reach a therapeutic goal. Different surgeons use different techniques to accomplish the same goal, and different DCs use different techniques to accomplish the same goal. There is no liability in selecting from several acceptable procedures and techniques available if the doctor is knowledgeable in their proper application. However, the procedures selected should be determined by the doctor's knowledge, experience, skill, and clinical judgment.

Defensive Actions

With the increasing number of malpractice suits and large judgments, doctor are obligated to practice a form of *defensive health care*. This requires the establishment of systematic and thorough procedures that will assure that the best interests of everyone concerned are considered.

Every doctor should develop a warning system that alerts him to malpractice risks. If he becomes aware that he or an assistant is being less than meticulous, it is important to take a few moments and recognize what is being done and how it can be corrected.

A direct correlation has been established between poor communications with patients and malpractice claims filed by those patients. When all questions are answered to the patient's satisfaction, the patient will likely be cooperative and appreciative. Before a procedure is applied to a patient who has never experienced it before, an explanation should be given in a calm step-by-step matter-of-fact fashion of what you are going to do and what the patient will experience.

Human Relations

Practitioners of average ability who exhibit good human relations are sued far less often than those who are exceptionally competent professionally but fail to understand or administer to human needs. Thus, the best insurance health-care personnel can have in preventing malpractice claims is the development of positive human relations. Attorneys conversant with malpractice suits report that the personality of the health provider in relating to the patient plays the paramount role in inhibiting or stimulating an injured patient to sue the doctor.

A doctor with average ability who exhibits good human relations is sued less frequently than those who are exceptionally competent professionally but fail to understand or administer to human needs. A doctor-patient relationship based on positive human relations regularly prevents a suit for real or imagined wrongs. Imagined wrongs, in fact, can easily be nourished if the proper atmosphere is not established and maintained.

Many people are timid in questioning a professional. While most patients want to know the details of their condition, they don't like to *ask* for the facts. Thus, positive human relations is good communications. Inform before you perform.

Controlling Patient Quality

Many practice management consultants feel that 95% of a practice's troubles will be caused by only 5% of its patients. If a few patients prove to be constantly troublesome despite quality office attitudes and services, it's better for the doctor to refer these patients to other doctors where the rapport might be improved. Keep in mind that unconscious body language and subtle voice reflections can communicate stronger than words.

Recognizing Basic Medicolegal Criteria

Training. All accredited chiropractic colleges teach that appropriate precautions must be taken prior to initiating patient care. This includes the recording and evaluation of the patient's clinical history, presenting complaint, subjective symptoms, objective findings, and necessary spinal, neurologic, roentgenographic, psychologic, and laboratory data. These findings must be correlated and a conclusion, diagnosis, or clinical impressions established.

Standards. Professional standards are greatly influenced by *current* educational criteria. Accredited chiropractic education includes systematic and thorough examination procedures that use methods, techniques, and instruments common to all health professions and methods of spinal and postural analysis that are fairly unique to chiropractic. Measures of physical, roentgenographic, and laboratory diagnosis are used to substantially profile the patient's condition, differentiate it from similar processes, and develop an accurate case record.

Reasonable Judgment. Reasonable judgment is based on rational procedures. The rule requiring physicians to use their best judgment does not hold physicians liable for an error of judgment *if* physicians do what they think is best after careful examination. Courts recognize that diagnosis is an art, and they usually forgive an error in judgment. On the other hand, they do not forgive a disregard for usual diagnostic procedures indicated by the patient's clinical signs and symptoms. It is recognized that physicians may make mistakes in the diagnosis of a case; but when there are common means to determine the cause of the ailment, physicians must use them.

Novel Approaches. Novel therapeutic approaches are dangerous practices if one is to avoid claims of malpractice. Thus, no diagnostic or therapeutic procedure should be applied unless it is based on credible instruction. When new procedures are used, patient releases and documentation of postgraduate training from a credible source (eg, accredited college) should be at hand in office files in the event it becomes necessary to prove quality of training.

Employing the Diagnostic Rationale

Diagnosis is the doctor's determination of the nature of a patient's state of health. The leading reason for studying signs, symptoms, and, for that matter, the case history, is to determine the pathophysiologic processes involved. Knowing "why" a certain sign or symptom exists is cardinal to identify the disorder and apply competent therapy. Clinical procedures should be initiated only after specific clinical decisions have been made.

Most malpractice cases involve a doctor's failure to carefully diagnose. Functional and pathologic processes are properly interpreted only when the clinical significance of the patient's sign and symptoms are recognized. The converse of this is the tendency to jump to conclusions based on a few facts. Before a physician can take rational therapeutic action, it must be preceded by careful observation, description, interpretation, verification, diagnosis, and periodic review.

D. D. Palmer, the founder of chiropractic, aptly stated that "Specific adjusting requires a knowledge of pathology, diagnosis, and where and how to adjust one vertebra. . . ." He also wrote that "In making a diagnosis, it should be the Chiropractor's business first to determine the nature of disease by learning what functions are abnormally performed; what part of the body is affected."

Diagnosis is the primary means by which physicians can suggest a course of action judged to be in the best interests of the patient. Although a specific act may not say that the chiropractor has the right to diagnose, several courts have held that chiropractors have the duty and obligation to diagnose, at least to the degree necessary to determine whether the case is likely to be amenable to chiropractic methods as stipulated in the chiropractic practice act.

Courts have held that the use of any therapy must be directed by the nature and scope of the patient's disorder as determined by the diagnosis. Before a doctor applies any form of therapy, it is implied that (1) the patient's malfunction or diseased state has been determined by the doctor so that the criteria for proper application can be applied and (2) the doctor understands the mechanisms involved and their predictable effects on the pathologic processes.

Determining Treatment Methods

A doctor must determine the most valid approach to treatment—keeping the welfare of the patient paramount. Courts have held that physicians should use all available means at their command to properly determine the nature of the patient's disorder before acting with regard to it.

A licensed doctor implicitly represents that he will provide only those services that are lawful to provide under his license and which he is competent to render. A doctor's failure to comply with statutory duties subjects him not only to the penalties provided by law but also to civil suit for injuries "caused" by that failure.

Competent professional service is usually judged in comparison to that level of skill generally practiced within the profession. A member of a school of practice other than that to which the defendant belongs is generally not competent to testify as an expert to define a standard of treatment in a malpractice case. One exception is where there is proof by competent evidence that the *methods of treatment are the same* despite the difference in the litigation is an expert's opinion to a *reasonable certainty* that the incident caused the injuries.

A "specialist" will generally be held to the standard prevailing within that specialty. Diplomates should be aware that this status almost assures them of a more rigorous standard by which their professional actions will be judged.

Several courts have ruled that the direction and scope of any procedure applied must be determined by the nature and scope of the disorder presented (ie, the diagnosis). Treatment methods, as diagnostic methods, are determined by the scope of practice authorized by state law and credible training, personal experience, and clinical judgment.

Case management and counsel often regard environmental, nutritional, and psychotherapeutic factors, as well as first aid, hygiene, sanitation, and structural and physiologic procedures designed to aid in health restoration and maintenance. Proper therapy includes preparatory procedures necessary to chiropractic adjustments, procedures to encourage healing, the development of body defenses, rehabilitative procedures, and counsel toward preventing aggravation of or recurrence of a disorder.

The Postexamination Conference

Once a differential diagnosis is arrived at, using appropriate procedures necessary to determine what type health care is best suited for the patient, the patient is treated or possibly referred to another physician. When a firm diagnosis by the doctor cannot be arrived at within a logical timeframe, consultation with an appropriate specialist should be arranged. To request the opinion of another physician reflects the referring doctor's concern for the patient's best interests. It is the duty of a doctor to discuss the findings of his examination with the patient and separate those conditions that fall within his expertise and scope of practice and those conditions that should be treated by another type of health-care provider.

To maintain good patient relations and rapport and to comply with legal requirements, examination findings should be discussed with the patient in language understood by the patient. This often includes a brief summary of the nature and extent of the patient's disorder, an overview of recommended therapies, alternative procedures, an explanation of possible benefits

and complications, anticipated length of therapy probably necessary, what the patient can hope for in terms of progress, and an explanation of office fees and policies. No ethical practitioner can or will imply any form of guarantee.

Monitoring Progress

Law requires that a diagnosis must follow examination and serve as the basis for any therapy selected. However, if the initial findings do not establish a diagnosis, a *working (tentative) diagnosis* is used while the data are still being considered and palliative therapy is applied. Even to arrive at an initial diagnosis is not necessarily to arrive at a fixed opinion. Diagnosis is a continuing process just as the stages of healing or degeneration are continuing processes.

The purpose of diagnosis is more than to identify, when possible, the cause of a patient's health problem and to direct therapy toward rehabilitation. Besides determining the nature of the disorder, diagnosis is a means to progressively monitor therapy and verify the accuracy of the original opinion. Thus, one of its objectives is to assess the effect of therapy.

Consultations and Referrals

After arriving at a diagnosis, all physicians should make realistic self-appraisals of whether the therapy indicated is within their ability and scope of practice. That is, it is the responsibility of doctors to judge whether they are competent to treat a case. If not, they should refer the patients to other practitioners in which they have confidence that the case will be treated competently.

In situations that are not "clear cut," alternative approaches, both within and without the profession, should be discussed with the patient about the relative risk involved and the speed of recovery anticipated with various approaches. The decision of the patient should be documented in detail in case records.

The law requires *any* physician to recognize his limits, refrain from treating people whose afflictions are beyond his skill, and refer that patient to an appropriate health-care provider. Referral should be made to that discipline which in the referring doctor's judgment can best resolve the problem(s) defined after the patient has been examined. A DC recommending another physician should only refer to doctors who are in good standing in the community and with their licensing board. To do otherwise would be difficult to justify. A DC is not liable for the negligence of another physician in good standing *unless* that chiropractor has the right to *control* the method or manner of treatment.

Failure to refer a patient when it would be in the best interests of the patient can constitute malpractice. Contrary philosophic arguments are useless in the court room. And a suggestion of referral alone is not always sufficient. Physicians must assure that their patients have followed their referral advice. In some states, making the patient solely responsible for ensuring that another practitioner will provide further care may be considered abandonment. A suggestion of referral should be followed-up, and, if necessary, its need reinforced.

A physician who improperly fails to refer a patient to a specialist may be held to the standard of care *applicable to the specialist* to whom the referral should have been made. Chiropractors are generally obligated to (1) recognize a medical problem as contrasted with a chiropractic problem; (2) refrain from further chiropractic treatment when a reasonable chiropractor should be aware that the patient's condition is not amenable to chiropractic treatment and the continuation of the treatment may aggravate the condition; and (3) refer the patient to a medical doctor when a medical mode of treatment is indicated.

In making a well-timed referral, a DC can avoid the risk of malpractice. Thus, doctors act wisely and with good conscience by suggesting a referral when they realize that resolution of a problem is beyond their ability and refusing to provide treatment requiring specialized training.

Keeping in Line with the Times

The courts have held that health practitioners are legally bound to keep abreast of the times and prepare themselves by fairly modern means to handle the work in which they are engaged. A physician's departure from approved methods *in general use*, if it injures a patient, will render the doctor liable despite his good intentions.

While physicians do not have to be the most skilled or learned in their area, they are obliged to keep abreast with developments by reading professional journals and standard reference texts, as health care is commonly recognized as a constantly changing science and art. Also, regular participation in continuing education programs is mandatory for license renewal in most states. Even when this is not a statutory requirement, courts have held that it is necessary for doctors to keep abreast with current standards of practice.

Working Within the Law

Chiropractors are licensed to practice their profession under the Chiropractic Practice Act legislated. Once licensed, there are certain events that doctors are legally obliged to report to certain authorities (usually the State Health Department) such as births and deaths, certain communicable diseases, child beating, drug addiction, elderly abuse, etc. In such cases, the doctor will usually be required to complete a standard form and mail it to the proper authorities. These forms should be in stock within each office.

A charge of practicing medicine without a license *does not* constitute malpractice. While it is usually considered a misdemeanor, it may be a parallel complaint if a DC or CA has exceeded the scope of practice as defined by law. It may color the entire litigation. The plaintiff patient in a malpractice case normally must prove his case against a chiropractor by expert testimony of one or more other DCs. Medical testimony is generally inadmissible in proving negligence of a chiropractor. However, if an act exceeding a DC's scope of practice is closely related to the injuries suffered by the plaintiff, the DC can be judged by the accepted standards of medicine. This would likely subject the DC to highly prejudiced testimony.

Maintain Accurate Clinical Records

A doctor's first line of defense in safeguarding against a false accusation is established by adequate *rapport, records, reports*, and *referrals* to appropriate practitioners. Quality health care is the effect of accurate observation and analysis, logical synthesis of information, and appropriate and justifiable action, thus decisions must be based on retrievable information that is accurate and complete.

Accurate and neatly prepared records are the best defense a practitioner can provide against a charge of malpractice. In questions of liability, the question of fact is paramount. Since many oral contracts are involved in health practice, the doctor's case records may be the only tangible evidence at hand. Office records are tangible evidence that a doctor can offer to justify an action or an appropriate treatment. Although the law does not specify exactly what records are necessary, the rule of "area standards" usually applies.

Basic Objectives. Office records should be consistent with accepted standards of professional practice. While the patient's history record should show the patient's status at the time of the initial visit, progress records should portray the patient's state of health at subsequent points in time. As a safeguard if serious pathology (eg, cancer) is coexistent with a disorder being treated, a disclaimer should be documented.

Progress Records. Progress notations constitute a permanent record of what was done and offer a chronology of patient status, changes in treatment, or changes to previously given instructions. Such records justify continued care and ensure continual reevaluation of the patient and/or treatment program. They also assure that the patient can be informed of his or her progress according to the doctor's findings and advised of the therapeutic, rehabilitative, and maintenance care judged necessary.

Entries. Both the DC and the CA should initial all record entries made within a patient's chart. When a doctor dictates notations, the recording assistant's initials should precede the doctor's initials. This is especially important in offices where several staff members make entries to a patient's record.

Vicarious Liability

Assistants new to an office sometimes become discomposed by the doctor's close observation of their actions, but this is his incumbent duty. Doctors are responsible for the office actions of their employees. He is legally obligated to assure that office procedures are as "fail-safe" as possible. Thus, careful supervision, direction, and control are necessary when assistants are acting for physicians. Legally, patients' complaints to a doctor's employees are notice to the doctor.

While the scope and depth of basic training and continued education of assistants are far beyond the scope of this manual, certain factors having special legal pertinence are described below to alert CAs to the motives involved.

The doctrine of *vicarious liability* holds an employer accountable for the acts of his employees. It is the doctor's duty to the patient that lays the foundation for vicarious liability.

The doctor's license requires him to hire competent people and oversee their actions. Unless the doctor can prove that an employee owed a separate duty to the patient and that the assistant relied on self-judgment in the treatment of the patient, the actions of the assistant will be considered those of the doctor. A doctor cannot create an independent-contractor relationship by simply designating employees as such.

In the context of vicarious liability, the doctor-employer has the right to decide the manner, method, and means of a CA's assignments. But in instances where employees act wholly outside the scope of their authority and beyond the doctor's right of control, the doctor is not liable for their actions. An office operations procedures manual provides an excellent reference source for new employees and an invaluable tool in defining the scope of employee's authority and duties.

The Risks of Delegation. State laws on delegation are often vague. They must be appreciated as interpreted by the State Board of Examiners. An assistant's training, skill, and competence are no defense if the state's statutory criteria have not been met. That is, if an assistant is not legally allowed by state law to administer therapy even under the doctor's supervision, the doctor lacks defense. In fact, the doctor-employer could be charged with unprofessional conduct and his license revoked for "aiding and abetting an unauthorized person in performing a procedure without a license."

Respondeat Superior. Under the legal doctrine of *Respondeat Superior,* physicians can be held responsible for the actions of their assistants if the acts are within the scope of the assistants' duties. When an employer-employee relationship is established, the doctor is liable for a careless or unskilled act of an assistant just as any employer is responsible for the actions of employees.

Patient Education. Assistants must frequently discuss certain health-related information with patients. At these times, they must be keenly alert that they do not transgress the Chiropractic Practice Act by directly or indirectly offering information that might be construed as recommending a type of treatment or making a diagnosis. The courts have strictly held that assistants may gather and record diagnostic data but they may not *interpret* the data. Nor should assistants comment to patients or answer inquiries concerning symptoms, diagnosis, care, or progress. These are the sole prerogatives of a licensed practitioner.

Inadvertent Diagnostics. If a patient should ask an assistant, "I have arthritis, don't I?" and an assistant casually responds with, "Well, it looks like it," the CA would be in an embarrassing situation if the doctor arrives at a different diagnosis. The CA might be considered guilty of rendering a diagnosis. All such inquiries should be referred to the doctor.

Inadvertent Therapeutics. A patient may telephone the office and be told that the doctor is out of the office but will return the call shortly. It is not uncommon for some patients then to ask the assistant if a certain type of home treatment recommended by the doctor should be continued although the treatment increases discomfort. Although the assistant might be aware that such side effects are quite common and transitory, it would be a gross error for her to advise the patient one way or another that would alter the recommended therapy. If the patient's condition should worsen, the doctor might be liable to suit and the assistant charged with practicing chiropractic without a license.

Handling Delinquent Accounts. Staff personnel should not be responsible for making any derogatory remark about a patient because of a delinquent account. Harassing telephone calls, collection dunning, or threats (overt or implied) should be strictly avoided. Besides such actions being antagonistic to encouraging the patient to make payment, they might precipitate a lawsuit for slander, harassment, or malpractice. A disabled patient may find it impossible to meet financial obligations until he can return to work. In these situations, a conference to discuss the possibility of agreeable installment payments is often the best solution.

Legal Relationships. Vicarious liability is not limited to actions of chiropractic assistants who treat patients under the supervision of the doctor. Liability also may extend to partners and those who do not administer treatment. While a doctor is not responsible for the actions of a substitute doctor if prudence is used in the selection, the physician is responsible for the actions of an associate if the associate is a partner in a group practice or a member of an incorporated practice. In legal associations, group members have traditionally been held responsible for the actions of other members in the group.

DANGEROUS SITUATIONS

Emergency Cases

It is well-advised that all health-care personnel become fully acquainted with the "Good Samaritan" statutes affecting emergency care in their respective states. Primary-care health practitioners are also obliged to be aware of the emergency medical system in their community.

Knowledge of basic cardiopulmonary resuscitation (CPR) and emergency cardiac care (ECC) standards should be acquired and kept current. These basic standards have been firmly established. Because of nationwide community training programs, basic techniques have become usual and customary procedures. The courts will undoubtedly expect all health professionals to possess the basic knowledge and skill involved.

While offering temporary first-aid in a life-threatening situation does not in itself create a formal doctor-patient relationship in a circumstance of dire emergency, the services rendered must meet the standards of being usual and customary for the situation. After emergency treatment has been started, the doctor must follow through to see that the injured party is placed in appropriate hands and not abandoned.

Warranties: Actual and Implied

According to law, doctors may promise to accomplish particular results or effect a cure by a contract with their patients. However, if the physicians involved in such contracts fail to produce the *exact* warranted results, they are liable for breach of contract even if they used the highest possible professional skill, knowledge, and care. Thus, such contracts are most rare and usually considered unprofessional if not unethical within the healing arts.

Ethical Warranty. In the typical doctor-patient contract, the doctor agrees only to perform certain procedures. Ethical practitioners will warrant only that (1) they possess the degree of skill and knowledge usual and customary within their profession, (2) they will use that skill and knowledge in examining and treating their patients, and (3) they have at least the skill and knowledge commonly required to safely and accurately perform any procedure conducted.

Contracted Courses of Treatment. There is a tendency for some chiropractors to have the patient sign an agreement to take a specific number of treatments for an agreed fee. Such contracts or agreements may not specifically promise a cure or improvement in the patient's condition. In fact, they may specifically disclaim such promises. Nevertheless, some patients tend to infer that the doctor is promising a cure or improvement simply by establishing a specific number of treatments in advance. Legal counsel advises that anything that may infer a promise to cure or improve should be avoided. The public has been conditioned to expect that health-care treatment will be successful.

Binding Contracts

Case-Basis Fees. As there is no known statistical basis currently acceptable to compute a case-basis fee for chiropractic services, case-basis fees are not usual and customary in the chiropractic profession. Whenever such a procedure is used, the physician involved may assume unnecessary legal risks as a warranty may be implied despite contractual language disclaiming any warranty. In addition, if results do not meet the patient's expectations, he may feel strong resentment for being involved in a "long-term" contractual arrangement and seek a legal escape from the commitment such as a malpractice suit or a claim of breach of promise.

The argument of these "term" relationships is that they provide patient motivation for a contracted length of time in which results can manifest. Nevertheless, as risks far outweigh advantages, it is better to get patient cooperation by other means. If a patient voluntarily meets his scheduled appointments, the doctor automatically knows where his degree of rapport with the patient is at each visit.

Extended-Payment Plans. Installment payment plans, on the other hand, with or without an advanced payment, do not carry such a liability if they are carefully designed for the benefit of the patient and provide that the patient is free to stop treatment with an *equitable refund* of any unused fee.

Careless Case Dismissal

After a doctor-patient relationship has been established, the physician is legally obliged to attend to the case as long as the patient desires or until the doctor gives adequate notice of his intention to withdraw from the case. Five common reasons for a doctor withdrawing from a case occur when (1) the doctor feels that another type of health service would better fit the patient's present needs, (2) the patient refuses to cooperate with the doctor's instructions, (3) the patient requests services by another physician, (4) the patient discharges the doctor, or (5) the doctor retires from practice or moves to a distant location.

When a physician desires to withdraw from a case, the doctor must give the patient *reasonable* notice so that the patient may obtain other health-care attention if the patient desires (Fig. 12.6). The timing for "reasonable notice" depends on the circumstances of the case and the availability of other physicians in the community. The physician is no longer legally obliged to follow the progress of the patient after the doctor-patient relationship has been formally terminated. Original case records, however, should be kept at least until the statute of limitations has run its course.

When the doctor withdraws from a case or the patient discharges the doctor to seek services elsewhere, the withdrawing doctor protects himself best by sending a registered letter with return receipt requested to the patient explaining why he is withdrawing from the case and offering his recommendations. This letter should be sent as a matter of record even if the reasons have been discussed in person. This "letter of record" also protects physicians from charges of abandonment if they are discharged by a parent or guardian.

Physicians should take caution during withdrawal from a case to protect themselves from charges of abandonment or liability when a patient acts contrary to professional advice. As a safeguard, the responsibility for discharge should be shifted whenever possible to the patient prior to discharge (Fig. 12.7). This contingency is

Dear Mrs. Smith:

As your condition requires professional health-care attention, I suggest that you place yourself under the care of another doctor as soon as possible. I find it necessary to inform you that I am withdrawing from professional attendance of your health care as you have refused to follow my advice and treatment.

If you desire, I shall be available to you for professional attention for a reasonable time after you receive this letter; however, such time shall not exceed 10 days as this will be ample time for you to select another doctor of your choice. If necessary, I will suggest the names of doctors in your area that I feel are competent.

With your approval and authorization, I will make available to the doctor of your choice your case and pertinent clinical records and findings.

Very truly yours,

_____

Figure 12.6. Sample letter to a patient from a doctor withdrawing from a case because of poor patient cooperation.

Dear Mr. Jones:

This will confirm our conversation of yesterday in which you discharged me from attending you as your doctor in your present illness. It is my professional opinion that your condition requires continued treatment. If you have not already done so, I recommend you select a specialist of your choice without delay.

Upon your request and authorization, I will furnish the doctor of your selection with a summary of my records of your case relative to the diagnosis and treatment program you have received at this office.

Very truly yours,

_____

Figure 12.7. Sample letter to a patient from a doctor responding to a patient's voluntary withdrawal.

necessary because the mental condition of a person suing has a great deal to do with the character of the suit. The date of withdrawal and the facts involved should be documented in the patient's records.

When withdrawing from a case, a physician is obligated to provide the patient with reasonable notice that he will be ceasing treatment. If a doctor wishes to stop a patient's care for refusing to follow his advice, making unreasonable demands, consistently breaking appointments, or failing to pay office fees, a private conversation should be held with that patient, followed by an explanatory registered letter with a return receipt requested. When a patient unwisely decides to end treatment for a disorder requiring attention, it is prudent for the doctor to discuss the potential consequences of this action with the patient. An explanatory registered letter to this effect is also helpful.

Accusations of Abandonment

Besides negligence, abandonment charges are another cause for malpractice. Abandonment is the unilateral termination of the professional relationship between a patient and the physician when the patient is in need of health care. Once a patient enters a

practice, the attending doctor is responsible for that patient's care until it is no longer needed or the doctor is properly relieved of this duty. That is, when a patient seeks treatment from a chiropractor and the DC provides the care, the doctor has an implied duty to continue treatment for the duration of the patient's illness or disability.

A refusal to treat a patient, certain complaints of a patient, or certain types of cases is not abandonment by itself. If patients are informed of practice restrictions before the doctor-patient relationship is firmed, refusal to make exceptions is not abandonment. If a doctor intends to limit his practice in any way, especially in an uncustomary way, it should be thoroughly explained to patients before they are accepted into the practice. Physicians are free to limit their practices about the location where services are rendered, the range of services offered, and the order they serve patients.

Courts maintain that a patient must prove five elements to recover against a doctor for abandonment. The plaintiff must show (1) that the doctor owed a duty to the patient; (2) that the doctor's act was unilateral; (3) that the patient was in need of continued treatment; (4) that injury was sustained; and (5) that the injury was caused by the physician's abandonment.

Abandonment suits against doctors have

at least quadrupled during the last two decades. The subject of abandonment involves so many complex variables that it is impossible to discuss each circumstance in detail, but certain principles should be acknowledged. For example, an abandonment suit may result if the doctor withdraws from a case without adequate warning to the patient or if the doctor fails to respond to an emergency call for help from the patient or for the patient from a relative and the patient later dies or suffers distress from the lack of professional attention. A doctor can usually justify whatever action he has taken; however, it is difficult to defend apparent inaction.

It is good policy to warn current and perspective patients that their problem should be checked promptly if the disorder worsens. If there is any doubt about the emergency nature of a situation, the doctor should see the patient or refer the patient to an emergency-care facility.

Other typical situations occur. For example, physicians may be charged with abandonment if they fail to appoint a substitute doctor when they are away from the office for an extended period (eg, convention, vacation). Doctors who refuse to treat a patient after the doctor-patient relationship has been established may be liable to charges of abandonment. Liability is also present when doctors fail to provide adequate follow-up care (eg, after referral), and an adverse event happens to the patient that would probably have been prevented by reasonable follow-up skill and care.

A physician must see a hospital-entered patient at regular intervals or be subject to charges of abandonment. Likewise, if a bed-ridden patient is not seen at regular intervals by his doctor and the patient takes a turn for the worse that could have been prevented by reasonable attention and attendance, the physician may be charged with abandonment.

Prior to vacationing, a doctor should insure he will not abandon a patient: (1) He must make provisions for a competent, compatible substitute with a similar treatment philosophy and style to care for his patients during his absence. (2) He must timely inform his patients that he will be un-

available on certain dates and that he has provided for continuity of competent care through the services of another doctor. (3) He must assure that he is not leaving one or more patients unattended who are in a critical condition.

Infection and Contagious Diseases

Besides notifying proper health authorities when appropriate, it is the duty of physicians attending patients afflicted with contagious diseases to warn and advise members of the family about the nature and danger of the disease so they may avoid acts that might spread the infection. Physicians who fail to give such warning are negligent and liable for damages to any person injured as a direct or approximate result of such negligence.

Physicians who know that they have an infectious disease and continue to contact patients must appraise their patients of this fact and/or take proper precautions. If this is not done and the disease is communicated to a patient, the involved physician may be responsible for the damage caused by his contact. State regulations vary considerably in this area of law.

Unethical Conduct

Ethical conduct will not be discussed here as it is well established in chiropractic education and the codes of various professional organizations. Although unethical behavior is not considered illegal conduct, it can under certain circumstances be used against a defendant in a malpractice case to establish a history of unprofessional deportment.

There infrequently is a type of female patient that will sue a male physician on grounds that the doctor made some type of personal advance during examination or treatment. Such patients are often those who have a fetish about being examined by a doctor of the opposite sex or those who feign that an advance was made in hopes that a financial award can be had. Precarious situations can be avoided by an assistant instructing female patients in the proper method of wearing a gown, explaining the procedures to be conducted, properly draping a disrobed patient, being present during a pelvic examination, and being alert to passing remarks of a patient that may reflect imagined sexual overtones.

Failure to Report or Advise

Health-care professionals have neither choice nor discretion when it comes to whether to report suspicions of abuse to a child or the elderly. Physicians who fail to report suspicions of abuse face *criminal* punishment, malpractice exposure, and possible other disciplinary sanctions.

In situations where there is a physical disorder that might impair safe operation of a motor vehicle or other types of machinery, the patient must be warned of any danger and a notation made in the patient's file that such warning was given.

CRIMINAL BEHAVIOR

Besides the civil actions of malpractice or unethical conduct described, a physician may become involved in a criminal act. The most common of these infrequent prosecutions are those involving misrepresentation, fraud, gross negligence, assault and battery, malicious injury, manslaughter, murder, and illegal abortion.

Misrepresentation

The doctrine of *caveat emptor* (let the buyer beware) does *not* apply in the doctor-patient relationship. If an erroneous statement accepted by another leads to a misunderstanding, anxiety, or fear of a condition that is different from reality, it can be held as a misrepresentation.

Misrepresentation usually occurs unintentionally, without any intent to defraud, such as in the use of terms that have a different meaning in chiropractic than is com-

monly held. For example, many chiropractors use the word "break" to indicate a type of cervical adjustment technic, the site of significant vertebral disrelationship, or an area of transition in a scoliotic curve. The average lay person, however, would interpret the term to mean a fracture.

Sometimes misrepresentation unintentionally occurs when a doctor tries to explain scientific facts by analogy: eg, "replace the bone," "straighten the spine," and "sprained muscles." Likewise, different words sound the same and become the grounds for inadvertent misrepresentation. For example, a vertebral "listing" may imply a spinal tilting to a layperson when the DC may be referring to a normal position.

Fraud

Fraud results when there is a deliberate act of intentional misrepresentation, deceit, deception, concealment, cheating, or dishonesty. Physicians must be on guard against entering fraudulent data within office literature, medicolegal reports, insurance reports, or depositions. The same is true when they act as witnesses in court in a misguided attempt to aid a patient or to receive undeserved compensation. Charges of fraudulent behavior are also found in offering exaggerated enthusiasm in a prognosis to a patient considering therapy, portraying hyperbolized consequences to motivate a patient through fear to continue care, or making unjustified claims in advertising.

Gross Negligence

Criminal negligence is established when gross inattention or indifference to a patient's welfare, disregard to a patient's safety, foolhardy methods, or serious lack of average competency can be proved to have resulted in harm to a patient.

In some states, it is a criminal offense for a physician to practice while under the influence of liquor or other drugs that would impair judgment. If the fact of intoxication is established, it is sufficient of itself to take the case to court. Health-care personnel can have no excuse for being under the influence of a drug while attending their work, and it would be extremely difficult to defend against a charge of gross negligence.

Attempting to examine or adjust through clothing could also be used in a charge of negligence. It would be difficult to establish that it is usual or customary or to defend a resulting diagnostic error.

Assault and Battery

While the definitions of assault and battery vary from state to state, it is generally held that failure to secure proper authorization before examination or treatment can result in criminal prosecution for assault (threat to touch in a harmful way) and battery (unlawful touching) even if there is no evidence of negligence and the results were beneficial.

No one has the right to touch another without the person's permission or the consent of a spouse, parent, or guardian if appropriate to the circumstances (eg, unconsciousness, incompetency, immaturity). Thus, liability might apply during a health fair or school screening clinic for scoliosis where examination is made without parental consent. Such situations of liability are also found in unprofessional "demonstrations" conducted at social gatherings and lay lectures. Even consent is invalid if the full scope of the procedures (eg, pelvic examination) or the risks involved (eg, adjustment of an arthritic hip) are not explained beforehand.

Malicious Injury

Injury from malice is also considered a criminal offense in most states. If it can be proved that injury was willfully and maliciously performed, there can be little doubt about the doctor's liability. In such situations, the involved doctor may be liable not only for the actual damages sustained but also for punitive damages. Such suits are usually the result of using excessive force on an uncooperative or obnoxious patient.

Manslaughter and Murder

These charges are rare occurrences in the doctor-patient relationship. They can result when gross negligence results in the death of a patient. Two examples on record are the death of a patient after a DC recommended that a diabetic patient stop insulin therapy and the death of a child with diphtheria where the DC failed to monitor the blood picture or seek consultation while the patient's clinical picture deteriorated.

COURT ACTIONS

Defensive Appearances

Initial Steps

If a patient claims he has been injured, no office personnel should make an admission of guilt. The doctor's malpractice insurance company should be contacted immediately for advice. If the doctor does not have malpractice coverage, he should immediately retain an attorney for advice and defense. If a patient's attorney should threaten suit, the complaint should be requested in writing. Neither the doctor nor his assistants should discuss the situation further with the patient or his attorney unless directed to do so by the doctor's attorney or insurance company. All office personnel should be polite but uninformative until proper counsel has been obtained. Office records should *never* be altered. Even the correction of a misspelling must be avoided. Jury decisions invariably arrive from emotional impressions more than they do from technical legal arguments.

Pretrial Preparation

An able assistant can be helpful to a doctor involved in a suit. If a doctor is called to testify in his defense, his attorney will instruct him of the pretrial preparation necessary. It is important that the doctor explains all usual and unusual aspects of the case and describes possible misconceptions in the charge. It is critical that his court testimony includes nothing that would surprise his attorney. An assistant may be able to aid the doctor's recall.

Certain basic procedures should be taken beforehand to offer the most optimal defense in court. Thorough preparation will save considerable embarrassment. For example, the doctor should review current texts and journals relative to usual and customary procedures in the type of case involved. He should carefully review all records, reports, x-ray films, laboratory data, letters, etc, concerning the case. As assistant can coordinate these records in an orderly fashion so that quick reference can be made to case history, examination findings, diagnosis, the therapy rendered, and patient response. The doctor can then review the questions his attorney anticipates asking all witnesses and their probable answers.

Record Check

A good defense cannot be made unless all records are accurate, complete, and comprehensive. The basic data that are usually required in a court appearance include entering, diagnostic, therapeutic, prognostic, and financial data. For this reason, the need for accurate detailed records has been emphasized in previous chapters.

Entering data should at least include the patient's name, age, address, occupation, and a description of what events occurred to the patient that brought him or her to seek your professional attention. Preferably, the patient's complaint should be in the patient's quoted words. A *dated* questionnaire that is completed and signed *by the patient* can be helpful evidence if a suit is filed.

Diagnostic data should include a detailed description of the doctor's examination findings that are concluded by his initial diagnosis. If x-ray films are used as evidence in the trial, an attorney may request an assistant who aided in taking the films to appear in court to identify the patient and the x-ray films.

Therapeutic, prognostic, and financial information is also important. For example, therapeutic data consist of the therapy applied and progress data, including dated entries for all patient visits and treatments. While an accurate prognosis can rarely be rendered during the initial care of a case, it is not unusual for the doctor to record a prognosis on the patient's last visit prior to the trial. Failure to bring a copy of the patient's financial account may be used by the opposition to insinuate excessive fees that are not usual and customary in the area.

Depositions

When a doctor's and/or an assistant's testimony is necessary in court in defense of a patient, attorneys sometimes prefer to take the testimony before trial. This advance testimony is called a *deposition*, and it is usually held in the doctor's office or an attorney's office.

Attorneys for both the plaintiff and defendant are present at a deposition, as well as a court stenographer. Prior to testimony, those to testify will be sworn in and questioned by both attorneys. Never give the plaintiff's counsel a tour of the office or allow him to take any brochures, booklets, or other material from wall displays. Also be alert that nothing said *is off the record!*

During a deposition in your office, the facilities function the same as a court of law and legal rules may not be broken. A courtroom atmosphere is maintained. Therefore, personnel should be warned not to interrupt the proceedings. Personal messages and telephone calls should be held until the proceedings are adjourned.

Chapter 13

Introduction to Clinical Duties of a Chiropractic Assistant

The scope of practice for doctors of chiropractic is determined locally by existing statutory enactment and judicial determination in the separate states. The same is true for chiropractic assistants: scope of duties and responsibilities are determined locally by existing statutory enactment and judicial determination. The procedures described here are general. They may or may not be applicable in a particular state at this time.

THE ASSISTANT IN A CLINICAL ROLE

Interpersonal Relationships in the Clinical Setting

Interpersonal relationships are defined as interactions taking place between individuals and other individuals and groups. There are two types of interaction—actions and reactions or cause and effect. When these interactions unite individuals and groups into teams whose members mutually support one another to accomplish their goal, good interpersonal relationships are devel-

oped. Since the goal of health service is to restore a patient to physical and mental health, good interpersonal relationships among office personnel and between office personnel and patients are essential.

Teamwork

It would be a mistake to think that good interpersonal relationships apply only in treatment units. Application must be throughout, including the reception area and the business desk. Through good interpersonal relationships, the patient receives the total physical and mental care that only team effort can provide. Authoritative studies have shown that patients sense and react to the harmony or lack of harmony shown by members of a health-care team as they perform their duties. Personnel who work well with their group and others experience a feeling of harmony and job satisfaction that is communicated to patients. Because of this feeling, patient care improves. When a patient feels secure and accepted and has confidence in the team effort of personnel caring for him, he is motivated to help himself toward recovery. Thus, good interpersonal relationships help all areas concerned with patient care.

Personal Guidelines

Development of good interpersonal relationships is not always easy. They are easier to describe than to achieve, and there are few never-fail formulas that apply in all situations. Some guidance can be given, however, for developing good interpersonal relations:

1. *Understanding Oneself.* The foundation for good relations with others is a state of good relations with oneself. Self-understanding and self-acceptance based on a realistic self-image and a genuine feeling of self-esteem justified by performance should not be confused with smugness. They are ingredients of an effective relationship with others. Just as each person is unique, each must accept the right of another person to differ within socially acceptable limits. Thus, in any instance in which relationships are less than the best, each person must first look within to see if a contribution has been made to the faulty relations.

2. *Understanding the Line of Authority.* Each CA team should clearly understand her responsibilities and authority. She should observe the prescribed organizational relationships both in accomplishing one's own assignment and in helping others. Each person functions effectively when working within the prescribed limitations. Every event must have goal lines and clearly defined boundaries.

3. *Understanding the Need for Patient Orientation.* Since patients experience a distinct feeling of loss of control over what is happening to them during health care, all personnel having face-to-face contact with them should be considerate of the emotions involved. Patients need kindness, sympathy, and simple courtesy, as well as competent technical care cheerfully given. If patients know what to expect from health-service personnel and what the office expects of them, they will be less apt to become apprehensive, critical, or demanding. Orientation is essential for cooperation.

Legal Aspects of Clinical Health Care

The public has special trust and confidence in the healing professions and in the institutions and organizations that provide health care and treatment. Since laws are written primarily to safeguard the public welfare, those that apply to the provision of health services have special significance. The fact that incompetence in providing health services might result in the loss of health or even of life is recognized.

Any activity involving remedial treatment of a patient is a medical act, and many paraprofessional activities are conditioned or dependent on the order and direction of the doctor-employer. The practice of chiropractic is strictly controlled by licensing, but chiropractic practice acts may permit delegation of certain health-care activities if certain conditions are met. The legal right to perform acts defined as medical acts is conditioned on (1) training and skill, which give the ability to understand the cause and effect of the act performed; (2) the act being performed on the order of a doctor; and (3) the direction and supervision of the act remaining the responsibility of the physician. The paraprofessional's right to perform various duties is also conditioned by the order, direction, or supervision of a licensed physician. In general, diagnosing, prescribing, and treating are medical acts in the generic sense.

Functions and activities for which paraprofessionals will be responsible are even more difficult to summarize than professional functions. Examples of established functions that a nonprofessional performing a clinical function would be expected to do include:

1. Environmental and physical management of the patient, providing suitable surroundings and personal hygienic measures for safety and comfort.

2. Factual observation, reporting, and recording of overt clinical signs and symptoms.

3. Performance of selected clinical procedures, with an understanding of cause and effect, in support of the doctor's orders.

4. Assistance in examinations, treatments, and diagnostic tests and procedures under the direction and supervision of the doctor.

A listing of typical duties of a chiropractic technical assistant is shown in Figure 13.1

Clinical Negligence

There is no uniform code of health-care law, but there are laws that have special significance in care and treatment areas. A basic rule of law applying in the provision of health services is the *rule of negligence*, explained in the previous chapter. Every one, professional and nonprofessional, has an absolute duty to conduct himself and his property to avoid injury to the person or property of others.

Although the spirit of service to others is a key principle in the performance of health-care duties, there are responsibilities extending beyond being kind and thoughtful in the provision of services. When services are provided, there is an obligation to use due care to assure that the patient is not injured by negligence, which can be defined simply as failure to exercise due care in relation to a person to whom care is due. But law is not usually so simply defined. A more complicated legal definition of negligence is "the doing or failure to do the act, pursuant to a duty, that a reasonable person in the same or similar circumstances would or would not do and the acting or nonacting is the proximate cause of injury to another person or his property."

Law holds every individual responsible for his acts of negligence. Negligence is commonly held to be an unintentional injury, but once an act has been performed and injury results, the performance of the act and the consequence of the act are facts. Thus, negligence is one of the most common causes for lawsuits against health-care personnel. Examples of the effects of negligence include injuries caused by faulty equipment, burns from applications of heating devices, improper use of traction, therapy errors, falling, and careless handling of instruments.

The law of negligence applies in almost all medicolegal problems that arise when, in the course of treatment, something is done that interferes with the rights and privileges of a patient. Under our form of government, however, there is legal recognition of unforeseeable, unavoidable, or inevitable accidents. Responsible authority provides for investigation to establish the facts of an accident or incident, and the facts are usually obtained when five questions are asked: when, where, who, what, how? These questions are not asked to establish guilt or innocence but to establish the *facts* on which a legal decision can be made.

Laws Governing Licensure

Professional practice acts are laws controlling the practice of legally recognized professions. The purpose of these acts is to protect the public from persons unqualified to practice. In general, professional practice acts (1) define the chiropractic profession; (2) provide standards that control the preparation for practice; (3) provide for licensure; and (4) through licensure, define by law who shall be licensed to practice and under what terms.

A license is a legal document permitting a person to offer to the public one's skills or knowledge in a field where such practice would otherwise be unlawful without a license. Licensure provides for rights and obligations. Thus, a major responsibility of a person licensed to practice a profession is that this person must act with the skill and care normally expected of a person claiming professional competence.

There is no uniform federal professional practice act, so requirements for licensure under professional practice acts vary from state to state. This is because under the Constitution each state is responsible for passing its own laws regulating the control of professions, trades, and occupations.

Currently, licensure as a chiropractic assistant is not necessary in the various states; however, several states are contemplating licensing of CAs. A desired goal is that each school conducting CA courses will be accredited by an appropriate accrediting agency that is recognized by a state licensure board for chiropractic assistants.

TYPICAL TECHNICAL ASSISTANT DUTIES

Diagnostic Assistance

- Assists in the doctor's diagnostic procedures.
- Records the doctor's examination findings.
- Records general body measurements.
- Records height and weight data.
- Gathers vital signs, general vision data.
- Collects blood and urine samples.
- Conducts in-office laboratory tests.
- Prepares patient x-ray identification markers.
- Conducts assigned x-ray patient positioning and exposures.
- Conducts x-ray film processing.

Therapeutic Assistance

- Conducts certain physiotherapeutic applications.
- Conducts massage and muscle therapy.
- Explains and distributes diet and exercise regimens.
- Teaches routine home-therapy and rehabilitative procedures.

Clinical Administrative Functions

- Processes work and school leaves or absences.
- Processes narrative and medicolegal reports.
- Processes state health reports (ie, reportable diseases).
- Processes external laboratory requests.
- Maintains laboratory data files.
- Checks outside laboratory invoices.
- Maintains roentgenography files.
- Checks clinical supply shipments.
- Maintains clinical supply inventory control.
- Sterilizes clinical instruments.
- Maintains cleanliness and sanitation of clinical areas and equipment.

Patient Relations

- Orients patients to pertinent equipment and procedures.
- Explains the necessity of patient cooperation for optimal recovery.
- Teaches good health habits and hygiene.
- Performs assigned counsel to patient's family when necessary.

Figure 13.1. Some typical responsibilities of a technical assistant. These functions are performed under the supervision of a licensed practitioner, in conformity with state laws and regulations.

GENERAL CHARACTERISTICS OF TECHNICAL ASSISTANTS

Paraprofessional care is doing needful and helpful things for and with a sick or injured person to restore him to the best possible state of physical and mental health. These needful and helpful things include environmental, hygienic, therapeutic, and supportive measures to protect the patient against contracting any additional pathologic condition, physical or emotional. Body, mind, and spirit must all receive consideration.

Several different members of an office team may assist a patient, each of whom contributes something toward the patient's welfare. Each member must understand and respect the role of others. Each must know where she fits in, what she is to do, to whom she is responsible, and how she is to do her part. Otherwise, proficient team function is impossible.

Basic Attributes

The technical assistant may perform any of a number of duties common to the provision of paraprofessional care for sick and injured individuals. To function effectively in this role, she must possess certain personal qualities. Many of these attributes are inherent (belonging to the nature of the individual), others must be cultivated and improved on, and all are interdependent. Basic traits of a reliable assistant include:

1. *Aptitude:* This is potential capacity for learning and performing a duty. The ability to anticipate needs of patients, to make appropriate decisions, and to adapt to various working conditions; intelligence; and a fairly high degree of manual dexterity show an aptitude for paraprofessional duties.

2. *Interest:* Interest in a duty assignment is a reflection of morale and leadership. It is a strong motivating force to perform satisfactorily. Interest leads one to improve on abilities and job-related knowledge. Experienced assistants should strive to stimulate and encourage less experienced individuals.

3. *Attitude:* Attitude is a manner of acting, feeling, or thinking that shows the individual's disposition or opinion. It is the action that speaks louder than words. A desirable attitude is one that leads to (a) cooperation and understanding among people working together; (b) concern and consideration for the welfare of patients; and (c) a sense of satisfaction in knowing one's job, with a resulting series of positive accomplishments. The gratitude of patients who have been helped to recovery is an extra but not minor dividend.

4. *Personal Hygiene:* Personal hygiene is usually considered personal cleanliness. It is that, but it is also anything that promotes positive or total health, which includes mental hygiene.

• *Cleanliness:* Scrupulous body cleanliness and clean well-fitting uniforms, shoes, and underclothing are essential. Body odors are offensive, yet the offender may be unaware of her offense. Daily bathing, use of body deodorants, and good oral hygiene are assurance against such odors. It is also good practice to wear a freshly laundered uniform daily, especially in patient-care areas.

• *Mental Hygiene:* Mental hygiene is the practice of good habits of the mind. Good mental habits can be cultivated. These habits are as necessary to health as safe food and water are to body systems. A mentally healthy adult enjoys life, works well with others, and takes disappointments as a part of living. Tolerance and respecting the rights of others reflect good mental hygiene.

Classification of Procedures

1. *Routine Procedures:* Procedures performed on a repetitive basis, requiring little or no modification to meet individual needs of a patient.

2. *Basic Procedures:* Procedures developed to meet hygienic, comfort, and therapeutic needs of patients. Some of these procedures involve direct patient care such as positioning and measuring temperature, pulse, and respiration. Some involve indi-

rect patient care such as ensuring cleanliness, preparing supplies and equipment, and maintaining clinical records and reports.

3. *Simple and Complex Procedures:* The term "simple" must be considered in relation to the total situation. Four factors decide a procedure's simplicity or complexity. It is a simple procedure if (a) abilities required to perform the procedure are based on a limited knowledge of scientific facts, (b) it can be performed by following a defined protocol step by step, (c) it is performed for a patient whose clinical state is relatively stable, and (d) the instructional needs of the patient are minimal.

A variation in any of these four factors contributes to the complexity of a procedure. For example, preparing a patient for therapy can be a routine, basic, simple procedure, or it can be an exceedingly complex procedure, depending on the condition of the patient. In a simple situation, the assistant would be assigned to carry out the procedure with minimal assistance and supervision. In a complex situation, the assistant would be assigned to help the doctor (or another assistant) with some phases of care and would carry out other phases with supervision and direction.

ACCIDENT PREVENTION IN THE OFFICE

Safety means freedom from danger or hazard. It is attained through accident prevention. This, in turn, calls for maintaining safeguards for patients, personnel, and visitors. The safety of the patient must always be considered when providing patient care. This involves ensuring a safe environment, practicing safe work methods, and using equipment properly. Accident prevention is a responsibility shared by *all* members of the health-care team.

The main causes of accidents are negligence by personnel, careless work habits, improper use of equipment, and use of faulty equipment. Most of these hazards can be avoided if *all* personnel observe safety rules, practice safety measures, and recognize and eliminate or report potential hazards.

Promoting a Safe Environment

Following are ways to promote safety in the office environment:

1. Keep floors clean, dry, and free of objects that might cause a person to fall.

2. Keep corridors clear and well lighted.

3. Keep working areas well lighted and uncluttered.

4. Use care in handling sharp and pointed instruments and glassware.

5. Do not use chipped or cracked glassware.

6. Wrap glass connectors and glass tubing in a towel or protective gauze before twisting, pulling, or pushing them into rubber or plastic tubing. The glass connection and the tubing into which it is inserted should be of appropriate and matching diameters. Moisten (not by mouth) both insertion points for ease in assembling. Clean tap water is the common lubricant for unsterile equipment. A sterile solution is *required* for sterile assemblies.

7. Never pour any material from an unlabeled container, and never pour stock solutions or cleaning compound solutions in containers bearing labels of other substances. Keep poisons in locked cabinets and properly labeled.

8. Use proper body mechanics in moving and lifting objects. Report unsafe conditions to the doctor. Safety in handling patients and in carrying out treatments is imperative.

9. Monitor and give constant supervision to patients receiving treatment.

10. Know how to use and care for equipment properly. Read all directions in the operator's manual accompanying the equipment.

11. Use precaution when using electrical equipment. Examine the cords and plugs of electrical appliances before using them. Ar-

range electrical cords so that there is no danger any one will trip over them. Keep electrical equipment dry. Do not use faulty equipment; tag it, and report (and document) that it needs repair.

12. Know and obey fire regulations. Practice fire prevention. Enforce smoking rules for patients and personnel. Never dim lights by covering them with a towel or paper product. Be careful when using flammable fluids such as ether or oxygen. Discard used oil or wax cleaning cloths in metal containers. Report gas odors immediately. Know the location and operation of fire extinguishers. Know how to report immediately the detection of any smoke of unusual fumes.

MEASURING AND REPORTING CLINICAL DATA

The manner in which a patient is received in the examining or therapy area of the office is an important contributing factor to his attitude and therefore toward his recovery. A feeling of confidence must first be established. Entering an office sometimes stimulates a considerable amount of dread and apprehension in a patient. Admission procedures should be as brief and reassuring as possible. Personnel should show interest in the patient as an individual and make it apparent to him that his care is planned on a personal basis.

The patient's clinical record is prepared and maintained according to office policy. A clinical record includes the forms on which are recorded the medical record of a patient during one current, continuous episode of a disease, injury, or other condition. The accumulation of forms is properly referred to as the patient's clinical record file or chart. It serves as a basis for planning patient care, providing communication between physicians and members of other professional groups, and presenting documentary evidence of the course of illness and treatment.

Clinical records remain in the custody of their owner, the doctor, while the patient is under his care. They are always handled so that only authorized persons officially concerned will have access to them.

Assistants (either administrative or clinical) often enter information and assemble the forms in the prescribed order in the chart holder. They see that diagnostic and test reports are attached or inserted in the record file on receipt, after these reports have been seen by the doctor. Each form is placed in an approved sequence. As further laboratory reports, consultation reports, or other forms are completed, they are added to the record. Each form used must have complete and legible identifying data.

Observation of Patients

Observation of a patient is taking notice of signs and symptoms that may suggest the patient's physical or mental condition. Observation is essential at all times in a clinical setting, from the patient's admission until his discharge. The doctor depends on technical personnel to observe and recognize, report and record the patient's condition accurately during contact. Effective observation by assistants helps (1) to enhance the doctor's observation, (2) to aid the doctor in making a diagnosis and in prescribing treatment, (3) to decide the effects of a prescribed course of treatment, and (4) to modify care to fit the needs of a patient.

1. *Signs and Symptoms.* Clinical signs and symptoms are evidence of a patient's condition and any disability.

• *Signs* are objective evidences that can be detected by one of the senses (sight, hearing, touch, smell, or taste). They can be noticed by an observer as well as by the individual experiencing them. For example, a rash can be seen, a swollen area can be seen and felt, a snoring respiration can be heard, the odor of a patient's body can be smelled.

• *Symptoms* are functional rather than structural evidence. They may be objective and therefore noticeable by an observer, as well as by the individual experiencing them—or they may be strictly subjective (the individual's own sensations). Examples of subjective symptoms are pain, itching, nausea, vertigo, and ringing in the ears. Categories of functional and structural signs and symptoms are shown in Table 13.1

2. *Causes of Symptoms and Signs.* There are two main groups of symptoms and signs to know to become efficient: (1) those caused by the disease or injury with which the patient suffers and (2) those relating to health care; i.e., those caused by the therapy.

3. *Training and Developing Power of Observation.* To increase skill in observing the patient's condition, the technical assistant should (a) increase her background knowledge, (b) take an active interest in the patient, (c) develop a sympathetic understanding of the whole patient, and (d) strive to be a good listener, attentive and accurate. The assistant can increase her knowledge by conscientious and accurate use of all senses and by accumulating a fund of information from books and from the doctor concerning symptoms to expect in various patient conditions. She can give attentive interest when the patient states how he feels. She can also try to anticipate the patient's emotional and physical needs and discomforts and do what can be done appropriately to relieve him. Lastly, she can be accurate and conscientious in the performance of

procedures that uncover signs of illness such as noting pulse rate and rhythm, respiration rate and rhythm, and blood pressure levels.

4. *Reporting and Recording Observations.* Detailed reporting should be done away from the patient and out of his sight and hearing if possible, in order to reduce patient anxiety or misunderstanding. Comments made in the patient's presence should be appropriate to what the patient needs to know or hear about his condition. Plain, everyday, factual language is used in reporting and recording. The patient is always identified by name, and the time the observation was made is noted.

• Any clinical measure provided should be reported, including a statement whether the measure seemed to help or not.

• Complaints and signs of pain should be reported as precisely as possible. Such things as location, plus any statement from the patient that the pain is sharp, dull, aching, throbbing, constant, or knife-life, are important. If the patient is quoted, his exact words should be used. The patient should be asked how long he has had the pain. In observing him, particular note should be

---

Table 13.1. Functional and Structural Categories of Symptoms and Signs

Symptoms resulting from physiologic changes:

• *Altered function:* eg, convulsions, tremors, arrhythmias, various visual disturbances, paresthesia, and aberrant articular movement.

• *Decreased function:* eg, atrophy, flaccid paralysis, depression, bradycardia, constipation, numbness, dehydration, hypothermia, and articular fixation.

• *Increased function:* eg, hypertrophy, spastic paralysis, anxiety, tachycardia, diarrhea, pain, edema, fever, and articular instability.

Symptoms resulting from structural changes:

• Bone and joint infection with resultant soft-tissue reactions, subperiosteal calcification, decalcification, bone destruction, and infiltration processes.
• Congenital anomalies.
• Deformity—witnessed as abnormal changes in angulation, displacement, or loss of continuity.
• Degenerative processes.
• Endocrine and metabolic imbalances.
• Malignant and benign tumors.
• Trauma.

made of: (1) Position assumed to relieve the pain. Is he bent over, unwilling to take a deep breath or to straighten an arm or leg? (2) Measures previously used to relieve the pain. Did a specific therapy relieve him for a period? Did any change of position relieve him?

• *Observations to be made.*

It is important to note signs of health, indications of returning strength, and a feeling of well-being, as well as noting disabilities and signs of progressing distress.

Recording Initial Case History Data

In many offices, a clinical assistant is used to develop the patient's initial case history. Her notations will later be embellished by the doctor. The elements of a comprehensive patient history are often set up as follows:

A. Presenting symptom
B. Present illness
C. Health history
D. Accident history
E. Family history
F. Personal history (patient profile)
    Activities
    Diet and nutrition
    Education
    Hobbies and special interests
    Occupation and its environment
    Postural considerations
    Residences
G. Systems review

A typical medical history profile structure is described in greater detail in Table 13.2. Standard symptom descriptors for recording a patient's presenting symptom accurately are shown in Table 13.3.

MAINTAINING A HYGIENIC ENVIRONMENT

Disease and Injury

Health is a state of physical and mental well being in which the body can function fully with comfort and the ability to renew and restore itself. On the other hand, disease is any departure from health; it is any disorder of a body system that interferes with the normal operation of a body process. For the purposes of this chapter, *disease* (or sickness) will be defined as any departure from health caused by pathogenic organisms or another factor not involving an external physical force; *injury* (wound) will be defined as any departure from health due to an external physical force or environmental condition.

Broadly speaking, the recognized causes of disease are pathogenic organisms, improper or insufficient nutrition, degeneration of tissues and organs, congenital anomalies, and neoplasms. Predisposing factors increasing the probability of an individual becoming ill are age, inadequate self-care, emotional factors, sensitivity reactions, and lowered resistance. Diseases can be classified by their cause, duration, or severity. For example:

1. *Acute disease.* A disease characterized by a rapid onset and quick changes in its progress and symptoms. An acute disease is not necessarily a serious disease. The common cold, for example, is an acute disease that can be severe, moderate, or mild.

2. *Chronic disease.* A continuous or recurrent persistence of a disease.

3. *Primary disease.* A disease developing independently of any other disease.

4. *Secondary disease.* A disease that develops because of a primary disease or an effect of an injury. In a secondary disease, the body may have much less capacity to deal effectively with annexed function impairment.

Classification of Injuries

Injuries and wounds can be classified by type, location, and cause. The extent of injury is described as severe, moderate, slight, superficial (involving surface tissue only), or deep (involving tissues below the subcutaneous layer). When there is no break in the continuity of the skin or mucous mem-

Table 13.2. Medical History Profile Structure

Presenting Symptom	The presenting symptom (chief complaint) consists of a brief statement, preferably in the patient's own words, concerning his reason for seeing the doctor. It also portrays the patient's sense of priorities about his problems. The presenting symptom is the major problem for which the patient is seeking help. It is the response to such questions as, "What seems to be the matter?" or "How can I help you?"
Present Illness	This is a detailed description of the patient's current problems developed chronologically. After the presenting symptom has been discussed, the doctor should proceed to ask, "What else has been troubling you lately?" The interviewer's goal is to encourage the patient to relate all his or her problems so he can arrive at a comprehensive description of the present illness. The quality of this judgment is determined to a great extent by how thoroughly the beginning and course of the problem is understood, where the problem is located and its radiation, the problem's quantity and quality, what circumstances aggravate or aid the problem, and what manifestations are associated. Answers to these questions should be available for each complaint.
Accident History	Detail of where, when, and how each accident or severe strain occurred should be recorded. Ascertain the care administered, the scope and degree of trauma, the diagnostic tests taken and the care administered. In an automobile accident, for instance, it is important to know from which side the force came, the position of the patient at the time of impact and after. Was a seat belt or shoulder harness fastened? Did the patient's head strike anything? Was there unconsciousness? What were the immediate symptoms? What were the later manifestations? These and similar questions must be deeply probed.
Family History	Genetic factors are sometimes involved in diabetes, renal disease, hypertension, mental illness, heart disease, cancer, and allergies. Inquiries should be directed toward the health status of grandparents, parents, and siblings. Ages and causes of death are important. Determine if one or more members of the family is experiencing or has experienced symptoms similar to those presented by the patient.
Health History	In this assessment, inquiries should be directed toward childhood diseases, major illnesses, hospitalizations, operations, pregnancies (deliveries and abortions), allergies (air-borne, contact, medications, food), drugs, immunizations and reactions to such.
Personal History	This is a brief narrative of the patient's way of life: (1) life history, including usual day's activities, (2) education, (3) marital status, (4) occupational mental and physical stress, (5) personality and temperament, (6) hobbies and special interests, (7) habits, (8) religion, (9) diet, and (10) unusual financial burdens. The purpose is to form a mental picture of the patient's present life-style: home, work, and recreational activities to see if anything therein may be the cause of or contributing to the patient's health status and to gain insight into the impact of the patient's problems on his or her daily activities and vice versa.
Systems Review	The purpose of the systems review is (1) to determine malfunction in areas not covered in the present illness; and (2) serve as a check for a manifestation of the present illness that was previously overlooked or forgotten by either patient or doctor. What is pertinent depends on the patient's chief complaint, present illness, uniqueness of the patient, and degree of suffering. Whenever symptoms suggest involvement of a particular system or organ, questions should be directed to determine if any other possible symptoms normally associated with such a dysfunction are or have been present.

Table 13.3. Standard Symptom Descriptors*

Characteristic	Examples	
Alleviating-exacerbating factors	Cold Coughing Drinking Eating Exercise Heat	Lying Medication Nothing Rest Sitting Sleeping
Associated factors	Breathlessness Bruising Chills Dizziness Emotional tension Fever Headache	Loss of appetite Nausea Pain Palpitations Sleeplessness Sweating Swelling
Character	Aching Blocking Burning Coldness Color (red, blue, green, yellow, etc) Cramping Crushing Deep Dull Expanding Giving way Itching	Lightning pains Pressure-like Restriction Sharp Shifting Squeezing Stabbing Superficial Texture (soft, hard, thick, watery, etc) Throbbing Tingling Twinges
Course	Fluctuating Intermittent Progressive Rapid	Relieved completely Slow Stable Subsiding
Duration: *Complaint duration*	Recent (hours, days, weeks)	Long term (months, years, childhood)
Episode duration	Seconds Minutes Hours	Days Weeks Months
Location-radiation	From anterior chest to left arm From left flank to groin From lower back to left calf	From right upper quadrant to right scapula From left shoulder to left hand From upper neck to eyes
Number of episodes	Decreasing Increasing Frequent	Intermittent Occasional Date of last episode

Table 13.3. *continued*

Characteristic	Examples	
Occurrence	Morning	During sleep
	Afternoon	During exercise
	Evening	During meal time
Onset	Abrupt	Insidious
	Gradual	
Precipitating factors	Alcohol	Position change
	Environmental change	Resisted movements
	Foods	Weather change
Resulting life-style changes	Dependency	Recreation
	Diet	Sexual relations
	Exercise	Sleep
	Hygienic habits	Social relationships
	Personality	Work

brane, the injury is referred to as a "closed wound." When skin or mucous membrane is cut or penetrated, the injury is called an "open wound."

Injuries can be classified according to involved anatomical parts of the body as head wounds (subdivided into skull, face, and jaw wounds); chest wounds; abdominal wounds; wounds of the extremities (arms or legs); wounds of joints; and spinal or pelvic wounds. The part of the body most severely injured determines the primary classification of multiple wounds.

Classification by causes of injury or wound are abrasion, contusion, strain, sprain, dislocation, subluxation, fracture, incision, laceration, penetrating wound, perforating wound, puncture wound, and rupture.

Microorganisms

All things existing in nature are classified into three general groups: animal, vegetable, and mineral. Animal and vegetable groups are living and therefore classed as *organisms* (any living thing). Plants and animals too small to be seen singly except with the aid of a microscope are called *microorgan-*

isms. Varying in size, shape, and their effect on mankind, they become visible to the naked eye when they form colonies or groups.

Microorganisms belonging to the animal kingdom are called *protozoa;* those belonging to the vegetable group are the *bacteria, viruses, fungi (yeasts and molds), rickettsia,* and *spirochetes.* Protozoa cause such diseases as malaria and amoebic dysentery; spirochetes, syphilis. Most infectious diseases of man are caused by bacteria and viruses.

Microorganisms are found almost everywhere; in the air, on uniforms, on hands, on furniture, on feet, on flies and other insects, in bedding, and on the floor. They enter the body with every breath and every mouthful of food. Fortunately, many of these are nonpathogenic (unharmful) to man in small quantities. Furthermore, natural body defenses protect to a certain extent against the harmful types. As microorganisms are constantly present in our natural environment, complete absence of microorganisms on items commonly used is impossible. The goal is to have as few present as possible by using preventive measures against infection and disease.

There are many methods of destroying microorganisms, but some are more effective than others. Washing with soap and water or exposure to light, fresh air, heat, and chemicals are effective only with some microorganisms, not all. The only known methods assuring complete destruction of microorganisms are germicides, steam under pressure, burning, exposure to a gas such as ethylene oxide, and sometimes exposure to a bleach. Sometimes a substance will destroy a microorganism but not its toxin. Spores are extremely difficult to destroy.

Classification of Pathogenic Organisms

1. *Bacteria.* Bacteria are minute, one-celled organisms that may occur alone or in large groups called colonies. Each bacterium is independent and may live and reproduce by itself. Since bacteria are in air, water, food; on man-made objects or normally clean skin; and in the mouth, throat, and intestines of healthy human beings, the possible sources of disease and wound infection are almost countless. Pathogenic organisms responsible for diseases other than wound infections are usually inhaled or swallowed. Most bacteria flourish in moist, slightly alkaline, surroundings at temperatures near that of the human body. Under less favorable conditions they may continue to exist, without multiplying, for a long time. Usually, all but the tough spore-forming bacteria are eventually destroyed by exposure to sunlight or by drying. Boils, wound infection, lobar pneumonia, and strep throat are common bacterial infections.

2. *Viruses.* Viruses are protein bodies that are much smaller than bacteria. They multiply only in the presence of living cells. They cause measles, mumps, influenza, herpes, a form of hepatitis, and many other infectious ailments.

3. *Rickettsia.* Rickettsia are organisms that are larger than viruses but smaller than bacteria. They are carried and spread chiefly by insects such as mites and ticks and cause diseases such as typhus and Rocky Mountain spotted fever.

4. *Fungi.* Fungi (yeasts and molds) are simple plant organisms that are larger than bacteria. They most often attack the skin, including the hair and nails, causing such chronic infections as ringworm and athlete's foot. Infections caused by fungi are called mycotic infections and can be serious when internal organs are invaded. Vaginal and rectal infections commonly have a yeast origin.

5. *Worms.* A few types of worms can live inside the human body and cause disease. Hookworms and tapeworms are examples of common intestinal parasites. They are usually ingested in raw or undercooked meats or by placing contaminated fingers or utensils in the mouth.

6. *Protozoa.* Protozoa are one-celled animals, a few of which cause illness in man. Common diseases caused by protozoa include systemic infections such as malaria and amebic dysentery and local infections such as trichomoniasis, which affects the external genitalia and distal urinary tract.

Body Defenses Against Pathogenic Organisms

The body has three lines of defense to combat invading organisms. In the healthy, these defenses show a remarkable ability to fight off invaders and to withstand their effects. However, such factors as impaired nerve function, malnutrition, injury, overexposure, fatigue, and chronic stress lower natural defense reserves.

1. The first line of defense, the skin, protects the body's surfaces. It acts like a wall to keep out most bacteria and other potential invaders. Bacteria entering the nose and mouth find another barrier, the mucous membrane coating the respiratory and digestive systems. Some cells of the membrane secrete mucus that entangles bacteria and molds, while others also have cilia that sweep the invaders out of the body.

2. The second line of defense is systemic immunity. Previous encounters of the body with many types of bacteria, viruses, and al-

lergens (eg, pollen) often produce a specific resistance (immunity) to those particular organisms. This acquired immunity is associated with the formation of antibodies by the body. Antibodies interfere with pathogenic invasion in several ways. They may neutralize toxins, kill the organism, make the organism more susceptible to attack by white blood cells, or cause the organism to clot into little clumps that the white cells of the blood can usually destroy. A healthy nervous system and good nutrition play an important role in maintaining the integrity of the immune system.

3. The third line of defense is the lymphatic system. Lymph bathes, cleans, and lubricates tissues at the extracellular level, then flows through vessels into lymph nodes (rich in white cells) and the venous system. The nodes act as filters for the removal of invading organisms.

Body Reactions to Disease and Injury

Inflammation and Healing

Inflammation is the local reaction of the body to irritation or injury. It occurs in tissue that is injured but not destroyed. It is a defensive and protective effort by the body to isolate and eliminate the causative agent and to repair the injury. A certain degree of inflammation takes place following any type of injury (extrinsic or intrinsic).

Inflammation can be caused by physical, chemical, or thermal agents, or by invading organisms. The signs of inflammation are redness, heat, swelling, pain, and disturbance of function. These five cardinal signs are produced by reaction of blood vessels and tissue in the injured area. When injury occurs, the blood vessels dilate, thus increasing the supply of blood to the injured area. The blood is warm and red, producing the first two signs, redness and heat. As the blood vessels dilate, their walls leak and blood serum escapes into the tissues. This results in swelling. The swelling produces pressure or tension on nerve endings caus-

ing pain. Disturbance of function can result from the effects of impaired circulation by the swelling or the pain (eg, protective spasm).

While changes in blood vessels produce the cardinal symptoms of inflammation, the body reacts further to injury in another way. White cells and fibrinogen (a clot-forming substance) leave the dilated blood vessels and move through the tissue fluids to the site of injury. These cells make a wall around the area to seal off the injurious agent. Within this area, the white cells work as scavengers (phagocytes), ingesting small particles of foreign matter, dead tissue debris, or bacteria if present.

As the source of injury is overcome or expelled, tissues return to normal. White cells disperse, and blood vessels return to normal size. Fluid accumulations disperse through the lymphatics and veins. If tissue has been severely destroyed, it is replaced by scar tissue. Thus, the dilation of blood vessels and the mobilization of white cells against the injuring agent are the two basic reactions in the inflammatory process. Proper therapy enhances these processes and attempts to control them from overreaction.

Healing is a process related to inflammation, for both are started by tissue injury (overt stimulation). It would be ideal if the body could heal itself by replacing all damaged tissues with an exact counterpart; then, an eye would be replaced with a new eye and a tooth with a new tooth. But very few tissues are replaced in kind. Examples of tissues that may replace themselves are liver tissue, kidney tubules, and connective tissue. Bone, which is one type of connective tissue, may replace itself if broken; that is, the broken bone is repaired by the formation of new bone tissue.

Healing in most tissues is, however, a process of replacement: the destroyed tissue is replaced by scar tissue (a fibrous type of connective tissue). If brain cells are destroyed, they are replaced by connective tissue. If heart muscle is injured, the damaged fibers are replaced by connective tissue. When a tooth is pulled or an eye is lost, the sockets are filled with connective tissue. Hence, replacement by scar tissue is the usual order in healing. The healing process takes place in one of two ways—by primary union or granulation.

Infections and Therapeutic Measures

Infection is the entry and development or multiplication of an infectious agent in the body. The agent can be any pathogenic organism. Factors contributing to the ability of the infectious agent to produce infectious disease include (1) the number and kind of invading organisms, (2) the ability of the body to resist infection, and (3) the virulence of the infecting organisms. *Virulence* is the ability of pathogenic organisms to overcome, at least temporarily, the defensive reactions of the body (phagocytosis, antibodies, and lymphatic involvement) that are mobilized when infection occurs. Virulent organisms can multiply rapidly within body tissues and to form toxins (poisonous waste products).

Different pathogenic organisms produce dissimilar toxins. Some toxins destroy tissue cells, some dissolve blood cells (hemolysis), and some are absorbed rapidly into the blood to cause toxemia, a generalized systemic reaction to infection.

The general therapeutic measures used in treating acute inflammation and infection are based on the need to (1) aid the body in mobilizing its natural internal defenses, (2) relieving pain, (3) promoting healing, (4) preventing complications, and (5) controlling the spread of infectious organisms if present. The typical measures used are rest, elevation of an involved extremity, use of cold or heat, professional therapy, promotion of elimination of waste products, and aseptic procedures to prevent and control the spread of infection.

1. *Rest.* Rest allows all the body's defensive effort to be directed toward healing and combating infection, rather than be veered by physical activity. This can hasten the defensive process of walling off an infected area, which will prevent the body from absorbing too much toxin. Rest conserves energy reserves and reduces movement of an inflamed and painful part.

2. *Elevation.* Elevation of an inflamed extremity allows the force of gravity to help drain swollen tissue spaces and blood vessels. The degree of elevation needed to promote tissue drainage of an extremity is above heart level. To provide this degree of elevation for the arm, the hand and elbow must be higher than the shoulder; for the leg, the foot and knee must be higher than the hip.

3. *Cold and Heat.* The effects of cold and heat are as follows:

• *Effect of cold.* Cold causes the blood vessels to constrict and tends to reduce edema. It reduces the pain of inflammation because it reduces the sensitivity of nerve endings in the skin. When applied immediately after an injury, it prevents or relieves swelling. The use of therapeutic cold is highly beneficial in the early stages of inflammation.

• *Effect of heat.* Heat applied to the body dilates capillaries and increases blood flow near the surface of the body (vice versa for deep tissues). The improved superficial blood supply increases the number of white cells in the area to combat pathogenic organisms and aid the formation and localization of pus. Due to increased circulatory flow, tissue nutrition and elimination of metabolic products are quickened.

4. *Professional Therapy.* The type of therapy used in combating inflammation and infection is determined by the doctor when the infecting organism is identified. Cultures, smears, or the development of particular signs or symptoms help in this identification. Besides anti-infective or anti-inflammatory therapy, specific therapies to improve nerve function and nutrition, normalize circulation (arterial, venous, lymphatic), relieve pain, enhance elimination, and assure rest (eg, support) are often indicated.

5. *Promotion of Elimination.* Toxic materials are eliminated largely by the kidneys. A daily urinary output of at least 1000 ml is necessary. An increased fluid intake (4000 ml or more) helps dilute toxins and protect the kidneys. Increased fluid intake also

helps bowel elimination, inhibits dehydration, and serves as a medium for supplemental nutrients.

6. *Aseptic Procedures.* Asepsis means freedom from disease-producing microorganisms.

Psychodynamic Pain Control

An assistant should strive to reduce excessive patient anxiety, which is produced by the pain itself or by the threat of pain. Anxiety reduces a patient's pain reaction threshold and triggers systemic responses. Just as anxiety can cause physical illness that may result in pain, so can pain produce anxiety. Patient anxiety can often be reduced simply by letting the patient talk, never leaving the patient in pain alone, helping the patient deal with stressful situations, and expressing empathy. Conversational distraction and diversion, reassurance, hope, and therapeutic suggestion can increase pain tolerance. Gaining the patient's trust and confidence is of vital importance in any pain therapy.

The Prevention of AIDS Transmission

Acquired immunodeficiency syndrome (AIDS) features total collapse of the body's immune system, thus making the body defenseless against a multitude of diseases—especially infections, pneumonia, and cancer. The *human immunodeficiency virus* (HIV) is commonly associated with AIDS. Transmission is essentially from blood to blood; viz, sexual contact, blood transfusion, mother to fetus, and needle sharing by drug addicts.

Evidence does not show ordinary social or occupational person-to-person contact to be a factor in transmission. Nor can the virus be communicated by airborne transmission or contact with laundry, food, beverages, or drinking containers. AIDS is considered a blood borne or sexually transmitted disease. However, because the disease is on the increase (and thus its risk), a CA that might become exposed to the blood of in-

fected patients should take special precautions. That is, the blood and body fluids of *all* patients should be considered suspect.

Whenever near contact with a patient's blood is anticipated, gloves should be used and changed after direct contact with each patient and handling each patient's specimens. This is especially true when performing venipuncture or dressing an open wound. Special care must be used in handling used acupuncture needles and pinwheels. All syringes should be the disposable type.

Any instrument that invades tissues or the vascular system or comes in contact with mucous membranes should be sterilized before reuse. HIV is rapidly inactivated by being exposed to common household bleach (sodium hypochlorite). A solution should be made daily in any ratio from 1:10 to 1:100. For instruments that might be corroded by bleach, commercial germicides are available.

CHIROPRACTIC PEDIATRICS

Pediatrics is that area of interest in chiropractic that deals with (1) the diseases of children and their treatment, and (2) the child's development and care. It is important for anyone involved in health care to realize that a child is not a "little adult."

An assistant should realize that illness has a distinct effect on the average child's personality and behavior. The developing personality can be affected by illness; eg, "being different" because of illness can definitely change a child's personality. The assistant can be of help once she understands the child's feelings.

A child patient needs much closer observation than an adult patient. It is well that assistants learn to recognize the types of behavior that suggest specific conditions or problem areas. This recognition includes *fear* and *withdrawal.* The assistant should also realize that the quiet good child may be suffering the greatest trauma. Among the common causes of behavioral problems are: (1) The child's response to examination and treatment as a threatening situation. (2) The belief that the illness is a punishment for previous "bad" behavior. The child may have been told that he will become sick if he does or does not do so and so. (3) Negative attitude of parents that affect the child and lead to tantrums, refusal to cooperate, and attempts to "run away." (4) The belief that sickness is a punishment from a revengeful God for some "sin." In such cases, you can expect different reactions on different days; sudden behavioral changes are common.

A proper psychologic approach is necessary to prevent as much trauma to the child as possible and to accomplish health-care objectives. Use as little force as possible and then only that which is absolutely necessary. The following approaches are often helpful in dealing with children:

• Never lie to a child; never threaten a child. Tell the child that the treatment or procedure is given to make him well. Offer some explanation even if the child is crying. Remember that a child's attention span is short, especially in the very young. Keep explanations brief and positive. Do not allow him to be in a position where he can say no.

• Do not tell a child of forthcoming treatments or other needs until immediately before they are performed, as the child will probably become anxious, but *do* inform him. Reward him for acceptable behavior by your approval. Do not talk down to a child, but be sure he understands you. Use the terms his family uses. Also, use his nickname, as he may not recognize his formal name.

• Attempt to keep him busy and distracted from unpleasant situations. Make games of procedures if possible. Consider each child an individual with rights of dignity and modesty, and respect these rights.

If misbehavior occurs despite everything you can do, his misbehavior must be dealt with, but certain rules can be used for guidance. Keep discipline firm, just, and consistent. Deal with misbehavior as it happens. If you ignore the breaking of rules, you weaken discipline and confuse the child. However, do nothing when extremely angry. Explain the reason for rules. It will help the

child (after 2-½ years) to understand that he is not just being pushed around—that each rule has a reason behind it. And be sure you have a good reason.

Keep your voice calm. It does no good to scream at a sick child (his illness is probably affecting his behavior) or to talk in a loud voice to a child who does not understand you. Avoid bribes; they let a child remain immature and be paid for it. Do not ridicule a child. Whenever possible, give the child a reason for changing undesirable behavior to good behavior. Make your suggestions positive rather than negative. Tell the child what to do, not what not to do.

When a child is being treated in the office, consider the feelings of the parents. If they are worried and tense, the child will soon sense it. Parents may be disturbed because of: (1) guilt feelings, (2) fear of the unknown, (3) fear of improper care for the child, (4) fear that the child will suffer, or (5) fear that the child may transfer his love to the people who now care for him during this time of need. These worries make parents often illogical, unreasonable, and demanding. Although this puts an extra load on both assistant and doctor, they must understand people and their problems and be empathetic with them.

Stages of a child's growth and development are not marked with sharp lines. Mental development, for example, begins long before it is discernible. The degree of its progress is influenced by the child's environment and his social development. No child will fit within any absolute pattern, but certain norms can be established. A child will change and develop continuously, but the growth can be uneven, with wide fluctuations within the normal. For example, most children will crawl before they walk, but they will not all crawl at the same age.

The inheritance of an individual can vary widely from that of his parents, since each parent cell supplies half of the 46 chromosomes that begin the new cell. Also, some characteristics are dominant and other are recessive. It is unlikely for a family of high intelligence to have a child with low intelligence or vice versa. A child is also likely to have personality traits similar to those of his parents.

Environment, too, is different and variable. An infant deprived of love and affection from birth will have a slower mental growth than one that is read to, loved, "mothered," and kept comfortable. A child brought up in a family where a foreign language is spoken may seem stupid when he enters a school where English is spoken. Even the health of the mother before the child's birth affects his development. There are also physical differences between the sexes and between people of various nationalities and races. Thus, many factors must be considered by personnel who furnish health care to children.

Here are some tips an assistant can teach parents to help their children: stress good posture habits, suggest regular exercise, and encourage a well-balanced diet and periodic health check-ups.

CHIROPRACTIC GERIATRICS

Geriatrics is that area of interest in chiropractic concerning the diseases of the elderly and their treatment.

Chronological age does not make a person young or old. Some people are young in spirit at age 85; others are old at 25. However, the chronological age of 65 is arbitrarily considered the dividing point between the middle age and old age. This is the age when retirement from active employment generally takes place and when Old Age and Survivors Insurance (Social Security) benefits begin.

The Aging Process

The process of aging begins at birth and stops only with death. It is a very gradual process, yet changes occur in a fairly predictable pattern, with the rate of change varying from one individual to another. It is a period that is often marked by mental confusion and vagueness. An assistant must consider this confusion and help the patient as much as possible. She also must be aware that the old person's body has undergone many other changes. The physiologic

changes seen in the geriatric patient can be generally classified as loss of elasticity in tissues and a general slowing down of physiologic processes. Table 13.4 shows typical consequences of old age.

Age may be a factor in musculoskeletal injuries. As a group, older persons are susceptible to fractures. Their vision and hearing may be impaired, increasing the possibilities of accidents. Atrophy of bone occurring as part of the aging process also may increase susceptibility to fracture. Besides, aged people may be poorly coordinated, have a decline in postural ability, and have difficulty walking. With age, one's level of proficiency progressively deteriorates (but to a highly variable degree).

Aged persons may also have disorders predisposing them to musculoskeletal injuries, eg, "drop attacks," cerebral ischemia, osteoporosis, cancer of the bone, arthritis, "dizziness," postural hypotension, muscular weakness, or neurologic disorders affecting locomotion. While disorders such as these predispose a person of any age to injury, the elderly person is particularly at risk because of other concomitant factors accompanying aging. Older women are especially prone to fractures. Men most commonly sustain fractures in their younger years, up to age 45. Musculoskeletal injuries range in severity from relatively minor soft tissue injuries to severe, crushing fractures.

The Assistant's Approach

An assistant who helps with geriatric patients must be emotionally stable and even-tempered: a condition known as *maturity*. The aged may be talkative, secretive, hostile, rude, and childish, but the assistant must not take their remarks personally. She must try to understand their behavior and react in a nonjudgmental tradition.

The assistant must express sincere interest and affection for the geriatric patient. Old people recognize and detest insincerity. All office personnel should be kind, tolerant, and patient. These qualities come only when you have gained true respect for yourself; only self-respect can be given to others. One cannot pour from an empty container.

Table 13.4. Normal Consequences of Old Age*

	Examples	
Decreased Organic Function		
Skin	Decreased subcutaneous fat Increased wrinkling	Sweat gland atrophy
Eyes	Decreased accommodation Decreased pupil size Lens discoloration	Lens opacities Presbyopia
Ears	Decreased perception of high 　frequencies	Intolerance to loud noises
Cardiovascular system	Decreased cardiac output Decreased elasticity of heart 　and peripheral vessels	Decreased heart rate 　adaptation to stress
Respiratory system	Decreased ciliary activity, 　hyposensitivity	Decreased cough reflex Decreased lung elasticity
Gastrointestinal system	Decreased calcium absorption Decreased colon motility	Decreased hydrochloric acid Decreased salivation
Genitourinary system	Decreased renal circulation Decreased sexual response Decreased urine osmolality Prostate enlargement (with 　outflow obstruction)	Vaginal mucous membrane 　drying and atrophy
Nervous system	Fewer hours of REM sleep Slower psychomotor 　performance	Slower righting reflexes
Musculoskeletal system	Decreased bone mass Decreased lean muscle mass Decreased ligament elasticity	Decreased muscle tone (lack of 　conditioning) Increased spondylosis
Endocrine system	Decreased estrogen secretion Glucose intolerance (decreased 　peripheral utilization)	Increased ADH response
Immune system	Absent thymic secretion	Decreased T cell function
Decreased Tolerance to Stress		
Mental/emotional	Decreased adaptability to 　change Decreased recall of current 　events	Decreased self-esteem Decreased vitality Increased tendency to 　depression
Physical	Easy exhaustion Excessive reaction to trauma	Intolerance to temperature 　extremes
Impaired Immunity		
	Increased susceptibility to 　infection	Increased susceptibility to 　neoplasms

Table 13.4. *continued*

	Examples
Miscellaneous	Increased atypical signs and symptoms	Increased susceptibility to multiple diseases
	Increased iatrogenic reactions from drugs	

*Adapted from Krupp et al, with minor changes.

A capable assistant will also have empathy (a projection of one's own personality into the problems and personality of another; a feeling *with* someone). If an assistant can imagine that she has lost her job, lost her friends, lost her sensory perceptions, lost her home, lost her ability to speak fluently, lost her health, and lost her self-esteem, then she can begin to understand the disagreeable stubborn outbursts of some elderly people. She must realize that hostility may be an expression of insecurity. She must also recognize the embarrassment that follows failure to do even a simple task by herself.

The admission of an aged person to a busy practice can be disruptive. Routines geared to the adult or younger patient will not meet the needs of the geriatric patient. Adapting routines and personnel habits is not without difficulty, but if the office is to fulfill its responsibility of providing health care to the elderly, it must be done. Older patients cannot and should not be rushed, particularly in the morning. An older patient will take almost twice the time as the younger patient. As an assistant, you must be aware of the time involved and plan accordingly.

Following are some helpful rules for caring for the aged:

- Do treat each as an individual.
- Do call by name such as Mr. Brown and Mrs. Green.
- Do be tolerant, patient, gentle, and kind.
- Do speak slowly and distinctly.
- Do help the patient to help himself.
- Do be extremely observant.
- Do be optimistic.
- Do not call old people "grandma" or "grandpa."
- Do not stick to procedure just for authoritative reasons.
- Do not shout.
- Do not do "everything" for the patient.
- Do not ignore minor complaints.
- Do not try to change life-long habits or life-style.

It will often seem easier and quicker to do something for the elderly patient rather than let him do it for himself, because it takes him so long. However, oversolicitous care and too much waiting on a patient forces him into a dependent role—a role he does not want and one that is incompatible with a healthy outlook on life. Avoid the temptation to take over. The aim of proper assistance is to permit the patient to do as much for himself as he can, with only a minimum of assistance from personnel. His small accomplishments mean a lot to him. Grant him what independence and self-esteem is possible. It is an act of love for a fellow human being.

Chapter 14

Typical Clinical Functions of a Chiropractic Assistant

This final chapter first explains how to physically assist the disabled patient and the patient in severe pain. Duties of a clinical assistant as assisting in patient examination, recording vital signs, and helping with various laboratory tasks are then described. The chapter concludes with an explanation of applying adjunctive therapy under supervision, explaining nutritional and dietary prescriptions, and assisting in the x-ray department.

ASSISTING THE DISABLED PATIENT

Office design must be planned carefully if the practice includes a large number of orthopedic cases. Affected patients often find it difficult to support themselves and move about because musculoskeletal disorders affect the locomotor and structural systems of the body. Devices to help the patient support himself and move about may include hallway handrails, grab bars by toilets, cushioned chairs with armrests, and so forth.

Applied Biomechanics

An assistant must know how to use her muscles to instruct patients how to use theirs. The combination of good posture and the use of proper body mechanics benefits both personnel and patients. This includes making the most efficient use of muscles, promoting optimal biomechanics, and avoiding strain and fatigue.

1. *Posture.* Posture is body alignment; the relative position of body parts standing, sitting, lying, or participating in any other type of activity. Posture determines the distribution of body weight and the consequent pull on muscles and joints. It affects the size and shape of body cavities, which, in turn, affect the position of the viscera. Circulation, respiration, digestion, and joint action are directly affected by posture. Body alignment favoring normal function and requiring the least strain reflects good posture.

• *In the standing position.* The back should be straight, feet firmly on the floor, about 4 to 6 inches apart to give an adequate base of support, with the toes pointing straight ahead or slightly toed out; head and rib cage held high; chin, abdomen, and buttocks pulled in; and knees slightly bent.

• *In the sitting position.* The back should be straight, with weight resting equally on the buttocks and under surface of the thighs (not on the base of the spine).

2. ***Body Mechanics.*** This is the coordinated use of body parts to produce motion and maintain balance. The use of biomechanical efficiency promotes the efficient use of muscles and conserves energy. The following principles apply to any moving or lifting activity (objects or patients):

a. Face the direction of movement.

b. Use the large muscle groups of the legs, arms, and shoulders to lessen strain on the back and lower abdominal muscles.

c. Bring the object to be lifted or carried as close to the body as possible before lifting. This keeps both centers of gravity close together.

d. Bend the knees and keep the back straight when leaning over a work level.

e. Kneel on one, knee, or squat, and keep the back straight when working at floor level.

f. Push, pull, slide, or roll a heavy object on a surface to avoid unnecessary lifting.

g. Obtain help before attempting to move obviously unmanageable weight.

h. Work in unison with an assistant. Give helpful instructions, and agree to a signal to start lifting.

To avoid back strain, the application of the principles of body mechanics provides a safe, efficient, and comfortable means of moving and positioning patients who cannot properly assist themselves. Preparation for these procedures includes:

• Knowing what the patient can do and should be encouraged to do in order to assist. Check doctor's orders.

• Telling the patient exactly what is to be done and what he can do to help.

• Obtaining necessary equipment and arranging it conveniently near the patient.

• Obtaining necessary assistance before trying to move a difficult-to-manage patient.

The General Scope of Orthopedics

Orthopedics is the specialty that includes the investigation, preservation, restoration, and development of the form and function of the limbs, spine, and associated structures by therapeutic means. The basis of orthopedic assistance is understanding and applying the principles of biomechanics. While the application of these principles is a basic requirement in all health care, additional emphasis is needed when working with orthopedic patients.

The challenge in caring for the orthopedic patient is in devising ways to carry out basic care while understanding and working with orthopedic mechanical devices such as braces and traction devices used in aiding and treating the healing process of subluxations, joint disorders, muscle and nerve injuries, and other affections of the neuromusculoskeletal system. The injured part and associated structures must sometimes be immobilized, while at the same time circulation must be maintained and muscles exercised to prevent atrophy.

The average orthopedic patient is a long-term case. Following a period of intensive treatment, he must undergo a period of supervised convalescence to insure optimum recovery. He can be expected to resent the necessary restrictions imposed upon him and to become impatient or discouraged. Therefore, every orthopedic patient must be taught and encouraged to become as self-reliant as possible, while at the same time he must understand the limits ordered by the doctor to insure healing and regain optimal function.

The doctor of chiropractic is likely to encounter orthopedic conditions caused by subluxations, sprains, and strains of either a postural or traumatic nature. Besides injury to bones and joints, there are complicating factors of injury to muscles, tendons, blood vessels, and nerves. Degenerative diseases, congenital deformities, developmental defects, and postdisease or posttrauma paralysis and disorders often respond exceptionally well to chiropractic care.

Musculoskeletal and neurologic disorders often present similarities. Both can be long-term illnesses, both cause motion impairment, both require concern to prevent immobility complications, and both require the regaining of or compensation for musculoskeletal impairment or loss.

Innovative orthopedic devices are constantly being put into use. They are all directed toward a twofold aim: (1) to provide support for the injured part until it heals and (2) to prevent deformity and stiffness of injured tissues. Support for an injured part is often provided by bandages; adhesive or elastic strapping; slings; splints, including plastic inflatable ones; foam supports; braces; or casts.

To prevent stiffness, the patient must be encouraged to use the affected part as much as possible within the limits prescribed by the doctor. Rehabilitative physical therapy is usually begun as soon as possible and may be continued for an extended period following the initial healing of the affected part. The patient may need some type of mechanical support (e.g., cane, crutch, sling, brace, corset) for several weeks after he becomes ambulatory.

Pain, immobility, and changes in self-image can result in discouragement and depression in the patient suffering a severe musculoskeletal disorder. Because of her frequent contact with the patient, the chiropractic assistant can be an essential positive influence during periods of distress and do much to foster hope and motivation. But rehabilitation cannot be a haphazard process based on "hope" alone. Successful rehabilitation is not possible without the doctor's planning and scheduling. The CA must be alert to assist the doctor in achieving the goal(s) of the treatment plan.

A clinical assistant may be called on to perform periodic muscle strength, joint motion, and neurovascular checks and to monitor traction set-ups to assure correct application.

Assisting with the Orthopedic Patient

It is important that the patient has confidence in the assistant that no "accident" will happen when aided to move. The assistant must always be "safety conscious." When aiding, moving, or supporting a patient, especially one with an orthopedic disorder, keep three points in mind at all times: (1) be gentle, (2) provide adequate support, and (3) avoid sudden movements. Tell the patient ahead of time what is expected and how you are going to help. Handle the patient as carefully as you would a large pane of glass. Keep in mind those movements and positions contraindicated for a specific patient's complaint because adverse movements or positioning can easily produce unnecessary pain or tissue injury and interfere with the healing process. If you cause unnecessary or unexpected discomfort, it will be difficult to regain the patient's confidence.

In helping a disabled patient, offer your help on the affected side. It is this side where you can best contribute your strength and stability.

Patient Education

An able clinical assistant is a good teacher who helps patients learn about their condition, its treatment, and how the patient can cope effectively during the recovery process. The CA can help the patient learn the correct use of equipment, exercises, procedures to be done at home, and other aspects of self-care. Of course, this must be done with the doctor's approval and supervision. Teaching duties may include helping the patient learn proper body alignment during bed rest, range-of-motion (ROM) exercises to maintain joint mobility and strengthen muscles, correct positioning of limbs to prevent deformities and complications, and instructions about personal sanitation.

General Emergency Protocols Following Injury

The assistant can be helpful to the doctor when specific "don'ts" are kept in mind:

• Don't tell the patient your opinion of his condition. The situation may look bad to you, but in reality it may not be that serious.

• Don't diagnose the condition.

• Don't allow other patients or friends of the patient in the examining or treating room.

• Don't provide information about the patient to *anyone but the doctor.*

The chiropractic assistant should be aware of her professional and legal responsibilities. This will be determined by state law, personal training and experience, and office policy.

When an injured patient is brought into the office and the doctor is not immediately available, the following procedures should be followed if directed by the doctor:

1. If the injury has just taken place and is an emergency, have the patient lie down, then:

• Place a cold pack on the injured area. Gently elevate the part if this does not increase patient discomfort (eg, fracture, dislocation).

• Check for shock.

• If there is bleeding, place a compression bandage on the wound.

• Assure the patient is breathing properly. If not, call for emergency professional assistance or start artificial respiration if you are so trained and authorized.

• Remove necessary sports equipment or clothing from the patient so the doctor may examine the area that is injured on his arrival. If the patient is a football player injured during a game, *do not remove the helmet.*

• Record the patient's description (or that of a witness) of how the accident took place and the exact location of the injury.

• Calm the patient's fears.

2. If the patient is unconscious when brought into the office, check the following immediately:

• Respiratory rate
• Character of pulse
• Pupil size and reaction

• Presence of blood; do not overlook blood in an ear
• Presence of clear fluid drainage from the nose or an ear
• Deformity of any area of the body.

With the doctor's authorization, an assistant can help the patient suffering minor injury until the doctor is available. Especially in uncomplicated injuries, the simple mnemonic device I-C-E is helpful to remember. If refers to *ice, compression,* and *elevation.*

Keep in mind that the first step is ice or cold in some form, never heat. Injuries are accompanied by bleeding. When it's internal, it is called a bruise or contusion. Cold retards bleeding and helps to prevent subsequent swelling. Usually, the routine is to maintain the cryotherapy for several minutes, four times a day, for 2 or 3 days. As heat should be avoided initially because it encourages bleeding and swelling, the patient should avoid hot baths. A fast tepid shower is permissible. The next step, compression, simply means wrapping the wound in a sterile pressure bandage. It protects the area and helps to reduce swelling. The last step, elevation, helps to reduce the painful pooling of fluids with the help of gravity. In the event there is severe swelling or pain, the patient should see a doctor immediately.

In any emergency, the rules of first aid apply. Do not try to do the spectacular. Only do what you have been trained or authorized to do until professional help can be gained. Some common conditions for which you may be helpful until the doctor arrives are listed below.

Epistaxis (Nosebleed)

Common causes of nosebleed are facial injuries, sinusitis or other abnormalities inside of the nose, high blood pressure, fractured skull, and "bleeding" diseases. Keep in mind that your role is not to diagnose, just offer temporary first aid until professional attention is available.

To stop or retard nosebleeds, apply pressure by gently pinching the nostrils or roll up a sterile gauze pad and place it over the upper lip of the patient and press it against the nose. Keep the patient in the sitting position so blood that trickles down the throat will not be aspirated into the patient's lungs. Keep the patient quiet. Apply ice over the nose compress.

Internal Bleeding

Internal bleeding is usually not visible. Bleeding from the mouth, rectum, vagina (nonmenstrual) is serious and an indication of serious internal problems. Common causes of internal bleeding are from a perforating ulcer, a fracture piercing blood vessels, or a lacerated liver or spleen.

The following signs are common: The pulse is weak and rapid, the skin is cold and clammy, the eyes are dull and the pupils may be dilated and respond slowly to light, blood pressure falls, the patient is usually thirsty and anxious, and nausea may be present.

First aid should consider treating the patient for shock. Oxygen is often given by the doctor because the loss of blood will deprive the tissues of the oxygen necessary for survival.

Closed Soft-Tissue Injury

This type of injury is often caused by a blunt object striking the body with enough force to damage tissues below the skin, but the skin is not broken. Small blood vessels are ruptured, and they leak into tissues to cause pain and swelling. Blood is highly irritating to nerve endings. First aid is to apply cold over a pressure bandage and possibly elevate the part.

Open Soft-Tissue Wounds (PAIL)

Use sterile techniques whenever caring for any open wound.

- *P—Puncture Wounds.* These are usually caused by a knife, nail, ice pick, or another pointed object. If the object is still in the patient, do not remove it. The object might have cut a large blood vessel, and removal may start a massive hemorrhage. It should be removed in surgery. First aid is

the control of bleeding, bandaging, and have the doctor treat or refer.

- *A—Abrasions.* These are a traumatic loss of the top layer of skin, frequently called a "mat burn" or "brush burn." They are usually painful, and blood and lymph may ooze from the wound. First aid is to clean the wound, apply a sterile dressing, and then bandage the area. The doctor may recommend coating abrasions with an approved soothing antiseptic ointment.

- *I—Incised or Avulsion Wounds.* These occur where a piece of skin is torn off or left hanging. First aid treatment is to stop the bleeding, dress, and bandage. Any large tissue that has been torn loose should be sent with the patient to the hospital for other surgical treatment. Pack the tissue within an ice compress.

- *L—Laceration.* This is a cut in the skin by a knife, razor, or other sharp object that leaves either a rough or smooth edge. The wound might be deep enough to cut muscles and blood vessels. The wound usually has to be sutured. First aid is to stop the bleeding, apply a sterile dressing over the wound, and bandage the area.

Fractures

A fracture is any break in the continuity of bone. The causes are direct or indirect blows, twisting forces, severe muscle contraction, overloading of weakened bone, and bone disease. Types of fracture include "greenstick," transverse, spiral, oblique, comminuted, and impacted. The signs of fracture are deformity, tenderness, grating, swelling, discoloration, inability to use the part, and possibly exposed fragments of bone. First aid is to splint the area. The joint above and below the fracture site should be immobilized.

UNDERSTANDING THE PATIENT IN PAIN

Because many painful disorders are chronic in nature, pain management must be carefully planned by the doctor. General measures used to reduce pain and inflammation associated with neuromuscular disorders include resting the affected joint or extremity such as by bed rest or bracing; employing physical measures such as moist heat, massage, trigger-point therapy; therapeutic exercise; and professional therapy such as manipulation, reflex techniques, meridian therapy, and muscle-relaxing procedures.

Severe musculoskeletal pain causes the patient to be restless and change position frequently. The patient also attempts to protect the anatomical region from which the pain arises by either *muscle splinting* or *pseudoparalysis*. Muscle splinting is active, often involuntary, muscle contraction that immobilizes the part. Pseudoparalysis mimics paralysis but is not accompanied by loss of sensation.

Muscle splinting differs from muscle spasm in that relaxation of the affected muscles occurs at rest. Prolonged pain in bone, muscle, tendons, and joints with resultant long-term muscle splinting and pseudoparalysis may lead to eventual osteoporosis in affected and possibly adjacent bones, and joint contractures may develop.

Musculoskeletal disorders frequently feature associated muscle cramps or spasms. These are powerful involuntary muscular contractions shortening the flexor muscles. The result is extreme, often incapacitating, pain stimulated by ischemia or hypoxia of muscle tissue. They are often associated with myositis, fibrositis, and arthritis.

False Notions About Pain

An assistant should have a general understanding of the pain phenomenon because she will be frequently involved in attempts to understand and reduce the pain patients suffer. To do this, she must realize that there are three commonly held delusions about pain:

1. *It is a fallacy that all persons who are critically ill or gravely injured experience intense pain.* People who are critically ill (eg, with terminal cancer) or are gravely in-

jured do not inevitably experience severe pain. Some do; others do not.

2. *It is a fallacy that the greater the pain, the greater the amount of tissue damage.* Intensity of pain is not directly proportional to the severity or extent of tissue damage.

3. *It is a fallacy that pain is symptomatic of incurable illnesses:* "If I have severe pain, it's probably too late for the doctor to help me." Pain is an important symptom indicating treatment is necessary, and most painful conditions are treatable and curable.

The Components of Pain

In general, the sensation of pain may be said to have three component parts: (1) *reception* of the pain stimulus by pain receptors (free nerve endings in the skin and certain other tissues) and *conduction* of the pain impulses by nerves; (2) *perception* of pain in the higher brain centers; and (3) *reactions* to pain such as physical, emotional, and psychologic responses. Pain is a complex "mind-body" experience involving the *total* person rather than only the mind or solely the body. Indeed, the mental and physical experiences of pain are inseparable.

Types of Pain

There are many ways of discussing or explaining the various types of pain or severe discomfort. For example, pain may be referred to in terms of:

1. *Time of occurrence:* posttherapy pain.

2. *Duration or length of time experienced:* chronic pain, acute pain.

3. *Intensity:* mild pain, severe pain.

4. *Causative agent:* self-inflicted pain, spontaneous pain.

5. *Mode of transmission:* referred pain, projected pain.

6. *Ease of transmission:* inhibited pain, facilitated pain.

7. *Location:* superficial pain, deep pain, central pain.

8. *Source:* gallbladder pain, sacroiliac pain, headache.

9. *Manner experienced:* sharp pain, burning pain, dull pain.

10. *General causation:* organic pain, psychogenic pain, pretended pain.

Pain Classifications

Pain syndromes can be classified into three major groups: (1) superficial pain, (2) deep pain, and (3) central pain. Each group has certain unique characteristics.

Superficial Pain

Superficial pain usually has a prickling quality or a burning quality having a sudden onset. It is relatively uncomplicated since it is directly perceived and can be readily localized. Associated symptoms may include hyperalgesia, paresthesia, analgesia, tickling, or itching. It may also be associated with brisk movements, a quick pulse, and a sense of invigoration. Nausea is not associated. The quality of pain is a sharp sensation felt near the surface. Its duration is typically shorter and its localization tends to be more precise than that of deep pain. Superficial pain is often experienced as a point, surface, or line. Hyperalgesia of a primary nature occurs at the site of the original noxious stimulation.

Deep Pain

Deep pain arises from structures far below the surface. Three varieties may occur: (1) true visceral (splanchnic) and deep somatic pain, which is felt at the point of noxious stimulation and may or may not be associated with referred pain; (2) referred pain, which is pain experienced at a site other than the area of stimulus; and (3) pain from secondary skeletal muscle contraction. True visceral pain arises from a diseased organ. Deep somatic pain is characterized by its segmental distribution and originates from a lesion of vertebra, muscle, or other neuromuscular origin. Referred pain is projected from a viscus or other deep structure to the surface of the body. Secondary skeletal muscle contraction causes pain from spreading excitation within the spinal cord.

The associated symptoms of deep pain are autonomic responses such as sweating, nausea, vomiting, and at times low blood pressure, bradycardia, syncope, faintness, and perhaps shock. Abdominal muscular rigidity may be associated. Nausea is found with renal disorders, intestinal colic, and angina. The quality of pain is primarily dull, but it may be boring, crushing, throbbing, or cramping; and in mild cases, soreness or a deep ache may be perceived. The duration is often quite long, and localization is usually diffuse over a fairly broad area. Secondary hyperalgesia may exist and occur at a site far from the origin of the referred pain and/or tenderness. A superficial hyperalgesia may be associated. Muscle contraction and tenderness often occur, and a segmental spread of pain is frequently noted. The pain may remain confined to the original spinal segment, but it may spread into one or more neighboring skin segments (dermatomes).

Central Pain

Central pain is that for which no peripheral cause exists at the time the pain is perceived by the patient. Causalgias, phantom limb pains, and central pains are sometimes spoken of collectively as "central pain syndromes," though their etiologies differ. *Causalgia* (from injury to a peripheral nerve) is sometimes listed separately from central pain (from lesions within the CNS that affect pain pathways), but the fact remains that causalgia, phantom limb pain, and central pain are all related because all three are autonomic reflex pain syndromes. The etiology of causalgia is usually a penetrating wound or injury damaging peripheral nerves where the wound or injury does not completely divide the nerves. *Phantom limb pain* follows amputation of a limb. The common cause of *central pain* is a lesion within the CNS directly affecting pain pathways.

Because a patient's pain has special meaning to him, he may expect that those caring for him will intuitively understand his subjective view of the situation and respond appropriately. If your view of a patient's pain fails to coincide with his, a breakdown in communication occurs. Your response must consider the sociocultural, personality, and psychogenic factors involved.

Several elements join and contribute to a patient's nature of pain. Some general factors are (1) the integrity of the patient's nervous system, (2) the patient's state of consciousness, (3) previous experience, training, or conditioning of the patient, (4) the patient's age, (5) the patient's racial or ethnic background, and (6) the patient's state of fatigue, debility, or lack of sleep.

During the taking of a patient's history, assessment of the nature of a patient's pain is important. This assessment should record such items as the history of the origin and occurrence of pain; localization of the pain in the body; extension, radiation, and depth of pain; duration of pain; onset or pattern of pain; day pains; night pains; and character or quality of the pain.

The doctor is aware that the cause of pain must be sought. Pain is a symptom, not a disease itself. However, accurate recording of the nature of a patient's pain is helpful to the doctor in seeking its cause. Descriptive terms of direction and location are reviewed in Table 14.1. Keep in mind that a patient's description of his pain is influenced by his perception of the pain and what the pain means to him.

Assisting the Patient in Pain

Pain control demands all the imagination, knowledge, skill, and humanity the assistant has at her command. The clinical care of any patient experiencing pain (acute or chronic) must be based on an understanding of the pain being treated, the individual being treated, and the mode of treatment. The assistant's attitude itself can be an agent of pain production or an agent of pain relief in many instances. Plan with the patient in pain, listen to his suggestions, encourage his help, and always let him know if you are going to do something that may be uncomfortable.

Pain is a "cry for help" that should be respected regardless of its origin. The whole patient (body, mind, and spirit) should receive attention and care, not just the symptom itself.

There is a vicious cycle of suffering in

Table 14.1. Terms of Direction and Location

Anterior	Toward or nearer the front or belly side of the body; ventral.
Caudad	Toward the feet.
Cephalad	Toward the head or cranial vertex.
Contralateral	On the opposite side.
Distal	Away from the point of reference or origin.
Dorsal	Posterior.
Inferior	Situated or directed below; caudad.
Ipsilateral	On the same side (homolateral).
Lateral	Away or farther from the median or midsagittal plane; right or left of the midline; toward the side.
Medial	Toward or nearer the midline, median, or midsagittal plane.
Palmar	Referring to the palm or volar surface of the hand.
Plantar	Referring to the sole or volar surface of the foot.
Posterior	Toward or nearer the back or backside of the body; dorsal.
Proximal	Near the point of reference or origin.
Superior	Situated or directed above; cephalad.
Ventral	Anterior.
Volar	Referring to the palm of the hand or sole of the foot.

pain that the assistant should try to break whenever possible:

- Fear of being hurt leads to
- Apprehension that leads to
- Physical tension that leads to
- An increased degree of pain that leads to
- Increased suffering and anxiety that leads to a reinforced fear of being hurt.

A CA should strive to reduce excessive patient anxiety, which is produced by the pain itself or by the threat of pain. Anxiety reduces a patient's pain threshold and triggers systemic responses. Just as anxiety can cause physical illness that may result in pain, so can pain produce anxiety. This anxiety can often be reduced simply by letting the patient talk, never leaving the patient in pain alone, helping the patient deal with stressful situations, and expressing your empathy. Conversational distraction, diversion, reassurance, and hope increase pain tolerance. Gaining the patient's trust and confidence is indispensable in any pain therapy.

ASSISTING DURING PHYSICAL EXAMINATIONS

A physical examination is made by the doctor on the patient's admission to the practice. The paraprofessional assisting with this procedure aids the doctor and patient and obtains firsthand information about the patient's condition that may be used in reinforcing the doctor's health-care plan.

The assistant's role in the physical examination has a dual purpose. It is both patient-oriented and doctor-oriented. The assistant is concerned with the psychologic, social, and physiologic needs and responses of the patient prior to, during, and after the examination. Another purpose is to enhance the doctor's efficiency by preparing the patient, providing the supplies and equipment needed, helping the doctor during the actual physical examination, and conducting some tests and measurements independently.

When a female patient is being examined, a female assistant is expected to be present in the room at all times. If a male is being examined, a female assistant leaves the room during the examination of his genitalia.

The following terms describe a doctor's general method of examining patients:

1. *Inspection.* This means observation of the patient's expression, habitus, skin condition, posture, gait, body structure, and presence of scars or swellings. Internal surfaces of body openings are observed through instruments such as a speculum or scope. An ophthalmoscope is used to view the posterior area of the eye. An otoscope is used to view the eardrum.

2. *Palpation.* Palpation is the diagnostic use of touch and feeling. Changes in bone surface quality and position, skin texture, superficial muscle integrity, and normal body contours, and the detection of masses and enlarged organs not obvious by inspection may be perceived by palpation.

3. *Auscultation.* Listening for sounds indicating changes from normal is the act of auscultation. Areas of sound production in the body include the heart, lungs, blood vessels, gastrointestinal tract, and joints. The doctor may use his ears with or without the aid of a stethoscope.

4. *Percussion.* Percussion means tapping body surfaces. This may be combined with auscultation and palpation to differentiate hollow air-containing structures from solid or fluid-containing structures. A percussion hammer is used to test reflexes.

5. *Mensuration.* Height, weight, body dimensions, limb circumferences, temperature, pulse, respiration, spirometry, muscle strength, joint ROM, and blood pressure are common measurements included in a physical examination.

Basic Clinical Instruments

Basic clinical equipment on the examination tray should contain stethoscope, ophthalmoscope, otoscope, nasal speculum, laryngeal mirror, flashlight, penlight, tongue depressors, percussion hammer, pin wheel,

tape measure, skin pencil, rubber gloves, lubricant, paper tissues and towels, cotton
balls, thermometer, tuning fork, goniometer,
and any other equipment requested by the
doctor in routine examinations. Any instrument that may contact a patient's blood or
mucous membranes must be sterilized before and after use.

General Objectives

The physical examination is the most valuable diagnostic procedure used by the chiropractic physician to obtain information
about the functional and structural state of
an individual. The data gathered can be used
by the doctor for a variety of purposes.
Physical examinations are performed as a
general health assessment measure, whenever a person seeks health-care attention
for an illness or disorder, and are usually required for entry into most schools and for
the issuance of insurance policies.

Major goals of a physical examination include: (1) determining an individual's level
of health or physiologic function; (2) arriving at a tentative diagnosis of a health problem or disease; (3) confirming a diagnosis of
dysfunction or disease; (4) indicating specific body areas or systems for additional
examination or testing; and (5) evaluating
the effectiveness of a prescribed procedure
or therapy.

Typical Protocol

After the doctor has discussed the intended
examination with the patient and obtained
informed consent, escort the patient to the
examining room. Reassure him about any
equipment to be used with simple explanations. Take and record any measurements of
the patient directed by the doctor (eg,
weight, height, vital signs). Then help the patient on the examining table in the position
requested by the doctor. See Table 14.2.

Cover the patient with a sheet if he or she
is recumbent. Expose various parts of the
body as the doctor's examination progresses, draping with the sheet or a towel to
avoid unnecessary exposure of the pubic
area or female breast.

A common order of examination is head,
chest, abdomen, extremities, genitalia, rectum, and spine, but this depends much on
the patient's complaint and clues derived in
the patient's case history and systems review. Thus, the doctor checks the anatomical and physiologic function of the patient
from head to toe in performing the physical
examination. This may be done by body systems or by body parts such as head, throat,
chest, extremities, and so forth. Hand the
patient tissues and remind him to turn his
head away from the doctor when he is requested to cough during a chest or hernia
examination.

Despite the method used, the doctor will
observe, feel, listen, test, and measure for
evidence of normal or unusual function of
the part or system examined. As an example, the physician would examine the following organs and systems for evidence of
proper functioning:

- *Musculoskeletal system*—symmetry of
parts, mobility, coordination, etc.

- *Integument*—intactness of skin, presence of scars or rashes, color, warmth, texture, etc.

- *Eyes, ears, nose, and throat*—receptiv-
ity of sense organs, equilibrium, patency of
sense organ passages and cavities, etc.

- *Cardiovascular system*—heart rate,
rhythm, and force; adequacy of circulation
systematically and peripherally, etc.

- *Respiratory systems*—respiratory rate,
rhythm, adequacy of ventilation and gas exchange.

- *Digestive system*—adequacy of digestive organs and function.

- *Nervous system*—normal and pathologic reflexes, adequate motor and sensory
innervation, development of intellectual and
psychologic processes, etc.

- *Genitourinary tract*—adequacy of
urine control and elimination, patency of
membranes and passages, appropriate development of reproductive organs, etc.

Table 14.2. Terms of Position

Adams position	Standing with the heels together, the knees locked, and the spine fully flexed forward.
Anatomical position	Standing erect with the arms at the sides and the palms of the hands facing forward. The anatomical position is the position of reference when terms of direction and location are used.
Antalgic position	Any physical attitude assumed to gain some relief of pain.
Knee-chest position	Resting on the knees and upper chest (also called the genupectoral position).
Knee-elbow position	Resting on the knees and elbows (also called the genucubital position).
Lateral recumbent position	Lying on either the right or left side, with the hips and elbows flexed.
Lithotomy position	Lying in a supine position with the hips and knees flexed at right angles, with the feet usually supported by stirrups (also called the dorsosacral position); a variant of Simon's position.
Physiologic position	Standing in a habitual posture.
Prone position	Lying face down.
Simon's position	Lying supine position with the hips slightly raised and flexed, the knees are flexed, and the thighs are widely separated.
Sims' position	Lying in a lateral recumbent position with one arm behind the back; the thighs are flexed, the upper more than the lower (also called the semiprone or English position).
Supine position	Lying upon the back, face up (also called the dorsal position).

• *Endocrine glands*—adequacy of hormonal activity shown by certain characteristics of body function or development, size of glands, etc.

Various routine measurements are often taken and recorded by a trained assistant. Evaluation of temperature, pulse and respiratory rate, blood pressure, height and weight, and general visual acuity and hearing are common when indicated. Other procedures that the physician might require as part of the general physical examination include a blood profile, a urinalysis, spirometry, various x-ray films, an electrocardiogram, and electromyography.

During the examination, it is important for the doctor to consider the general physical and mental condition of the patient. Care is given not to create anxiety or hold orthopedic maneuvers beyond the tolerance of the patient, keeping in mind the possibility of underlying pathologic conditions.

Aid the patient in dressing if necessary, and make him comfortable after the examination. Clean and reset the instrument tray before the next examination.

While vital signs, color blindness examination, general visual acuity tests, and some other tests described can be conducted by a trained assistant, most examination procedures are performed by the examining physician. A full examination seldom exceeds 45 minutes because most tests require only a few seconds and the positions smoothly evolve through standing, sitting, supine, side lying, prone, Sims', knee-chest lithotomy positions and then conclude with final upright and sitting examinations. By witnessing the steps taken by a particular doctor during examination, the assistant can aid the doctor and anticipate the needs of both doctor and patient.

Summary Review: Typical Preparation Checklist

Following is a general performance checklist in preparing for and assisting the doctor with a general physical examination:

1. Assemble the equipment and supplies needed for the examination.

2. Check the patient's records, and obtain his cooperation.

3. Take any physical or functional measurements of the patient directed by the doctor and record the results in the patient's chart.

4. Prepare the patient for the doctor's examination: (a) Have the patient void, and save the specimen. (b) Have the patient undress and put on an examining gown. (c) Position the patient on the examining table in the position directed by the doctor. (d) Drape the patient.

5. Assist the doctor during the examination (hand him appropriate supplies and equipment as needed).

6. Assist the patient during the examination, giving reassurance and comfort.

7. Change the patient's position for appropriate examination, drape the patient, and have necessary instruments ready.

8. Provide for patient's comfort at conclusion of the examination by removing drapes, assisting in dressing, etc.

9. Carry out doctor's orders for additional tests or examinations.

10. Collect, clean, and return equipment used; dispose of and replace all supplies used.

Assisting with a Spinal Examination

Besides standard physical, laboratory, and roentgenographic examinations, the doctor of chiropractic includes a postural and spinal analysis, an innovation in the field of physical diagnosis and examinations.

General considerations in the spinal analysis include body type, occupational and outdoor activities, past trauma, and gross mechanical disorders. Then a detailed differential diagnosis of mechanical lesions considers pain, tenderness, hyperesthesia, anesthesia, joint and tissue mobility and locking, bone displacement or subluxation, muscle tone, soft-tissue changes, skin changes, reflexes, and associated roentgenographic findings.

The examination of intervertebral segments will usually include both active and passive tests. Active tests include active movements and auxiliary tests associated with active movements such as flexion, extension, rotation, and lateral bending. Auxiliary tests include joint-compression tests and evaluations for vertebral artery insufficiency. Passive tests include palpation, passive range of intervertebral movement, and movement of the pain-sensitive structures in the vertebral canal and intervertebral foramen. These findings are coordinated with other examination findings to arrive at a diagnosis.

Assisting with a Vaginal (Pelvic) Examination

A calm, matter-of-fact attitude will reassure the patient and help her relax. Necessary equipment includes vaginal speculae (different sizes), lubricant, clean latex gloves, basin of detergent solution, and a stool so the doctor may sit. If a PAP smear is to be taken, assure that the proper supplies are at hand.

Position the patient in a dorsal recumbent or lithotomy (feet in stirrups) posture. In the lithotomy position, the buttocks must be even with the break in the table. Drape the patient with a sheet while assisting her into position. Use the sheet as a diamond, one corner over chest, one corner wrapped around and tucked under each leg, and the fourth corner over the pubic area, to be folded back when the doctor is ready to do the examination.

Adjust the light and drape. Have lubricant ready to apply to the speculum and to the doctor's gloved fingers. Stand by the patient's side while the examination is made instead of attempting to look over the doctor's shoulder. After the examination, aid the patient to wipe off lubricant with tissues. Help her into a comfortable position and to arrange her clothing.

RECORDING VITAL SIGNS

Temperature, pulse, respiration (TPR) and blood pressure (BP) are called vital signs (VS) because they are important signs of the body for indicating the vitality of the patient. The evaluation of these signs and their interrelationship aid the doctor in arriving at a diagnosis and prescribing treatment. They also help to decide the amount and type of care necessary. For greater accuracy, these signs are checked while the patient is at rest. Any marked deviation from a normal range is a signal of distress expressed by the body. TPR and BP measurements of every patient are taken and recorded on admission. Subsequently, they are measured on the doctor's orders. Vital signs should be recorded immediately by the person who takes them.

Temperature

Body temperature is determined by the balance maintained between the heat produced and the heat lost through normal body processes. The heat produced is distributed by the circulating blood and dissipated through the skin, lungs, and excreta. When the balance of core temperature is disturbed, deviations in surface temperature result and serve as a guide to the physician.

A person's temperature tends to be lower in the early morning after a night of rest and higher in the evening after a day of activity.

The range is between 97° and 99°F when measured by a mouth thermometer. The average normal temperature is 98.6°F. An abnormal (elevated) temperature is called a fever. It is one of the first indications of infection or other disease process. Deviations that persist below the average normal temperature (subnormal) may be caused by shock, starvation, or a long-lasting illness (eg, tuberculosis). It indicates that body resistance is low.

Temperature Measurement

Temperature is measured by a clinical thermometer; viz, a glass shaft with the stem calibrated in 0.2°F. Within the stem is a hollow tube extending from a bulb end. The bulb contains mercury that, when warmed, expands and rises in the tube.

Two types of thermometers, oral and rectal, are commonly used. Each is identified by the shape of the bulb. The standard oral thermometer has a long slender bulb, but occasionally an oral thermometer with a short stubby bulb is supplied. The standard rectal bulb is specially designed to prevent damage to the mucosa when inserted into the rectum.

In reading the thermometer, the thermometer is held by the stem end. Notice the ridge side, with numbers below the ridge and lines indicating 0.2 fractions above. With the ridge at eye level, rotate the thermometer slowly forward and backward until the column of mercury is seen. Read the highest level of the column to the nearest 0.2°. Note that an arrow points to the average normal temperature mark.

In shaking down the thermometer, grasp the stem end firmly. Stand in a clear space to avoid striking anything with the thermometer. With a sharp downward wrist motion, shake the thermometer. Check the mercury column, and repeat the shaking procedure, if necessary, to lower the column to near the 95° mark. Always check and shake down the thermometer if necessary before using it.

Thermometers are fragile and must be handled carefully for safety and economy. Each patient should be provided with a clean, sanitized thermometer each time his temperature is taken.

Oral Temperature

Oral temperature is the most convenient method and can be used for adult responsive patients. Wait 15 minutes before taking the temperature if the patient has just had a hot or cold drink or has been smoking. Ask the patient to remove any chewing gum from the mouth. Instruct the patient to be seated. Check a clean, dry thermometer. Shake down to 95° if necessary. Normal oral temperature is 98.6°F or 37.0°C.

Handle thermometers by stem end only. Place bulb end under the patient's tongue where it will be near large blood vessels. Instruct the patient to close the lips firmly around the stem and to breathe through the nose. Leave thermometer in place for 3 minutes. Remove thermometer, and wipe with a tissue from stem to bulb to remove saliva. Read and record, using a decimal number; eg, 98.4°. Place the thermometer in a "used" oral thermometer holder.

Rectal Temperature

Rectal temperature is the most accurate method. It is used for all infants and young children and for adults who are irrational or who have difficulty breathing with the mouth closed. It is not used on patients who have had rectal surgery or have had a rectal disorder. Normal rectal temperature is 99.6°F or 37.5°C.

Screen the patient, then turn him on his side (Sims' position) and expose the buttocks. Life the upper buttock to expose the anus. Insert the well-lubricated bulb of the thermometer slowly and fully about 1½ inches into the anus. Hold thermometer in place for 2–3 minutes. Remove the thermometer. Wipe downward with tissue. Rectal temperature is usually 1° higher than that of oral temperature. Place rectal thermometer in "used" rectal thermometer holder.

Axillary Temperature

When temperature cannot be taken orally or rectally, it can be measured under the arm where the thermometer bulb can be surrounded by body tissue. An oral thermometer is used to record axillary temperature. Normal is 97.6°F or 36.5°C.

Pat the armpit dry with a tissue or towel. Place the bulb of the thermometer in the center of the armpit. Fold the patient's arm across his chest with his fingers near the opposite shoulder. Leave the thermometer in place for 10 minutes. Read, and record; eg, 100.2° (A). Axillary temperature is usually 1° lower than that of oral temperature. Place the thermometer in "used" oral thermometer holder.

Care of Equipment

Remove contaminated thermometers from "used" holders. Cleanse thermometers with gauze saturate with green soap. Cleanse each thermometer with a twisting motion from stem to bulb end. Rinse under tepid running water. Place thermometers in a basin of Wescodyne® solution, 150 ppm, for 30 minutes. Wash and dry thermometer holders. Place layer of cotton in the bottom of each. Remove thermometers from Wescodyne solution, rinse under running cool water and dry. Shake down thermometers if necessary and return them to their respective "clean" holders. Return small tray with holders to proper space on large tray used for diagnostic instruments. Boil all containers on thermometer tray and change the Wescodyne solution as directed by the doctor.

The Pulse

Changes in the character of the pulse may be caused by: (1) any factor interfering with heart function, (2) the volume of circulatory blood, and (3) the elasticity of the artery wall. Characteristics and rate of the normal pulse vary slightly in healthy individuals. Generally, the normal pulse is regular in rate, rhythm, and force (strength). The average range is from 60 to 80 pulse beats per minute. Normal variations occur; eg, an increased rate is associated with exercise and nervousness.

The term "thready" describes a weak, rapid pulse. "Arrhythmia" means both irregular intervals between beats and beats of unequal force. An irregular pulse must be counted for a full minute. A regular pulse may be counted for 20 seconds and the rate multiplied by 3.

Taking the Pulse

The pulse may be measured wherever an artery lying near the surface of the body can be pressed against firm tissue. Pulse is usually taken by applying slight pressure to the radial artery on the thumb side of the wrist. A watch with a second hand is used to time the pulse rate.

Radial Pulse Measurement

The patient should be relaxed and lying on a cot or sitting. The arm used (preferably the left arm) is extended in supination (palm up) and supported on the chair arm. (1) Place the tips of your first, second, and third fingers over the pulse point. Do not use the thumb as the thumb has its own pulsation that can be confusing. Press your fingers moderately to feel the pulse. Do not press firmly enough to shut off the circulation in the artery. Count the pulse. Remember, any irregularity in a pulse requires a full minute count. While counting, note the pulse's force and rhythm. (2) Record count and any irregularity.

Apical-Radial Pulse Measurement

This procedure is ordered by the doctor for an individual patient who has a questionable radial pulse rate due to a heart or circulatory disorder. A stethoscope is used for counting the apical pulse. In this procedure, there is simultaneous counting by two people of the apical beat of the heart and the radial pulse. The difference between the apical and the radial pulse, when counted simultaneously, is called the *pulse deficit.*

Explain the procedure and relax the patient. Uncover the left anterior chest area. Locate the apical beat of the heart below the left nipple (5th intercostal space). Listen for clear heart sounds through the stethoscope. Tell the other assistant to locate radial pulse. Begin simultaneous count on a signal such as "start." Count for a full minute. The apical count will normally be the same or slightly higher than the radial count.

Repeat the procedure to recheck if abnormal or subnormal. Record the apical and radial counts immediately in the patient's chart. Describe any unusual observation.

Respiration

The complete cycle of inhalation (breathing in) and exhalation (breathing out) is one respiration. Normal respiration is carried on automatically without effort and is regular in rate, rhythm, and depth. The normal range in adults is from 16 to 20 respirations per minute. Since respirations can be consciously controlled to some extent, they are counted when a patient is unaware of the procedure, if possible. Any disease or injury affecting the lungs, chest wall, or oxygen-carrying ability of the blood will usually affect the respiratory rate or the effort needed to inhale and exhale. If breathing movements are painful, the patient may be reluctant to take a breath of sufficient depth to aerate his lungs. He must be reminded and helped to take periodic deep breaths at regular intervals if possible.

The Respiration Rate

After counting the pulse and while the fingers are still on the wrist, measure the respiratory rate. If the patient thinks his pulse is still being counted, he has less tendency to control breathing consciously. Watch the rise and fall of the chest or upper abdomen. Count each rise, and continue to watch and count for 1 minute. Note the depth, rhythm, and ease of each respiration besides the rate per minute. Record both normal and unusual findings. If a normal rate is not recorded, it may later be inferred that the measurement was not taken.

Blood Pressure

The term *blood pressure* usually means the pressure of blood within the arteries. BP is written as a fraction, with systolic pressure the numerator and diastolic pressure the denominator; eg, in a BP reading of 120/80, 120 is the systolic pressure and 80 is the diastolic pressure. For adults, the average range of systolic blood pressures is 100–140; average range of diastolic pressure is 60–90. An abnormally high BP is associated with arteriosclerosis (hardening and narrowing of the arteries) and hypertension (vasospasm). An abnormally low blood pressure is associated with weakened heart action and lowered circulating blood volume as in shock.

Pulse Pressure

Pulse pressure is determined by subtracting the diastolic from the systolic pressure. Thus if the BP is 120/80, the pulse pressure is 120 minus 80 or 40. Pulse pressure indicates how well the heart and blood vessels are coordinated.

Blood Pressure Measurement

Blood pressure is recorded by a sphygmomanometer (the air-pressure device) and a stethoscope (the listening device). The cuff of the manometer contains a rubber bladder. When this cuff is wrapped around the upper arm and inflated with air, the air pressure registers on the manometer gauge, which is calibrated in millimeters of mercury. Measuring blood pressure accurately requires practice—the individual must apply the cuff properly, manipulate the air bulb, and simultaneously listen through the stethoscope and watch the gauge. Talking and other distractions during the procedure decrease the chance of an accurate measurement.

Necessary equipment includes (1) stethoscope, (2) sphygmomanometer, (3) container of 2 × 2-inch gauze pads in alcohol, and (4) record sheet and pen.

Check manometer. The cuff must be completely deflated and the gauge must register zero before starting. With an alcohol sponge, wipe the bell (or diaphragm) and ear pieces of the stethoscope firmly. Place the patient in a relaxed and comfortable position, sitting next to a table. Support the arm to be used at the level of the patient's heart. Expose the patient's upper arm. Remove garment if sleeve is tight. Place the wide portion of the cuff against the inner surface of the upper arm; wrap cuff firmly and smoothly, tucking in the narrow end to secure it. A snap-fastened cuff or a self-adherent (velcro closure) cuff may be available. Clip gauge of aneroid-type manometer to the cuff or place a mercury manometer on a firm, level, adjacent surface outside the patient's field of vision.

Locate the pulse of the brachial artery by palpating at the bend of the elbow with your fingertips. Place the bell or diaphragm of the stethoscope over the pulse point. Be sure the earpieces face forward when inserted in your ears. Tighten the thumbscrew of the air bulb with one hand while holding the stethoscope in place with the other. Inflate the cuff by pumping the bulb. Listen, look, and inflate the cuff about 20 mm above where the pulse sounds were last heard. It is at this point that air pressure causes the wall of the artery to collapse. Slowly loosen the thumbscrew of the bulb, and allow air to escape gradually. At the same time, watch the gauge. When the first distinct sound is heard, remember the number on the gauge. This is the *systolic pressure*. Continue to release the air pressure slowly. Look, listen, and remember the number on the gauge at which the last distinct sound is heard. This is the *diastolic pressure*. Record your findings.

With some patients, sounds may be heard to extremely low levels—all the way to the bottom of the gauge. If this occurs, note the level on the gauge at which the sound changes from a distinct tone to a dull, muffled beat. The diastolic pressure is recorded at the level at which the sound changes.

Open the valve completely, releasing all air. If any doubt exists about the reading, repeat each step to recheck. If doubt still exists, ask the doctor to recheck the BP. Never hesitate to request this recheck.

Record the measurements in the patient's chart. Remove cuff from patient's arm. Roll the cuff from the narrow to the wide portion before replacing in the case. Before closing the case, be sure tubing is not pinched or kinked. Wipe earpieces of the stethoscope including the lumen and the bell (or diaphragm) with an alcohol sponge before returning equipment to storage area.

ASSISTING WITH BASIC LABORATORY TESTS

Hematology

The study and practical application of clinical hematology reveal considerable information concerning physiologic and pathologic changes in the body. From an examination of a patient's blood, practical meaning will be derived by the doctor relative to the patient's symptoms and demonstrable signs.

Some tests are strictly routine such as a complete blood count (CBC). Even an apparently healthy person having a physical examination will have his blood cells counted, his hemoglobin measured, and possibly be tested for diabetes. After the examination and the study of the patient's history, the chiropractic physician may suspect signs of illnesses requiring further blood tests.

Just a few drops of blood can speed diagnosis and evaluation of disease. New tests are developing rapidly to measure changes in the blood due to illness that improve the accuracy and efficiency of chiropractic care. The use of these tests enables the doctor to individualize his therapeutic approach.

Chiropractic physicians often use an in-office modular testing system. The DC may either do the tests in his office or elect to send the sample to a commercial laboratory for analysis. The latter procedure is the most common.

Finger Puncture

The most simple procedure in blood sampling is the finger puncture. The equipment necessary includes a lancet, alcohol pledgets, dry sterile cotton, pipettes, and microscope slides.

To insure a proper amount of blood in the hand, have the patient place his hand in the dependent position. Cleanse the palm or surface of the selected fingertip with an alcohol swab. Dry the finger with sterile cotton. With a sterile disposable lancet, quickly prick the finger to a depth of from 2 to 3 mm. Wipe off the first drop of blood to eliminate

tissue fluids. The second drop is used for the examination. After the blood has been obtained, have the patient place a new sterile swab against the puncture site until bleeding has stopped. Place a band-aid over the puncture site.

Venipuncture

The best method for blood procurement is venipuncture. Venipuncture is the entering of a vein with a needle to obtain a blood specimen for laboratory tests. State legislation determines whether a technical assistant may do venipuncture.

The recommended site for venipuncture is the antecubital area of either forearm, just below the bend of the elbow. In this area, branches of two major superficial veins (median basilic or median cephalic) are prominent and usually accessible through a skin puncture. Alternate sites may be selected by the doctor for venipuncture such as accessible superficial veins in the dorsal area of the hand, wrist, or foot. This is required when arm veins have collapsed (eg, chronic diabetics).

The equipment necessary on a venipuncture tray includes disposable sterile needles with syringes, sizes 5 to 20 ml, individually wrapped; blood specimen collection tubes and vials from the laboratory. Vials for unclotted blood specimens contain an anticoagulant (always verify what type of tube is to be used); flexible latex tubing, about 18-inches long for a tourniquet; gauze, 2 × 2-inch squares in a container of prescribed skin germicide or foil packet; sterile package of dry 2 × 2-inch gauze; rubber or plastic protective sheet; and a towel. Never use a short length of tubing for the tourniquet. Although it can be stretched for application, it may be too constricting.

Following is the basic procedure:

1. Wash hands.

2. Place an identifying label on the blood-collecting tube.

3. Assure that the needle's bevel and the syringe graduations are visible on the same side. Test assembly by pulling the plunger back and forth to ensure that the needle is

not plugged and that the syringe works smoothly. Push the plunger all the way into the barrel toe to expel all air. Then replace the needle protector tube before setting the syringe assembly aside temporarily.

4. Position the patient so that his fully extended arm is supported at cot or table level. Roll his sleeve well above the elbow. Place protective sheet and towel under the extended elbow and forearm.

5. When applying a tourniquet, use soft-walled latex tubing about 18 inches in length. Place the tubing around the limb about 2 inches above the site of venipuncture (Fig. 14.1, top). Be certain that the tails of the tubing are turned away from the proposed site of injection. Apply tourniquet pressure firm enough to stop venous flow but not so tightly that radial pulse cannot be felt. Tell the patient to open and close his fist several times to increase circulation. Never leave a tourniquet tightened for more than 2 minutes at any one time.

Technique of Obtaining Blood by Venipuncture

1. Select a prominent vein in the antecubital area. Palpate the vein with fingertips and estimate tissue support (Fig. 14.1, bottom). The vein selected should not roll unduly. Ask the patient to close his fist and keep it closed until further advised.

2. Cleanse the skin over the selected area with germicide-saturated gauze, using firm circular movements from center outward. Allow the skin to dry. Discard gauze in waste basin.

3. Pick up syringe. Remove needle protector tube, and insure that the plunger is all the way down in the barrel. Grasp syringe with needle bevel up. Place forefinger on needle hub to guide it during insertion through the skin and into the vein.

4. Position yourself to have a direct line of vision along the axis of the vein to be entered.

5. With your free hand, draw the patient's skin below the cleansed area downward to hold the skin taut over the selected puncture site. Place the needle point, bevel up, parallel to and about a half inch below the venipuncture site.

6. Holding needle at approximately a 30° angle, insert it through the skin, lower it slightly, and then move it forward parallel to the vein for about a half inch.

7. Direct the needle point into the vein with a slight sideward movement. A faint "give" will be felt. On entry into the lumen of the vein, blood will appear in the syringe. Advance the needle slightly, watching for increased blood flow. Take care to prevent penetrating the vein through the other side by keeping the needle at the same angle.

8. If venipuncture is successful, obtain the blood specimen. Hold the syringe and needle steady with one hand, and use the other hand to aspirate by gently pulling on plunger to obtain the required amount of blood.

Note: If venipuncture is unsuccessful, withdraw the needle slightly and insert again to direct the needle point into the vein before withdrawing the needle from the skin. On repeated failure, release the tourniquet, withdraw the needle, and place a dry sterile 2 × 2-inch gauze square over the needle site as the needle is withdrawn. Notify the doctor before attempting to enter another vein.

9. When releasing the tourniquet, ask the patient to relax and open his clenched fist. The tourniquet is removed after obtaining the specimen but before withdrawing the needle from the vein.

10. Place a dry sterile 2 × 2-inch gauze square over the needle site and withdraw the needle. Ask the patient to keep his arm extended and to press the gauze against the puncture area for 2 or 3 minutes.

11. Collect the required blood specimen from the syringe as soon as possible, before blood starts to clot. Remove the needle from the syringe and run the blood down an inner side of the collection vial, using gentle pressure on the plunger to avoid foam and injury to blood cells. If the vial contains anticoagulant, insert stopper and gently invert sev-

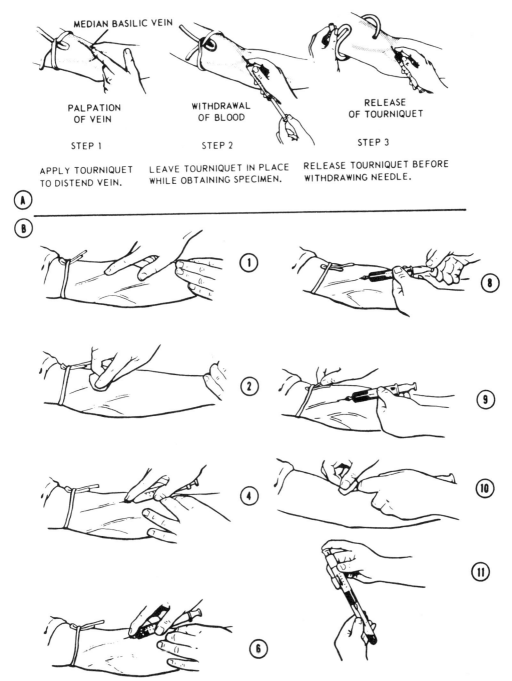

Figure 14.1. Top (A), applying a tourniquet for venipuncture; bottom (B), steps in obtaining blood by venipuncture.

eral times to mix. Never shake the blood collection vial.

12. If more than one specimen is needed, tubes must be changed without removing the needle. See Figure 14.2. Adjust patient's sleeve and leave him in a comfortable position.

Alternate Measure: Vacutainer

An alternate method of venipuncture is shown in Figure 14.3.

Care of Equipment

1. If a disposable syringe is not used, immediately aspirate cold water into the reusable syringe and needle. Use care to protect yourself from needle puncture.

2. If disposable equipment is used, place needle protector on needle and snap needle off shaft to prevent reuse. Hold the disposable syringe in a folded towel and break the syringe before discarding it in a waste receptacle.

3. Remove tourniquet and protective sheet from under the patient's arm. Check the puncture site. Usually, no dressing is needed after the initial pressure period. If blood continues to ooze from the puncture site, apply a dry sterile 2 × 2-inch gauze pad and adhesive tape or a sterile adhesive compress strip. Be sure to record venipuncture and the specimen collected in the patient's chart.

Urinalysis

Sometimes both routine and microscopic examination of the patient's urine should be carried out. These tests have been simplified to such an extent that within a minute or two the doctor can have five quantitative analyses as well as the specific gravity of the urine. The equipment needed includes reagent test strips; urinometer and cylinder; urine specimen cups; and a microscope, centrifuge, and glass slides if a microscope examination is to be made.

Procedure

During the routine examination of urine, note its color and report as either yellow, straw, or amber. Note turbidity and report as clear, hazy, or cloudy. Note quantity and specific gravity. Fill the cylinder about 80% full with the patient's urine. Gently insert the urinometer into the sample with a spinning motion so no bubbles cling to the urinometer scale. Read the urinometer at the point where the scale parallels the meniscus of the urine column.

In a quantitative analysis, dip the reagent strip into the urine sample. Read the results by comparing the colors to the chart furnished in this order: pH, protein, glucose, ketones, and occult blood.

Microscopic Examination

In a microscopic examination, the urine must be centrifuged for 5 minutes prior to examination. After this is completed, decant the supernatant liquid, and place a drop of the sediment on a clean glass slide. Cover with a cover slip, and microscopically examine the urine. Report findings such as casts, bacteria, pus cells, blood cells, and epithelial tissue.

Glossary of Common Tests and Their Abbreviations

Albumin/Globulin Ratio	— A/G Ratio
Blood Urea Nitrogen	— BUN
Calcium/Phosphorus Ratio	— Ca/P Ratio
Complete Blood Count	— CBC
C-Reactive Protein	— CRP
Serum Creatinine	— Creatinine (SER)
Urine Creatinine	— Creatinine (UR)
Erythrocyte Sedimentation Rate	— ESR
Fasting Blood Sugar	— FBS
Lactic Acid Dehydrogenase	— LDH
Mononucleosis agglutination	— MONO

IF IN VEIN WITH NEEDLE BEVEL UP:

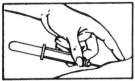

(1) USE THUMB AND 2D FINGER OF LEFT HAND TO GRASP BOTTOM OF HOLDER.

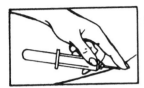

(2) GENTLY PRESS PAD OF LEFT-HAND INDEX FINGER OVER NEEDLE BEVEL, AS IT IS POSITIONED IN VEIN, TO STOP BLOOD FLOW.

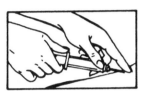

(3) PLACE RIGHT-HAND THUMB AGAINST HOLDER FLANGE, KEEPING IT AWAY FROM TUBE, USING THUMB TO PUSH AGAINST FLANGE. WRAP RIGHT-HAND FINGERS AROUND TUBE AND PULL TUBE OUT WITH PRESSURE FROM FINGERS.

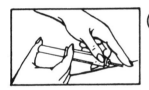

(4) STORE FILLED TUBE SAFELY. PICK UP NEW TUBE, PLACE TWO RIGHT-HAND FINGERS BEHIND HOLDER FLANGE AND USE RIGHT-HAND THUMB TO PUSH TUBE ALL THE WAY ONTO PUNCTURE NEEDLE. RELEASE LEFT-HAND FOREFINGER FROM VEIN TO LET TUBE FILL WITH BLOOD.

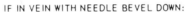

IF IN VEIN WITH NEEDLE BEVEL DOWN:

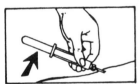

(1) WITH LEFT HAND, RAISE TUBE HOLDER, TO PRESS NEEDLE BEVEL AGAINST LOWER VEIN WALL AND OCCLUDE BLOOD FLOW.

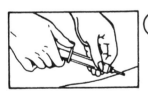

(2) PLACE RIGHT-HAND THUMB AGAINST HOLDER FLANGE, KEEPING IT AWAY FROM TUBE. USING THUMB TO PUSH AGAINST FLANGE, WRAP RIGHT-HAND FINGERS AROUND TUBE AND PULL TUBE OUT WITH PRESSURE FROM FINGERS.

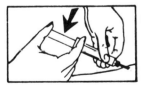

(3) STORE FILLED TUBE SAFELY, PICK UP NEW TUBE. PLACE TWO RIGHT-HAND FINGERS BEHIND HOLDER FLANGE AND USE RIGHT HAND THUMB TO PUSH TUBE ALL THE WAY ONTO PUNCTURE NEEDLE. LOWER TUBE HOLDER TO RE-POSITION NEEDLE IN VEIN LUMEN, LET TUBE FILL WITH BLOOD.

Figure 14.2. Method of changing tubes; top, needle with bevel up; bottom, needle with bevel down.

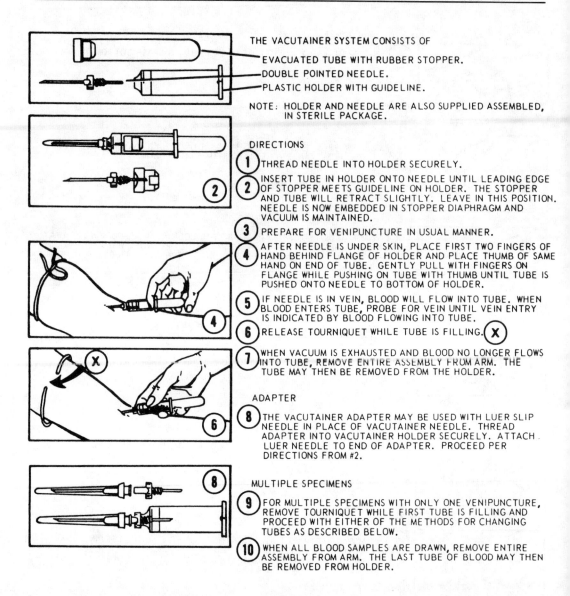

THE VACUTAINER SYSTEM CONSISTS OF

EVACUATED TUBE WITH RUBBER STOPPER.

DOUBLE POINTED NEEDLE.

PLASTIC HOLDER WITH GUIDELINE.

NOTE: HOLDER AND NEEDLE ARE ALSO SUPPLIED ASSEMBLED, IN STERILE PACKAGE.

DIRECTIONS

1 THREAD NEEDLE INTO HOLDER SECURELY.

2 INSERT TUBE IN HOLDER ONTO NEEDLE UNTIL LEADING EDGE OF STOPPER MEETS GUIDELINE ON HOLDER. THE STOPPER AND TUBE WILL RETRACT SLIGHTLY. LEAVE IN THIS POSITION. NEEDLE IS NOW EMBEDDED IN STOPPER DIAPHRAGM AND VACUUM IS MAINTAINED.

3 PREPARE FOR VENIPUNCTURE IN USUAL MANNER.

4 AFTER NEEDLE IS UNDER SKIN, PLACE FIRST TWO FINGERS OF HAND BEHIND FLANGE OF HOLDER AND PLACE THUMB OF SAME HAND ON END OF TUBE. GENTLY PULL WITH FINGERS ON FLANGE WHILE PUSHING ON TUBE WITH THUMB UNTIL TUBE IS PUSHED ONTO NEEDLE TO BOTTOM OF HOLDER.

5 IF NEEDLE IS IN VEIN, BLOOD WILL FLOW INTO TUBE. WHEN BLOOD ENTERS TUBE, PROBE FOR VEIN UNTIL VEIN ENTRY IS INDICATED BY BLOOD FLOWING INTO TUBE.

6 RELEASE TOURNIQUET WHILE TUBE IS FILLING. (X)

7 WHEN VACUUM IS EXHAUSTED AND BLOOD NO LONGER FLOWS INTO TUBE, REMOVE ENTIRE ASSEMBLY FROM ARM. THE TUBE MAY THEN BE REMOVED FROM THE HOLDER.

ADAPTER

8 THE VACUTAINER ADAPTER MAY BE USED WITH LUER SLIP NEEDLE IN PLACE OF VACUTAINER NEEDLE. THREAD ADAPTER INTO VACUTAINER HOLDER SECURELY. ATTACH LUER NEEDLE TO END OF ADAPTER. PROCEED PER DIRECTIONS FROM #2.

MULTIPLE SPECIMENS

9 FOR MULTIPLE SPECIMENS WITH ONLY ONE VENIPUNCTURE, REMOVE TOURNIQUET WHILE FIRST TUBE IS FILLING AND PROCEED WITH EITHER OF THE METHODS FOR CHANGING TUBES AS DESCRIBED BELOW.

10 WHEN ALL BLOOD SAMPLES ARE DRAWN, REMOVE ENTIRE ASSEMBLY FROM ARM. THE LAST TUBE OF BLOOD MAY THEN BE REMOVED FROM HOLDER.

NOTES

1. TUBES WITH POWDERED ANTICOAGULANTS SHOULD BE TAPPED NEAR THE STOPPER TO DISLODGE ANY ANTI-COAGULANT THAT MAY BE BETWEEN STOPPER AND WALL OF TUBE.

2. ALL TUBES WITH ANTICOAGULANTS SHOULD BE FILLED TO THE EXHAUSTION OF THE VACUUM TO ENSURE PROPER RATIO OF ANTICOAGULANT TO BLOOD.

3. ALL TUBES WITH ANTICOAGULANTS SHOULD BE MIXED THOROUGHLY BY GENTLE INVERSION SEVERAL TIMES. DO NOT SHAKE VIGOROUSLY. SOLUBILITY OF SOME ANTICOAGULANTS IS SLOW (E.G., SODIUM FLUORIDE). THEREFORE LONGER MIXING MAY BE REQUIRED. IF MULTIPLE SAMPLES ARE DRAWN, TUBES MAY BE MIXED WHILE SUCCEEDING TUBES ARE FILLING.

Figure 14.3. Vacutainer method of blood specimen collection.

Papanicolaou test for malignancy	— PAP
Rheumatoid Factor (screening test)	— R_3

CHIROPRACTIC PHYSIOLOGIC THERAPEUTICS

The use of physiotherapeutic measures to facilitate the chiropractic adjustment is valuable in many cases. These procedures offer specific functional benefits as well as help to reduce stiffness in joints, relieve tension, relax muscle spasm, enhance circulation, control pain, and excite sluggish nerves and muscles.

The chiropractic assistant is frequently directly involved and of special help to the doctor in applying a variety of apparatus and specialized equipment. While many forms and designs of equipment are available, only a few forms of application will be used in the typical office, depending on the doctor's experience and preference.

The doctor prescribes the therapy, and an assistant is often called on to administer the therapy under the direct supervision of the doctor. The practitioner is well acquainted with the underlying fundamentals and physics involved to properly prescribe the appropriate modality, intensity, duration, and technique, as well as to effectively analyze procedures and evaluate treatment. The assistant must be thoroughly aware of application technique, indications, and contraindications that vary with a patient's age and condition and individual tolerance.

In a few states, application may be done only by a licensed doctor or a registered physiotherapist. However, even when the doctor begins the therapy, an assistant is often called on to remain with the patient during therapy and monitor the process. Therefore, a well-trained assistant should be acquainted with each modality within the office to the degree of her responsibility.

The Rationale

Physiotherapy techniques are used before and after the chiropractic adjustment to normalize function, to prevent and minimize pain and deformities resulting from trauma or disease, and to maintain what has been gained in the treatment. Superficial heat, cold, diathermy, microwave, ultrasound, meridian therapy, percussion, ultraviolet light, galvanic and sinusoidal currents, traction, hydrotherapy, and therapeutic massage and exercise are among the common therapies used in chiropractic that may benefit the patient when properly applied.

Chiropractic physiotherapy can be defined as the therapeutic application of forces and substances that induce a physiologic response and use and/or allow the body's natural processes to return to a more normal state of health. Modalities do not "cure" any disease. They influence functional reactions.

The rational use of physiologic therapeutics first requires an understanding of their mechanism of action and their predictable effects on the pathophysiologic processes involved. Second, an understanding of the abnormal or diseased state must be determined by the doctor; i.e., the abnormal processes involved at the time of therapy are the primary criteria for proper application.

A particular disease or disorder may at various times in its course entail a number of abnormal physiologic reactions and processes. Thus, treatment must vary with the abnormal process and be adapted to the patient and the condition at the moment rather than fixed by an unalterable routine or concept. Disease is not a thing; it is a process. The primary intent of chiropractic physiotherapeutics is to help the body adapt to and/or normalize the abnormal processes of a diseased state.

When an abnormal functional process manifests in a patient, therapy must be directed at either stopping or reversing the process as it currently exists so the body can return to a more normal state. To understand this, the operator must have at least a general understanding of the pathophysiologic processes involved.

The Stages of Healing

Whether a tissue becomes primarily injured through frank trauma or microtrauma, or is undergoing a change as a secondary reaction to a neuropathic process initiated elsewhere, the following stages usually occur (1) hyperemia, (2) passive congestion, (3) consolidation of the protein exudate, and (4) formation of a fibrinous coagulate, organization through fibroblastic activity, fibrosis, ischemia, and therefore, possibly more fibrosis and/or atrophy.

The processes often exist in different ratios within the same tissue at the same time, but one usually dominates and treatment should be directed primarily for it. A change in therapy becomes necessary as the dominant feature alters.

The four stages of involvement, the common procedures used, and their major effects are:

1. *State of hyperemia or active congestion.* Ice packs offer a vasoconstrictive effect as well as several others (Fig. 14.4). Positive galvanism produces vasoconstriction and toughening of tissues. Ultrasound has a dispersing effect and increases membrane permeability. Rest with possible support is often recommended to avoid irritation and prevent further injury during this stage.

2. *State of passive congestion.* Alternating hot and cold applications, preferably in a 3:1 ratio every few hours, has a revulsive effect as does light massage, particularly effleurage. Passive manipulation is also revulsive. It helps to maintain muscular tone and tends to free coagulates and avoid early adhesions. Mild range of motion exercises

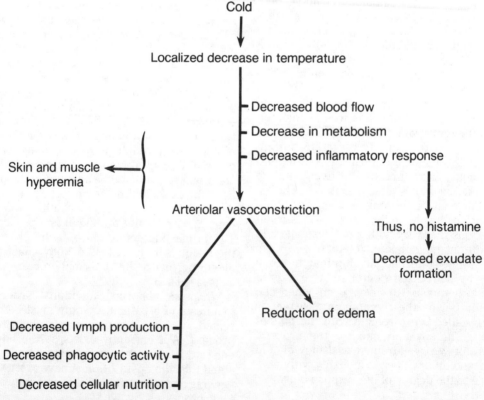

Figure 14.4. The physiologic effects of cold.

and surging sinusoidal stimulation have the same effects as passive manipulation. Ultrasound increases gaseous exchange in the tissues, disperses fluids, liquifies gels, and increases membrane permeability (Fig. 14.5).

3. *Stage of consolidation and/or formation of fibrinous coagulate.* Local moderate heating, preferably of a moist nature, produces a mild vasodilation and increases membrane permeability (Fig. 14.6). Moderate active exercise, motorized alternating traction, moderate range-of-motion manipulation, and surging or pulsating sinusoidal current are all revulsive. They tend to free coagulates and early adhesions, and tend to maintain muscular tone and ligament integrity. Ultrasound at this stage produces hyperemia, liquefaction of gels, dispersion of gases and fluids, increased membrane permeability, and softening of tissues.

4. *Stage of fibroblastic activity and fibrosis.* Prolonged deep heating such as diathermy prolongs vasodilation, increases membrane permeability, and increases tissue

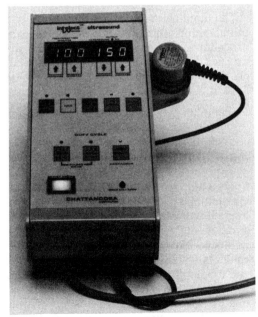

Figure 14.5. The Intelect 205 ultrasound unit (shown with permission of the Chattanooga Corporation).

chemical activities. Deep massage such as petrissage or other soft-tissue traction without weight bearing maintains muscle and ligament integrity, stretches fibrotic tissues, breaks adhesions, and enhances tissue elasticity. Motorized alternating traction has the same effects (Fig. 14.7).

In any state, too vigorous a therapy may be so traumatic that a return to an active stage of inflammation may occur. This must be avoided and steady progress favored. Also, excessive variety, time, intensity or other types of overtreatment that may counteract the beneficial effects of rational physiotherapy must be guarded against.

Prior to any treatment, always inform the patient what you are going to do, how you are going to do it, what feelings they can expect, and why it is necessary. This avoids patient anxiety and enhances cooperation. To do this, you must have a sound understanding of the what, when, where, and why involved with each modality.

Types of Applications

Common ancillary procedures used in chiropractic include:

Baths (therapeutic)	Meridian therapy
Cryotherapy	Microwave diathermy
Douches	Percussion/vibration
Electrodiagnosis	Phonophoresis
Enemas	Shortwave diathermy
Exercise	Sinusoidal current
Galvanic current	Soft-tissue manipula-
Heat	tion
High-volt therapy	Traction
Interferential current	Ultrasonic diathermy
Iontophoresis	Ultrasound
Massage	Ultraviolet light

Besides the applications listed above, mechanical supports are often necessary to rest and protect a part during healing. Some types are shown in Figure 14.8.

An assistant should be alert that any therapeutic agent possesses a potential for effectiveness and a potential for danger. Each modality has its specific indications, contraindications, and special precautions

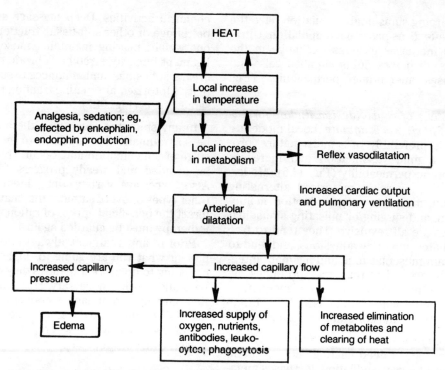

Figure 14.6. The physiologic effects of local heating.

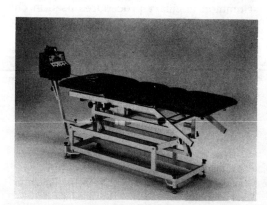

Figure 14.7. Traction table (Model TRE-24, shown with the permission of the Chattanooga Corporation).

that must be observed if the therapy is to be applied safely and effectively. This requires a knowledge of the biophysics involved, the physiologic responses involved and their modification by the technique used, and their pros and cons in achieving a specific therapeutic purpose.

The applications, indications, and contraindications for each of these devices and procedures are beyond the scope of this manual. For reference, refer to Jaskoviak PA, Schafer RC: *Applied Physiotherapy*, Arlington, VA, American Chiropractic Association, 1986.

Maintenance of Equipment

It is customary for a technical assistant to see that all therapy equipment is clean and in good working order. Modalities and their attachments should be wiped clean after each use. Metal should shine, and wooden cabinets should be occasionally polished and frequently dusted. If an apparatus is not working properly, the doctor should be notified immediately. Likewise, signs of wear, especially of electrical cords, should be brought to the doctor's attention. Cleanliness and good operating order are the priority.

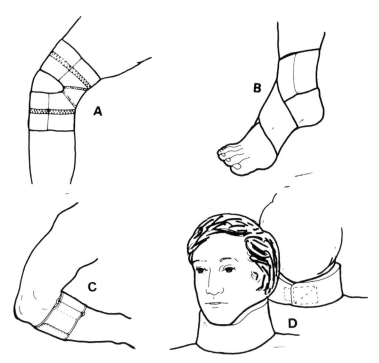

Figure 14.8. Various types of light supports: A, semiflexible knee support; B, ankle wrap support; C, tennis elbow elastic bandage; D, foam cervical collar (shown with permission of STC, Inc).

THERAPEUTIC NUTRITION AND DIETARY ASSISTANCE

People differ in how much they want to know about nutrition, but everyone needs to know a few facts about food and health as a basis for selecting foods to eat. We need food to get energy for work and play, to move, to breathe, to keep the heart beating, and just to be alive. The maturing young need energy from food to support growth. Food also provides a variety of substances: nutrients essential for the building, upkeep, repair of body tissues, and efficient function of the body.

Everyone needs the same nutrients throughout life but in different amounts. Proportionately greater amounts are required for the growth of a body than just for its upkeep. Boys and men need more energy and nutrients than girls and women. Large people need more than small people. Active people require more food energy than inactive ones. People recovering from illness need more than healthy people.

Foods vary in kind and amounts of nutrients they contain. No one food provides all the nutrients in the amounts required for growth and health. We need a variety of foods each day to assure getting all necessary nutrients.

Case Management Fundamentals

Nutrition is more than diet. Case management frequently necessitates preventive nutrition through dietary control and supplementation as an aid in countering cellular malnourishment and enhancing recuperative powers. Proper nutritional guidance must therefore consider supplementation; dietetic regimens; balanced quantities of nutrients; adequate ingestion, digestion, absorption, and transportation to and utilization by the cells.

Nutritional deficiencies can result from inefficient distribution such as in circulatory impairments; accumulation of injurious metabolic debris such as in azotemia or uric acid deposition; inadequate nutritional supply such as in dietary deficiencies; or ineffective cellular utilization of nutrients such as in hypoinsulinism, asphyxia, and enzyme deficiencies. Thus, malnutrition may be endogenous as well as exogenous.

Although the basic requirements for satisfactory human nutrition are fundamentally similar throughout life, various physiologic changes occur with the passing years that call for diet modification. Recognition and adaptation of these factors help retard the onset of symptoms and establish habit patterns that tend to enhance the pleasure of the prime of maturity.

If we recognize that growth and general health processes depend to a large extent on the food ingested, and assume this growth is counterbalanced by a destructive or aging process, then it is logical to consider nutrition as one of the more important factors in the prolongation of healthful life. Unquestionably, the nutrition of a person is important both for survival and for day-to-day comfort and activity. Although the aged body requires the same basic nutrients as the younger person, it usually requires less quantity and higher quality.

In contrast to chiropractic, attention under traditional medical care is rarely given to malnutrition until overt manifestations appear. This is undoubtedly due to the emphasis placed on nutrition in chiropractic colleges and state boards while it is rare to find formal nutritional curricula in a traditional medical college.

Effects of Food Processing and Storage

Although all natural foods contain the micronutrients necessary for their metabolism, they seldom have their original spectrum of micronutrients when they reach the table. While caloric values and the quantity and quality of protein, carbohydrate, and fat are relatively unchanged, at least six vitamins can be lost or partly destroyed by steaming, frying, processing, cooking, roasting, freezing, drying, boiling, storage, or irradiation. Many elements are lost through boiling. Industrialized food processing often results in a deficiency in vitamins and elements necessary for metabolism. Americans are the most overfed and undernourished people in the world.

Dietary supplementation is the price we must pay for the wide distribution of purified, stored, and processed foods. Without supplementation, we run the risk of unbalancing the diet in terms of micronutrients. While meat is a common source of protein, it is commonly ingested with an array of antibiotics, artificial sex hormones, and a round of additives that preserve, age, cure, tenderize, color, flavor, season, and scent to satisfy producers' profit motives. Fruits and vegetables commonly contain a degree of pesticide residue.

In any nutritional management or dietary regimen, consideration should be given to what people like to eat as well as what they should eat. The prescribing doctor should be cognizant of and adapt his thinking to include known social, religious, racial, ethnic, and psychologic factors involved in individual life-styles.

Teaching Healthy Dietary Habits

There are many conditions for which a special diet is indicated. This diet therapy may be a small or large part of the patient's treatment program. After the doctor prescribes a specific diet for a patient, it is often the assistant's responsibility to discuss the details with the patient, answer questions, and explain certain points based on a general knowledge of nutrition.

A prescribed diet usually means that certain foods must be taken and others omitted. The quantity of food may be regulated, and the interval between meals may be specified.

Although Hippocrates wrote a book on the subject over 2000 years ago, diet as a systematic form of therapy is relatively new. Even today, dietetics is an empiric science. There are, however, a few specific rules based on our knowledge of physiology, pathology, and biochemistry. General rules are difficult to establish because controlled diet experiments on human beings are difficult to control since individuals react differently to different foods. For this reason, physicians will generally modify a standardized diet according to their experience, preferences, and clinical judgment.

Some patients have difficulty in seeing the relationship between their dietary habits and their illness and do not take the doctor's instructions seriously. Such an attitude can be detrimental to a rapid recovery. Other patients frequently become neglectful in following instructions. They forget instructions or fail to follow suggestions. On the other hand, there are patients who take a diet so literally that failure to follow the letter of the diet becomes a source of stress.

The alert assistant should be able to answer routine questions regarding standardized diets prescribed by the doctor. She can do this intelligently only if she has a basic knowledge of nutrition and diet therapy. Before attempting to explain a diet to any patient, the assistant should study it carefully, familiarize herself thoroughly with the details, and have the doctor answer any questions that may arise. A CA should learn enough about the subject that she can talk intelligently and convincingly with a patient.

Sound nutritional considerations are important in the determination of future health. In the battle against many correctable conditions and needless disturbances, dietary guidance and supplementation afford a significant weapon in chiropractic care and can contribute substantially to the lives of the doctors' patients in both quantity and quality.

While there is little evidence that excess vitamin intake has any beneficial effect on health and well being other than as a micronutrient for organisms that feed on sewage, there is strong evidence that *marginal intakes can result in a state of poor health without causing overt symptoms of deficiency.*

Roger J. Williams, professor of biochemistry at the University of Texas and discoverer of pantothenic acid, said after enumerating various changes characteristic of aging: "I want to call attention to the idea that every one of these signs of old age probably is connected with failure of the cells related to cell and tissue nutrition.... The longer cells are furnished with the necessities of life, including good nutrition, the longer they will continue in good working order."

Nourishment of cells of the body presents a formidable problem in body logistics. The right food has to be distributed equitably. Since circulatory patterns are different in everybody, there is no assurance that every cell and tissue always gets exactly what it needs. The problem is further complicated: different cells of the body do not have the same nutritional requirements.

Dietary Supplementation

Animal requirements, on which most experiments are based, are not necessarily human requirements. Individual variations in requirements can be exasperatingly large even without any distinguishable pathology. Needs are quite different from one person to another, so for the aged. Although certain nutrients occur widely in foods, this does not mean that deficiencies will not occur. That depends on storage, processing, vagaries of diet, absorption rates, distribution rates, metabolism, clinical and subclinical disease processes, and all the other peculiarities of individuals and their requirements. To these we can add the impressions of emotional and physical stress.

Many authorities believe that some individuals are benefitted by a generous supply of supplements, presumably because their individual needs are out of line with average needs. Unfortunately, there is no means at present to gauge what individual requirements might be. For this reason, many biochemists recommend that perfectly safe, nontoxic nutrients can and should be taken in excess of the average need as insurance against possible deficiency.

There have been surprisingly few adequate studies of the effect of vitamin supplementation. A widely recognized one was a controlled 2-year study of 80 chronically ill hospitalized elderly patients that was conducted in England. Of the 80 patients, 95% showed some sign of nutritional deficiency and 90% had low levels of thiamine or ascorbic acid. Significant improvement in both physical and mental condition occurred with supplementation, and deficiency signs reappeared when supplementation was ceased—even while the patients were eating the regular "controlled" hospital diet.

Classical vitamin deficiency syndromes are infrequently seen in this country today. Subclinical deficiency is often hard to prove or disprove. To suggest that vitamin deficiencies cause most depletion states would be unscientific at this point, but to discard the fact they do cause some and contribute to many others would be unwise. A rational approach to the use of supplementation must weigh individual problems and needs.

ASSISTING IN THE X-RAY DEPARTMENT

It was a fortunate coincidence that the discovery of x rays by Roentgen and the rediscovery of chiropractic by Palmer both occurred in 1895. X rays have become a valuable diagnostic tool of the chiropractic profession since the early 1900s. When the doctor of chiropractic uses x rays for diagnostic purposes, he is employing one of the most valuable tools of the health professions. He is fully trained to use x-ray equipment safely and to interpret the results.

Why Doctors of Chiropractic Use Roentgenography

Diagnostic imaging enables the chiropractic physician to analyze bone integrity and structural balance. His diagnosis is often based in part on roentgenographic finding corroborated by other tests. X-ray films can often reveal the cause, extent, and seriousness of many body ills and degenerative processes as well as traumatic effects. In addition, x-ray films readily show skeletal relationships and postural deficiencies.

X-ray diagnosis aids the doctor of chiropractic in correcting a patient's disorder or disability, and enables him to offer the patient sound advice that can help avoid future illness or discomfort. As an aid for ac-

curate diagnosis, films are studied by the doctor and used as a guide in development of a treatment plan. Accurate and early diagnosis of health problems assures a favorable opportunity for correction.

The assistant who works in a chiropractic x-ray department must have a general knowledge of anatomy to properly assist in taking films of most parts of the body. She must also be familiar with the principles of exposure and of film processing. A DC who is not a roentgenologist will prefer an assistant who has had training in x-ray technique, but few are available to meet the need. Therefore, most doctors will teach their assistant, within the realm of state laws, how to operate the equipment safely, how to develop films, and how to position the patient for those particular procedures necessary. This assistant must also learn the rules regarding protection from harmful exposure, preparation of the patient, and filing and record keeping of films and reports.

If you were to go into an established x-ray laboratory to study x-ray technology, it probably wouldn't be long before you could go through the mechanics of making a radiograph. You could get the film and patient ready, place the x-ray tube just so, operate the controls exactly as you had been shown, and develop, fix, wash, and dry the film. But that would not mean that you had become an x-ray technician, for radiography is much more than a series of procedures. It is a science and an art. It is a science in that it embodies the sciences of physics, geometry, and chemistry. It is an art in that it requires practice and experience to attain the desired skill.

Depending on the state law governing the scope of the chiropractic assistant in the radiology, it is here that she may perform some important functions necessary to a smooth running facility. The importance of thorough knowledge in both the x-ray room and the darkroom is paramount for the elimination of unnecessary retakes, for whatever reason.

In radiology, the chiropractic assistant's foremost preoccupation is (1) patient safety, the reduction of unnecessary radiation, and (2) the assurance of quality film production.

Basic Principles of Radiology

X-rays are like light in that they radiate in straight lines in all directions from the focal spot of the tube unless stopped by an efficient absorber. For that reason, an x-ray tube is enclosed in a lead housing that stops most of the x-radiation except useful rays, which are permitted to leave the tube through a "window" and are called the *primary beam*. That pencil of radiation at the geometric center of this primary beam is called the *central ray*.

To produce an x-ray image of lasting value, it must be properly recorded on specialized film, and then processed to provide a visible image. It is helpful if the CA has been taught the principles of x-ray absorption, the effect of milliamperage and kilovoltage, the effect of tube-patient distance, the geometry of image formation, the technique of exposure, x-ray film and its sensitivity, why scattered radiation occurs, the use of intensifying screens and cones, controlling film density/contrast/detail, how to keep within a specified latitude (tolerance for error), and knowing how to properly develop and fix exposed film. This technical knowledge cannot be indoctrinated in a manual of this size. Emphasis here will be on monitoring exposure absorption, patient safety and preparation, film information (patient, part and position), common terms and designations, patient positioning routines, record keeping and filing, and film handling. Some personal knowledge is added about the removal of stains from white fabrics and proper care of the skin when working with x-ray chemicals.

Dangers of X-Radiation to Patients

Ionizing radiation, which encompasses x rays, has been well documented for its potential harmful effects. Included are the influence on the thyroid gland, eyes, testes, ovaries, and fetus. Of these, an embryo and the reproductive organs (testes and ovaries) are of special concern. It has been shown that certain aberrations to cellular structures are caused by excessive ionizing radiation.

The in-utero embryo has shown extreme radiosensitivity, particularly within the first 8–12 weeks of pregnancy. As a result, it is an absolute that the patient be questioned closely about the possibility of pregnancy. If the patient is pregnant or unsure on this point, it is well to find out from the ordering physician if the examination might not be delayed until such determination can be made. This is particularly so should the examination ordered expose the reproductive anatomy as part of the routine; ie, lumbar spine, pelvis, sacrum, or coccyx.

Much information has been gained to suggest that the most sensitive time of the embryo to ionizing radiation is the first 3–6 weeks after implantation: a time many women are not yet aware of their condition. It is recommended that in the female patient, the optimum time of x-ray examination is within 10 days of the first day of her last period. During this time, it is highly unlikely that pregnancy has occurred. This information (ie, date of last menstrual period [DLMP]) is recorded on the identification card imprinted permanently on the film. Doing so demonstrates the assistant's awareness and responsibility.

A radiograph is unnecessary unless the information gained by such an examination is useful in the total diagnosis of the patient's complaint. Only when a need is shown will the doctor order radiographic examination. Careless or needless exposure of a patient to the potentially harmful effects of ionizing radiation is both morally and professionally unethical.

Male Patients

In the male patient, protection of the gonads by lead shielding is always recommended for men to prevent aberration of spermatozoa. The extreme radiosensitivity of the testes demands their protection at all ages, whenever possible. This is typically accomplished with a gonad shield: a cup-like protective device encompassing the entire male gonads. Placement of the shield is best made by using briefs or underwear specifically designed for holding the shield. In this manner, once the shield is in place it will afford protection in all views, regardless of the position of the patient. The importance of these devices is so well documented that in many states their availability for use by the patient, if requested, is mandatory. They are available from commercial suppliers in both infant and adult sizes.

Female Patients

With females, there are no certain measures available for protection such as in the male. Due to the deeper anatomical location of the ovaries and uterus, even when adequately protected by lead placed directly over the organs, scatter and secondary radiation still finds its way to these structures. While attenuation of the ionizing radiation can be reduced in the male by upwards of 95% through gonad shields, it is estimated that only about 35% can be achieved in the female. These figures are applicable when the reproductive organs are in the direct field of exposure.

The problems of protection in the female is not only the anatomical location of the organs. To protect these structures totally, the attenuating device would also obscure the anatomical structures that prompted the need for the radiograph in the first place. Thus, to adequately shield might mean the loss of information sought for diagnosis. A compromise must often be sought between clinical need and absolute safety.

Personnel Monitoring

As important as the safety of the patient is, so is the accurate and detailed radiation exposure level of the department personnel. It is common knowledge that all people are exposed daily to minute amounts of radiation through the earth's atmosphere or as it is commonly known, background radiation. While in itself not a hazard to health, it becomes more important to people who work with or around other sources of radiation. Radiation has an accumulating biologic effect.

Both federal and state laws require personnel working with radiation to be monitored for any detectable amounts of exposure received on the job. Most installations meet this requirement by providing film badges to monitor exposure. These badges are provided in many forms (eg, clip-ons, pins, rings, etc), and each is always worn when working in, with, or near the x-ray room. Monthly determination of exposure is afforded so any failure of safe procedures becomes immediately known. Most badges measure primary, secondary, and scatter radiation despite origin.

A monthly determination provides a continuing measure of lifetime absorbed dose for each individual. These measurements are filed annually with the appropriate state or federal radiation agency and by that assures a continuation of measurement should personnel move from one installation to another. These procedures are necessary to ensure that personnel are well aware of their monthly, yearly, and life time radiation-absorbed dose levels and by that be protected and forewarned of unwanted exposure to ionizing radiation.

Patient Preparation

Diagnostic roentgenography in the chiropractic office will be confined for the most part to examination of the osseous structures, particularly of the spine, with chest examinations the second priority. Some more sophisticated procedures such as gastrointestinal, gallbladder, and kidney examinations are usually confined to those installations using a diplomate of the American Chiropractic Board of Roentgenology. As this manual is aimed at a general audience, our descriptions will deal primarily with the typical facility of a general practitioner.

In data gathering, the patient's name, address, age, and sex are absolute information. The name of the insurance carrier and Medicaid or Medicare numbers are important for billing purposes.

1. The recording of the patient's age and sex is important, particularly as they relate

to the reproductive capabilities of the patient. In general, a patient is considered within the reproductive years from puberty until the age of 45 in the female and the age of 50 in the male, unless prior surgical interruption is reported such as hysterectomy, permanently tied tubes, or vasectomy.

2. The age and gender of the patient are also important to the ordering physician or roentgenologist when interpreting the film(s). These factors alone are invaluable in helping to differentiate certain variations from normal: physiologic or pathologic. Many conditions have a predilection for certain age groups, and the patient's gender often explains varying textures of bone as seen on the film.

3. It is necessary that every patient be totally disrobed prior to x-ray examination. Removal of wigs, earrings, jewelry, watches, eye glasses, rings, bobby pins, dentures, etc, are essential. While many facilities may not require the removal of dentures until the actual time of exposure, it is nonetheless imperative that they not be overlooked.

When the patient undresses, an examination gown is given to the patient. Usually a special dressing room is provided. If the patient must undress in the x-ray room, the assistant should instruct the patient and then leave the room for a while to allow the patient privacy. The patient's modesty must be considered at all times. It is important to explain to the patient just what garments to remove and how to put on the examination gown. In some offices, crepe paper slippers are provided. The laundry should be instructed not to starch these gowns, not only because starched gowns are uncomfortable but also because they may produce a shadow on the film.

The male is also provided with the gonad shield and asked to put it on. Careful instruction is often necessary so that he understands that the entire organ complex be within the cup; ie, both the testes and the penis.

To understand the importance of complete disrobing, it is necessary to realize that everything has density. Density of varying thickness casts shadows on finished films. These shadows, particularly when subtle and overlaying certain anatomical parts, can obscure or distort the film to cause confusion and possibly misinterpretation during analysis. Should the item be of sufficient density, it might obliterate detail of structure and cause the doctor to miss variations such as hairline fractures, tumors, etc. These are inexcusable because they can easily be prevented by proper attention to patient preparation.

The presence on the finished film of extraneous materials as described above gives rise to what are called *artifacts*. Other artifacts may find their way onto the finished film, but these can be dealt with by proper film-processing procedures.

A woman should be instructed to place all her jewelry in her handbag and take this with her into the x-ray room. Tissues should be given to the patient to wrap dentures in if necessary. Splints or supports should not be removed without the order of the physician.

Attention to the physical and emotional needs of the patient is always important. Some patients need to be reassured that the radiographic examination entails little, if any, discomfort. Such assurance, plus a warm towel over the shoulders if the patient is chilled, will do much to enhance relaxation and therefore the examination itself. When the patient has pain with movement, be certain that transport and positioning of the patient is made with care and caution. It is well to remember that regardless of your experience and expertise, the patient knows when and where it hurts better than you. X-ray tables are notoriously hard and cold. Let the patient ease himself into the directed position, and, if possible, prewarm or provide a towel or sheet for protection against the chill. Any examination is easier and therefore better if the patient can and will cooperate and relax.

Explain to the patient what is going to be done and what is expected of him. Ask him courteously to lie still, to move up or down, to flex his leg, or to do whatever may be necessary. Always remember that he may be nervous and therefore not concentrating on your remarks. Do not become impatient if the patient carries out your instructions incorrectly.

The assistant should show concern for the patient's comfort. Whenever possible, a small pillow should be placed under the head. The x-ray room and the dressing room should be comfortably warm and free from drafts. A blanket should be within easy reach to cover the patient if he complains of being cold or if he must wait a few moments between having radiographs taken. All adjustments on the machine should be made before the patient is placed on the table.

Patients having radiographs are often injured, handicapped, or in pain. They may need help in getting to the x-ray room and getting on and off the x-ray table. A definite technique is required for an operator to lift a patient without strain. The body should be flexed at the hips, as this gives the operator more strength and puts less strain on the back muscles than if the back were bent. A footstool should be in front of the x-ray table, as the table is usually higher than many people can reach comfortably.

Patients with suspected fractures generally have severe pain and must be handled with extreme care. An important function of the assistant in placing the injured part on the table is to relax completely and follow the movements of the patient. That is, she should place both hands under the injured part, tell the patient how it should be placed, and then follow his movements with her hands and arms under the injured part. The CA's movements must be slow and steady in order not to jar the patient. This holds true for any painful area, not just fractured bones.

The patient may have to be turned on his side, and this can present a problem if he is in pain, handicapped, or very heavy. It is advisable to place such a patient on a sheet or blanket. When he is to be turned, grasp the ends of the sheet on the side opposite to which the patient is to be turned. Pull the sheet or blanket toward you to start the patient turning, and then gently push him in the desired direction.

If the patient is ill or in pain, he may feel faint when getting off the x-ray table. There-

fore, spirits of ammonia and a basin should be near if the patient has to vomit.

Film Information: Patient

Each radiograph must have certain information permanently affixed to it to meet medicolegal requirements concerning identification of the patient and where the radiograph was taken. The doctor's name or that of the facility where the procedure was performed is necessary. The patient's name or case history number and the date of the exposure are essential. As explained, the inclusion of the age and date of last menses (DLMP) is highly recommended.

Two common methods of film identification are (1) the use of lead letters and characters held in place by a master letter holder and (2) the use of a semiautomatic card imprinter:

• The lead-letter holder usually has the doctor's or facility's name and location preset, and merely the addition of the patient's name, age, case number, and DLMP are needed. This is done by "hand loading" the master holder with the appropriate letters and numbers into the channels provided. As the characters are lead, they will attenuate the x rays, and the finished film will show all information "fed" into the holder. The holder must of course be transferred from one cassette to another before each exposure. With the lead-letter technique, the holder will occasionally be positioned on the cassette where no patient attenuation will occur and therefore the characters may be "burned" out by a heavy mA dose of x rays; ie, more than their thickness could attenuate or diminish from reaching the film.

• A card imprinter is a device that allows light, set from a switch, to pass through a card with information typed or written on that is transferred directly to a pre-exposed film. The pre-exposed film requires that a lead blocker of the same size used by the card imprinter be placed in the cassette to prevent that portion of the film from being exposed. This portion of film will then be exposed by the light emitted from the card

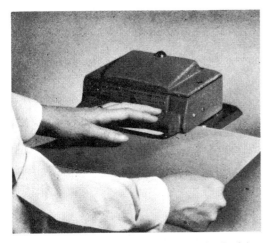

Figure 14.9. The photographic method of including data on a film is easy and fast.

imprinter (Fig. 14.9). Several distinct advantages of this method are had. First, the ability to write in or type the information onto the card is less cumbersome than handling many lead characters. Next, the card allows space for more information; eg, postaccident data, serial film number, referring doctor, etc. It also allows for all films of one examination to be imprinted at the time of development without changing the information plate from one cassette to another. The imprinter method also has the advantage of always being of the same quality on the finished film because of the lead blocker used in the cassette.

Film Information: Part and Position

Besides the identification of whose image it is, it is also necessary to identify what part of the patient is being visualized on the finished film. This information is essential, even sometimes critical, to proper film interpretation. A cardinal rule is to always mark the part closest to the film, and be certain that all designations such as right and left are referring to the patient's right or left.

Every film must have at least the designation of the patient's right or left. Other designations such as LPO, LAO, RPO or RAO

should be used when patient oblique views are taken (Fig. 14.10). The film is marked by placement of the appropriate marker on the cassette before exposure. These characters can be taped to the cassette with adhesive tape and be removed before reloading or reusing the cassette. Remember, *each* film must show the patient's right or left; and on oblique views, what part is closest to the film at the time of exposure (Fig. 14.11).

Radiographic Terms of Position

AP—refers to anterior-posterior (front to back); designates that the x-ray beam enters the front or anterior portion of the patient and exits at the posterior or rear of the patient. Refer to Figure 14.10.

PA—posterior (back) to anterior (front) projection; the opposite of an AP view.

R—right side of patient or part being examined.

L—left side of patient or part being examined.

RAO—right anterior oblique indicates the right anterior portion of the part examined is closest to the film, and the whole of the examined part is positioned obliquely to the central ray of the x-ray beam.

LAO—opposite of RAO; the left anterior portion of the part being examined is closest to the film.

RPO—the part examined is positioned obliquely to the central ray and film with the right posterior portion of the part closest to the film.

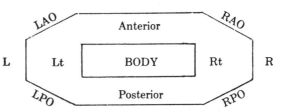

Figure 14.10. Descriptors used in recording patient position in roentgenography.

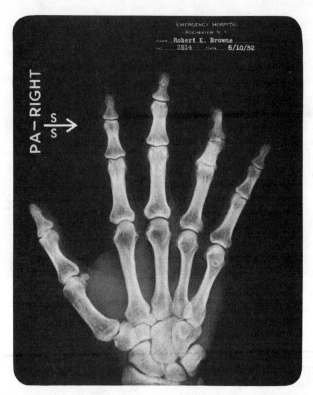

Figure 14.11. Radiograph showing proper use of identification and directional markings.

LPO—opposite of RPO; the left posterior portion of the part being examined is positioned closest to the film.

OBLIQUE—the slanting or off-centering of a part in reference to the plane of the film.

POSTURAL—the part examined is x-rayed with the patient standing upright in habitual posture.

PRONE—film taken with the patient lying on his stomach.

SUPINE—film taken with the patient lying on his back.

Patient Positioning Routines

There are three general factors in roentgenology that may be varied according to the preference of the doctor and the limitations of the equipment. These are: (1) use of an upright or recumbent position, (2) the focal-film distance and/or central ray angle used, and (3) film size.

The minimum FFD (film focal distance) or SID (source image distance) of 72 inches should be used along with an upright position for chest films, lateral cervical films, and, under most circumstances, oblique cervicals. Full spine films should use no less than a 72-inch distance; 84 inches is recommended. An acceptable film focal distance for recumbent films and for most upright studies except those specified otherwise is 40 inches. Variation to a longer distance than this is acceptable, but less than 40 inches should only be used for specific reasons (eg, a magnification technique).

Another important factor is film size. Good radiologic practice dictates that only those areas showing clinical necessity should be exposed to x rays. Besides that, the smaller the film size and the tighter the collimation, the sharper the radiographic detail and the less scatter radiation. This will lower patient dose and decrease scatter fog to the film. It is therefore recommended that the smallest film size compatible with clinical needs be used. The x-ray beam should be centered over the area to be exposed (Fig. 14.12).

Record Keeping and Filing

An exposed film is a permanent record of the patient's radiographic appearance at the time of examination. It serves not only as a graphic diagnostic aid at the time, but allows for determination by comparison to other films taken either before or after. Films are an integral part of the patient's file and as such require careful attention to their safekeeping. The medicolegal requirements are that all radiographs and their concurrent diagnostic findings remain with the doctor as part of his records for a minimum of 7 years. The information garnered from the film (ie, the report) is legally regarded as the patient's property and as such may be given to him or to whomever he may designate after signing a *record release.*

While stored films occupy office space, their usefulness for comparison with a subsequent film can be valuable. They offer a pictorial progression of a patient's condition. Many installations attempt to keep the films as long as space permits, after which they can be sold and the silver reclaimed.

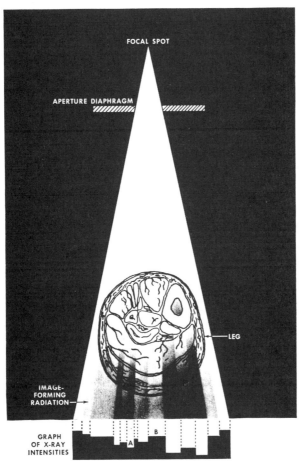

Figure 14.12. Diagram showing the passage of an x-ray beam through a leg and the resulting variation in intensity of image-forming radiation.

A system of filing films must be decided by the individual facility and, once initiated, maintained. Large institutions find that giving each patient a case number to be used on all records of that patient is useful. As impersonal as this approach may be, it is practical. Individual practitioners generally find it to their advantage to use patients' names for identification. Whichever method is selected, the record-identification system must be adhered to on all records of the patient. In the radiography department, the name or case number must appear on each film, as described earlier. It is also used when recording exposure information and when filing the films.

Most examinations require several films, often of varying sizes. For this reason, it is suggested that *all* films of a patient be filed in a single jacket. The outside of the jacket should show the name of the patient, case number if any, date of examinations, and name of the referring doctor if any. Storage must be in a clean dry area where extremes of temperature are not likely. Alphabetical or numerical filing methods are essential for easy retrieval. When multiple examinations are made over a period, filing by date in separate film jackets is advised. When retrieving, it is customary to advise the doctor of multiple jackets so he may choose which films he is interested in at the time.

Finished films may be stored flat or on end, whichever is easiest with the storage space available. The film jacket allows for its identification in either manner. Be certain that all jackets are maintained in good repair. A torn end may allow film damage during handling. As jackets are open ended, it is important to carry, file, and store films in a way that they will not slip from their envelopes.

A method of inventory control is necessary in a busy radiographic department, as is a record of film size use. To do both quickly, a record of exposure is used. Exposures should be recorded *immediately* after each examination to assure accuracy.

Film and Film Handling

X-ray film is highly sensitive and easily damaged. It is sensitive to x rays, light, some gases, heat, and moisture—even aging causes a gradual change. Its chemically coated surfaces are delicate and may be marred by careless handling.

Packaging. The protection of x-ray film begins in the factory where packaging is rigidly controlled. After the film is enclosed in individual paper folders, each lot of 25, 75, or 100 sheets is inserted in a moisture-proof container that is hermetically sealed and then boxed. The paper folder protects the film from abrasion during shipment as well as during removal from the box. The sealed inner container provides protection against moisture and fumes. As long as the seal is unbroken, the film retains its ideal moisture content—it will not absorb more or dehydrate.

Storage. A user must pay special attention to the storage of film. Film should be kept in a cool place, well protected from radiation. The supply should be adequate, yet small enough to provide a reasonably rapid turnover of stock to ensure "freshness." Proper turnover is easily controlled because each package is dated. The oldest, of course, should be used first.

Pre-Exposure Handling. Several types of film are manufactured for x-ray use. The choice depends on such factors as the part to be examined, the type of equipment employed, its capacity, etc. Despite type, x-ray film must be handled carefully to avoid physical strains due to pressure, creasing, buckling, and friction. See Figure 14.13. Do not draw film rapidly from cartons, exposure holders, or cassettes, or handle it in any manner that would produce static electric discharges. Carefulness will avoid one common cause of objectionable circular or tree-like black marks on radiographs. When removing film from a carton, the paper wrapper should be withdrawn with it to protect the film surface from abrasion.

Containers. There are two types of containers in which sheet films are held during exposure: the cassette and the exposure holder. The cassette houses a pair of intensifying screens between which the sheet of

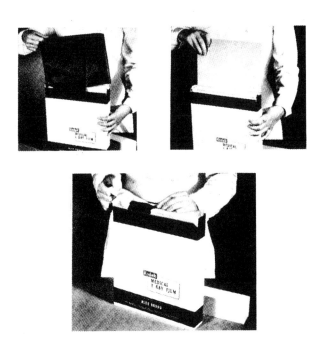

Figure 14.13. Remove the lid from the box and bend the scored flap downward when opening a box of x-ray film. This should be done in a darkroom using a certified safelight. Tear the sealed wrapping at the center and strip it toward one side of the box; then repeat for the other half. Remove the black paper cap, and withdraw both cardboard stiffeners to permit easy removal of the first few films.

film is placed. The exposure holder is a hinged cardboard folder containing a light-tight envelope to enclose the film for direct exposure techniques.

Inserting into Cassette. When holding a cassette, place the film without its inter-leaving wrapper in the cassette on the front screen (Fig. 14.14). Always handle the film between the thumb and one finger. This will prevent the film from kinking. Close the lid carrying the other screen gently, and then lock it with the back springs.

Film Processing

Processing of exposed film consists of de-veloping, stop bath, rinsing, fixing, and washing. A few years ago, this was a tedi-ous, smelly chore when cramped in a small darkroom working over large tanks of chemical solutions. Most offices today use automated temperature-controlled units for film processing and drying. Past problems with film fog; preparing and maintaining de-

veloper, rinse, and fixer solutions; and visu-ally determining development have been eliminated through technologic advances.

Removal of Stains from White Fabrics

Although staining clothing with processing solutions has been greatly reduced by the use of automated equipment, accidents can occur. Prevention is the best method of en-suring unspotted uniforms. This requires care in handling solutions so they will not splash or drip on clothing. A protection apron is helpful, but even the most careful worker may occasionally have to deal with a spot or two. Unfortunately, no stain re-moval system is ideal.

If a solution has been splashed on cloth-ing, the garment should be rinsed as soon as possible in cold water. The stain can be pre-vented entirely if the chemical is removed thoroughly before it has a chance to decom-

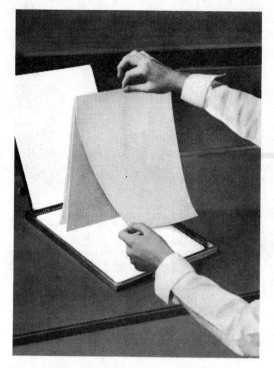

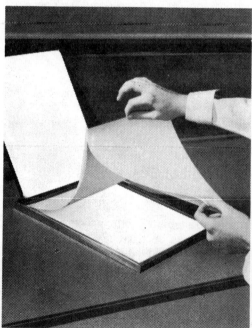

Figure 14.14. Loading a cassette containing intensifying screens: Open the cassette. Remove the film and its paper folder from the box. Hold the film gently between the thumb and forefinger of one hand, and lift the lower edge of the paper in the same manner with your other hand. Lower the film surface nearest you onto the screen. Do not kink the film. Remove the interleaving paper. Close and lock the cassette. Cassette loading must be done in a darkroom using a safelight.

pose, which may otherwise occur on standing or in the laundering process. Even if the stain has formed, the garment should be rinsed before laundering to prevent possible intensification.

Once the stain has formed, its nature will determine the method of removal. Yellow or brown stains due to oxidized developer can be removed by treatment with reducer and stain remover. This procedure uses an acid permanganate solution followed by a bisulfite bleach. While effective in removing developer oxidation stains, it may weaken the fabric and should be applied only to white garments.

Yellow, brown, or black stains formed by used fixer are due to decomposition of the "hypo" and formation of silver sulfide. Slight stains can be removed by a fresh solution of liquid x-ray fixer diluted as usual and containing hardener. Removal requires immersing the affected area from a few minutes to overnight, depending on the intensity of the stain.

A more rapidly acting bleach, and one effective with more dense stains, is made by adding citric acid to liquid fixer at the rate of 2 ounces per gallon of diluted fixer. This will effectively attack dense stains, although an occasional stain is not removed. Any stain remover should be applied with caution to colored fabrics because the dye might be affected.

When the cause of a stain is uncertain, the following successive treatments are suggested: (1) immerse the garment in fresh liquid x-ray fixer; (2) if this is ineffective, add citric acid (2 ounces per gallon of diluted fixer); and (3) after thorough rinsing, apply reducer and stain remover.

Care of the Skin

Because anyone can become sensitized to processing solutions, contact should be kept at an absolute minimum. Avoid getting developer solution on the skin. If the fingers happen to be dampened occasionally, the solution should be removed immediately by rinsing the hands in a stop bath solution and then rinsed again with tap water and dried. When cloth hand towels are used, they should be changed frequently to avoid their becoming contaminated with chemicals and transferring them to the skin.

If the skin becomes stained with developer, a helpful remedy is the application of a potassium permanganate solution, followed by a rinse, first in sodium bisulfite solution and then in warm tap water. The first solution consists of 1/4 ounce of potassium permanganate dissolved in 32 ounces of water. The second is made of 10 ounces of sodium bisulfite dissolved in 32 ounces of water. The solutions should be kept in labeled bottles ready for use.

Bibliography

Adler A: *The Practice and Theory of Individual Psychology.* New York, Harcourt, 1924.

Allport GW: *Personality.* New York, Holt, 1937.

American Chiropractic Association: Chiropractic Coverage in Your Health Insurance, E-3. Des Moines, Iowa, American Chiropractic Association, 1977.

American Chiropractic Association: Consumer's Guide to Chiropractic Health Care. Des Moines, Iowa, American Chiropractic Association, 1977.

American Chiropractic Association: *The Doctor's Assistant.* Des Moines, Iowa, American Chiropractic Association, Handbook Series No. 200, 1970.

American Chiropractic Association: *Focus '77 Lecture Notes.* Des Moines, Iowa, American Chiropractic Association, 1977.

American Chiropractic Association: *Indexed Synopsis on Public Health and Related Matters.* Des Moines, Iowa, 1976.

American Chiropractic Association: *Office Manual on Insurance Relations.* Des Moines, Iowa, American Chiropractic Association, No. 300, 1967.

American Chiropractic Association: *The Professional Image.* Des Moines, Iowa, American Chiropractic Association, Handbook Series No. 500, 1970.

American Dental Association: *Guidebook for the Dental Office Staff.* Chicago, American Dental Association, ADA Council on Dental Practice, 1981.

American Management Association: *Leadership in the Office.* Chicago, American Management Association, 1963.

American Medical Association: *Allied Health Education,* ed 11. Chicago, American Medical Association, 1982.

American Medical Association: *The Business Side of Medical Practice.* Monroe, Wisconsin, American Medical Association, 1979.

American Medical Association: *Employment and Use of Physician's Assistants,* revised edition. Monroe, Wisconsin, Department of Health Manpower, 1978.

American Medical Association: *Group Practice.* Denver, American Medical Association, Center for Research in Ambulatory Health Care Administration, 1978.

American Medical Association: *Medical Collection Study Course.* Chicago, American Medical Association, 1981.

American Medical Association: *Medicolegal Forms.* Monroe, Wisconsin, American Medical Association, 1981.

American Medical Association: *Planning Guide for Physicians' Medical Facilities,* ed 3. Chicago, American Medical Association, 1973.

American Medical Association: *Winning Ways with Patients.* Monroe, Wisconsin, American Medical Association, 1979.

American Optometric Association: *Preparing for Optometric Practice.* St. Louis, American Optometric Association, no date shown.

American Society of Mechanical Engineers: *American Standard Abbreviations for Scientific and Engineering Terms.* The American Society of Mechanical Engineers, 1986. Place of publication not shown.

Angyal A: *Foundations for a Science of Personality.* New York, Commonwealth Fund, 1941.

Army Medical Department Handbook of Basic Nursing. Washington, DC, U.S. Government Printing Office, Technical Manual 8-230, 1970.

ASME: *American Standard Abbreviations for Scientific and Engineering Terms.* The American Society of Mechanical Engineers, 1966.

Balint M: *The Doctor, His Patient, and the Illness.* New York, International Universities Press, 1957.

Balliett G: *Getting Started in Private Practice.* Oradell, New Jersey, Medical Economics, 1978.

Basmajian JV (ed): *Grant's Method of Anatomy,* ed 9. Baltimore, Williams & Wilkins, 1975.

Bayan EC: Chiropractic Malpractice. *ACA Journal of Chiropractic,* October 1980.

Beck LC: *The Physician's Office.* Princeton, New Jersey, Excerpta Medica, 1977.

Beck LC, et al: *Restrictive Covenants in Medical and Dental Practices.* Bala Cynwyd, Pennsylvania, The Health Care Group, date not shown.

Bell System: *Your Telephone Personality.* Pacific Telephone. Place and date of publication not shown.

Bell System. *Your Voice Is You: An Aid to Better Telephone Speech.* Bell Telephone System. Place and date of publication not shown.

Berne E: *Transactional Analysis in Psychotherapy.* New York, Grove Press, 1961.

Bickle MD, Houp KW: *Reports for Science and Industry.* Chicago, Henry Holt and Company, 1955.

Bitter GG: *Computers in Today's World.* New York, John Wiley & Sons, 1984.

Bliss BP, Johnson AG: *Aims and Motives in Clinical Medicine: A Practical Approach to Medical Ethics.* Brooklyn Heights, New York, Beekman, 1975.

Bredow M: *The Medical Assistant,* ed 2. New York, McGraw-Hill, 1964.

Drennan MJ III: Conclusion of Survey Looks at Personal Characteristics. *ACA Journal of Chiropractic,* 20:4, April 1983.

Bryan JE: *Public Relations in Medical Practice.* Baltimore, Williams & Wilkins, 1954.

Buck ML: *How to Build a More Rewarding Medical Practice.* Englewood Cliffs, New Jersey, Executive Reports Corporation, 1970.

Burke WJ, Zaloom BJ: *Blueprint for Professional Service Corporations.* New York, Thomas Y. Crowell, Dun and Bradstreet Library, 1970.

Canning RG, Leeper NC: *So You Are Thinking About a Small Business Computer.* Englewood Cliffs, New Jersey, Prentice-Hall, 1983.

Caruthers HG: *Selective Composition of Narrative Reports.* Phoenix, Arizona, Caruthers Foundation, 1967.

Cashman TJ, Shelly GB: *Introduction to Computers and Data Processing.* Fullerton, CA, Anaheim Publishing, 1980.

CBE Style Manual Committee: *CBE Style Manual,* revised ed 5. Bethesda, Maryland, Council of Biology Editors, 1983.

Center AH: *Public Relations Practices: Case Studies.* Englewood Cliffs, New Jersey, Prentice-Hall, 1975.

Chance MD: *Examination and Insurance Report for Back Injuries.* Long Island, New York, Jonorm Publishing. Date not shown.

Chiropractor Held to Standard of Care of Reasonable Chiropractor in Same Circumstances. *ACA Legal Briefs,* 2(3), Summer 1988.

Claypool J: *How to Get a Good Job.* New York, Granklin Watts, 1982.

Coelho GV, et al (eds): *Coping and Adaptation Interdisciplinary Prospectives.* New York, Basic Books, 1974.

Colby KM: *A Primer for Psychotherapists.* New York, Ronald Press, 1951.

Collins JE: *Claims Procedure in Compensable Industrial and Liability Injuries.* Lafayette, Indiana, Tribune Printing, 1961.

Corbin RK, Perrin PG: *Guide to Modern English.* Chicago, Scott, Foresman and Company, 1955.

Cotton H: *Medical Practice Management,* revised edition. Oradell, New Jersey, Medical Economics, 1977.

Cross H, Bjom J: *The Problem-Oriented Private Practice of Medicine—A System for Comprehensive Health Care.* Modern Hospital Press, 1970.

Cusanelli TF: *Facility Program.* Elmhurst, New York, date not shown.

Daly TR: Chiropractic Referral to Medical Radiologists: Liability "Red Herring." *ACA/FYI,* p 4, July 1988.

Daly TR: Chiropractors and X-rays. *ACA/FYI,* p 3, April 1988.

Daly TR: The Uniform Health Care Information Act. *ACA/FYI,* p 3, February 1989.

Diagnostic Radiation and Female Patients of Child-Bearing Age. *Patient Rx Newsletter,* 11(3), May 1989.

Dolan JP, Holladay LJ: *First-Aid Management,* ed 4. Danville, Illinois, Interstate Printers and Publishers, 1967.

Doris L, Miller BM: *Complete Secretary's Handbook.* New York, Prentice-Hall, 1968.

Douglas P: *Communication Through Reports.* Englewood Cliffs, New Jersey, Prentice-Hall, 1957.

Doudna DJ, et al: *Guide to Insurance for Professionals.* Arlington, Virginia, American Chiropractic Association, date not shown.

Drucker PF: *Managing for Results.* New York, Harper & Row, 1964.

Duvall SM: *The Art and Skill of Getting Along with People.* Englewood Cliffs, New Jersey, Prentice-Hall, 1961.

Eastman Kodak Medical Division: *The Fundamentals of Radiography,* ed 8. Rochester, New York, Eastman Kodak Company. Date not shown.

Eder M, Tilscher H: *Chiropractic Therapy: Diagnosis and Treatment,* English translation edition edited by Gengenbach MA: Rockville, Maryland, Aspen Publishers, 1990.

Egerter BC: *Professional Practice Management.* New York, Pageant Press, 1957.

Ehrlich A: *Ethics and Jurisprudence.* Champaign, Illinois, Colwell Systems, 1975.

Ehrlich A: *Guidelines to More Efficient Practice Management.* Champaign, Illinois, Colwell Systems, 1977.

Elmstrom G: *Advanced Management for Optometrists.* Chicago, Illinois, The Professional Press, 1974.

Elsman M: *How to Get Your First Job.* New York, Crown Publishers, 1985.

Evans HW: *Terminology Textbook for Chiropractic Students and Practitioners.* Bowling Green, Kentucky, published by author, 1954.

Eysenck H: *Learning Theory and Behavioral Therapy.* New York, Pergamon Press, 1960.

Farber L: *Personal Money Management for Physicians,* ed 3. Oradell, New Jersey, Medical Economics, 1981.

Finnegan R: Outpatient Medical Records—the Future. *Medical Records News,* 41:142–149, 1970.

Flack MW: *The Chiropractic Doctor and His Assistant.* Indianapolis, Indiana, published by author, 1969.

Fordney MT: *Insurance Handbook for the Medical Office,* ed 3. Philadelphia, W. B. Saunders, 1989.

For Executives Only. Chicago, Dartnell, 1967.

Fredenburgh FA: *The Psychology of Personality and Adjustment.* Menlo Park, California, Cummings Publishing, 1971.

Freiberger SJ, Chew P Jr: *A Consumer's Guide to Personal Computing and Microcomputers,* ed 2. Rochelle Park, New Jersey, Hayden Book Company, 1988.

Freud A: *The Ego and the Mechanisms of Defense.* New York, International University, 1946.

Freud S: *Collected Papers.* London, Hogarth Press, 1950.

Friedman EM: *Sharpening Laboratory Management Skills.* Oradell, New Jersey, Medical Economics, 1978.

Fromm E: *Man for Himself.* New York, Rinehart Press, 1950.

Gaedeke RM, Tootelian DH: *Small Business Management.* Glenview, Illinois, Scott, Foresman and Company, 1980.

Garrison FH: *History of Medicine,* ed 4. Philadelphia, W.B. Saunders, 1929.

General Electric Company: *A Guide to Radiological Anatomy.* Milwaukee, Wisconsin, Technical Services, X-Ray Department, General Electric Company, 1952.

Gerber PC, Petrie KJ: What's the Economic Outlook for Medical Practice? *Physician's Management,* August 1984.

Gettys RC, Zasa RJ: *Medical Group Practice Management.* Cambridge, Massachusetts, Ballinger Publishing, 1977.

Glasser W: *Reality Therapy.* New York, Harper & Row, 1965.

Goldenson M: *The Encyclopedia of Human Behavior: Psychology, Psychiatry, and Mental Health.* Garden City, New York, Doubleday, 1970.

Goldsmith SB: *Ambulatory Care*. Germantown, Maryland, Aspen Systems, 1977.

Gootnick D: *Getting a Better Job*. New York, McGraw-Hill Paperbacks, 1978.

Gordon BI: *Simplified Medical Records System*. Acton, Massachusetts, Publishing Sciences Group, 1975.

Gorlick SH: *The Whys and Wherefors of Corporate Practice*. Oradell, New Jersey, Medical Economics, 1982.

Graham FE: Group vs Solo Practice—Arguments and Evidence. *Inquiry*, June 1972.

Gregg JR: *The Business of Optometric Practice*. White Plains, New York, Advisory Enterprises, 1975.

Gregg JR: *How to Communicate in Optometric Practice*. Philadelphia, Pennsylvania, Chilton Book Company, 1969.

Hassard H: *Medical Malpractice: Risks, Protection, Prevention*. Oradell, New Jersey, Medical Economics Book Division, 1966.

Hendrickson RM: Solo vs Group Practice. *Prism*, November 1974.

Hepburn WH, Snyder L: Legal Medicine. In Piersol GM (ed): *Encyclopedia of Medicine and Surgery*. Philadelphia, F.A. Davis Company, Vol 8, 1949.

Heuser GD: *The Management of a Chiropractic Practice*. Published by author, no site or date of publication shown.

Hodge JR: *Practical Psychology for the Primary Physician*. Nelson-Hall, Chicago, 1975.

Hollinshead WH, Jenkins DB: *Functional Anatomy of the Limbs and Back*, ed 5. Philadelphia, W.B. Saunders, 1981.

Holmgren JH: *Purchasing for the Health Care Facility*. Springfield, Illinois, Charles C. Thomas, 1975.

Holtz H: *Beyond the Resume: How to Land the Job You Want*. New York, McGraw-Hill, 1984.

Homewood AE: *The Chiropractor and the Law*. Toronto, Ontario, Chiropractic Publishers, 1965.

Horney K: *Neurosis and Human Growth*. New York, Norton, 1950.

Horsley JD, Carlova J: *Your Family and the Law*. Oradell, New Jersey, Medical Economics, 1975.

Hospital Risk Control Update. *ECRI*, p 5, December 1986.

Howe HF (ed): *The Physician's Career*. Chicago, American Medical Association, 1970.

Institute for Business Planning: *Professional Corporation Desk Book*. Englewood Cliffs, New Jersey, Institute for Business Planning, 1975.

Ireland SH: *How to Prepare Proposals*. Chicago, Dartnell Corporation, 1967.

Iverson C, Dan BB, Glitman P, et al: *American Medical Association Manual of Style*, ed 8. Baltimore, Williams & Wilkins, 1989.

James W: *The Principles of Psychology*. New York, Dover Publications, Vols I and II, 1950.

Janse J: *Principles and Practice of Chiropractic*. Lombard, Illinois, National College of Chiropractic, 1976.

Jaquet PF: *An Introduction to Clinical Chiropractic*. Geneva, Switzerland, published by author, 1974.

Jaskoviak PA, Schafer RC: *Applied Physiotherapy*. Arlington, Virginia, American Chiropractic Association, 1986.

Jerome WT III: *Executive Control—The Catalyst*. New York, John Wiley & Sons, 1961.

Johnson AC: *Chiropractic Drugless Therapeutics*. Palm Springs, California, published by author, 1965.

Jourard SM: *The Transparent Self*. Princeton, New Jersey, D. Van Nostrand, 1964.

Jung CG: *On the Nature of the Psyche*, translated by R.F.C. Hull. Princeton, New Jersey, Princeton University Press, 1969.

Junghanns H: *Clinical Implications of Normal Biomechanical Stresses on Spinal Function*, English language edition edited by Hager HJ. Rockville, Maryland, Aspen Publishers, 1990.

Kabbes EF: *Medical Secretary's Guide*. West Nyack, New York, Parker Publishing Company, 1967.

Kennedy R: *Office Manual*. Published by author, site and date of publication not shown. Once available from Pasadena Chiropractic College Bookstore.

Kern RT: The Insurance Form Trap. *The ACA Journal of Chiropractic*, March 1983.

Kern RT: Worker's Compensation and Employer Liability. *The ACA Journal of Chiropractic, December 1977*.

Kimball C: *The Biopsychosocial Approach to the Patient*. Baltimore, Williams & Wilkins, 1981.

Kimber DC, et al: *Textbook of Anatomy and Physiology*, ed 11. New York, Macmillan, 1942.

Kinn ME, Derge EF, Lane K: *The Medical Assistant—Administrative and Clinical*, ed 6. Philadelphia, W.B. Saunders, 1988.

Klass R: *The Physician's Business Manual*. New York, Appleton-Century-Crofts, 1983.

Lalla GT: *A Guide to Professional Practice Management*, Vols I and II. St. Paul, Minnesota, published by author, 1979. Once available from Northwestern Chiropractic College Bookstore.

Lalla GT, Lalla PD: *Clinic Procedure Manual*. St. Paul, Minnesota, published by authors, 1979. Once available from Northwestern Chiropractic College Bookstore.

Lawrence-Leiter & Company: *Practice Management Manual*. St. Louis, Missouri, American Optometric Association, 1965.

Lawson JD, et al: *Leadership Is Everybody's Business*. San Luis Obispo, California, Impact Publishers, 1977.

Levoy RP: *The Successful Professional Practice*. Englewood Cliffs, New Jersey, Prentice-Hall, 1970.

Lockenour J: Document or Die. *The Eagle*, pp 16–17, Spring 1989.

Luckmann J, Sorensen KC: *Medical-Surgical Nursing: A Psychophysiologic Approach*. Philadelphia, W.B. Saunders, 1974.

Manning FF (ed): *Medical Credit and Collections*. Cambridge, Massachusetts, Ballenger, 1977.

Manning FF: *Medical Group Management*. Cambridge, Massachusetts, Ballinger Publishing, 1977.

Mappes TA, Zembaty JS: *Biomedical Ethics*. New York, McGraw-Hill, 1981.

Marder D: *The Craft of Technical Writing*. New York, Macmillan Company, 1960.

Marks G, Beatty WK: *The Story of Medicine in America*. New York, Scribners, 1974.

Maslow AH: *Motivation and Personality*. New York, Harper & Row, 1954.

Masters NC, Shapiro HA: *Medical Secrecy and the Doctor-Patient Relationship*. New York, International Publications Service, 1966.

Mattera MD: *How to Hire, Train, and Manage Your Employees.* Oradell, New Jersey, Medical Economics, 1982.

Maurer EL: personal notes on chiropractic assistance in general practice chiropractic roentgenography. Kalamazoo, Michigan, 1978.

McKee JI, Vaughn DT: The Organization and Management of a Private Physical Therapy Practice. *Physical Therapy,* October 1971.

Medicaid, Medicare: Which Is Which?: Washington, DC, U.S. Government Printing Office.

Medical Group Management Association: *Manual on Insurance.* Denver, Colorado, Medical Group Management Association, 1974.

Menninger KA, et al: *The Vital Balance.* New York, Viking Press, 1963.

Menninger KA: *Man Against Himself.* New York, Harcourt & Brace, 1938.

Milkie GM: *Office Policy/Procedure Manual for Paraoptometric Personnel.* St. Louis, Missouri, American Optometric Association, 1974.

Minimize ER Risks with Smooth Operations and Good PR. *Hospital Risk Management,* 9(6):97–98, August 1987.

Mockridge N: *Types of Medical Practice: Making Your Choice.* Oradell, New Jersey, Medical Economics Books, 1982.

Montgomery RL, Singleton MC: *Human Anatomy Review.* New York, Arco Publishing, 1974.

Mortillaro LF: A Coordinated Personnel System for Hiring Chiropractic Assistants and Chiropractic Technicians. *ACA Journal of Chiropractic,* June 1980.

Mosier A, Pace FJ: *Medical Records Technology.* Indianapolis, Indiana, Bobbs-Merrill, Allied Health Series, 1975.

Moulton RD: Helping the Patient to Understand His Emotional Experiences. *ACA Journal of Chiropractic,* February 1964.

Moya F: *Fundamentals of Management for the Physician.* Springfield, Illinois, Charles C. Thomas, 1974.

National Chiropractic Association: *Professional Relations Manual.* Webster City, Iowa, National Chiropractic Association, 1955.

Nelson JR: *Writing the Technical Report.* New York, McGraw-Hill, 1952.

Nemec J: *Highlights of Medicolegal Relations.* Bethesda, Maryland, U.S. Dept. of H.E.W., Pub. No. (NIH) 76-1109, SN: 017-052-00170-1, 1976.

New York Chiropractic College: *Practice Management Guide.* Glen Head, New York, 1983. Class notes in tenth trimester.

Nicholson M: *A Dictionary of American English Usage.* New York, Oxford University Press, 1957.

Odiorne GS: *How Managers Make Things Happen.* Englewood Cliffs, New Jersey, Prentice-Hall, 1961.

Orlikoff J: Avert Malpractice Action with Improved Patient Communications. From column, "Risk Management Strategies." In *Hospital Risk Management,* p 142, October 1985.

Ornstein RE: *The Psychology of Consciousness.* New York, Viking Press, 1972.

Parker J: *Textbook of Office Procedure and Practice Building for the Chiropractic Profession.* Fort Worth, Texas, Parker Chiropractic Research Foundation, 1970.

Parsons EJ: *In the Doctor's Office.* Philadelphia, J.B. Lippincott, 1945.

Pennsylvania Insurance Management Company: The Healing Touch: Managers Can Lend a Hand. In *Hospital Risk Control Update,* PIMCO, pp 6–7, December 1986.

Pennsylvania Insurance Management Company: Responding to Patients' Complaints. In *Hospital Risk Control Update,* PIMCO, p 2, December 1987.

Perrin PG: *Writer's Guide and Index to English.* Chicago, Scott, Foresman and Company, 1972.

Poe GF: How to Reach Your Patients and Prospects with Your Health Message. *ACA Journal of Chiropractic,* January 1964.

Pollack RS: *Clinical Aspects of Malpractice.* Oradell, New Jersey, Medical Economics Company, 1980.

Poor Communication and Documentation Practices Lead to Lab Liability. *ECRI,* p 9, December 1986.

Quigley WH: Understanding and Aiding the Older Citizen. *ACA Journal of Chiropractic,* July 1967.

Ramsey P: *The Patient as a Person: Explorations in Medical Ethics.* New Haven, Connecticut, Yale University Press, 1974.

Reiser DE, Schroder AK: *Patient Interviewing: The Human Dimension.* Baltimore, Williams & Wilkins, 1980.

Robinson ES: *The Art of Being Successful.* Glendale, California, Educational Research Society, 1959.

Robinson ES: *Professional Economics Course.* Glendale, California, published by author, 1955.

Rogers CE: *Client-Centered Therapy.* Boston, Houghton, 1951.

Roper N: *Man's Anatomy, Physiology, Health and Environment,* ed 5. New York, Churchill Livingston, 1976.

Rosse C, Clawson DK: *The Musculoskeletal System in Health and Disease.* New York, Harper & Row, 1980.

Sandor AA: Medicine and the Law. *Journal of the American Medical Association,* 163(6):459.

Sante LR: *Manual of Roentgenological Technique,* ed 20. Ann Arbor, Michigan, Edward Brothers, 1962.

Schafer RC: *Basic Principles of Chiropractic: The Neuroscience Foundation of Clinical Practice.* Arlington, Virginia, American Chiropractic Association, 1990.

Schafer RC: *Chiropractic Health Care,* ed 3. Des Moines, Iowa, The Foundation for Chiropractic Education and Research, 1978.

Schafer RC: *Chiropractic Management of Sports and Recreational Injuries,* ed 2. Baltimore, Williams & Wilkins, 1986.

Schafer RC: *Clinical Biomechanics,* ed 2. Baltimore, Williams & Wilkins, 1987.

Schafer RC: *Clinical Malpractice.* Des Moines, Iowa, National Chiropractic Mutual Insurance Company, 1983.

Schafer RC: *Consumer's Guide to Chiropractic Health Care.* Des Moines, Iowa, American Chiropractic Association, 1977.

Schafer RC: *Developing a Chiropractic Practice—An Introduction to Tactical Chiropractic Economics.* Arlington, Virginia, American Chiropractic Association, 1984.

Schafer RC: *Dictionary of Chiropractic Terminology*

and *Style*. Des Moines, Iowa, prepublication copyright 1978.

Schafer RC (ed): *Basic Chiropractic Procedural Manual*, ed 4. Arlington, Virginia, American Chiropractic Association, 1984.

Schafer RC (ed): *Indexed Synopsis of ACA Policies on Public Health and Related Matters*. Des Moines, Iowa, American Chiropractic Association, 1978.

Schafer RC (ed): *Public Relations Manual*. Des Moines, Iowa, American Chiropractic Association, G-13, 1977.

Schafer RC, et al: *Dynamics of Personal Success*. Denver, Advancement Motivation Systems, 1970.

Schafer RC, et al: *How to Become Financially Independent*. Denver, Success Associates International, 1970.

Schafer, RC, et al: *Power Tactics of Personal Achievement*. Denver, Advancement Motivation Systems, 1971.

Schafer RC, et al: *Science of Motivational Management*. Denver, Success Associates International, 1970.

Schafer RC, et al: *Strategic Motivational Management*. Denver, Strategic Leadership Systems, 1971.

Schafer RC: *The Magic of Self-Actualization*. Montezuma, Iowa, Behavioral Research Foundation, 1977.

Schafer RC: Motivational Patient Communications. *ACA Journal of Chiropractic*, December 1974.

Schafer RC: *Opportunities in Chiropractic Health Care*, ed 2. VGM Career Horizons, Skokie, Illinois, National Textbook Company, 1984.

Schafer RC: *Physical Diagnosis: Procedures and Methodology in Chiropractic Practice*. Arlington, Virginia, American Chiropractic Association, 1988.

Schafer RC: Professional Public Relations. *ACA Journal of Chiropractic*, April 1979.

Schafer RC: Relating to the Public. *ACA Journal of Chiropractic*, October 1975.

Schafer RC, Davis I: Relating to the Public. *ACA Journal of Chiropractic*, October 1975.

Scheflen AE: Human Communication. *Behavioral Sciences*, Vol 13, 1968.

Schmitz RM: *Preparing the Research Paper*, ed 4. New York, Rinehart and Company, 1957.

Schwab J: *Handbook of Psychiatric Consultation*. New York, Appleton-Century Crofts, 1968.

Schwartz HS: *Mental Health and Chiropractic*. New Hyde Park, New York, Sessions Publishers, 1973.

Schwartz HS: Toward a Broader Concept of Chiropractic. *ACA Journal of Chiropractic*, December 1964.

Scoggins MLC: Preparing the Patient for X-Ray Examination. *The American Journal of Nursing*, January 1957, pp 76–79.

Sellars D: *Computerizing Your Medical Office*. Oradell, New Jersey, Medical Economics, 1983.

Shepard RS: *Human Physiology Examination Review*. New York, Arco Publishing, 1975.

Shidle NG: *The Art of Successful Communication*. New York, McGraw-Hill, 1965.

Shulman M: Demystifying Health Insurance Language. *Patient Care*, December 15, 1982.

Skillin ME, et al: *Words Into Type*, rev ed. New York, Appleton Century-Crofts, 1974.

Skousen M: *Complete Guide to Financial Privacy*, ed 3. Alexandria, Virginia, Alexandria House, 1982.

Smith WD: *The Hippocratic Tradition*. New York, Cornell University Press, 1979.

Soukhanov AH (ed): *Webster's Medical Office Handbook*. Springfield, Massachusetts, G & C Merriam Company, 1979.

Source Book of Health Insurance Data, ed 22. Washington, DC, prepared for the Health Insurance Association of America by the Health Insurance Institute, 1981.

Souther JW: *Technical Report Writing*. New York, John Wiley & Sons, 1957.

Southwest Research Institute: *Publications Handbook*. San Antonio, Texas, Southwest Research Institute, 1967.

Space Guidelines for Ambulatory Health Centers. Washington, DC, U.S. Government Printing Office, U.S. Department of H.E.W., Publication No. (HSA) 75-6014, 1974.

Spotting Patients Who May Be Trouble for Hospitals and MDs. *Hospital Risk Management*, p 79, June 1985.

Stegeman W: *Medical Terms Simplified*. St. Paul, Minnesota, West Publishing, 1976.

Stekel W: *Compulsion and Doubt*. New York, Liveright, 1949.

Stekel W: *Technique of Analytical Psychotherapy*. New York, Liverright, 1950.

Sweeney DR, et al: *Office Managers—Often an Essential Ingredient in an Effective Practice*. Bala Cynwyd, Pennsylvania, The Health Care Group, date not shown.

Tancredi L (ed): *Ethics of Health Care*. Washington, DC, Institute of Medicine, National Academy of Sciences, 1974.

Teach MDs Good Patient Communications to Avoid Lawsuits. *Hospital Risk Management*, 8(12):157–161, December 1986.

Thomas CL (ed): *Taber's Cyclopedic Medical Dictionary*, ed 14. Philadelphia, F.A. Davis, 1981.

Thomas JW: *Your Personal Growth*. New York, Frederick Fell, 1971.

Timberlake B: New Trends in Third Party Payor Health Plans. *ACA Dateline*, January-February 1983.

Time-Life Books: *Understanding Computers*. Alexandria, Virginia, Time-Life Books, Vol I–IX. Publication date not shown, approximately 1987.

Trelease SF: *How to Write Scientific and Technical Papers*, ed 3. Baltimore, Williams & Wilkins, 1958.

United States Department of Agriculture: Conserving the Nutritive Values in Foods. In *Home and Garden Bulletin* No. 90. Washington, DC, USDA, 1976.

United States Department of Agriculture: Food Is More Than Just Something to Eat. In *Home and Garden Bulletin* No. 216. Washington, DC, USDA, 1976.

United States Department of Agriculture: Nutrition: Food at Work for You. In *Home and Garden Bulletin* No. 1. Washington, DC, USDA, 1976.

Vaux K: *Biomedical Ethics*. New York, Harper & Row, 1976.

Veatch RM: *Case Studies in Medical Ethics*. Cambridge, Massachusetts, Harvard University Press, 1977.

Vogel PA: *A Physician's Guide to Narrative Report Writing and the Insurance Examination*. Miami, Florida. Published by author. Date not shown.

Wagner KR: Organizing and Translating Goals into Objectives. *Medical Group Management*, January-February 1976.

Walker HK, et al: *Clinical Methods: The History, Physical, and Laboratory Examinations*. Boston, Butterworths, 1976.

Walker RC: *Over My Shoulder: Reflections on Beginning a Private Practice in Physical Therapy*. Cedar Rapids, Iowa, published by author, 1977.

Warriner JE, Griffith F: *English Grammar and Composition: A Complete Handbook*. New York, Brace and Company, 1957.

Webster's New Collegiate Dictionary. Springfield, Massachusetts, G & C Merriam Company, 1980.

Weinerman ER: Problems and Perspectives in Group Practice. *Group Practice*, April 1969.

White RW: *The Study of Lives*. New York, Altherton Press, 1963.

Wiehe R: *Professional Office Procedures*. Lincoln, Illinois, published by author, 1968.

Wilson J: *How to Get Paid for What You've Earned*. Oradell, New Jersey, Medical Economics, 1974.

Winfrey R: *Technical and Business Report Prepara-*

tions, ed 3. Ames, Iowa, Iowa State University Press, 1967.

Wolberg L: *Technic of Psychotherapy*. New York, Grune & Stratton, 1967.

Wolf S: Emotions in the Autonomic Nervous System. *Archives of Internal Medicine*, 126, December 1970.

Wood LA (ed): *Nursing Skills for Allied Health Services*. Philadelphia, W.B. Saunders, 1978, vol 3.

Woodford FP (ed): *Scientific Writing for Graduate Students*. Bethesda, Maryland, Council of Biology Editors, 1968.

Yanda RL: *Doctors as Managers of Health Teams*. New York, AMACOM, 1977.

Your Medicare Handbook. Washington, DC, U.S. Government Printing Office, HEW Pub. No. (SSA) 77-1055.

Ziegler AB: *Doctor's Administrative Program*. Oradell, New Jersey, Medical Economics, 1979–1982, Vols 1–8.

Zirkle TE: *Professional Corporations in Perspective*. Monroe, Wisconsin, American Medical Association, 1977.

INDEX